FIRST AID FOR THE® Family Medicine Boards

Second Edition

TAO LE, MD, MHS

Associate Clinical Professor
Chief, Section of Allergy and Clinical Immunology
Department of Medicine
University of Louisville

MICHAEL D. MENDOZA, MD, MPH

Assistant Professor
Medical Director, Highland Family Medicine
Department of Family Medicine
University of Rochester Medical Center

DIANA COFFA, MD

Clinical Assistant Professor
Assistant Medical Director
Family Health Center, San Francisco General Hospital
Department of Family and Community Medicine
University of California, San Francisco

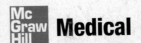 **Medical**

New York   Chicago   San Francisco   Lisbon   London   Madrid   Mexico City
Milan   New Delhi   San Juan   Seoul   Singapore   Sydney   Toronto

First Aid for the® Family Medicine Boards, Second Edition

4 5 6 7 8 9 10   DSS   18 17 16

ISBN 978-0-07-173726-5
MHID 0-07-173726-X

NOTICE

Medicine is an ever-changing science. As new research and clinical experience broaden our knowledge, changes in treatment and drug therapy are required. The authors and the publisher of this work have checked with sources believed to be reliable in their efforts to provide information that is complete and generally in accord with the standards accepted at the time of publication. However, in view of the possibility of human error or changes in medical sciences, neither the authors nor the publisher nor any other party who has been involved in the preparation or publication of this work warrants that the information contained herein is in every respect accurate or complete, and they disclaim all responsibility for any errors or omissions or for the results obtained from use of the information contained in this work. Readers are encouraged to confirm the information contained herein with other sources. For example and in particular, readers are advised to check the product information sheet included in the package of each drug they plan to administer to be certain that the information contained in this work is accurate and that changes have not been made in the recommended dose or in the contraindications for administration. This recommendation is of particular importance in connection with new or infrequently used drugs.

This book was set in Electra LH by Rainbow Graphics.
The editors were Catherine A. Johnson and Cindy Yoo.
The production supervisor was Jeffrey Herzich.
Project management was provided by Rainbow Graphics.
RR Donnelley was printer and binder.

Library of Congress Cataloging-in-Publication Data

First aid for the family medicine boards / [edited by] Tao Le. — 2nd ed.
     p. ; cm.
Includes index.
ISBN-13: 978-0-07-173726-5 (pbk.)
ISBN-10: 0-07-173726-X (MHID)
1. Family medicine—Examinations, questions, etc. 2. Physicians—Certification—United States. 3. American Board of Family Medicine. I. Le, Tao.
[DNLM: 1. Family Practice—United States—Outlines. 2. Specialty Boards—United States—Outlines. WB 18.2]
RC58.F54 2012
610.76—dc23

2012007802

DEDICATION

To our families, friends, and loved ones, who endured and assisted in the task of assembling this guide, and to the contributors to this and future editions, who took the time to share their knowledge, insight, and humor for the benefit of residents.

"]

Contents

Contents

CONTRIBUTING AUTHORS

Bethany Calkins, MD
Fellow, Department of Palliative Care
University of Rochester Medical Center

Freeman T. Changamire, MD, ScD
Assistant Professor, Department of Family Medicine
Tufts University School of Medicine

Leticia Cantu, MD
Resident, Department of Family Medicine
The Methodist Hospital–Family Medicine Residency Program

Jack Chase, MD
Hospitalist, Eden Hospital
East Bay Physicians Medical Group
Associate Physician, Department of Family and Community
    Medicine
University of California, San Francisco
San Francisco General Hospital Urgent Care Center

Kellene V. Eagen, MD
Physician, Housing and Urban Health Clinic
San Francisco Department of Public Health

Magdalen Edmunds, MD, MPH
Staff Physician
LifeLong Medical Care, Berkeley, California

Narges Farahi, MD
Clinical Instructor, Department of Family Medicine
University of North Carolina

Sachiko Kaizuka, MD
Staff Physician
Sacopee Valley Health Center
Porter, Maine

Kerry Kay, MD, MPH
Staff Physician
Asian Health Services, Oakland, California

Pebble M. Kranz, MD
Senior Instructor, Department of Family Medicine
University of Rochester Medical Center

Andres Marin, MD
Staff Physician, La Clinica de la Raza
Oakland, California

Ryohei Otsuka, MD
Fellow, Geriatric Medicine
University of Rochester

Brett Spitnale, MD
Staff Physician
Palo Alto Medical Foundation

Suzannah Stout, MD
Physician, Silver Avenue Family Health Center
San Francisco Department of Public Health

Kristen Thornton, MD
Senior Instructor, Department of Medicine and Family
    Medicine
University of Rochester School of Medicine and Dentistry

K. Pallav Kolli, MD
Imaging Editor
Fellow, Department of Radiology and Biomedical
    Imaging
University of California, San Francisco

SENIOR REVIEWERS

Preface

First Aid for the® Family Medicine Boards provides residents and clinicians with the most useful and up-to-date preparation guide for the American Board of Family Medicine (ABFM) certification and recertification examinations. This edition represents an outstanding effort by a talented group of authors and includes the following:

- A new full-color design for more effective study.
- A practical exam preparation guide with resident-tested test-taking and study strategies.
- Concise summaries of thousands of board-testable topics.
- Hundreds of high-yield tables, diagrams, and color illustrations.
- Key facts in the margins, highlighting "must know" information for the boards.
- Mnemonics throughout, making learning memorable and fun.
- Timely updates and corrections through the First Aid Team's blog at **www.firstaidteam.com.**

We invite you to share your thoughts and ideas to help us improve *First Aid for the® Family Medicine Boards*. See How to Contribute, p. xiii.

Tao Le
Louisville

Michael Mendoza
Rochester

Diana Coffa
San Francisco

Acknowledgments

This has been a collaborative project from the start. We gratefully acknowledge the thoughtful comments, corrections, and advice of the residents, international medical graduates, and faculty who have supported the authors in the revision of the second edition of *First Aid for the® Family Medicine Boards*.

Thanks to senior reviewers Shieva Khayam-Bashi, MD and Christine Dehlendorf, MD for their feedback on this project. For support and encouragement throughout the process, we are grateful to Thao Pham, Selina Franklin, and Louise Petersen. For editorial support, an enormous thanks to Carol Ayres and Karla Schroeder.

Thanks to Albert Yu, MD, and Richard Wilson, MD, for their feedback. Thanks to our publisher, McGraw-Hill, for the valuable assistance of their staff.

Tao Le
Louisville

Michael Mendoza
Rochester

Diana Coffa
San Francisco

Acknowledgments

This has been a collaborative project from the start. We gratefully acknowledge the thoughtful comments, suggestions, and advice of the residents, information and medical educators, and faculty who have supported the authors in the revision of this second edition of CURRENT for the Family Medicine Boards.

Thanks to senior reviewers Shiva Khayam-Bashi, MD and Christine Delgadillo, MD for their feedback on this project. For support and encouragement throughout the process, we are grateful to Thuy Phung, Selina Franklin, and Louise Petersen. For editorial support, enormous thanks to Carol Ames and Karen Schroeder.

Thanks to Albert Yiu, MD, and Richard Wilson, MD, for their feedback. Thanks to our publisher, McGraw-Hill, for the valuable assistance of their staff.

D. B. T.
Louisville

Michael Mendoza
Rochester

Philip Sadja
San Francisco

How to Contribute

To continue to produce a high-yield review source for the ABFM exam, you are invited to submit any suggestions or corrections. We also offer **paid internships** in medical education and publishing, ranging from three months to one year (see below for details). Please send us your suggestions for:

- Study and test-taking strategies for the ABFM
- New facts, mnemonics, diagrams, and illustrations
- Low-yield topics to remove

For each entry incorporated into the next edition, you will receive up to a $20 gift certificate as well as personal acknowledgment in the next edition. Diagrams, tables, partial entries, updates, corrections, and study hints are also appreciated, and significant contributions will be compensated at the discretion of the authors. Also, let us know about material in this edition that you feel is low yield and should be deleted. Please submit entries, suggestions, or corrections to the First Aid Team's blog at:

www.firstaidteam.com

Please include your name, address, institutional affiliation, phone number, and e-mail address (if different from the address of origin). You can also e-mail us directly at:

firstaidteam@yahoo.com

NOTE TO CONTRIBUTORS

All entries become the property of the authors and are subject to editing and review. Please verify all data and spellings carefully. In the event that similar or duplicate entries are received, only the first entry received will be used. Include a reference to a standard textbook to facilitate verification of the fact. Please follow the style, punctuation, and format of this edition if possible.

INTERNSHIP OPPORTUNITIES

The author team is pleased to offer part-time and full-time paid internships in medical education and publishing to motivated physicians. Internships may range from three months (eg, a summer) up to a full year. Participants will have an opportunity to author, edit, and earn academic credit on a wide variety of projects, including the popular *First Aid* series. Writing/editing experience, familiarity with Microsoft Word, and Internet access are desired. For more information, submit a résumé or a short description of your experience, along with a cover letter, to **firstaid@ usmlerx.com**.

Guide to the ABFM Examination

Introduction

For residents, the American Board of Family Medicine (ABFM) certification exam represents the culmination of 3 years of hard work, and for those taking the recertification exam, 7–10 years after that. However, the process of certification and recertification does not merely represent yet another in a series of expensive tests. To your patients and their families, it means that you have attained the level of clinical knowledge and competency required to provide good clinical care.

In this chapter, we talk more about the ABFM exam and provide you with proven approaches to conquering the exam. For a detailed description of the exam, visit **www.theabfm.org.** The ABFM also provides information about specific study strategies that have worked for candidates who failed the exam initially and went on to pass successfully. These are detailed at www.theabfm.org/cert/fail-safe.pdf.

ABFM—The Basics

WHEN IS THE EXAM OFFERED?

The exam is offered during 2 months each year, typically in April and in November. Applicants must register for one of the limited dates that are offered in each of those months. Generally, more dates are available in the spring session than in the winter session.

HOW DO I REGISTER TO TAKE THE EXAM?

You can register for the ABFM exam online at www.theabfm.org. Individuals who complete residency training after June 30 or who do not pass the exam in the summer may be eligible to take the test during the winter.

Those who are certifying for the first time must have a user name and password supplied by their residency program. The registration deadline is typically January, with increasing late fees for each subsequent month. The latest date to register is generally in June. The registration fee in 2012 was $1300.

Check the ABFM Web site for the latest information on registration deadlines, fees, and policies. Note that the deadlines and schedules for the Certificates of Added Qualifications vary.

WHAT IF I NEED TO CANCEL THE EXAM OR CHANGE TEST CENTERS?

The ABFM currently provides partial refunds if a cancellation is received a certain number of days before the scheduled exam (in 2011, there was no cancellation fee 30 days before the exam). You can also change your test center and test dates before a specific deadline. Check the ABFM Web site for the latest on refund and cancellation policies as well as current procedures.

HOW IS THE ABFM TEST STRUCTURED?

The ABFM certification/recertification exam is currently a 1-day computer-based test administered at approximately 350 test centers around the country. For questions about the computer-based format, see the ABFM Web site tutorial and FAQs. The test is distributed by subject matter, as described on the ABFM Web site at www.theabfm.org/cert/CertRecertExaminationOutline.pdf. The exam itself is divided into a morning and an afternoon session. The morning session consists of 3 sections: 120 multiple-choice questions (120 minutes), an optional scheduled 15-minute break, and then two 45-question special modules (45 minutes) selected by the candidate on the day of the exam. The modules are described in detail on the Web site; briefly, they are Ambulatory Family Medicine, Child and Adolescent Care, Geriatrics, Women's Health, Maternity Care, Emergent/Urgent Care, Hospital Medicine, and Sports Medicine. The morning session is followed by an optional 70-minute break. The afternoon session consists of 2 sections: 80 multiple-choice questions (95 minutes), an optional scheduled 15-minute break, and another 80 multiple-choice questions (95 minutes). Twenty of the exam questions are being tested and are not included in the scoring—but you will not know which questions these are! Overall, you will have approximately 1 minute to answer each question.

WHAT TYPES OF QUESTIONS ARE ASKED?

All questions are **single-best-answer** types only. You will be presented with a scenario and a question followed by 5 options. Most questions on the exam are vignette based. A substantial amount of extraneous information may be given, or a clinical scenario may be followed by a question that could be answered without actually requiring that you read the case. As with other board exams, there is no penalty for guessing. Questions can pertain to the diagnosis, treatment, or prevention of disease.

KEY FACT

Most questions on the ABFM exam are case based.

HOW ARE THE SCORES REPORTED?

Both the scoring and the reporting of test results have varied, but may take up to 3 months. Your score report will give you a "pass/fail" decision, the overall number of questions answered correctly with a corresponding percentile, and the number of questions answered correctly with a corresponding percentile for more than 40 different subject areas. Results from all candidates who took the test on the same date are presented alongside your results for each subject area. In 2010, the pass rate for the certification exam was 82%; for the recertification exam, the pass rate was 67%.

The Recertification Exam

The recertification exam is 1 part of the Maintenance of Certification for Family Physicians (MC-FP). The exam must be completed every 7 or 10 years, depending on your situation. Additional components of the MC-FP include Self-Assessment Modules (SAMs), Performance in Practice Modules (PPMs), and continuing medical education. Please check the ABFM Web site for additional details.

Test Preparation Advice

The good news about the ABFM exam is that it tends to focus on the diagnosis and management of diseases and conditions that you have likely seen as a resident—and that you should expect to see as a family physician. Assuming that you have performed well as a resident, *First Aid* and a good source of practice questions may be all you need to pass. However, you might also consider using *First Aid* as a **guide** and using multiple resources, including a standard textbook, journal review articles, and a concise electronic text such as *UpToDate*, as part of your studies. Original research articles are low yield, and very new research (ie, research conducted less than 1–2 years before the exam) will not be tested. In addition, a number of high-quality board review courses are offered around the country. Such courses are costly, but can help those who need some focus and discipline.

Ideally, you should start your preparation early in your **last year of residency**, especially if you are starting a demanding job or fellowship right after residency. Cramming during the period between the end of residency and the exam is **not advisable.**

As you study, concentrate on the **nuances of management,** especially for difficult or complicated cases. For **common diseases,** learn both common and **uncommon presentations;** for **uncommon diseases,** focus on the **classic presentations** and manifestations. Draw on the experiences of your residency training to anchor some of your learning. When you take the exam, you will realize that you've seen most of the clinical scenarios in the course of your 3 years of clinic and hospital medicine.

Depending on the modules you choose in the morning session, you may want to focus on specific chapters and sections in the *First Aid for the Family Medicine Boards:*

- **Ambulatory Family Medicine:** Community Medicine, Cardiology (hypertension, dyslipidemia, CHF), Endocrinology (diabetes), Gastroenterology, Pulmonary Medicine, Dermatology, and Reproductive Health (gynecology).
- **Child and Adolescent Care:** Pediatric and Adolescent Medicine, Reproductive Health (gynecology), and Hematology and Oncology (anemia, leukemias).
- **Geriatrics:** Geriatrics, Community Medicine, Cardiology, Neurology (cerebrovascular disease), Dermatology (herpes zoster), and Psychiatry.
- **Women's Health:** Reproductive Health, Geriatrics (osteoporosis, incontinence), Psychiatry, Pediatric and Adolescent Medicine (eating disorders, female athletic triad), Surgery (breast cancer), and Community Medicine (domestic violence).
- **Maternity Care:** Reproductive Health (obstetrics), Psychiatry, and Community Medicine (domestic violence).
- **Emergent/Urgent Care:** Emergency/Urgent Care, Psychiatry, Surgery, Pediatric and Adolescent Medicine (common acute conditions), and Community Medicine (bioterrorism).
- **Hospital Medicine:** Cardiology, Pulmonary Medicine, Endocrinology (DKA, HHNS), Gastroenterology (GI bleeding, end-stage liver disease, diverticulitis, pancreatitis), Hematology and Oncology (oncology), Infectious Disease, Pulmonary (lower respiratory disease), Nephrology (acute renal failure), Neurology (cerebrovascular disease, seizure, syncope), Surgery, and Emergency/Urgent Care.
- **Sports Medicine:** Sports Medicine.

KEY FACT

The ABFM tends to focus on the horses, not the zebras.

KEY FACT

Use a combination of *First Aid*, textbooks, journal reviews, and practice questions.

OTHER HIGH-YIELD AREAS

Focus on topic areas that are typically not emphasized during residency training but are board favorites. These include the following:

- Basic biostatistics (eg, sensitivity, specificity, positive predictive value, negative predictive value).
- Adverse effects of drugs.

Test-Taking Advice

By this point in your life, you have probably gained more test-taking expertise than you care to admit. Nevertheless, here are a few tips to keep in mind when taking the exam:

- Arrive 30 minutes early for your test. You want to be relaxed and ready to start on time, not rushed and stressed by traffic. Bring snacks and dress in layers so that you will be comfortable all day.
- Avoid a heavy lunch! Many test-takers have reported that it can be difficult to focus on the exam after a heavy meal.
- For long vignette questions, read the question stem and scan the options, and **then** go back and read the case. You may get your answer without having to read through the whole case.
- There's no penalty for guessing, so you should **never** leave a question blank.
- Good pacing is key. You need to leave adequate time to get to all the questions. Even though you have 1 minute per question on average, you should aim for a pace of 45 seconds per question. If you don't know the answer within a short period of time, make an educated guess and move on. You can flag that question to come back to if you have time at the end.
- It's okay to **second-guess** yourself. Research shows that our "second hunches" tend to be better than our first guesses.
- Don't panic over "impossible" questions. These may be **experimental questions** that won't count in your score. Again, take your best guess and move on.
- Note the age and race of the patient in each clinical scenario. When race or ethnicity is given, it is often relevant. Know these well, especially for more common diagnoses.
- Questions often describe clinical findings instead of naming eponyms (eg, they cite "tender, erythematous bumps in the pads of the finger" rather than "Osler node" in a febrile adolescent).
- As described above, visit the Web site www.theabfm.org/cert/fail-safe.pdf for study strategies specific to the ABFM certification/recertification exam.

 KEY FACT

Never, ever leave a question blank! There is no penalty for guessing.

Testing and Licensing Agencies

American Board of Family Medicine
2228 Young Drive
Lexington, KY 40505-4294
859-269-5626 or 888-995-5700
Fax: 859-335-7501 or 859-335-7509
www.theabfm.org

Educational Commission for Foreign Medical Graduates (ECFMG)
3624 Market Street, Fourth Floor
Philadelphia, PA 19104-2685
215-386-5900
Fax: 215-386-9196
www.ecfmg.org

Federation of State Medical Boards (FSMB)
P.O. Box 619850
Dallas, TX 75261-9850
817-868-4000
Fax: 817-868-4099
www.fsmb.org

CHAPTER 2

Community and Preventive Medicine

Freeman Changamire, MD, ScD

Preventive Medicine

- **1° prevention** includes disease prevention measures, such as counseling for at-risk behaviors, immunizations, and chemoprevention, that are taken **before the disease develops.**
- **2° prevention** is defined as **early detection and treatment of asymptomatic disease,** including risk assessment.
- **3° prevention** is management of chronic diseases to **prevent or minimize complications.**
- Characteristics that make a disease appropriate for screening include the following:
    - The disease leads to **significant morbidity and mortality.**
    - **Effective treatment** is available.
    - The disease is **detectable** in the asymptomatic period.
    - Testing is accurate and simple.
    - Treatment administered during the asymptomatic period yields a better outcome than treatment in the symptomatic period.
- Characteristics of appropriate risk factors for screening are as follows:
    - There is a **high prevalence** of the risk factor in the population to be screened.
    - A large percentage of those with the risk factor are unidentified.
    - The associated **disease** should have a **high incidence** in the population to be screened.
    - The disease should have **serious consequences.**
    - Treatment that can modify the risk factor should be readily available.
    - **Risk modification should ↓ disease incidence.**

ADULT IMMUNIZATIONS

Table 2.1 outlines common adult immunizations and their indications. For information on immunization of pediatric populations, refer to the Pediatric and Adolescent Medicine chapter.

CANCER SCREENING

The following guidelines are based on recommendations from the United States Preventive Services Task Force (USPSTF) and the American Academy of Family Physicians (AAFP).

Skin Cancer

The USPSTF concludes that the current evidence is insufficient to assess the balance of benefits and harms of using a whole-body skin examination by a primary care clinician or patient skin self-examination for the early detection of cutaneous melanoma, basal cell cancer, or squamous cell skin cancer in the adult general population.

Cervical Cancer

- Routinely screen for cervical cancer with a Pap smear all women ≥ 21 years of age who have been sexually active and have a cervix (**strongly recommended**). Repeat screening at least every 3 years.
- Routine screening is **not** recommended for women > 65 years of age with a history of adequate ⊖ screening and who are otherwise **not at high risk.**

TABLE 2.1.   Recommended Adult Immunization Schedule

Vaccine	Schedule
Tetanus, diphtheria, pertussis	Give the complete primary series if the patient has not been previously vaccinated. First dose: Tdap; second dose: Td 4 weeks later; third dose: Td 6 months later. Tdap can substitute for only 1 of the 3 Td doses in the series. Booster doses of Td should be given every 10 years thereafter.
Human papillomavirus	ACIP recommends vaccination of females 9–26 years of age with either HPV2 or HPV4 (3 doses). HPV4 was licensed for use in males in 2009.
Varicella	If the patient has a history of chickenpox, consider immune. Otherwise, vaccinate with 2 doses given 1–2 months apart.
Zoster	Single dose recommended for adults ≥ 60 years of age regardless of whether they report a prior episode of herpes zoster.
Measles, mumps, rubella	If the patient was born before 1957, consider immune. If the patient was born after 1957, 2 doses should be given at least 1 month apart. For rubella specifically, ensure that women of childbearing potential have immunity.
Influenza	Routine annual influenza vaccination recommended for all persons aged ≥ 6 months, including all adults.
Pneumococcal (polysaccharide)	Give to all patients > 65 years of age. Give to all patients who are immunocompromised or who have chronic diseases. Revaccinate patients ≥ 65 years of age if they received their 1° vaccine > 5 years ago or are at high risk.
Hepatitis A	Vaccinate any person seeking protection or people of the following indications: MSM, chronic liver disease, persons traveling or working in endemic areas. Two doses should be given at least 6 months apart.
Hepatitis B	Vaccinate any person seeking protection or people of the following indications: persons at high risk for STDs, health care personnel, end-stage liver disease patients, HIV-infected patients, chronic liver disease patients. Three dose series of Hep B should be given.
Meningococcal	Give to adults with asplenia, first-year college students in dormitories, military personnel.

The evidence is insufficient to recommend for or against the routine use of new technologies or HPV testing to screen for cervical cancer.

Ovarian Cancer

Do not routinely screen for ovarian cancer by ultrasound, measurement of tumor markers, or pelvic examination. Although the specificity for screening strategies is high, the positive predictive value is low because of the low prevalence of ovarian cancer in the general population. Further, the invasive nature of testing that follows a positive screening test led the USPSTF to conclude that the potential risks outweigh the potential benefits.

Breast Cancer

- **Screen women 50–74** years of age for breast cancer every 2 years with mammography.
- **Individualize** your decision to start regular, biennial screening mammography for women < 50 years of age based on patient context, including the patient's values regarding specific benefits and harms.
- **Do not routinely screen** women ≥ 75 years of age with mammography.

Prostate Cancer

- **Consider screening men ≥ 50** years of age if the patient is expected to live at least 10 years.
- Begin screening at an **earlier age if patients are at ↑ risk** (eg, African-American men or those with a first-degree relative with prostate cancer).
- The USPSTF and the AAFP conclude that the current **evidence is insufficient** to assess the balance of benefits and harms of prostate cancer screening in men < 75 years of age.
- **Do not screen** for prostate cancer in men ≥ 75 years of age (USPSTF and AAFP recommendation).

Colon Cancer

- **Screen adults ≥ 50** years of age for colon cancer with an annual fecal occult blood test, sigmoidoscopy every 3–5 years, or colonoscopy every 10 years (**strong recommendation**).
- Screen **earlier if there is ↑ risk** for colorectal cancer—eg, if the patient has a personal or strong family history of colorectal cancer, adenomatous polyps, or a family history of a hereditary syndrome (familial adenomatous polyposis, hereditary nonpolyposis colon cancer).
- Do not screen for colorectal cancer in adults > 85 years of age.

ADULT HEALTH MAINTENANCE

A 45-year-old man comes to your office for a routine annual physical exam. He is a nonsmoker who is generally healthy and has no current medical complaints. In an average week, he exercises by jogging 30 minutes 2 times a week. However, he has a family history of high blood pressure, and his older brother recently had an MI at 48 years of age. The patient asks if there is anything that can be done to prevent this from happening to him. What do you suggest?

Recommend checking his BP today, ordering a lipid panel, and discussing the benefits of a healthy diet and aspirin therapy.

Tables 2.2 through 2.4 present recommended clinical preventive services for different adult populations based on the latest recommendations from the USPSTF and the AAFP.

See cancer screening and immunization recommendations above.

TABLE 2.2.   **Recommended Clinical Preventive Services for All Adults**

AGE	CONDITION	RECOMMENDATION
≥ 18	Accidental injury.	Counsel as appropriate for age.
	Alcohol misuse.	Screen and counsel behavior to ↓ misuse.
	CAD.	Recommend aspirin for men 45–79 years of age and women 55–79 years of age when the potential benefit due to reduction in MIs outweighs the potential harm due to an ↑ in GI bleeding.
		Not routinely recommended for persons > 80 years of age.
	DM type 2.	Screen asymptomatic adults with sustained elevated BP > 135/80.
	Depression.	Screen for depression.
	Hypertension.	Screen for high blood pressure.
	Obesity.	Screen for obesity by measuring height and weight. Offer counseling and behavioral interventions to promote sustained weight loss for obese adults.
	Physical activity.	Recognize that physical activity is desirable and advise accordingly.
	Healthy diet.	Counsel adults with hyperlipidemia and other risk factors for CVD and diet-related chronic disease.
	Secondhand smoke.	Counsel parents who smoke about the harmful effects of smoking on children's health.
	STIs, including HIV.	Counsel adults at ↑ risk for STIs about the risks for STIs and how to prevent them.
	Tobacco use.	Screen for tobacco use and provide tobacco cessation interventions as appropriate.
	Tuberculosis.	Screen by PPD patients at high risk for TB.
≥ 65	Hearing difficulties.	Screen and counsel.
	Visual difficulties.	Screen with the Snellen acuity test.

TABLE 2.3.   **Recommended Clinical Preventive Services Specific for Adult Men**

AGE	CONDITION	RECOMMENDATION
≥ 35	Lipid disorders.	Screen with a fasting lipid profile or nonfasting total and HDL cholesterol.
≥ 65	Abdominal aortic aneurysm.	Offer one-time screening by ultrasonography for individuals 65–75 years of age who have ever smoked.

TABLE 2.4.   **Recommended Clinical Preventive Services Specific for Adult Women**

AGE	CONDITION	RECOMMENDATION
≥ 18	Osteoporosis.	Counsel patients to maintain adequate calcium intake.
18–25	Chlamydia.	Screen sexually active women.
Pregnancy	Bacteriuria, asymptomatic.	Screen with urine culture at 12–16 weeks' gestation or at the first prenatal visit.
	Chlamydia.	Screen asymptomatic pregnant women.
	Gonorrhea.	Screen women at ↑ risk for infection.
	HBV.	Screen at the first prenatal visit.
	HIV infection.	Screen all pregnant women.
	Neural tube defects.	For women with no history of a previous pregnancy affected by a neural tube defect, prescribe folic acid at a dosage of 0.4–0.8 mg/day from 1 month before conception through the first trimester of pregnancy. For women with a history of a previous pregnancy affected by a neural tube defect, the dose should be ↑ to 4 mg/day. Prescribe 0.4 mg/day of folate supplementation in women of childbearing potential.
	Rh(D) incompatibility.	Order Rh(D) blood typing and antibody testing at the first prenatal visit; repeat antibody testing for all Rh(D)-⊖ women at 24–28 weeks' gestation.
	Rubella.	Screen by ensuring immunity via history, serology, or vaccination.
	Syphilis.	Screen all pregnant women.
	Tobacco use.	Provide smoking cessation counseling for all pregnant smokers.
	Iron deficiency anemia.	Screen routinely in asymptomatic pregnant women.
	Breastfeeding.	Counsel on interventions to promote and support breastfeeding.
≥ 45	Lipid disorders.	Screen with a fasting lipid profile or nonfasting total and HDL cholesterol.
60–64	Osteoporosis.	Screen selected women at risk for fractures.
≥ 65	Osteoporosis.	Screen all women for osteoporosis.

DENTAL CARE

Prevention of Dental Caries in Preschoolers

A total of 19% of children 2–5 years of age and 52% of children 5–9 years of age experience dental caries. Ethnic minority and economically disadvantaged children are at ↑ risk. Despite recommendations, few preschool-aged children ever visit a dentist.

Guidelines for the dental care of preschool children are as follows:

- Prescribe currently recommended doses of **oral fluoride supplementation** to preschool children > 6 months of age whose 1° water source is fluoride deficient (USPSTF recommendation).
- You may use **topical fluoride varnishes,** which are easier to use, accepted widely by patients, and have ↓ potential for toxicity, as adjuncts to oral supplementation.
- Monitor for dental fluorosis, a mild adverse effect of fluoride supplementation primarily of cosmetic significance.

Endocarditis Prophylaxis

Offer antimicrobial prophylaxis for dental and other procedures to patients with cardiac conditions with the highest risk of adverse outcome from infective endocarditis.

Endocarditis prophylaxis is recommended for the following cardiac conditions:

- **Cardiac valvulopathy** in a cardiac transplant recipient.
- **Congenital heart defect completely repaired** within the previous 6 months with prosthetic material or device, whether placed by surgery or by catheter.
- **Repaired congenital heart disease** with residual defects at the site or adjacent to the site of a prosthetic patch or device.
- **Unrepaired cyanotic congenital heart disease,** including palliative shunts and conduits.
- Previous history of **infective endocarditis.**
- **Prosthetic heart valves.**

Do not offer antimicrobial prophylaxis to patients with any other form of congenital or acquired heart disease such as bicuspid aortic valve, acquired aortic or mitral valve disease (including mitral valve prolapse with regurgitation), or hypertrophic cardiomyopathy.

Offer antimicrobial prophylaxis to patients with the cardiac lesions cited above when they undergo procedures, such as the following, likely to result in bacteremia with a microorganism that has the potential to cause endocarditis:

- All **dental procedures** that involve manipulation of gingival tissue or the periapical region of teeth or that perforate the oral mucosa.
- **Procedures of the respiratory tract** that involve incision or biopsy of the respiratory mucosa.
- Procedures in patients with **ongoing GI or GU tract infection.**
- Procedures on infected skin, skin structure, or musculoskeletal tissue.

Nutrition

OBESITY

The prevalence of obesity in the adult population of the United States is now about 34%, and the prevalence of childhood obesity is about 17%.

- Obesity is associated with ↑ **risk of both cardiovascular and overall mortality.** In addition, there are clear associations between obesity and ↑ morbidity.
- Obesity ↑ the risk of cardiovascular disease, hypertension, stroke, type 2 DM and insulin resistance, dyslipidemia, cancer (including cancers of the colon, kidney, and gallbladder), sleep apnea, gallbladder disease, GERD, and knee osteoarthritis.
- Obesity is also associated with ↓ quality of life, including ↓ mobility and social stigmatization.
- By contrast, a reduction of 5%–7% of body weight is associated with ↓ incidence of diabetes, ↓ BP, and improved dyslipidemia, **cancer, and overall mortality.**

Screen all adult patients for obesity and offer intensive counseling and behavioral interventions to promote sustained weight loss to obese adults.

Body Mass Index (BMI)

 A 32-year-old woman comes to your clinic for her annual exam. She is 5'4" and weighs 203 pounds. Her only concerns are that she has irregular menses and would like to lose some weight. She has heard that guar gum might help her lose weight and wonders if there is anything else you might recommend. What is her BMI, and what do you advise her to do?

This patient has a calculated BMI of 35 kg/m². You encourage her to lose weight, explaining that doing so will ↓ her risk of premature death, and consider screening her for diabetes and dyslipidemias. After explaining that guar gum has not been shown to be effective for weight loss, you also recommend a diet and exercise regimen.

The **calculation for BMI** is:

$$BMI = \text{weight (kg)} / \text{height (m}^2)$$

See Table 2.5 for the categories of BMI.

Treatment Methods

Consider the following modalities in the treatment of obesity:

- **Diet and exercise counseling with behavioral strategies** to help patients change eating patterns and become physically active. This may lead to small/moderate degrees of weight loss (1–6 kg) typically sustained for at least 1 year.
- **Medications:** Weight loss resulting from medications (see Table 2.6) is modest (average 3–5 kg), and discontinuation of medications may lead to rapid weight gain.
    - Medication may be considered for patients with BMI > 30 when diet and exercise attempts have failed and/or when the patient has comorbidities.
    - Weight loss medications in combination with lifestyle changes result in a greater weight reduction than use of medication alone.
- **Surgery:**
    - Consider patients for **gastric bypass and vertical banded gastroplasty** if they have a BMI > 40 or BMI > 35 with comorbidities, have failed to respond to previous nonsurgical weight loss attempts, and are well informed and motivated.
    - Discuss with them postoperative complications, which may include a mortality rate of 0.2%, wound infection, reoperation, vitamin deficiency, diarrhea, and hemorrhage.
    - Refer for **bariatric surgery** to high-volume centers with experienced surgeons.
    - Prepare patients and offer appropriate support, including psychological screening and a diet and exercise program, for successful surgical weight loss.

KEY FACT

A BMI ≥ 30 is associated with ↑ risk of both cardiovascular and overall mortality. Intentional weight loss of 25 pounds has been associated with a ↓ in cardiovascular disease, cancer, and overall mortality.

TABLE 2.5. BMI Categories

Definition	BMI (kg/m²)
Overweight	25–29
Obese	30–39
Morbidly obese	40–49
Super-obese	50–59

KEY FACT

Medications for the treatment of obesity allow for sustained weight loss only if they are continued.

TABLE 2.6.   Medications Used to Treat Obesity

MEDICATION	MECHANISM	NOTES
Sympathomimetic Drugs		
Phentermine and diethylpropion	Sympathomimetic agents.	Can ↑ BP. Use up to 12 weeks only (Schedule IV drugs with abuse potential).
Ephedrine and ephedra (not recommended)	Ephedrine is a sympathomimetic amine. Ephedra ↑ thermogenesis.	No longer on the market because of safety concerns.
Drugs That Alter Fat Digestion		
Orlistat	Inhibits pancreatic lipase.	Can be used on a long-term basis, with average weight loss approximating 9 kg. Side effects include abdominal cramps, flatus, and oily spotting.
Antidepressants		
Fluoxetine	Acts as an appetite suppressant.	Not FDA approved for weight loss; must use ≥ 60 mg/day.
Bupropion	Acts as a norepinephrine modulator.	Not FDA approved for weight loss.

MALNUTRITION

Table 2.7 outlines the clinical manifestations and treatment of severe malnutrition.

TABLE 2.7.   Presentation and Treatment of Severe Malnutrition

	MARASMUS	KWASHIORKOR
Definition	Total calorie malnutrition.	Protein malnutrition.
Etiologies (in developed countries)	COPD, CHF, cancer, AIDS.	Trauma, burns, sepsis.
Symptoms/exam	Weight loss/**wasting.**	Normal weight. Edema, ascites.
Treatment	Correct fluid and electrolyte abnormalities; treat infections; give vitamins and minerals. Start with 1 g protein/kg and 30 kcal/kg, preferably enterically.	Treatment is the same as that for marasmus.
Complications	Immunosuppression, poor wound healing, impaired growth and development, muscle atrophy leading to organ dysfunction.	Same as those for marasmus.

VITAMINS AND MINERALS

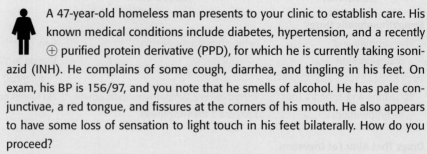

A 47-year-old homeless man presents to your clinic to establish care. His known medical conditions include diabetes, hypertension, and a recently ⊕ purified protein derivative (PPD), for which he is currently taking isoniazid (INH). He complains of some cough, diarrhea, and tingling in his feet. On exam, his BP is 156/97, and you note that he smells of alcohol. He has pale conjunctivae, a red tongue, and fissures at the corners of his mouth. He also appears to have some loss of sensation to light touch in his feet bilaterally. How do you proceed?

You check hematocrit, peripheral blood smear, and B_{12} and folate levels and treat him accordingly.

KEY FACT

If neurologic deficits are present, diagnose and treat vitamin B_{12} deficiency quickly to prevent irreversible symptoms.

KEY FACT

Give 400 IU of vitamin D supplementation per day to breast-feeding babies beginning in the first 2 months of life.

Vitamin Deficiencies

Vitamin deficiencies may be more common in developed countries than is generally believed. Vitamins are needed for basic metabolism, but since most of them cannot be synthesized, they must be present in our diets. The presentation and treatment of water- and fat-soluble vitamin deficiencies are summarized in Tables 2.8 and 2.9.

TABLE 2.8. **Presentation and Treatment of Water-Soluble Vitamin Deficiencies**

VITAMIN	ETIOLOGY	SYMPTOMS/EXAM	TREATMENT
B_1 (thiamine)	The most common cause is alcoholism.	Anorexia, muscle cramps, paresthesias. Dry beriberi leading to neuropathy and Wernicke-Korsakoff syndrome; wet beriberi leading to high-output heart failure.	Oral thiamine.
B_2 (riboflavin)	Usually occurs with other deficiencies.	Nonspecific symptoms (eg, mouth soreness, glossitis, cheilosis, weakness, irritability) plus seborrheic dermatitis and anemia.	Oral vitamin B_2.
B_3 (niacin)	Associated with alcoholism.	Nonspecific symptoms (see above); **pellagra** (dermatitis, diarrhea, dementia).	Oral nicotinamide.
B_6 (pyridoxine)	Associated with medication interactions (INH, OCPs) or with alcoholism. Fat malabsorption syndromes may contribute.	Nonspecific symptoms (see above); peripheral neuropathy, anemia, and seizures. Levels can be measured (normal > 50 ng/mL).	Oral or intramuscular vitamin B_6.
B_{12} (cyanocobalamin)	Found in vegans, gastrectomy patients, and those with pernicious anemia.	Megaloblastic anemia, glossitis, anorexia, diarrhea. Peripheral neuropathy, balance problems, dementia (reversible if treated within 6 months).	Vitamin B_{12} administered intramuscularly.

TABLE 2.8. **Presentation and Treatment of Water-Soluble Vitamin Deficiencies** *(continued)*

VITAMIN	ETIOLOGY	SYMPTOMS/EXAM	TREATMENT
C (ascorbic acid)	Found in urban poor, elderly, alcoholics, cancer patients, smokers, and those in renal failure.	**Scurvy:** Poor wound healing, easy bruising, bleeding gums, subperiosteal hemorrhage, and anemia leading to edema, oliguria, neuropathy, and intracerebral hemorrhage.	Oral vitamin C.
Biotin	Caused by eating large quantities of raw eggs.	Myalgias, dysesthesias, anorexia, and nausea leading to dermatitis and alopecia.	Oral biotin.
Folic acid	Caused by inadequate dietary intake.	Megaloblastic anemia, neural tube defects.	Oral folic acid.

Vitamins and Disease Prevention

Vitamins recommended for prevention of chronic disease are summarized in Table 2.10.

TABLE 2.9. **Presentation and Treatment of Fat-Soluble Vitamin Deficiencies**

VITAMIN	ETIOLOGY	SYMPTOMS/EXAM	TREATMENT
A (retinol)	Found in urban poor, elderly, and those with fat malabsorption syndrome.	Night blindness, xerosis, Bitot's spots (white patches on the conjunctivae) leading to keratomalacia, endophthalmitis, and blindness.	High-dose vitamin A.
D	Found in elderly patients, those with insufficient sun exposure, those suffering from malnutrition or malabsorption, breast-feeding infants, and anticonvulsant users.	**Children:** Rickets (restlessness, craniotabes, costochondral beading, bowlegs, kyphoscoliosis). **Adults:** Osteomalacia.	High-dose oral vitamin D.
E	Associated with severe malabsorption.	Areflexia, peripheral neuropathy, gait abnormality, ophthalmoplegia, ↓ proprioception.	Oral vitamin E.
K	Caused by poor diet, malabsorption, antibiotic use.	Clotting factor deficiencies (II, VII, IX, X).	Vitamin K SQ.

TABLE 2.10. Vitamin Supplements to Prevent Chronic Disease

VITAMIN	DOSE	PREVENTION
Folic acid	400–1000 µg/day in women of childbearing age.	Neural tube defects.
D	800 IU/day (with 1–2 g of calcium).	Fractures, osteoporosis.

Be cautious in offering several vitamins, including A, C, and E, with antioxidant functions for protection against cancer, heart disease and Alzheimer's disease since studies report equivocal results for these effects, and several vitamins have been shown to be detrimental at high doses.

HERBAL MEDICINES

More than 40% of the U.S. population use some type of complementary or alternative medicine. Effects of herbal supplements are difficult to evaluate 2° to problems in isolating the active component. Some have been demonstrated to be safe and effective (see Table 2.11). Others have been found to have deleterious effects. Use the following herbal remedies with caution:

- **Black licorice:** Causes hypertension.
- **Chromium:** ↓ blood sugar.
- **Garlic, ginger, gingko, ginseng, feverfew, CoQ10:** Prolong INR.

TABLE 2.11. Safe and Effective Herbal Medications

HERBAL MEDICATION	DISEASE/CONDITION	NOTES
Garlic powder	High cholesterol.	Has modest effect; prolongs INR.
Ginger root	Nausea, motion sickness.	Prolongs INR.
Glucosamine	Osteoarthritis.	Use with caution in the presence of seafood allergy.
Horse chestnut	Venous insufficiency.	
Peppermint oil	IBS.	
Saw palmetto	BPH.	Give at a dose of 160 mg BID or 320 mg qd.
St John's wort	Depression.	Use with caution in light of multiple drug interactions.

> **KEY FACT**
>
> Be aware of herbal remedies that interact with warfarin (Coumadin) including **g**arlic, **g**inger, **g**ingko, **g**inseng, feverfew, and CoQ10.

Travel Medicine

A 30-year-old businessman presents to your office seeking advice about his upcoming job relocation to Calcutta. He is leaving in 5 weeks and will be staying in India for 6 months. The man has no significant past medical history and is generally in good health. He has his immunization record with him but is concerned that he may need some boosters or perhaps some additional vaccinations. His biggest concerns, however, are of contracting malaria and having his stay in India tainted by bouts of diarrhea. How do you address his concerns?

Review his immunization records, looking specifically for the date of his last tetanus booster and whether he has been immunized against HAV and HBV; offer general travel advice regarding food, water, and insect repellant; and provide prescriptions for both malaria prophylaxis and traveler's diarrhea, with strict and clear instructions on when and how they should be taken.

Travel is associated with potential morbidity and even mortality from infectious sources, modes of transportation, environmental exposures, and adverse medical outcomes from illnesses independent of travel. Offer the following guidelines and recommendations to those contemplating or planning travel to reduce the risk of adverse events.

PRETRAVEL ASSESSMENT

- Determine the patient's **health status** (eg, infants, elderly, pregnant women, or those with chronic illnesses or underlying medical conditions).
- Identify potential **medical needs** (eg, allergy to vaccine components, medication use, immunosuppression).
- Evaluate the patient's **travel itinerary** (eg, planned destinations, climate and altitude, rural vs. urban environment, duration of stay, accommodations, purpose of travel).

GENERAL GUIDELINES

- **Food:** Advise patients that **fruits are safe only when peeled** and that **vegetables need to be fully cooked** to prevent contamination from fecally passed organisms in the soil. Unpasteurized dairy products and inadequately cooked fish or meat should be avoided.
- **Water:** Counsel patients to **avoid ice cubes** and that water is safe only after it has been boiled. Chlorination will kill most viral and bacterial pathogens, but protozoal pathogens such as *Giardia lamblia* can survive. Carbonated drinks, beer, wine, and drinks made from boiled water are safe.
- **Insect repellents:** Advise travelers to use at least **20% DEET** on clothing and exposed skin to prevent mosquito-borne infections such as malaria, yellow fever, and dengue fever. Protection with DEET lasts for several

hours but is mitigated by swimming, washing, sweating, wiping, and rain. Travelers may also choose to treat clothing and bed netting with **permethrin,** which can effectively repel mosquitoes for more than a week, even with washing.

- **Medications:** Advise travelers to bring adequate supplies of regularly used medications, since equivalent drugs may not be available at their destinations. Medications should be stored in carry-on luggage in the event that checked baggage is lost in transit.
- **Other:**
  - Counsel patients to **avoid swimming in fresh water** in areas where schistosomiasis is prevalent. Swimming in chlorinated or salt water is safe.
  - Give patients safe-sex counseling and advice regarding sun protection.

> **KEY FACT**
>
> Guidelines for travelers with regard to food and water: "Boil it, cook it, peel it, or forget it!"

RECOMMENDED VACCINATIONS

Address 3 **categories of vaccinations:**

- **Routine or standard immunizations:** Review childhood immunization programs and age-appropriate updates, regardless of travel (see Table 2.1).
- **Required immunizations:** Offer **yellow fever** vaccine for travel to certain parts of sub-Saharan Africa and tropical South America. Offer the **meningococcal** vaccine for travel to Saudi Arabia during the Hajj (required by the Saudi Arabian government).
- **Recommended immunizations:** Offer HAV, HBV, typhoid fever, meningococcal meningitis, Japanese encephalitis, rabies, and tick-borne encephalitis, depending on the trip-related risk and exposure to such diseases.

MALARIA PROPHYLAXIS

> **KEY FACT**
>
> Advise travelers to minimize exposure between dusk and dawn since mosquitoes that transmit malaria usually feed at night.

Address malaria prophylaxis with all patients planning travel to endemic regions. Malaria is transmitted by the female *Anopheles* mosquito and is most commonly caused by the organism *Plasmodium falciparum*; other species include *P vivax*, *P malariae*, and *P ovale*. Symptoms can begin from 8 days after initial infection to several months after departure from the malarious region. The 2 most important components of malaria prevention are **avoidance of mosquitoes and chemoprophylaxis** (see Table 2.12).

TRAVELER'S DIARRHEA

> **KEY FACT**
>
> Avoid the use of bismuth subsalicylate in patients with aspirin allergy, renal insufficiency, and gout and in those taking anticoagulants, probenecid, or methotrexate.

Approximately 40%–60% of travelers to developing countries develop diarrhea. Of these cases, 85% are caused by bacterial pathogens, the most common of which is **enterotoxigenic *E coli*** (ETEC). Parasites account for 10% and viruses for 5% of cases. Counsel patients traveling to developing countries on the following preventive measures:

- Advise travelers to pay attention to food and beverage selection (see the guidelines listed above).
- You may offer **bismuth subsalicylate,** the active ingredient in Pepto-Bismol, which has been shown to ↓ **the incidence of traveler's diarrhea** from 40% to 14%. Discuss side effects, which include blackening of the tongue and stool, nausea, constipation, and, rarely, tinnitus. **Avoid use in children** with viral infections because of the risk of Reye syndrome.
- Do not routinely offer prophylactic antibiotics to travelers.

TABLE 2.12.   Drugs Used for Malaria Prophylaxis

Drug Name	Indication	Administration	Safe for Children?	Safe in Pregnancy?	Side Effects
Atovaquone/ proguanil (Malarone)	Prophylaxis in areas with chloroquine-resistant or mefloquine-resistant *P falciparum*.	Daily dosing. Begin 1–2 days before travel and continue for 7 days after leaving the malarious area.	Yes, if weight is > 11 kg.	**No.**	Abdominal pain, nausea, vomiting, headache, rash.
Chloroquine phosphate (Aralen and generic)	Prophylaxis only in areas with chloroquine-sensitive *P falciparum*.	Weekly dosing. Begin 1–2 weeks before travel and continue for 4 weeks after departure from the malarious area.	Yes.	Yes.	GI disturbance, dizziness, blurred vision, headache, insomnia, pruritus.
Doxycycline	Prophylaxis in areas with chloroquine-resistant or mefloquine-resistant *P falciparum*.	Daily dosing. Begin 1–2 days before travel and continue for 4 weeks after departure from the malarious area.	Yes, if ≥ 8 years of age.	**No.**	Photosensitivity skin reactions.
Mefloquine (Lariam and generic)	Prophylaxis in areas with chloroquine-resistant *P falciparum*.	Weekly dosing. Begin 1–2 weeks before travel and continue for 4 weeks after departure from the malarious area.	Yes.	Yes, in the second and third trimesters.	Nausea, dizziness, vertigo. Lightheadedness, bad dreams, paranoid ideation, seizures, psychosis in patients with significant psychopathology.
Primaquine	Good choice for prophylaxis in areas where *P vivax* is the main species.	Begin 1–2 days before travel and continue daily until 7 days after departure.	Yes, if not G6PD deficient.	No.	In G6PD normal persons, GI upset if taken on empty stomach is common. In G6PD deficiency, primaquine can cause fatal hemolysis. Rule out **G6PD deficiency by appropriate lab test** before use.

SYMPTOMS/EXAM

- Patients may present with malaise, anorexia, nausea, vomiting, and abdominal cramps, followed by sudden onset of watery diarrhea 4–14 days after arrival, with symptoms lasting 1–5 days.
- Patients typically do not present with symptoms of colitis such as blood or pus in the stool +/– low-grade fever.

TREATMENT

- **Replace fluids:** The 1° and most important treatment! Replete both fluid **volume** and **electrolytes.**
- Give **antibiotics** for those presenting with moderate to severe diarrhea characterized by more than 4 unformed stools daily; fever; or blood, pus,

Replace fluids in patients with diarrhea using a solution of ½ teaspoon of salt, ½ teaspoon of baking soda, and 4 tablespoons of sugar in 1 L of water.

or mucus in the stool. Use a fluoroquinolone such as **ciprofloxacin or azithromycin** in areas of increasing resistance to fluoroquinolones.

■ Do not use antimotility agents for mild to moderate cases; use only in severe cases in conjunction with antibiotics. Discontinue if abdominal pain worsens or if diarrhea persists after 2 days.

■ You may use **bismuth subsalicylate,** which has antisecretory and antimicrobial properties, to ↓ stool frequency and shorten the duration of illness (15 mL or 2 tablets every 30 minutes for up to 8 doses).

■ Advise patients to seek medical care in the presence of high fever, severe abdominal pain, bloody diarrhea, or vomiting, and when antibiotics have not been helpful.

Domestic Violence

CHILD ABUSE

Defined as a recent act or failure to act by a parent or caretaker that results in the death, serious physical or emotional harm, sexual abuse, or exploitation of a child < 18 years of age. In the United States, the incidence of child abuse and neglect ranges from 15–42 per 1000 children. All 50 states have laws requiring physicians to report suspected child abuse to Child Protective Services.

Table 2.13 outlines common risk factors for child abuse. Suspect child abuse in the presence of the following:

■ A history that is **inconsistent with the child's injuries.**
■ A history that is **vague** or that changes in repeated versions.
■ A history that is **inconsistent with the developmental stage** of the child.
■ An **implausible** history.
■ Multiple injuries in various stages of healing or different types of coexisting injuries.
■ Evidence of poor caretaking.
■ Behavioral disturbances in the child.
■ Arguing, roughness, or observed **violence** in interaction with a parent.
■ **Aloofness** or lack of emotional interaction between the parent and child.

TABLE 2.13. **Risk Factors for Child Abuse**

PERPETRATORS	ENVIRONMENT	VICTIMS
Most commonly fathers, mothers' boyfriends, female babysitters, and mothers (in descending order of frequency).	Financial difficulties.	Young age.
	Divorce or interpersonal conflict.	Past history of abuse or repeated injuries.
	Illness.	Speech and language disorders.
Young or single parents.	Professional problems.	Learning disabilities.
Parents with lower levels of education.	Social isolation.	Conduct disorders.
Those with unstable family situations.	Distant or absent extended family.	Congenital anomalies.
Those with a history of abuse.	Acceptability of violence as a means of problem solving.	Mental retardation or other handicaps.
Those with a history of substance abuse.		Chronic illnesses.
Those with psychiatric illness.		Hyperactivity.
		Adopted children.
		Stepchildren.
		Prematurity and low birth weight.

- Inappropriate parental response to the severity of injury.
- A **delay** in seeking medical care.
- Partial confession by the parent.

Be cognizant of the **4 major types** of child abuse: **physical abuse** (inflicting physical pain or injury); **sexual abuse** (nonconsensual contact of any kind); **emotional or psychological abuse;** and **child neglect.**

Consider **physical abuse** in the following circumstances:

- Bilateral, symmetric injuries seen on the buttocks, genitalia, back, and back of hands (vs. accidental injuries, which are seen on the shins, forearms, and hips).
- Fractures to the metaphyses caused by pulling or wrenching (eg, chip fractures, where the corner of the metaphysis of a long bone is torn off, with damage to the epiphysis).
- Characteristic burns caused by abuse are cigarette burns, immersion burns affecting the buttocks and perineum, clearly demarcated scald lines without evidence of splash marks, and stocking-glove burns on the hands or feet.

Injury to the head is the most common cause of death from physical abuse. Children can present with convulsions, apnea, ↑ ICP, subdural hemorrhages, retinal hemorrhages, or coma. Do a **complete skeletal survey** in children < 2 years of age when physical abuse is suspected. Children with a history of "easy bruising" should receive a screen for a bleeding diathesis, including CBC, PT, PTT, and bleeding time.

Consider **sexual abuse** in the following circumstances:

- Vaginal, penile, or rectal pain as well as erythema, discharge, bleeding, chronic dysuria, enuresis, constipation, or encopresis.
- Inappropriate behaviors such as sexualized activity with peers or objects or seductive behavior also suggest a history of sexual abuse.

Recommendations for Screening

- Be alert for signs and symptoms associated with abuse and neglect.
- The AAFP and the USPSTF have concluded that there is insufficient evidence to recommend for or against screening of parents or guardians for the abuse of children.

INTIMATE-PARTNER ABUSE

Defined as **intentional controlling by or violent behavior from** a person who was or is in an intimate relationship with the victim. This behavior may be **physical abuse, sexual assault, emotional abuse, economic control, and/or social isolation.**

- Women are more likely than men to be the victims of chronic physical abuse.
- Violence in gay and lesbian relationships appears to be as common as in heterosexual relationships.
- Most states do not currently require mandatory reporting of domestic violence against competent adult women. Table 2.14 outlines risk factors for intimate-partner abuse.

KEY FACT

A history that is inconsistent with the patient's injuries is the hallmark of physical abuse.

T A B L E 2 . 1 4 .   Risk Factors for Intimate-Partner Abuse

RISK FACTORS	WHEN TO SUSPECT
Female gender.	Inconsistent explanation of injuries.
Young age.	Delay in seeking treatment.
Low socioeconomic status.	Multiple somatic complaints.
Pregnancy.	Gynecologic conditions such as premenstrual syndrome, STDs, unintended
Mental health problems.	pregnancy, or chronic pelvic pain.
Substance abuse on the part of victims or perpetrators.	Lateness for prenatal care visits.
Separated or divorced status.	Frequent ER visits.
History of childhood abuse.	Patient noncompliance.
	Central distribution of injuries (breasts, abdomen, genitals).

Recommendations for Screening

- Be alert for signs and symptoms of intimate-partner violence.
- The USPSTF found insufficient evidence to recommend for or against the routine screening of women for intimate-partner violence.

Occupational Medicine

 A 57-year-old smoker comes to see you complaining of feeling out of breath when he takes walks with his wife. He wonders if he is just getting old. He denies any chest pain or other cardiac symptoms. You discover that he has worked in shipbuilding for > 30 years, and on pulmonary exam you note some fine crackles. He also has clubbing of his fingernails. What are your next steps?

Suspecting COPD as well as possible asbestosis, you obtain a CXR and PFTs.

Work-related injuries and illnesses are prevalent and are associated with significant morbidity, mortality, and cost, both to the individual and to society.

- Pulmonary diseases predominate occupational illnesses. The etiologies and presentation of common occupational pulmonary illnesses are outlined in Table 2.15.
- Common nonpulmonary occupational illnesses include carpal tunnel syndrome, low back pain/injury, and contact dermatitis.

EVALUATION OF ILLNESS

Use the following guidelines to evaluate occupational illness:

- Take a **brief history** of possible work-related injuries or illnesses, including symptoms/review of systems; current and past jobs held; and the temporal relationship of the symptoms to jobs or work schedule.
- Include other components of the history such as **evaluation of products used** or manufactured at the workplace, examination of Material Safety Data Sheets (MSDSs) and assessment of the degree of protective measures taken (eg, protective clothing, appropriate ventilation).

KEY FACT

Occupational exposures that can present with fever include toxic organic dust syndrome, hypersensitivity pneumonitis, and metal fume fever (zinc exposure).

TABLE 2.15.   Common Occupational Pulmonary Disorders

ILLNESS	AGENTS/POTENTIAL EXPOSURE	CLINICAL PRESENTATION
Asthma	Isocyanates, flour, dyes, metals, wood dust, latex. Rubber or plastic production, bakers.	Rhinoconjunctivitis, wheezing.
Silicosis	Crystalline silica mining, quarrying, sandblasting, masonry, foundry work, ceramics.	May be asymptomatic, with an abnormal CXR (nodules or fibrosis), or may present with cough and dyspnea.
Asbestosis	Textiles, shipbuilding, cement, insulation, plumbing, pipefitting, renovation of asbestos-containing buildings.	After 20–30 years, presents with dyspnea on exertion. Fine bibasilar crackles and clubbing may also be seen. CXR shows interstitial fibrosis and pleural plaques. **Can lead to mesothelioma.**
Toxic organic dust syndrome	Moldy hay.	Fever, cough, wheezing, dyspnea.
Hypersensitivity pneumonitis (extrinsic allergic alveolitis)	Farmer's lung, hot tub lung, humidifiers, birds/poultry, grain processing, lumber milling/construction.	**Acute:** Fever, malaise, cough, dyspnea, chest tightness (no wheeze!) 4–6 hours after exposure. **Chronic:** Weight loss, fatigue, dyspnea, clubbing. Consider in the presence of recurrent "pneumonias."

- **Exam:** The physical exam should include evaluation of the lungs, skin, any painful musculoskeletal region as well as an examination of the extremities for clubbing.
- **Dx:** Diagnostic testing will often include a CXR and PFTs.

The following groups may be of aid if on-site investigation is necessary:

- **The Occupational Safety and Health Administration (OSHA):** Within the Department of Labor. Creates and enforces workplace safety and health regulations.
- **The Environmental Protection Agency (EPA).**
- **The National Institute for Occupational Safety and Health (NIOSH):** Part of the Centers for Disease Control and Prevention (CDC) and within the Department of Health and Human Services (DHHS). Conducts research and makes recommendations for the prevention of work-related illnesses and injuries.
- American College of Occupational and Environmental Medicine (ACOEM).
- The Association of Occupational and Environmental Clinics (AOEC).
- **Private certified industrial hygienists.**
- **Poison Control Centers.**

IMPAIRMENT VS. DISABILITY

- **Impairment:** Defined as loss or abnormality of psychological, physiological, or anatomical structure or functioning of a body part or organ system, which can be shown by medically acceptable clinical and laboratory diagnostic techniques.
- **Disability:** An impediment that prevents an individual from interacting with the environment at the specific level determined by the legal system. Defined by the Social Security Administration as "the inability to engage

in any substantial gainful activity by reason of any medically determinable physical or mental impairment which can be expected to lead to death or which has lasted or can be expected to last for a continuous period of not less than 12 months."

In your assessment, you may state just the objective findings and degree to which the patient's functional capacity is limited. You do not need to and are not expected to make a disability determination.

Public Health

SMOKING CESSATION

Prevalence of cigarette smoking among adults in the United States was estimated by the CDC to be 21% in 2008. Smoking causes as many as 400,000 deaths/year and is the most common preventable cause of death.

Smoking cessation is known to confer the following **health benefits:**

- **MI:** ↓ mortality risk. The risk of recurrent coronary events is progressively ↓ to near that of a nonsmoker by 3 years postcessation.
- **Stroke:** Associated with a ↓ risk over time.
- **Pulmonary disease:** ↓ progression in the decline of FEV_1 in patients with COPD. Also associated with a ↓ risk of pulmonary infections such as bacterial pneumonia and TB.
- **Malignancy:** ↓ risk of lung, kidney, bladder, stomach, and cervical cancers, among others.
- **PUD:** ↓ risk of developing PUD; accelerated rate of healing.
- **Osteoporosis:** ↓ risk of bone loss and fracture (begins 10 years after quitting).

KEY FACT

Three years after smoking cessation, the risk of recurrent MI ↓ to that of a nonsmoker.

Cessation Methods

- Evaluate the patient's cigarette use, assess his or her interest in quitting, and find out about previous attempts at quitting.
- Once the patient is ready, offer strategies such as setting a "quit day" and help define alternative oral behaviors to substitute for the cigarette (eg, gum, throat lozenges).
- Many behavioral methods have been advocated to encourage patients to work toward quitting. Discuss and agree upon methods for cessation (see Table 2.16) in advance of the quit day.

POSTEXPOSURE PROPHYLAXIS (PEP)

Measures for PEP, which are also key to infection control, are as follows:

- **TB:** Offer tuberculin skin testing (TST) to close contacts of individuals with active TB. A reaction > 5 mm is considered ⊕. A ⊖ test should be repeated 10–12 weeks later. Those with a ⊕ test should be treated with INH for latent TB infection.
- **HAV:** Transmitted by fecal-oral spread. PEP consists of concurrent administration of **immune globulin (IgG) and the first dose of the HAV vaccine.** Consider PEP in the following individuals who have had close contact with an individual with serologic confirmation of infection:
  - Unvaccinated household and sexual contacts.
  - Those who have shared needles with the infected individual.

TABLE 2.16.   Methods for Smoking Cessation

METHOD	DESCRIPTION	EFFICACY
Group counseling	Lectures, groups, exercises, strategies.	Associated with a 20% 1-year quit rate.
Nicotine replacement (gum, patch, nasal spray, inhaler)	Suppresses withdrawal symptoms: depressed mood, insomnia, irritability, restlessness, weight gain.	When used with a behavioral program, gum and patch methods double the quit rate.
Bupropion	Enhances central noradrenergic and dopaminergic function when administered at a dosage of 150 mg daily.	Greater efficacy than nicotine replacement. Buproprion used together with nicotine patches has been shown to have > 50% efficacy.
Varenicline	Partial agonist of the nicotinic acetylcholine receptor. Case reports of suicidal thoughts and aggressive and erratic behavior have been reported.	As effective as or more effective than bupropion.
Hypnosis and acupuncture		No evidence to support the efficacy of these procedures.

- Staff, attendees, or residents of day care and nursing home facilities.
- Food handlers.
- **HBV and HCV:** Blood borne or transmitted sexually. An estimated 600,000–800,000 needlestick injuries occur annually in hospitals in the United States. Guidelines for PEP are as follows:
    - OSHA-required evaluation of health care workers exposed to needle-stick or mucous membrane contact must include identification of the source individual and testing of his/her blood for HBV, HCV, and HIV.
    - Offer **hepatitis B immune globulin (HBIG)** and start the vaccine series to an unvaccinated individual who has been exposed to HBV.
    - There is no proven effective PEP for HCV. Obtain liver enzymes, HCV RNA, and serologic testing at the time of exposure as well as 4 weeks later.
- **HIV:** Exposure to HIV can occur in health care settings as well as through sex, needle sharing, or blood transfusions. The seroconversion rate of health care workers after a needlestick injury is estimated to be < 1%. The risk of conversion is influenced by the type of exposure as well as by the viral load of the source. For sexual transmission, receptive anal intercourse confers the highest risk of infection. Use the following guidelines:
    - Conduct the OSHA-required evaluation similar to that described for the hepatitis viruses for health care worker exposures.
    - Make the decision to administer PEP after carefully considering risks and benefits because PEP for HIV is more inconvenient and is associated with possible toxicity.
    - Handle PEP in nonoccupational exposures in a similar manner, although management of individuals with ongoing behavioral risk is difficult.
    - Start PEP as soon as possible (within 72 hours of exposure) when deemed appropriate.
    - Start a 4-week course of a dual nucleoside or nucleotide reverse transcriptase inhibitor (NRTI) regimen (**basic 2-drug regimen**) consisting

KEY FACT

No proven effective postexposure prophylaxis is available for HCV.

of zidovudine (AZT) plus lamivudine (3TC) or emtricitabine (FTC) OR tenofovir (TDF) plus 3TC or FTC, as recommended by the CDC.

- Add a protease inhibitor for severe or high-risk exposures (**expanded 3-drug regimen**).
- Obtain HIV serology testing at the time of exposure as well as at 6 weeks, 12 weeks, and 6 months.

BIOTERRORISM

Biological weapons are a credible threat to the public. Organisms and toxins that are sturdy, readily grown in large quantities, and easily disseminated over large areas—such as anthrax, smallpox, plague, botulism, tularemia, Ebola/Marburg viruses, and Lassa/Junin viruses—are the most dangerous.

Anthrax

Bacillus anthracis, a spore-forming gram-$\oplus$ rod, is transmitted to humans through direct contact with infected animals or with animal products through skin exposure, inhalation, or ingestion.

Symptoms/Exam

- **Cutaneous anthrax** presents as small, painless papules, which enlarge to become vesicles that ulcerate, with eschar formation within 2 days. Fever and hematologic abnormalities may also be seen.
- **Inhalational anthrax (woolsorter disease)** is acquired from inhalation of spores that result in hemorrhagic necrosis of thoracic lymph nodes and hemorrhagic mediastinitis. This initially presents with flulike symptoms and then progresses to severe respiratory distress and to bacteremia and meningitis. You may see a widened mediastinum on CXR.
- **Pharyngeal and GI anthrax** is acquired from consumption of infected meat. Presents with fever, pharyngitis, neck swelling, and eschars in the oropharynx or with severe abdominal pain, hemorrhagic ascites, and melena.

Diagnosis

Obtain a Gram stain and culture of lesions, PCR, or serologic testing.

Treatment

Treat with ciprofloxacin or doxycycline for cutaneous anthrax. Use a multidrug regimen for inhalational anthrax. You may also use ciprofloxacin and doxycycline for **chemoprophylaxis.**

Smallpox

A highly contagious disease that is caused by the variola virus. No cases have been reported since its global eradication in 1979. Smallpox is transmitted via inhalation and is generally not widespread owing to the severity of the disease. The incubation period is 7–19 days.

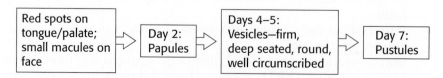

FIGURE 2.1.   **Progression of smallpox infection.**

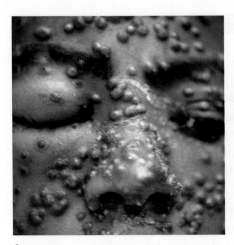
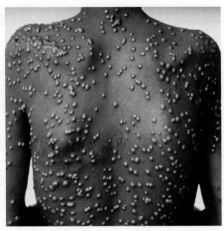
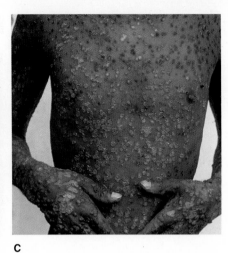

A   B   C

FIGURE 2.2.   Smallpox lesions. Multiple pustules becoming confluent on the face (**A**). Multiple pustules on the trunk, all in the same stage of development (**B**). Multiple crusted healing lesions on the trunk, arms, and hands (**C**). (Reproduced, with permission, from Wolff K, Johnson RA. *Fitzpatrick's Color Atlas & Synopsis of Clinical Dermatology*, 6th ed. New York: McGraw-Hill, 2009, Fig. 27-8.)

SYMPTOMS/EXAM

- Infection begins with 2–4 days of fever, headache, backache, and vomiting. The rash progresses as illustrated in Figure 2.1.
- The rash then spreads centrifugally, and, as lesions evolve, they may become confluent or umbilicated (see Figure 2.2). Lesions then crust over by day 14.

DIAGNOSIS

Diagnosis is made clinically by the criteria described in Table 2.17. If all 3 major criteria are met, report to local health authorities immediately and consult infectious disease specialists. Confirm diagnosis through culture of the virus from skin lesions and serologic tests.

TREATMENT

No known effective treatment. Place individuals with suspected smallpox in respiratory and contact isolation. Vaccinate exposed individuals during the incubation period to prevent spread.

COMPLICATIONS

Prognosis depends on the type of smallpox. Variola major strains have a mortality rate of approximately 20%, whereas minor strains have a mortality rate of < 1%. Death is usually related to toxic shock. Bacterial superinfection of rash is also a frequent complication.

TABLE 2.17.   Diagnostic Criteria for Smallpox

MAJOR CRITERIA	MINOR CRITERIA
Febrile prodrome.	Centrifugal distribution.
Classic smallpox lesions.	First lesions on oral mucosa/palate, face, or forearms.
Lesions in the same state of development.	The patient appears toxic or moribund.
	Slow evolution (each stage lasting 1–2 days).
	Lesions on palms and soles.

TUBERCULOSIS

Latent Tuberculosis Infection (LTBI)

A 43-year-old homeless man presents to your clinic to establish care. He has occasional wheezing but otherwise has no complaints. His medical problems include diabetes, hypertension, and tobacco use. He wonders if he should be tested for TB, since some of the men who lived at his previous shelter were recently diagnosed with active TB infection. He has had no fevers, night sweats, or cough. What do you advise?

On the basis of his homeless status and diabetes, he should be screened annually for latent TB infection. Since he may have had contact with active TB, induration ≥ 5 mm would constitute a ⊕ test for him. He would then require a CXR to rule out active disease and need 9 months of INH therapy to ↓ the risk of reactivation.

LTBI represents a large subset of infections caused by *Mycobacterium tuberculosis*, which infects 19%–43% of the world's population. The lifetime risk of acquiring reactivation TB with LTBI is roughly 10%–20%, with 2%–5% developing active TB in the first 2 years. If cases of LTBI are not detected and treated, new cases of TB will continually develop from this group (Figure 2.3).

DIAGNOSIS

- Use **TST** via PPD to detect LTBI. A delayed-type hypersensitivity reaction mediated by T lymphocytes results in induration of the skin 48–72 hours after inoculation.
- Obtain **annual screen** with PPD (in asymptomatic individuals) for:
  - Those with HIV infection.
  - Health care workers, prison guards, and mycobacteriology laboratory personnel.
  - Those with a medical condition that ↑ the risk of active TB (eg, diabetes, use of immunosuppressive medications, end-stage renal disease, alcoholism, conditions associated with rapid weight loss or chronic malnutrition).
  - Homeless individuals and IV drug users.
  - Those who reside in a long-term care facility.
- Obtain a **one-time screen** for:
  - Those with a single potential exposure to TB (repeat PPD in 6–12 weeks if the exposure is recent).
  - Those with an incidentally discovered fibrotic lung lesion.
  - Immigrants and refugees from countries with a high prevalence of TB.
- False-⊖ skin tests may be seen in cases of:
  - Anergic states such as HIV and malignancy.
  - Newly diagnosed pulmonary TB or severe extrapulmonary TB.
  - Corticosteroids or immunosuppressive therapy.
  - Concurrent viral infection.
  - Poor nutrition.
- Because different types of exposures and varying baseline immune status result in a wide distribution of PPD reactions, criteria have been developed to minimize the number of false ⊕s (see Table 2.18).

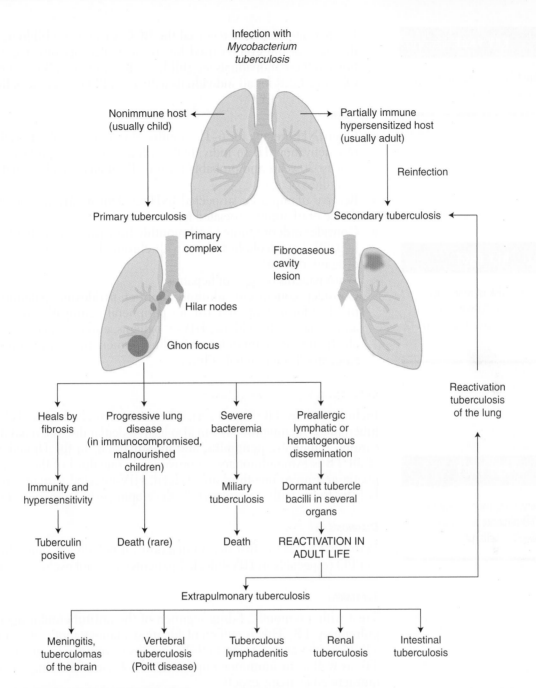

FIGURE 2.3. **Evolution of pulmonary tuberculosis.** (Reproduced, with permission, from Chandrasoma P, Taylor CR. *Concise Pathology,* 2nd ed. Originally published by Appleton & Lange. Copyright © 1995 by The McGraw-Hill Companies, Inc.)

TABLE 2.18. **Criteria for a Positive PPD**

≥ 5-MM INDURATION	≥ 10-MM INDURATION	≥ 15-MM INDURATION
Recent contact.	Immigrants who have come from a high-prevalence country within the past 5 years.	No risk factors.
HIV infection.	IV drug users.	
Chronic steroid use.	Residents/employees of high-risk facilities (hospitals, jails, nursing homes, shelters).	
Organ transplantation/ immunosuppression.	Those < 4 years of age.	
	Those < 18 years of age who have been exposed to a high-risk adult.	
Inactive TB on x-ray, untreated.		

- For persons who have received the BCG vaccine as children, interpret on the basis of the criteria used for unvaccinated persons. Large PPD reactions in these individuals are still likely to represent TB infection.
- Obtain a CXR for all individuals with a ⊕ PPD to exclude active disease.

TREATMENT

- Offer INH therapy for 6–12 months (9 months ideally) to reduce the risk of reactivation TB in individuals with a ⊕ PPD. Its protective effect lasts at least 20 years and probably for life. Treat all individuals with a ⊕ PPD, regardless of age.
- Reserve rifampin for suspected INH-resistant strains in view of the ↑ incidence of rifampin-associated liver toxicity.
- Consider ordering initial and monthly liver panels in patients at ↑ risk for hepatitis (eg, alcoholics, those with chronic liver disease, HIV-⊕ patients, drug interaction).
- Warn patients of signs of hepatitis.
- Consider concurrent administration of pyridoxine (vitamin B_6, 25–50 mg/day) for patients at ↑ risk for peripheral neuropathy, paresthesias, and ataxia, such as the elderly, HIV-⊕ patients, children, people with diabetes, alcoholics, pregnant or breast-feeding women, those with chronic liver disease, and those in renal failure.

Extrapulmonary Tuberculosis

Includes miliary TB (Figure 2.4), tuberculous lymphadenitis, skeletal TB, and tuberculous meningitis. TB can also lead to ocular disease, renal disease, pericarditis, salpingitis, peritonitis, and intestinal TB. In the United States, 5.4% of all TB is extrapulmonary. Approximately one-third of these cases are lymphatic and up to one-third are skeletal. HIV-infected patients are at particularly high risk, with as many as 60% developing extrapulmonary TB.

DIAGNOSIS

Perform TST as the first step in diagnosis, if not already done. Remember, a ⊖ PPD (especially in HIV-infected patients) does not exclude the diagnosis.

TREATMENT

Treat with a 6-month, 4-drug regimen of the **antitubercular agents** used for pulmonary TB. This is sufficient for most manifestations of extrapulmonary TB. Consider an extension to 9–12 months in miliary, meningeal, or skeletal TB, as well as in immunocompromised hosts (see following sections) as recommended by many experts.

Miliary Tuberculosis

Defined as the disseminated hematogenous spread of *M tuberculosis* (Figure 2.5). ↑ risk is seen with older age and comorbidities that alter cellular immunity (eg, diabetes, HIV, renal failure).

SYMPTOMS/EXAM

Presentation is highly variable, ranging from fevers, night sweats, and failure to thrive/generalized malaise to specific organ system dysfunction (see Table 2.19).

DIAGNOSIS

- CBC reveals hematologic derangements in either direction. ↑ ESR and hyponatremia are also commonly seen.

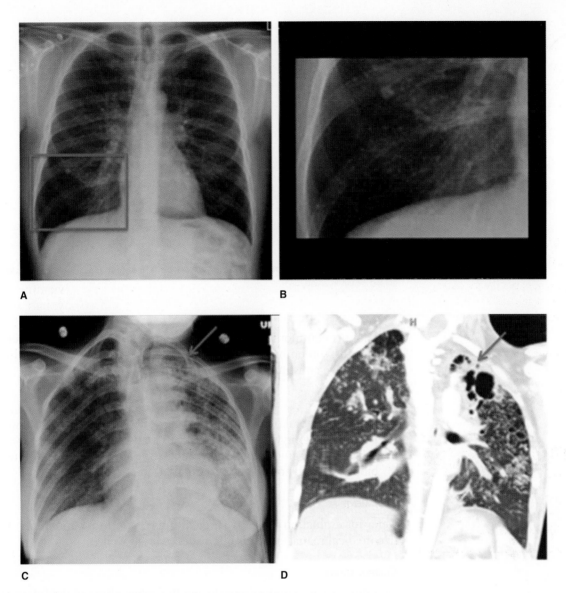

FIGURE 2.4. Pulmonary tuberculosis. (A) Frontal CXR demonstrating diffuse, 1- to 2-mm nodules due to miliary TB. **(B)** A zoomed-in view corresponding to the area delineated by the red box in Image A. **(C)** Frontal CXR demonstrating left apical cavitary consolidation *(red arrow)* and patchy infiltrates in the right and left lung in a patient with reactivation TB. **(D)** Coronal reformation from a noncontrast chest CT in the same patient as Image C, better demonstrating left apical cavitary consolidation *(red arrow)* and other areas of parenchymal abnormality corresponding to the endobronchial spread of TB. (Reproduced, with permission, from USMLERx.com.)

- A miliary pattern is seen on CXR in more than two-thirds of cases.
- Obtain an AFB smear and culture of accessible and suspicious body fluids.

Tuberculous Lymphadenitis

- **Sx:** Commonly presents as a single nontender lymph node (most often cervical—scrofula).
- **Dx:** Obtain an FNA or excisional biopsy. The latter is also a necessary aspect of treatment.

Skeletal Tuberculosis

SYMPTOMS/EXAM

- About one-half of cases involve the spine (Pott disease), but other common manifestations include tuberculous arthritis and extraspinal tuberculous osteomyelitis.

KEY FACT

Scrofula is tuberculous lymphadenitis of a cervical lymph node.

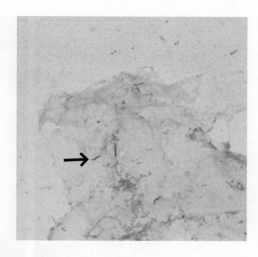

FIGURE 2.5.   *Mycobacterium tuberculosis* **on AFB smear.** (Courtesy of the Centers for Disease Control and Prevention, Atlanta, GA.)

■ Patients commonly present with progressive localized pain over weeks to months, sometimes associated with muscle spasm and rigidity. Fewer than 40% have constitutional symptoms.

DIAGNOSIS

■ Obtain vertebral plain films to look for osteolytic lesions.
■ Further imaging with CT or MRI can be useful.
■ Refer for CT-guided biopsy of infected lesions. For tuberculous arthritis, biopsy of the synovium or periarticular bone is necessary.

TREATMENT

Refer for evaluation for early surgical intervention to ↓ morbidity. Conservative medical management is often successful as well.

COMPLICATIONS

Monitor for cord compression during the active phase of the infection, which may result in paraplegia.

TABLE 2.19.   **Organ System Involvement in Miliary Tuberculosis**

ORGAN SYSTEM	CLINICAL MANIFESTATIONS
GI	Abnormal LFTs, hepatomegaly, cholestatic jaundice, pancreatitis, cholecystitis.
CNS	Meningitis, tuberculomas.
Skin	Tuberculosis cutis miliaris disseminata.
Cardiovascular	Pericarditis (rare).
Adrenal	Adrenal insufficiency (rare).
Renal	Sterile pyuria.

Tuberculous Meningitis

- **Sx:** Patients may present with headache, fevers, meningismus, vomiting, and other neurologic signs.
- **Dx:** Obtain an AFB stain and culture of CSF. Hydrocephalus is noted in a minority of patients on CT scan.
- **Tx:** Give corticosteroids for the first 6–8 weeks of therapy to ↓ mortality in both children and adults.

Epidemiology and Biostatistics

LEADING CAUSES OF DEATH

Table 2.20 outlines the principal causes of mortality, grouped by age.

TEST PARAMETERS

Common terms used in statistical methodology are as follows:

- **Incidence:** Defined as the **number of new cases** of a disease in a defined population over a specific period of time.
- **Prevalence:** Defined as the **number of existing cases** of disease in a given population over a specific period of time or a particular moment in time.
- **Sensitivity (Sn)—"PID" (Positive in Disease):** The probability that a test will be ⊕ in someone with the disease when compared with a gold standard; in other words, the test's **ability to correctly identify individuals who truly have the disease.**
- **Specificity (Sp)—"NIH" (Negative in Health):** The probability that a test will be ⊖ in someone who truly does not have the disease when compared with a gold standard; in other words, the test's **ability to correctly identify individuals who truly do not have the disease.**

In general, if a disease has a **low prevalence**, choose a **more specific test**, and if it has a **high prevalence**, choose a **more sensitive** test.

- **Positive predictive value (PPV):** The proportion of persons testing ⊕ who have the condition; in other words, **of all the people who test ⊕, the probability that they truly have the disease** (or the probability of disease in patient with a ⊕ test result).
- **Negative predictive value (NPV):** The proportion of persons testing ⊖ who do not have the disease; in other words, **of all the people who test ⊖, the probability that they truly do not have the disease** (or the probability of not having disease when test result is ⊖).
- **Likelihood ratio (LR):** Defined as the proportion of patients **with a disease** who have a certain test result over the proportion of patients **without**

KEY FACT

Remember: A sensitive test rarely misses patients with disease and is used if there are major consequences of missing the disease. Good diagnostic tests must be sensitive to rule out disease. **Sensitive tests pick true ⊕s.**

KEY FACT

Remember: A specific test picks true ⊖s and is useful to confirm or rule in a diagnosis. A specific test should have few false ⊕s. It is an ideal test if there are major consequences for true ⊕s.

KEY FACT

		Disease	
		+	−
Test	+	*a*	*b*
	−	*c*	*d*

$Sn = a / a + c$
$Sp = d / b + d$
$PPV = a / a + b$
$NPV = d / d + c$

KEY FACT

If prevalence is high, PPV ↑ and NPV ↓.

TABLE 2.20. Leading Causes of Death by Age Group

AGES 1–24	AGES 25–64	AGES 65 AND OLDER
Unintentional injuries	Malignant neoplasms	Heart disease
Suicide and homicide	Heart disease	Malignant neoplasms
Malignant neoplasms	Unintentional injuries	Cerebrovascular disease
Heart disease	HIV	COPD
Congenital anomalies	Suicide and homicide	Alzheimer disease

the disease who have the given test result (remember: "WOWO"—with over without).

- Pretest odds of a disease × LR = posttest odds of a disease.
- Positive LR = sensitivity / (1 – specificity) or true ⊕s/false ⊕s; for example, a high-probability V/Q scan has an LR of 14. This means that a ⊕ V/Q scan is 14 times more likely to be seen in patients **with** pulmonary embolism than in those **without** pulmonary embolism.
- Negative LR = (1 – sensitivity)/specificity; it shows how much the odds of disease are decreased if the test result is negative.

- **Lead-time bias:** Lead time is the time by which a screening test advances the date of diagnosis from the usually symptomatic phase to an earlier presymptomatic phase. The time between diagnosis and death will always ↑ by the amount of lead time (see Figure 2.6). To avoid lead-time bias, the lead time must be subtracted from the overall survival time of screened patients.
  - **Example:** A new screening test for pancreatic cancer is able to detect disease in a presymptomatic stage. Unfortunately, because the poor overall prognosis for the disease remains the same, screened patients know about their disease sooner and live with the disease longer but will still die of pancreatic cancer.
- **Length-time bias:** Because cases vary in the length of their asymptomatic phase, screening will overdetect cases of slowly progressing disease (longer asymptomatic phases) and miss rapidly progressive cases.
- **Relative risk (risk ratio):** Used in cohort studies and randomized controlled trials. Defined as the incidence of a disease in exposed individuals divided by the incidence of disease in unexposed individuals.
  - **Example:** Individuals with a high dietary fiber intake and those with a low fiber intake are evaluated for colon cancer to determine if fiber intake is a risk factor for colon cancer. Results may be a statement such as "Individuals who do not have a high-fiber diet have been shown to have a relative risk of 1.7 of developing colon cancer."
- **Odds ratio:** Used in case-control studies. Defined as the odds that an individual with a specific condition has been exposed to a risk factor divided by the odds that a control has been exposed.
  - **Example:** Individuals with colon cancer are compared with matched controls without colon cancer in terms of fiber intake. Results may be a statement such as "Individuals with colon cancer were *x* times less likely to have had a high-fiber diet than those without colon cancer."

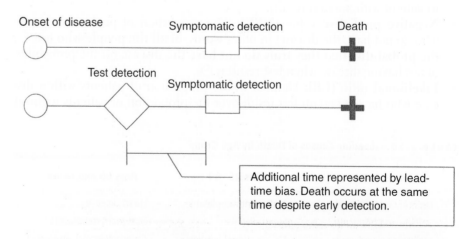

FIGURE 2.6. Lead-time bias. (Reproduced, with permission, from Le T, et al. *First Aid for the Internal Medicine Boards,* 2nd ed. New York: McGraw-Hill, 2008: 80.)

- **Absolute risk:** Calculated by subtracting the incidence of a disease in non-exposed persons from the incidence of disease in exposed persons (usually in percentage points).
- **Number needed to treat (NNT):** The number of patients needed to treat to prevent one additional bad outcome. NNT is the inverse of absolute risk.

MAJOR STUDY TYPES

Table 2.21 outlines the types of studies conducted in epidemiologic and biostatistical analyses.

THREATS TO VALIDITY

- **Confounding factor** is a variable that is associated with both the predictor variable and the outcome variable but does not have a causal relationship with either.
- **Recall bias** is self-reporting by subjects that is often influenced by knowledge of the study hypothesis.
- **Misclassification bias** occurs when a person without disease is "misclassified" into the disease group or vice versa.
- **Random misclassification** occurs when subjects are randomly placed in the wrong group, biasing results to the null hypothesis.
- **Nonrandom misclassification** occurs when subjects are selectively placed in the wrong group, biasing results either toward or away from the null hypothesis. Also referred to as **systematic or differential misclassification.** May introduce bias.
- **Selection bias** occurs when subjects are selected into or drop out of a study in a way that falsely changes the degree of association.

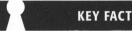

KEY FACT

	Disease	No Disease
Exposed	A	B
Unexposed	C	D

Relative risk: $\dfrac{A / (A + B)}{C / (C + D)}$

Odds ratio: $\dfrac{AD}{CB}$

TABLE 2.21. Categories of Studies

Study Type	Definition	Example	Advantages	Disadvantages
Randomized controlled trial	Subjects are **assigned** to an exposure, and disease outcomes are observed.	Assigning patients with hypertension to receive either a diuretic or an ACEI.	Controls for unforeseen confounders.	Expensive.
Cohort study	Exposed subjects are identified and then **followed** for disease outcomes.	Identifying obese children and then following them for the development of type 2 diabetes.	The most robust observational study type; can evaluate multiple exposures.	May take a long time to develop disease outcomes.
Case-control study	Cases and noncases of the disease are identified **before** defining the exposure.	Identifying children with certain birth defects and then looking for possible prenatal exposures.	Inexpensive; fast; ideal for rare diseases.	Prone to biases.
Cross-sectional study	Exposures and disease outcomes are **identified at the same time** within a **specific population** of subjects.	Checking for childhood diabetes while obtaining data on obesity in all children seen in specific community health clinics.	Survey data.	Cannot detect temporal relationship between exposure and outcome.

HYPOTHESIS TESTING

- **Null hypothesis** is the theory that the exposure or intervention being studied is not associated with the outcome of interest.
- **p-value** is a quantitative estimate of the probability that a study's outcome could occur by chance alone. A study with a $p < 0.05$ means that the probability of the results occurring by chance alone is < 1 in 20 and is thus "statistically significant."
- **Type I error (α):** The probability of detecting a difference when none exists and thus rejecting the null hypothesis.
- **Type II error (β):** The probability of failing to detect a difference when one exists and thus failing to reject the null hypothesis.
- **Power:** The probability of avoiding a type II error in a study; in other words, the probability that a study will not accept the null hypothesis and conclude that there was no difference when there really was one.

EVIDENCE-BASED MEDICINE

Evidence-based medicine can provide you with the tools for finding, understanding, and using the most up-to-date data from clinical research and making sound recommendations for patient care. The criteria by which evidence is graded are listed in Table 2.22; grades of evidence are described in Table 2.23.

TABLE 2.22.　Levels of Evidence (Oxford Centre for Evidence-Based Medicine)

LEVEL	DESCRIPTION
1a	Systematic review of randomized controlled trials.
1b	Individual randomized controlled trial.
1c	All-or-none.[a]
2a	Systematic review of cohort studies.
2b	Individual cohort study.
2c	Outcomes research[b] and ecological studies.
3a	Systematic review of case-control studies.
3b	Individual case-control study.
4	Case series.
5	Expert opinion.

[a]Met when all patients died before the treatment became available, but some now survive on it; or when some patients died before the treatment became available, but none now die on it.

[b]Looks at whether predicted outcomes (based on randomized controlled trials) are actually being observed in clinical practice.

TABLE 2.23. **Grades of Recommendation (Oxford Centre for Evidence-Based Medicine)**

GRADE	DESCRIPTION
A	Consistent level 1 studies.
B	Consistent level 2 or 3 studies or extrapolations from level 1 studies.
C	Level 4 studies or extrapolations from level 2 or 3 studies.
D	Level 5 evidence or troublingly inconsistent or inconclusive studies of any level.

CLINICAL TRIALS

Defined as studies in humans that answer specific health questions, including whether experimental treatments or new ways of using known treatments are safe and effective. Ideally conducted clinical trials provide one of the fastest and safest tools with which to change disease management and improve health in a population. Types of trials include the following:

- **Treatment trials:** Test experimental treatments, new combinations of drugs, or new approaches to surgery or radiation therapy.
- **Prevention trials:** Investigate better ways to prevent disease in a disease-free population or to prevent recurrent disease.
- **Diagnostic trials:** Investigate better tests or procedures for diagnosing a specific disease.
- **Screening trials:** Test the best way to detect disease and health conditions.
- **Quality-of-life trials:** Investigate for ways to improve comfort and quality of life for individuals with chronic diseases or illnesses.

Table 2.24 describes the phases through which drugs and treatments must proceed in clinical trials.

TABLE 2.24. **Phases of Clinical Trials**

PHASE	DESCRIPTION
Phase I	The experimental drug or treatment is tested in a small group of people (20–80) for the first time to evaluate **safety,** to determine safe **dosage ranges,** and to identify **side effects.**
Phase II	The experimental drug or treatment is tested in a larger group of people (100–300) to evaluate **efficacy** and further evaluate **safety.**
Phase III	The experimental drug or treatment is given to large groups of people (1000–3000) to confirm **efficacy,** to monitor for **side effects,** and to **compare** it with treatments already in use.
Phase IV	Postmarketing studies to determine additional information, including risks, benefits, and optimal use.

Other Topics

MEDICARE AND MEDICAID

The United States has 2 major publicly funded health insurance plans: Medicare and Medicaid. These plans are compared in detail in Table 2.25.

DISABILITY PROGRAMS

The United States government publicly funds 3 major disability programs: Social Security Disability Insurance (SSDI), Supplemental Security Income (SSI), and workers' compensation.

- **SSDI:** Like Medicare, SSDI is funded through payroll taxes. Once an individual meets both the definition of disabled (see the section on occupational medicine) and the eligibility criteria based on length of time employed and wages earned, he/she and dependents qualify for benefits. After 2 years on SSDI, the individual becomes eligible for Medicare benefits.
- **SSI:** Funded through general taxes rather than payroll or Social Security taxes. To be eligible, an individual must be > 65 years of age, blind, or disabled. In addition, only individuals with limited income and resources qualify.

TABLE 2.25. Comparison of Medicare and Medicaid

FUNDING SOURCE	MEDICARE	MEDICAID
Eligibility	Federal government. Those > 65 years of age (who have worked and therefore have contributed to Medicare through payroll taxes). Those < 65 years of age who are receiving Social Security disability. Patients receiving dialysis.	Federal and state governments (the federal government reimburses each state 50%–83% of costs). Pregnant women plus women and their children < 6 years of age if their family income is < 133% of poverty level. Children 6–17 years of age if their family income is < 100% of poverty level. The elderly poor. The disabled poor. Other optional groups vary by state.
Benefits	**Part A:** Inpatient services, skilled nursing facility, home health and hospice. **Part B:** Outpatient care, x-rays, durable medical equipment, laboratory work. **Part C (Medicare Advantage):** Allows enrollment in Medicare-eligible HMOs or PPOs; includes additional services such as dentures, eyeglasses, and drugs. **Part D:** Prescription drug benefit. **Medigap:** Private supplemental insurance.	Physician services; laboratory, x-ray, inpatient hospital care, family planning, prenatal, and maternity services. Nursing home care services. **Optional benefits:** Rehabilitation services, dental care, physical therapy, eyeglasses, intermediate-care facilities, inpatient psychiatric care for individuals > 65 or < 21 years of age.
Physician reimbursement	**Medicare-Approved Amount (MAA):** Government-determined payment for any given service. The physician can bill only up to the MAA. Medicare pays 80% of the MAA and the patient pays 20%.	Providers receive reimbursement directly from Medicaid and must accept that amount as payment in full.

- **Workers' compensation:** This program pays for medical expenses incurred from an injury or illnesses related to employment. A portion of the worker's wages is also paid out during the period of disability. Workers who are partially disabled can receive long-term payments of a portion of their salary.

HEALTH INSURANCE PORTABILITY AND ACCOUNTABILITY ACT (HIPAA)

In April 2003, the first-ever federal privacy standards to protect patients' medical records and other health information took effect. Developed by DHHS, these standards apply to health plans, doctors, hospitals, and other health care providers. In short, these new standards provide patients with access to their medical records and control over how their personal health information is used and disclosed. Patient protections include the following:

- **Access to medical records:** Patients should be able to see and obtain copies of their medical records and request that corrections be made.
- **Notice of privacy practices:** Covered health plans, doctors, and other health care providers must notify patients of their rights and how their personal medical information may be used.
- Limits on use of personal medical information.
- **Prohibition of marketing:** Patient authorization must be obtained before specific information may be used for marketing purposes.
- Confidential communications.
- **Complaints:** Patients have the right to file formal complaints regarding the privacy practices of a health plan or provider.

CHAPTER 3

Cardiology

Suzannah Stout, MD

Diagnostic Testing

PHYSICAL EXAM

Pulses

Table 3.1 addresses causes of increased and decreased pulses.

Heart Sounds

- **S1**: Closure of the mitral and tricuspid valves. ↓ with LV systolic dysfunction and mitral regurgitation. See Figure 3.1 for the relation of heart sounds to other parts of the cardiac cycle.
- **S2**: Closure of the aortic and pulmonary valves. Normally, the aortic component (A2) precedes the pulmonic component (P2).
  - **Physiologic splitting**: ↑ time between A2 and P2 with inspiration. P2 is delayed during inspiration as negative intrathoracic pressure pulls more blood volume into R side of the heart. Normalizes when the breath is held.
  - **Wide splitting**: Early closing of A2 or delayed P2. Causes include RBBB, pulmonic stenosis, pulmonary embolism (PE), or pulmonary hypertension.
  - **Paradoxical splitting**: A2 comes after P2 so ↑ splitting with expiration. Causes include AS, left bundle branch block (LBBB), use of a pacemaker, and LV systolic dysfunction.
  - **Fixed splitting**: Time between A2 and P2 doesn't vary with breath. Caused by atrial septal defect.
- **S3**: Low-pitched sound after S2 as ↑ blood volume flows into dilated ventricle. Best heard with the bell at the apex. Suggests ventricular enlargement and LV systolic dysfunction (CHF, dilated cardiomyopathy).
- **S4**: Low-pitched sound preceding S1 as atrial contraction forces blood into a stiff ventricle.

CARDIAC TESTING

Electrocardiography (ECG)

Definitions and guidelines pertinent to reading ECGs:

- **Dimensions:** One small box (1 mm) is 40 msec horizontally and 0.1 mV vertically.

TABLE 3.1. Alterations in Normal Pulses

	INCREASED	**DECREASED**	**NOTES**
Arterial	Aortic regurgitation (AR), persistent ductus arteriousus, high cardiac output (sepsis, hyperthyroid).	Peripheral vascular disease, low cardiac output.	**Water-hammer:** Radial rapid rise/fall, seen in AR.
Carotid		Delayed in aortic stenosis (AS).	**Pulsus bisferien:** Two pulse peaks, seen in AR and large PDA.
Jugular venous	Distention with volume overload (CHF), tamponade.		

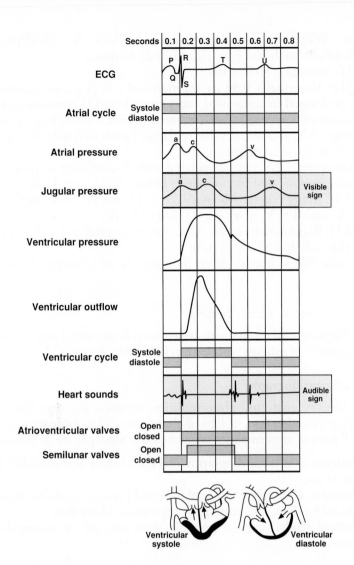

FIGURE 3.1. **Relation of heart sounds to other events in the cardiac cycle.** (Reproduced, with permission, from LeBlond RF, DeGowin RL, Brown DD. *DeGowin's Diagnostic Examination*, 9th ed. http://www.accessmedicine. com. Copyright © The McGraw-Hill Companies, Inc. All rights reserved.)

- **Rate:** The normal rate is 60–100 bpm. For discussion of abnormal rates (bradycardia and tachycardia), see Dysrhythmias section.
- **Rhythm:** In sinus, there are P waves before every QRS complex. The P is upright in I, II, and avF. For discussion of abnormal rhythms (atrial fibrillation, atrial flutter, ventricular rhythms), see Dysrhythmias section.
- **Axis:**
  - **Normal:** From −30 degrees to +90 degrees. **QRS** is net ⊕ in I and II.
  - **Left-deviated:** < −30 degrees. **QRS** is net ⊕ in I and net ⊖ in II. Associated with left anterior fascicular block (LAFB), left bundle branch block (LBBB), inferior MI, Wolff-Parkinson-White (WPW) syndrome with posteroseptal pathway, and COPD.
  - **Right-deviated:** > 90 degrees. **QRS** is net ⊖ in I and net ⊕ in II. Associated with RVH, lateral or anterolateral MI, WPW with left-lateral pathway, and left posterior fascicular block (LPFB).
- **Intervals:**
  - **PR:** Normal 0.12–0.20 sec. Increased in AV blocks (see AV Blocks section).
  - **QRS:** Normal 0.12 sec. Prolonged in bundle branch blocks, ventricularly paced rhythms (ventricular tachycardia or fibrillation, pacemak-

ers), WPW, or aberrantly conducted SVTs. See Dysrhythmias and Bundle Branch and Fascicular Blocks sections.

- **QT:** Normal < 50% of RR.
- **QTc:** Abnormal > 0.44 sec for men and > 0.46 sec for women. Interval is **prolonged** in congenital conditions (long QT syndrome), metabolic abnormalities, drug use (antiarrhythmics, antibiotics, psychotropic drugs), MI, and mitral valve prolapse. Leads to ventricular arrhythmias such as Torsades de pointes.
- **Hypertrophy:** ↑ LV mass associated with ↑ incidence of poor outcomes, including systolic dysfunction, heart failure, CVA, and death.
  - **LVH:** Many criteria—R in aVL is > 11 mm (1.1 mV) **or** the sum of S in V_1 and R in V_5 or V_6 is > 35 mm (3.5 mV).
  - **RVH:** Right-axis deviation. One criterion is R:S > 1 in V_1. Another criterion is $RV_1 + SV_6 > 11$ mm.
- **Ischemia:** See Coronary Artery Disease: Acute Coronary Syndrome section.

Noninvasive Cardiac Stress Testing

Used to diagnose CAD in patients in whom it is suspected and in the prognosis/management of patients with known CAD (see Table 3.2).

Resting Echocardiography

Used to identify **anatomic abnormalities**; to assess the size, thickness, and function (ejection fraction, or EF) of chambers; and to evaluate valvular function. Wall motion abnormalities suggest CAD. Subtypes are as follows:

- **Transthoracic echocardiography (TTE):** Usually first modality tried due to ease of use.
  - **Doppler:** Characterizes blood flow and pressure gradients across valves. Useful for detecting stenotic or regurgitant blood flow.
  - **Bubble study:** Agitated normal saline injected intravenously to diagnose shunts.

TABLE 3.2. Stress-Testing Modalities

MODE	STRESS METHOD	PLUSES/MINUSES	CONTRAINDICATIONS
Stress ECG	Exercise treadmill	+ **Widely available.** – Less sensitive and specific than other modes, especially in women.	Patient can't exercise to 85% of max HR. Abnormal resting ECG (LBBB, WPW, ST depressions, LVH). On digoxin or has pacemaker. History of revascularization.
Stress echo	Exercise or pharmacologic (dobutamine)	+ Sensitivity and specificity are high (highest specificity). + Provides structural information. + Lower cost than perfusion imaging. – Interpretation is operator dependent.	Symptomatic aortic aneurysm or high risk of ventricular arrhythmia. Abnormal resting echo. LBBB can → false ⊕ septal defect.
Radionuclide myocardial perfusion imaging (sestamibi or thallium)	Exercise or pharmacologic (adenosine or dipyridamole)	+ Sensitivity and specificity are high (highest sensitivity mode). + **Can assess tissue viability with restriction study** (reversible vs. fixed defects). – Involves radiation exposure.	Contraindications to stress Rx: hypotension, sick sinus syndrome, second/third-degree heart block, or severe reactive airway disease. Use of caffeine within 24 hrs or theophylline within 72 hrs.

- **Transesophageal echocardiography (TEE):** An ultrasound probe in the esophagus that allows for better visualization of posterior cardiac structures.
  - **Indications:** Suspicion of left atrial thrombus, aortic dissection, or valvular vegetations.
  - **The sensitivity of TEE in endocarditis is 95%–100%** (vs. 40%–75% with TTE).

Cardiac Catheterization and Coronary Angiography

Indications:

- Stable angina with persistent symptoms despite medical management.
- **Acute coronary syndrome** (see section on Acute Coronary Syndrome).
- Previous revascularization with recurrent symptoms to look for reocclusion.
- Aortic disease with concurrent angina to determine if CABG might be performed at the time of valve replacement.
- Assessment of intracardiac pressures and oxygen saturations when pulmonary hypertension or shunts are suspected.
- Assessment of severity of aortic stenosis.
- **Interventions include angioplasty and stenting.**
- **Coronary CT angiography:** The role of CTA in diagnostic work-up and management of CAD is being studied but has not been clarified. It may play a larger role in the future.
- **Cardiac MRI:** Occasionally used as an adjunctive test in the assessment of RV and LV function, myocardial viability, cardiomyopathy, valvular heart disease, pericardial disease, and aortic disease.

Dysrhythmias

An 85-year-old woman presents to the ER with intermittent palpitations and lightheadedness for the last month. Her medical problems include hypertension, diabetes, CAD with a previous stent, and hypothyroidism. Her BP is 145/80 and her pulse is 120. An ECG shows atrial fibrillation. Review of her records shows a previous ECG with this finding 3 years ago, with normal ECGs in the interim. In the ER, you determine that there is no urgent indication for cardioversion, and you lower her heart rate with β-blockers. She has no evidence of ischemia by biochemical markers and her TSH is normal. An echocardiogram shows LVH but no other structural abnormalities or thrombus. How do you proceed?

You continue to control her heart rate with β-blockers and calculate her CHADS score, which shows she has a high risk of embolism. You begin warfarin anticoagulation with a target INR of 2–3.

BRADYCARDIA

Bradycardia is defined as a heart rate < 55–60.

ETIOLOGIES

- **Common:** Idiopathic degeneration, ischemic. Can be normal in highly conditioned athletes.
- **Rheumatologic:** SLE, RA, scleroderma.
- **Infectious:** Endocarditis, Chagas disease.
- **Infiltrative:** Sarcoidosis, amyloidosis, hemochromatosis.
- **Autonomic:** ↑ vagal tone (carotid sinus hypersensitivity).
- **Iatrogenic:** Heart transplant, β-blockers, calcium channel blockers (CCBs), clonidine, digoxin, antiarrhythmics.
- **Metabolic:** Electrolyte abnormalities (hypo- and hyperkalemia), hypothyroidism, hypothermia.

SYMPTOMS/EXAM

- Dizziness, weakness, fatigue, and syncope. May be asymptomatic.
- Exam reveals ↓ pulse. Look for signs associated with the underlying cause of the bradycardia.

DIAGNOSIS

- **ECG:** Heart rate < 60 bpm. Look for dropped beats or AV dissociation.
- Metabolic workup, telemetry, event monitors, tilt-table testing, and electrophysiology studies can be helpful.

TREATMENT

- For unstable patients, follow the ACLS protocol.
- **Medications: Atropine,** glucagon (for β-blocker overdose), calcium (for CCB overdose).
- **Transcutaneous or transvenous pacing.**
- **Permanent pacemaker:** Consider for those with documented symptomatic bradycardia, third-degree heart block, > 3-second pause, or a pulse < 40.

KEY FACT

Consider a permanent pacemaker for documented symptomatic bradycardia, third-degree heart block, > 3-second pause, or a pulse < 40.

NARROW QRS COMPLEX TACHYCARDIAS

Atrial Fibrillation (AF)

The **most common dysrhythmia in the general population** (0.5%–1.0%); prevalence ↑ with age. Usually found in the setting of structural heart disease with ventricular failure.

The most common etiologies are **hypertension and CAD.** Also common are valvular heart disease and heart failure. Less common etiologies include pulmonary disease (COPD, pulmonary embolism), ischemia, rheumatic heart disease, hyperthyroidism, congenital heart disease, sepsis, alcoholism, WPW syndrome, and cardiac surgery.

Types of AF (terms are less commonly used now to determine treatment):

- **Paroxysmal:** Episodes last < 7 days and usually < 24 hours.
- **Persistent:** Lasts > 7 days; responds to cardioversion but may recur afterward.
- **Permanent:** Present > 1 year; failed cardioversion.
- **Lone:** One episode of AF in the absence of structural heart disease.

SYMPTOMS/EXAM

- Often asymptomatic. Palpitations, fatigue, dyspnea, dizziness, diaphoresis, heart failure, or ↓ exercise tolerance may be seen.
- Look for evidence of coexisting heart disease.

DIAGNOSIS

- **ECG:** The most common cause of irregularly irregular rhythm is AF. The absence of P waves is diagnostic (see Figure 3.2).
- **Echocardiogram:** Used to predict stroke risk with structural abnormalities such as left atrial enlargement, valvular disease, LVH, and ↓ EF. TEE is more effective for visualizing left atrial thrombi.

TREATMENT

- **Rate control:** Preferred unless unstable. β-blockers and non-DHP CCBs (ie, verapamil, diltiazem) common. Administer digoxin in the presence of other comorbidities such as CHF; administer amiodarone if hypotension is an issue.
- **Cardioversion:**
  - Indicated if the patient is unstable or if the duration of AF is < 48 hours.
  - If > 48 hours: First anticoagulate to prevent embolization of an atrial clot. Then perform TEE-guided cardioversion.
  - Anticoagulate for at least 4 weeks postcardioversion.
  - If AF recurs after cardioversion, treat with rate control and anticoagulation.

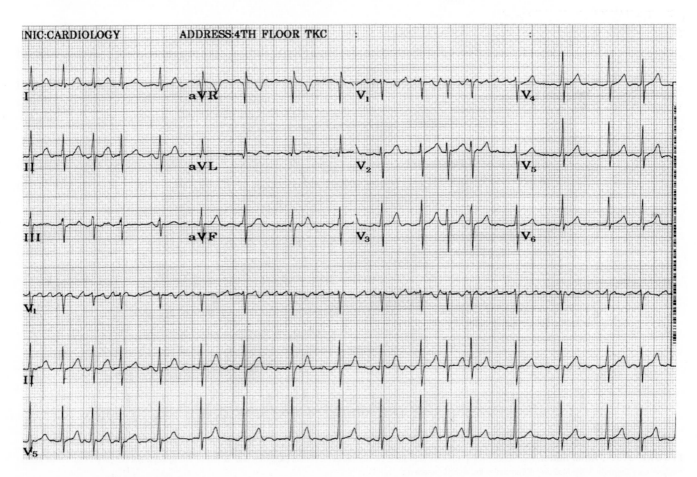

FIGURE 3.2.   Atrial fibrillation. (Reproduced, with permission, from Fuster V, O'Rourke RA, Walsh RA, Poole-Wilson P. *Hurst's The Heart,* 12th ed. http://www.accessmedicine.com. Copyright © The McGraw-Hill Companies, Inc. All rights reserved.)

- **Anticoagulation:** To determine the need for anticoagulation, estimate stroke risk with the **CHADS2 score:**
  - CHF
  - Hypertension $\left.\begin{array}{l}\\ \\ \\ \\ \end{array}\right\}$ 1 point each
  - Age > 75 years
  - Diabetes
  - Stroke/TIA (2 points)
    - **Score 0:** Aspirin 325 mg daily.
    - **Score 1–2:** Aspirin 325 mg or warfarin; based on the individual patient characteristics and discussion of risks/benefits.
    - **Score 3+:** Warfarin; target INR of 2.5 (range 2–3) in most patients. Target INR is 3.0 (2.5–3.5) with valvular disease, previous thromboembolism, or mechanical valve.
- **Rhythm control:** Not a mainstay of treatment. Flecainide, propafenone, amiodarone, sotalol, ibutilide.
- Some patients, particularly young patients and patients who have failed pharmacologic rhythm control, may be candidates for radiofrequency catheter ablation to restore normal sinus rhythm. This technique can have significant risks and the success is operator dependent, but its use is becoming more common.

Atrial Flutter

Uncommon in a structurally normal heart. Can occur with LV dysfunction and rheumatic heart disease. Other etiologies, exam findings, and treatment are similar to those associated with AF; significant differences are listed below.

EKG FINDINGS

- **Typical isthmus-dependent flutter (counterclockwise):** Atrial rate of 250–350. Can present with or without typical flutter waves.
- **Clockwise flutter:** Presents with a sawtooth pattern in leads II, III, and aVF. Flutter rate should be around 300. Consider the diagnosis in patients with a ventricular rate of 150, as flutter usually presents with 2:1 conduction (see Figure 3.3).

TREATMENT

- Approach to cardioversion, anticoagulation, and rate control is similar to that with AF.

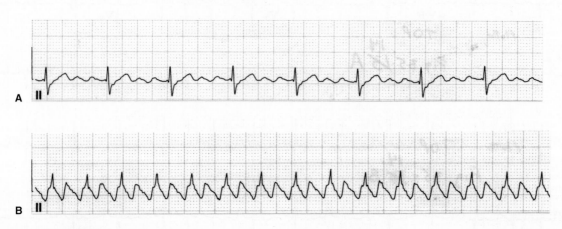

FIGURE 3.3. Atrial flutter. (Reproduced, with permission, from Stone CK, Humphries RL. *Current Diagnoses and Treatment: Emergency Medicine,* 6th ed. http://www.access-medicine.com. Copyright © The McGraw-Hill Companies, Inc. All rights reserved.)

- Watchful waiting for reversion to NSR is appropriate in stable patients with minimal atrial dilation and a known reversible cause such as hyperthyroidism or PE.
- Radiofrequency ablation is highly effective and is the preferred treatment.
- Alternatives include antiarrhythmics or pacemakers, which require long-term anticoagulation.

Other Supraventricular Tachycardias (SVTs)

- **Reentrant SVT:** The point of reentry can be:
    - **AV node:** Also called AVNRT. Most common, accounting for 60% of cases of reentrant SVT.
    - The bypass tract or other site. Also called AVRT.
- Sinus tachycardia
- Atrial tachycardia.
- Multifocal atrial tachycardia.
- Junctional tachycardia.

Symptoms/Exam

Asymptomatic or may present with palpitations, lightheadedness, presyncope, syncope, or chest pain. Exam should focus on auscultation for evidence of valvular disease or cardiomyopathy.

Diagnosis

ECG shows regular rhythm. QRS is generally narrow, although it may be wide if aberrant conduction is present. Varying morphologies of P waves seen in **multifocal atrial tachycardia.** Retrograde P waves may be seen in AVNRT, AVRT, and junctional tachycardia.

Treatment

Valsalva; unilateral carotid sinus massage (if no prior TIA, prior serious cardiac arrhythmia, MI within past 6 months, or carotid bruit). Adenosine if these maneuvers are unsuccessful. Cardioversion is indicated if the patient is unstable.

Ventricular Tachycardia (VT) and Ventricular Fibrillation (VF)

Causes include ischemia, infarction, cardiomyopathy, electrolyte abnormalities, and drug toxicities. Types of VT are as follows:

- **Monomorphic:** Uniform QRS pattern. Usually associated with myocardial scar.
- **Polymorphic:** Characterized by a bizarre and changing QRS. Often precipitated by ischemia. **Torsades de pointes** (in which the QRS complex oscillates around a baseline) is often associated with medications and electrolyte abnormalities that prolong the QT interval (see Figure 3.4).

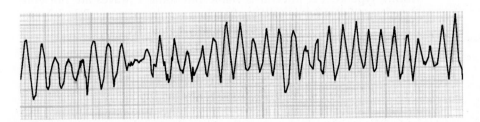

FIGURE 3.4.   Torsades de pointes. (Reproduced, with permission, from Knoop KJ, Stack LB, Storrow AB, Thurman RJ. *The Atlas of Emergency Medicine,* 3rd ed. http://www.accessmedicine.com. Copyright © The McGraw-Hill Companies, Inc. All rights reserved.)

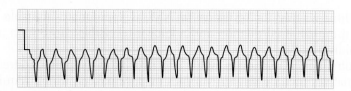

FIGURE 3.5. **Ventricular tachycardia.** (Reproduced, with permission, from Gomella LG, Haist SA. *Clinician's Pocket Reference*, 11th ed. http://www.accessmedicine.com. Copyright © The McGraw-Hill Companies, Inc. All rights reserved.)

SYMPTOMS/EXAM

Chest pain, dyspnea, syncope, **sudden cardiac death.**

DIAGNOSIS

- Wide QRS complex. **Must be distinguished from SVT with aberrant conduction.** Baseline ECG may show bundle branch block or intraventricular conduction delay with a similar QRS morphology.
- **Unstable patients:** Assume VT (see Figure 3.5).
- **Stable patients:** VT is evidenced by AV dissociation, complexes not typical of LBBB or RBBB, variation in QRS complexes, and fusion beats of simultaneously occurring ventricular and supraventricular beats.

TREATMENT

- **Unstable patients:** Cardioversion.
- **Stable VT:** First-line treatment is IV amiodarone.
- **Polymorphic VT** (including Torsades): Can be treated with magnesium infusion and overdrive pacing.
- A defibrillator should be placed if the cause is not transient or reversible.

Conduction Abnormalities

AV BLOCKS

Delayed conduction through the AV node → prolonged PR interval → eventual dissociation of atrial and ventricular rhythms if completely blocked. Increased with ↑ vagal tone, drugs (β-blockers, non-DHP CCBs), ischemic heart disease, cardiomyopathies, myocarditis, or congenital heart disease.

- **First-degree AV block:** Prolonged PR interval > 200 msec. Try to treat underlying cause (lower medication dose) but can be observed untreated.
- **Second-degree AV block:** Some atrial impulses fail to reach ventricles.
  - **Mobitz type I (Wenckebach):** Progressively longer PR interval followed by a nonconducted P wave. Usually block is at AV node and is benign.
  - **Mobitz type II:** PR interval is stable but some P waves are not conducted (not followed by QRS), often in a regular patterns, 2:1, 3:2, etc. More serious condition; block is usually below AV node and can → complete heart block. Pacemaker often required.
- **Third-degree AV block:** No atrial impulses reach the ventricles. Complete dissociation of the atrial (P wave) and the ventricular (QRS) rhythm. "Escape rhythms" drive the ventricle from below the block. Escape rhythm is slower than a sinus rhythm and two-thirds of the time has a narrow QRS (focus for the escape rhythm is still within the conduction system). **Requires a pacemaker.**

KEY FACT

VT must be distinguished from SVT with aberrant conduction, but in an unstable patient, treat as VT.

MNEMONIC

Mobitz type I: PR gets longer and longer, then **ONE** drops (longer, longer, drop, now you have a Wenckebach).
Mobitz type II: It's not **TWO** long until you need a pacer.

TABLE 3.3. **ECG Changes in Intraventricular Blocks**

Type	Axis	ECG	QRS	Miscellaneous
LAFB	Left	Upright QRS in I; $\ominus$ QRS in aVF.	Narrow	
LPFB	Right	$\ominus$ QRS in I; $\oplus$ QRS in aVF.	Narrow	
RBBB	Right or normal	rSR' in V_1–V_2; **rabbit ears.**	Wide	Can still read ischemia.
LBBB	Left or normal	**Broad R wave in I; broad, deep S in V_1; RS in V_6.**	Wide	Difficult to read ischemia.
Bilateral block		Third-degree heart block.	Wide and bizarre	

BUNDLE BRANCH AND FASCICULAR BLOCKS

An impairment in the fast conduction of current through the septum/ventricles from the AV node (see Table 3.3 and Figure 3.6). Can be from age-related degeneration of the conduction system, CAD, cardiomyopathies, or acute ischemia. Pacemakers should be considered in some situations.

WOLFF-PARKINSON-WHITE (WPW) SYNDROME

A persistent accessory pathway between the atria and ventricles. May be found incidentally, but even asymptomatic patients are at risk for tachyarrhythmias. More common in those with first-degree relatives with WPW.

DIAGNOSIS

- **Antegrade accessory pathway conduction:** Impulses conduct from the atria to the accessory pathway to the ventricles. Characterized by ventricu-

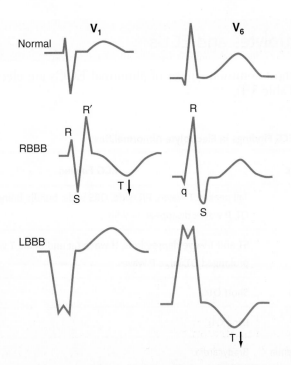

FIGURE 3.6. **ECG changes in right and left bundle branch blocks.** (Reproduced, with permission, from Fauci AS, Kasper AL, Braunwald E, Hauser SL, Longo DL, Jameson JL, Loscalzo J. *Harrison's Principles of Internal Medicine,* 17th ed. http://www.accessmedicine.com. Copyright © The McGraw-Hill Companies, Inc. All rights reserved.)

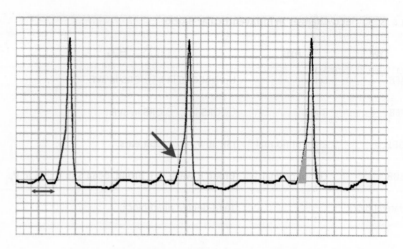

FIGURE 3.7. **Wolff-Parkinson-White syndrome.** (Reproduced, with permission, from Knoop KJ, Stack LB, Storrow AB, Thurman RJ. *The Atlas of Emergency Medicine,* 3rd ed. http://www.accessmedicine.com. Copyright © The McGraw-Hill Companies, Inc. All rights reserved.)

lar preexcitation with **short PR and delta waves** (slurred upstroke of QRS; best seen in lead V_4). Delta waves with net-$\ominus$ deflection can resemble Q waves (see Figure 3.7).

- **Retrograde accessory pathway conduction:** Impulses conduct from the ventricles to the accessory pathway to the atria. Resting ECG is often normal; no delta wave is seen.

TREATMENT

Electrophysiologic study; ablation of the bypass tracts.

COMPLICATIONS

Serious complications usually happen in the setting of AF. Avoid AV nodal blockers in patients with a delta wave, as this can cause 1:1 conduction of AF → VF and cardiac arrest.

Electrolytes and ECGs

Some of the most common causes of abnormal ECGs are electrolyte abnormalities (see Table 3.4).

TABLE 3.4. **ECG Findings in Electrolyte Abnormalities**

ELECTROLYTE	ECG FINDING
Hyperkalemia	Tall peaked T waves, PR wide, QRS wide, bundle branch blocks, short QT, P waves disappear → V-fib.
Hypokalemia	ST and T wave depressions, **U wave** (at end of the T wave), pseudo-prolonged QT, large P waves.
Hypercalcemia	Short QTc.
Hypocalcemia	Long QTc.
Hypermagnesemia	Bradycardia.
Hypomagnesemia	Long QT, prolonged PR, widened QRS.

Hypertension

High blood pressure = systolic BP $\geq$ 140 or a diastolic BP $>$ 90 on more than 2 occasions. Hypertension (HTN) is associated with MI, heart failure, stroke, and kidney disease and has a $\uparrow$ prevalence in ethnic minorities, women, and those with $\uparrow$ age.

TYPES OF HYPERTENSION

- **Essential:** Idiopathic.
- **2°:** Usually in severe, treatment-refractory HTN or in younger patients. Causes include:
  - Chronic kidney disease
  - Medications (steroids, OCPs, NSAIDs, antidepressants)
  - Renovascular (renal artery stenosis)
  - Alcohol, cocaine
  - Hyperaldosteronism
  - Polycythemia vera
  - Hyper/hypothyroidism
  - Coarctation of the aorta
  - Cushing disease
  - Sleep apnea
  - Pheochromocytoma
  - Hyperparathyroidism
- **Hypertensive urgency:** SBP $>$ 180–200 or DBP $>$ 120 without acute signs of end-organ damage.
- **Hypertensive emergency:** SBP $>$ 180 or DBP $>$ 120 with signs of acute end-organ effects:
  - Brain (confusion, lethargy indicate cerebral edema or hemorrhage).
  - Eye (blurry vision, papilledema).
  - Heart (chest pain or SOB may indicate aortic dissection, ACS, or pulmonary edema).
  - Kidney (oliguria, hematuria, or $\uparrow$creatinine indicates ARF).
- **Hypertensive encephalopathy:** Hypertension with signs of cerebral edema (altered sensorium, nausea, vomiting, headache).
- **Malignant hypertension:** Hypertension with retinal hemorrhages, exudates, or papilledema, usually with diastolic BP $>$ 120.

SYMPTOMS/EXAM

- **Sx:** Headache, chest pain, SOB, vision changes.
- Exam should include a cardiopulmonary exam and an investigation for chronic changes associated with chronic HTN:
  - **Fundoscopic exam for retinopathy** to look for arteriolar narrowing or sclerosis, AV nicking (see Figure 3.8), hemorrhages, and hard exudates.
  - PMI with left shift indicating LVH, signs of CHF.
  - Signs of stroke with severe HTN.
- Look for signs of 2° HTN such as renal artery bruits, significant difference in right/left or upper/lower extremity BPs, decreased or delayed femoral pulses, obesity, and physical findings of alcohol abuse or liver disease.

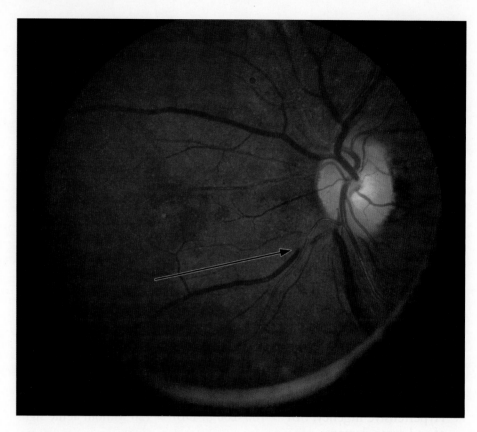

FIGURE 3.8. **AV nicking.** (Reproduced, with permission, from USMLERx.)

DIAGNOSIS

- **Elevated BP on 3 separate occasions with correct cuff size.**
- **Labs:** Hematocrit, UA, urine albumin-to-creatinine ratio, electrolytes, creatinine, glucose, calcium, ECG.
- Rule out 2° causes of hypertension (see above) in those with severe or refractory HTN (on 3 meds, including a diuretic), proven age of onset before puberty, age < 30 if nonobese and no family history of HTN, onset of stage 2 HTN after age 55, family history of early-onset hypertension, or an acute ↑ in BP over a previously stable baseline.
- Additional labs to consider based on suspected causes of 2° HTN: TSH, renal ultrasound, plasma aldosterone-to-renin ratio.

TREATMENT

- The goal is < 140/90, or < 130/80 in patients with **diabetes, renal disease, or cardiovascular disease.**
- Patients with prehypertension and stages 1 and 2 hypertension should be counseled about lifestyle modifications, including adherence to a low-sodium/DASH diet (rich in fruits, vegetables, and low-fat dairy), weight ↓, aerobic activity, and ↓ alcohol consumption.
- Assess factors that may modify treatment choices (see Table 3.5).

KEY FACT

The goal of hypertension treatment is a BP of < 140/90, or < 130/80 in patients with diabetes, renal disease, or cardiovascular disease.

TABLE 3.5.   Antihypertensive Medications

	THIAZIDES	β-BLOCKERS	ACEIS	ARBS	CALCIUM CHANNEL BLOCKERS
Drug examples	HCTZ, chlorthalidone.	Atenolol, metoprolol.	Captopril, enalapril, ramipril, lisinopril.	Irbesartan, losartan, valsartan.	Nondihydropyridines (non-DHPs): diltiazem, verapamil. Dihydropyridines (DHPs): amlodipine, felodipine, nifedipine.
Side effects	Hypokalemia, ED, ↑ insulin resistance, hyperuricemia, ↑ TG.	Bronchospasm, depression, fatigue, ED, ↑ insulin resistance.	Cough (10%), hyperkalemia, renal failure.	Less cough, hyperkalemia, renal failure.	Conduction defects (non-DHPs); lower extremity edema.
Indications for use as first-line drug	**Most patients** as mono- or combination therapy (stage 1 or 2 hypertension), **osteoporosis, kidney stones.** Recurrent stroke prevention.	**MI,** high CAD risk, rate control for afib/flutter CHF.	**DM, MI,** CHF, mild chronic renal failure.	DM, MI, CHF, chronic renal failure, ACEI-related cough.	Non-DHPs used for rate control for afib/flutter.
Contraindications	Gout.	Severe bronchospasm; high-degree (type II second- or third-degree) heart block, bradycardia.	Pregnancy. Moderate-severe renal failure; caution in renal artery stenosis.	Pregnancy. Moderate-severe renal failure; caution in renal artery stenosis.	High-degree heart block.

(Reproduced, with permission, from Le T, et al. *First Aid for the Internal Medicine Boards,* 1st ed. New York: McGraw-Hill, 2006: 49.)

Hyperlipidemia

A 58-year-old woman with low back pain and urinary incontinence comes to your office for a yearly physical exam. She is a smoker and has no family history of premature heart disease. Her BP is 150/95 and has been elevated in the past. Her lipid panel includes an HDL-C of 38, an LDL-C of 170, and a triglyceride level of 150. The woman has no CAD equivalents but has 3 risk factors: tobacco use, low HDL-C, and hypertension. You calculate her 10-year Framingham risk at 24% and determine that her LDL-C goal is 130. What do you do?

Counsel her about smoking cessation, exercise, and a low cholesterol diet. Six months later, her lipid profile is not significantly different. How do you proceed?

Initiate a statin.

Coronary risk ↑ proportionally with total cholesterol. Accordingly, the control of hyperlipidemia is critical to ↓ the incidence of CAD, CVA, CKD, and PVD. Mortality benefits have been noted both in patients without known CAD and in patients with established CAD.

SCREENING GUIDELINES

- The United States Preventive Services Task Force (USPSTF) recommends hyperlidemia screening:
  - Every 5 years in men > 35 years of age and women > 45 years of age.
  - At age 20 with CAD risk factors or significant family history.
- Screening is generally **not** recommended for patients > 75 years of age.
- Measurement of fasting lipids is optimal, but nonfasting total cholesterol-to-HDL-C ratio is an alternative.

RISK FACTORS

Risk factors influencing cholesterol goals are as follows (see also Table 3.6):

- **CAD equivalents:** DM, symptomatic carotid disease, abdominal aortic aneurysm, peripheral arterial disease, and renal insufficiency (creatinine > 1.5).
- **CAD risk factors:** Tobacco use, hypertension (> 140/90) or use of antihypertensives, HDL-C < 40, family history of premature CAD (male relative < 55 years of age, female relative < 65 years of age), and patient age (men > 45, women > 55). **HDL-C > 60 is a ⊖ risk factor.**

MANAGEMENT

Table 3.7 outlines drugs used in conjunction with lifestyle modifications to treat hyperlipidemia.

TABLE 3.6. **Risk Categories That Modify LDL Cholesterol Goals**

RISK CATEGORY	LDL GOAL	LEVEL AT WHICH TO INITIATE THERAPEUTIC LIFESTYLE CHANGES	LEVEL AT WHICH TO CONSIDER DRUG THERAPY
CAD or CAD equivalents (10-year risk > 20%)	< 100 mg/dL (optional goal of < 70 in very high risk)	≥ 100 mg/dL	≥ 130 mg/dL (drug optional for 100–129 mg/dL)[a]
2+ risk factors (10-year risk ≥ 20%)	< 130 mg/dL	≥ 130 mg/dL	10-year risk 10%–20%: ≥ 130 mg/dL 10-year risk < 10%: ≥ 160 mg/dL
0–1 risk factor	< 160 mg/dL	≥ 160 mg/dL	≥ 190 mg/dL (LDL-lowering drug optional for 160–189 mg/dL)

[a]Some authorities recommend use of LDL-lowering drugs in this category if an LDL cholesterol < 100 mg/dL cannot be achieved by therapeutic lifestyle changes.

(Adapted from the Third Report of the National Cholesterol Education Program, Panel on Detection, Evaluation, and Treatment of High Blood Cholesterol in Adults [(Adult Treatment Panel III) Executive Summary. Washington, DC: National Institutes of Health, NIH Publication No. 01–3670, May 2001, www.nhlbi.nih.gov/guidelines/cholesterol/index.htm.])

TABLE 3.7. Classes of Drugs Used in the Treatment of Hyperlipidemia

Drug	LDL	HDL	TG	Side Effects	Best for	Monitor
Statins (atorvastatin, simvastatin, pravastatin)	↓	↑	↓	GI distress, elevated LFTs[a], myositis.	Elevated LDL only; elevated LDL and TG.	LFTs[a] (CK if symptomatic).
Nicotinic acid (niacin)	↓	↑	↓	Flushing, gout, GI distress, elevated LFTs, pruritus, ↑ blood glucose.	Elevated LDL and TG; low HDL ("jack of all trades").	LFTs.
Bile acid-binding resins (cholestyramine)	↓	↑	↓	GI distress, ↓ absorption of fat-soluble vitamins and other drugs, ↑ TG.	Elevated LDL only.	
Fibrates (gemfibrozil)	↓	↑	↓	GI distress, myositis (especially in combination with statins).	Elevated TG.	LFTs.

[a]Follow-up studies show no increased transaminitis in statins over placebo, and some authorities advocate for no LFT monitoring for statin patients.

(Reproduced, with permission, from Le T, et al. *First Aid for the Internal Medicine Boards,* 1st ed. New York: McGraw-Hill, 2006: 23.)

HYPERTRIGLYCERIDEMIA

Epidemiologic data suggest that hypertriglyceridemia is independently associated with CAD. Suggested management according to the Adult Treatment Panel III (ATP III) includes the following:

- **Triglycerides 150–199 (borderline):** Nonpharmacologic interventions (weight loss, increased activity); pharmacologic treatment to achieve the LDL goal.
- **Triglycerides 200–499 (high):** Consider pharmacologic therapy directed toward ↓ triglycerides in high-risk patients or those with known CAD.
- **Triglycerides ≥ 500 (very high):** Pharmacologic treatment to ↓ triglycerides (fibrates, nicotinic acid) and prevent pancreatitis.

Coronary Artery Disease (CAD)

A 65-year-old man with a history of MI and a 3-vessel CABG 10 years ago comes to your office to establish care. He is a nonsmoker who is active and feels well, and he is currently on aspirin, a statin, and HCTZ. On exam, you note that he is obese, his BP is 160/80, and he has an S4. You check his lipids, and his LDL-C is 125. What further interventions are necessary?

You add an ACEI and a β-blocker for BP control and for 2° prevention of CAD, and ↑ his statin dose to improve his LDL-C toward his goal of 70. You also encourage him to continue to exercise and abstain from tobacco, and you discuss nutritional strategies to improve his cardiac health.

CAD is the leading cause of mortality in women and men in the United States. It is associated with other forms of cardiovascular disease, including cerebrovascular disease, peripheral artery disease, and aortic atherosclerosis. Risk factors for CAD include the following:

- **Age:** There is ↑ risk in women > 65 years of age or with premature menopause, and in men > 55 years of age.
- **Family history:** There is ↑ risk with a family history of CAD in a first-degree female relative < 55 years of age or a male relative < 45 years of age.
- **Smoking.**
- **Hypertension** with a BP > 140/90 or use of an antihypertensive.
- **HDL-C < 40** on several occasions (**an HDL-C > 60 is a ⊖ risk factor**).
- **Elevated LDL.**
- **Obesity** (BMI > 30) and **physical inactivity.**
- **Chronic kidney disease.**
- **Diabetes:** Patients with diabetes are at a level of risk equivalent to those with established CAD.

More novel risk factors include elevated CRP, elevated homocysteine, coronary artery calcification on cardiac CT, and LVH.

KEY FACT

Diabetes is a CAD equivalent.

PREVENTION

1° Prevention

Risk factor reduction includes the following:

- **Smoking cessation:** Yields an immediate ↓ in risk that reverts to a normal level after several years.
- **Diet:** Low in fat and high in whole grains, fruits, vegetables, and omega-3 fatty acids.
- **Hypertension:** The goal BP is < 140/90 or 130/80, depending on risk factors.
- **Hyperlipidemia:** Target LDL-C cholesterol levels should be based on the patient's 10-year risk for heart disease.
- **Diabetes:** Intensive control of type 2 diabetes has not been shown to ↓ cardiovascular events in most studies. Consider an A_{1c} target of < 7.0 for most new-onset type 2 diabetics and 7.0–7.9 in frail diabetics and those with long-standing disease (8–12 years).
- **Other risk factors** that should be addressed include obesity and physical inactivity. Low to moderate alcohol intake (1–2 drinks a day) has been postulated to slightly ↓ the risk of CAD.
- **Pharmacologic therapy: Consider aspirin** therapy for 1° prevention in nondiabetics when 10-year CVD risk > 20% and for diabetics when 10-year CVD risk > 10% and no ↑ risk of bleeding. Use of aspirin in patients with lower CVD risk is of uncertain benefit.

2° Prevention

Risk factor ↓ measures are the same as those outlined above:

- **Pharmacologic therapy:**
  - **Aspirin:** ↓ mortality with daily use (75–325 mg). If contraindicated, clopidogrel may be used.
  - **Clopidogrel:** ↓ mortality in patients with recent acute coronary syndrome or in those with a stent.
  - **Statins:** ↓ mortality and the risk of acute cardiac events. Goal for those with CAD is an **LDL < 100**, while some groups recommend an LDL goal of < 70.

- **β-blockers:** ↓ mortality. All patients with CAD should be on a β-blocker unless an absolute contraindication exists.
- **ACE inhibitors (ACEIs):** ↓ mortality and risk of MI and stroke. If not tolerated, an angiotensin receptor blocker (ARB) may be used.

STABLE ANGINA

Fixed artery stenosis limiting O_2 delivery in times of stress.

SYMPTOMS/EXAM

Classically presents with chronic, exercise-induced chest discomfort that is relieved by rest and nitroglycerin and does not change in severity or frequency. May be associated with dyspnea or nausea, and may radiate to the neck, jaw, or arms. Exam findings are nonspecific.

DIAGNOSIS

Start with stress testing with either nuclear perfusion imaging or echocardiography. **Cardiac catheterization is the gold standard.**

TREATMENT

- The same as 2° prevention of CAD. Antianginal medical therapy includes nitrates, β-blockers, and CCBs.
- **Indications for revascularization:**
  - Chronic stable angina with 3-vessel disease.
  - Two-vessel disease with prominent LAD involvement.
  - One- or 2-vessel disease with high-risk features such as LV dysfunction.
  - Significant left main artery disease (> 50% stenosis).
  - Refractory symptoms or chronic angina.

CARDIAC ISCHEMIA/ACUTE CORONARY SYNDROME

See the Emergency/Urgent Care chapter for an overview of symptoms, exam, and initial medical treatment of acute coronary syndrome (ACS)/MI. ACS encompasses 3 diagnoses: unstable angina, non-ST elevation MI (NSTEMI), and ST elevation MI (STEMI), which reflect different levels of damage to the myocardium from ischemia.

DIAGNOSIS

- ECG findings in ischemia (see Figures 3.9 and 3.10):
  - Prolonged QTc, T-wave flattening, T-wave inversions (TWI), or normalization of previous TWI → ST depressions → ST elevations → Q waves.
  - New LBBB.

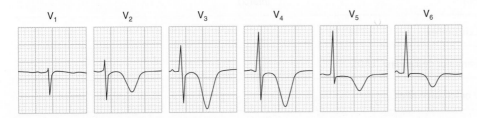

FIGURE 3.9.   Myocardial ischemia. (Reproduced, with permission, from Fauci AS, Kasper AL, Braunwald E, Hauser SL, Longo DL, Jameson JL, Loscalzo J. *Harrison's Principles of Internal Medicine,* 17th ed. http://www.accessmedicine.com. Copyright © The McGraw-Hill Companies, Inc. All rights reserved.)

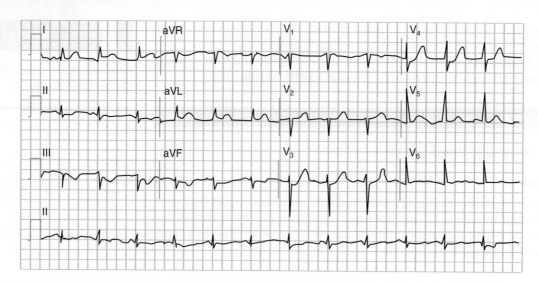

FIGURE 3.10. **Myocardial infarction (lateral, with inferior and anterior reciprocal changes).** (Reproduced, with permission, from Fauci AS, Kasper AL, Braunwald E, Hauser SL, Longo DL, Jameson JL, Loscalzo J. *Harrison's Principles of Internal Medicine,* 17th ed. http://www.accessmedicine.com. Copyright © The McGraw-Hill Companies, Inc. All rights reserved.)

- Heart block.
- Ventricular arrhythmias.
- Cardiac markers: Elevated troponin or CK-MB.
- Echo may show new wall motion abnormalities.

See Table 3.8 for summary of ECG changes characteristic of areas of the heart affected.

DIAGNOSIS OF ACS

See Table 3.9 for categorization of types of ACS based on serum markers and ECG findings.

TREATMENT

- Initial medical treatment for chest pain: morphine, O_2, sublingual nitrate, ASA.
- If ACS:
  - Add high-dose statin, β-blocker, ACEI.
  - Anticoagulate with heparin drip or low-molecular-weight heparin.
  - Clopidogrel.

TABLE 3.8. **Localization of Transmural Infarction**

LEADS	LOCATION	ARTERY	MISCELLANEOUS
II, III, aVF	Inferior	Right coronary artery (80%) or left circumflex (20%).	Perform right-sided ECG (look for ST ↑ in V_4R → RV infarct).
I, aVL	Lateral	Left circumflex.	
V_1–V_3	Anteroseptal	Left anterior descending (LAD).	
V_4–V_6	Apical/lateral	LAD or left circumflex.	
V_4–V_6R	RV	Right coronary artery (+ branches of LAD).	Seen on right-sided ECG.
V_1–V_2 depression V_7–V_9	Posterior	Left circumflex or right coronary artery.	Check posterior ECG. If ST ↓ in V_1 or V_2, look for ST ↑ in V_7–V_9.

TABLE 3.9. Diagnosis and Treatment of Acute Coronary Syndrome

	POSSIBLE ACS	ACS		
		UNSTABLE ANGINA	NSTEMI	STEMI
History	CP	Worsening of CP	CP	CP
ECG	Normal or nonspecific	Usually ischemic—contiguous T-wave inversion, ST depressions		ST ↑ > 1 mm in 2 contiguous leads, or new LBBB, new Q waves
Serum markers	⊖	⊖	⊕	⊕
Medications	+/− β-blocker, nitrates, etc.	MONA; β-blocker; statin		
Anticoagulation	ASA	ASA + heparin + clopidogrel +/− Gp IIb/IIIa inhibitors		

- May also require GIIb/IIIa receptor antagonist or nitrate drip (contraindicated in RV infarction).
- Percutaneous coronary intervention (PCI)/percutaneous transluminal coronary angioplasty (PTCA), either emergently (STEMI) or urgently (UA/NSTEMI). Stents are usually placed, or if extensive disease, CABG is performed.
  - Bare metal stents: Higher risk of restenosis, lower risk of thrombosis.
  - Drug-eluting stents: Lower risk of restenosis, higher risk of thrombosis.
- Thrombolytics such as tPA can be used to break up plaque if PCI/PTCA cannot be performed urgently.

MNEMONIC

Initial treatment for chest pain—

MONA

Morphine
O$_2$
Nitrate
ASA

Congestive Heart Failure (CHF)

A 65-year-old man comes to see you at your office after having been hospitalized several months ago with a new diagnosis of heart failure following presentation with dyspnea and edema. His history is notable for AF, hypertension, and hyperlipidemia. An echocardiogram during his hospitalization showed an EF of 20%, LVH, and no wall motion abnormalities. He was discharged from the hospital on furosemide, an ACEI, a statin, and a β-blocker. His O$_2$ saturation is normal and on exam he is euvolemic. He continues to have dyspnea when walking from the kitchen to the bathroom in his house. What do you do?

You add digoxin in an attempt to improve his symptoms, as he currently can be categorized as NYHA class III, and it may help with his AF. You could also consider adding spironolactone, which confers a mortality benefit in class III–IV CHF.

CHF is a condition in which the ability of the heart to maintain circulation is compromised. CHF is most often chronic but may also be acute or subacute. Risk factors generally include ischemic heart disease, valvular disease, tobacco use, hypertension, obesity, and diabetes. CHF may be classified by symptom severity (see Table 3.10), by stage of evolution, by type of dysfunction (systolic or diastolic), or by part of the heart primarily affected (right or left):

- **Stage A:** High risk for heart failure due to comorbidities (hypertension, CAD, DM) without symptoms or structural disease.

TABLE 3.10.   NYHA Classification of CHF by Symptom Severity

Class I	Class II	Class III	Class IV
Symptoms at levels identical to those of normal individuals.	Symptoms with moderate exertion.	Symptoms with mild exertion only.	Symptoms at rest.

- **Stage B:** Structural heart disease associated with the development of heart failure (LVH; enlarged, dilated ventricle; valvular disease; previous MI) without symptoms.
- **Stage C:** Structural heart disease with previous or current symptoms. This is the **largest group.**
- **Stage D:** Refractory heart failure despite medical therapy, requiring specialized interventions.
- **Systolic dysfunction:** Defined as ↓ EF evidenced on echocardiogram in the setting of signs or symptoms of heart failure.
    - **Left heart failure:** Most common. Etiologies include CAD (present in 70% of patients with systolic dysfunction), dilated cardiomyopathy, hypertension, AF, and valvular disease.
    - **Right heart failure:** If in combination with left heart failure, usually from increased pressures via pulmonary vasculature from LV systolic dysfunction. If isolated to right, from increased pulmonary pressures (from chronic lung disease such as severe COPD, bronchiectasis, PEs) or predominant RV infarction, will find less lung involvement and more peripheral edema, causing a preload-dependent state.
- **Diastolic dysfunction: Abnormal LV filling** and normal systolic function. Etiologies are as follows:
    - ↓ myocardial relaxation due to ischemia, hypertrophy, cardiomyopathies, and aging.
    - ↑ myocardial stiffness due to fibrosis, scarring, hypertrophy, and infiltration.
    - Endocardial fibrosis.
    - Constrictive pericarditis, tamponade.

KEY FACT

Most patients with CHF have combined systolic and diastolic dysfunction.

SYMPTOMS

- **Subacute or acute:** Usually related to excess fluid accumulation—dyspnea at rest or with exertion, orthopnea, paroxysmal nocturnal dyspnea, ascites.
- **Chronic:** Fatigue, edema, and anorexia may be more prominent.
- Diastolic dysfunction is often asymptomatic.

EXAM

- **Systolic:** Signs of excess fluid accumulation related to decreased EF of blood from the affected ventricle:
    - Left-sided: Lung crackles, S3, narrow pulse pressure.
    - Right-sided: Leg edema, ascites, elevated JVP, hepatojugular reflex.
- **Diastolic:** The same as systolic except for the presence of an **S4.** An S3 should **not** be present in isolated diastolic dysfunction.

DIFFERENTIAL

COPD, pneumonia, cirrhosis, nephrotic syndrome, pulmonary embolism.

DIAGNOSIS

- **Labs:** CBC, electrolytes, and creatinine (for initiation of diuretics, assessment of renal failure from renal hypoperfusion), TSH, fasting glucose, LFTs, CXR, and ECG (to rule out ischemia, arrhythmias).
- **Brain natriuretic peptide (BNP):** Released with myocyte stretch. If ↑, helpful in distinguishing between CHF and pulmonary causes of dyspnea. Not helpful in assessing severity. Tends to be ↓ in obese patients and ↑ in those with CKD or sepsis.
- **CXR:** May show cardiomegaly (cardiac-to-thoracic ratio > 50%), Kerley B lines, pleural effusions (see Figure 3.11).
- **Echocardiography:**
  - **Systolic dysfunction:** Demonstrates an **EF < 40%** with an enlarged, dilated left ventricle.
  - **Diastolic dysfunction:** EF is normal, but hypertrophy, RV enlargement, pericarditis, and infiltrative disease may be seen.

TREATMENT

- **Systolic dysfunction:**
  - Always start with lifestyle modifications: Smoking cessation, reduction of alcohol consumption, decreased salt intake, weight loss, and monitoring.

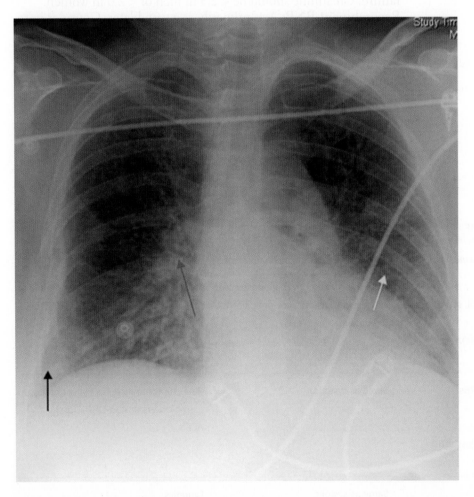

FIGURE 3.11.   CXR in CHF. (Reproduced, with permission, from Fauci AS, Kasper AL, Braunwald E, Hauser SL, Longo DL, Jameson JL, Loscalzo J. *Harrison's Principles of Internal Medicine,* 17th ed. http://www.accessmedicine.com. Copyright © The McGraw-Hill Companies, Inc. All rights reserved.)

- **Stepwise medication approach** (see Table 3.11 for treatment targeted to area of dysfunction):
  - **Diuretics:** Used acutely to relieve symptoms of pulmonary edema. Confers **no mortality benefit.**
  - **ACEIs:** Mortality benefit in **all classes of CHF.** If not tolerated, an ARB may be substituted.
  - **β-blockers:** Mortality benefits in **classes II, III, and IV** have been shown with carvedilol, metoprolol, and bisoprolol. Avoid starting in decompensated heart failure, but acceptable to continue during an exacerbation unless it is severe.
  - **Digoxin: May provide symptomatic relief, but confers no mortality benefit.** Helpful for rate control in patients with concurrent AF. **Symptoms of digoxin toxicity** (seen more often in those with renal insufficiency, hypokalemia, hypomagnesemia, use of non-DHP CCBs) include fatigue, disturbed color perception, anorexia, vomiting, abdominal pain, confusion. **Bradycardia,** prolonged PR interval, hyperkalemia are also often seen.
  - **Hydralazine with nitrates:** Can be used as an alternative to other treatments if contraindicated or as an addition for patients with moderate-severe symptoms on optimal therapy with ACEI, β-blocker, and diuretics.
  - **Spironolactone:** Confers a mortality benefit in **class III–IV heart failure.** Creatinine should be < 2.5 in men or < 2.0 in women.
  - **Recombinant BNP:** Acts primarily as a vasodilator. Consider in severe heart failure requiring ICU care.
- **Advanced treatments:**
  - **Mechanical therapy:** Consider a balloon pump for severe heart failure due to ischemia. Consider ventricular assist devices for very poor cardiac output as a bridge to transplantation.
  - **Implantable cardioverter-defibrillator (ICD):** For secondary prevention of sudden cardiac death (SCD) in those with a history of cardiac arrest, VF, or hemodynamically destabilizing VT. For primary prevention of SCD > 40 days after an MI, LVEF < 35, class II or III symptoms, and an expected survival > 1 year.

TABLE 3.11. **Targeted Treatment of CHF**

	SYSTOLIC DYSFUNCTION	ISOLATED RIGHT-SIDED DYSFUNCTION	DIASTOLIC DYSFUNCTION
Acute treatment	Loop diuretics. Oxygen, pain control, sodium/fluid restriction. Vasodilators (nitrates).	Slow use of diuretics (high doses can cause hypotension since preload-dependent).	Rate control (β-blockers or non-DHP CCBs). Slow use of diuretics (preload-dependent). ACE inhibitors.
Chronic treatment (mortality benefit)	ACE inhibitors or ARBs. β-blockers. Hydralazine/nitrates. Spironolactone in class III/IV. Exercise.	Same as systolic.	Rate control to increase filling time (β-blockers or non-DHP CCBs). ACEIs.
Chronic treatment (symptom relief)	Diuretics. Digoxin.	Same as systolic.	Diuretics.

- **Cardiac resynchronization:** Pacers used with severe systolic heart failure (class III or IV), sinus rhythm, and wide QRS. ↑ ventricular synchrony and cardiac output.
  - **Cardiac transplantation:** Reserved for end-stage heart disease that either limits survival to < 2 years or severely limits daily quality of life.
- **Isolated right-sided dysfunction:** Largely the same as left-sided systolic dysfunction management. Because of the risk of hypotension, avoid taking off too much fluid acutely with diuretics in preload-dependent state.
- **Diastolic dysfunction:**
  - Goals are to improve ventricular relaxation, ↓ heart rate, maintain sinus rhythm, and treat hypertension to achieve LVH regression.
  - Usually β-blockers and nondihydropyridine CCBs (verapamil, diltiazem). Other heart failure therapies are also used (see systolic dysfunction above).

KEY FACT

ACEIs, β-blockers, hydralazine, and spironolactone provide mortality benefit; diuretics and digoxin are used for symptomatic relief.

Valvular Heart Disease

An 81-year-old woman with a history of CAD, diabetes, hypertension, and hyperlipidemia comes to your office complaining of progressive fatigue, chest pain, dyspnea, and lightheadedness over the previous several years. She has had several episodes of syncope over the past few weeks without accompanying palpitations but with chest pain and dyspnea. Her BP is 170/90. She has a late-peaking systolic murmur at the left upper sternal border radiating to the carotids. PMI is displaced and sustained. Her ECG is normal, and her echocardiogram shows severe aortic stenosis with a valve area of 0.75 cm². How do you proceed?

You continue to work with her toward improved BP and lipid control but also refer her to a cardiologist and a cardiothoracic surgeon for consideration of a valve replacement.

See Table 3.12 for characteristic symptoms, exam findings, and treatment of different valvular pathologies.

PROSTHETIC VALVES

- **Mechanical valves:** Last 20–30 years; require lifetime anticoagulation because of thrombosis risk but have ↓ risk of structural failure.
- **Bioprosthetic valves:** Last 10–15 years; do not have as great a risk of thrombosis but do have ↑ risk of structural failure. Can be porcine, bovine, human heterograft, or autograft.
- Major complication is thromboembolism:
  - Risk for mitral valves > aortic valves.
  - Risk for mechanical valves > bioprosthetic valves.
  - Risk ↑ if patient has other thrombosis risk factors such as AF.
  - Larger thrombi (> 5 mm) require fibrinolysis or valve replacement. Heparin may be used with smaller thrombi.
  - See Table 3.13 for recommendations on when to use anticoagulation with prosthetic valves.

KEY FACT

Bioprosthetic valves are preferable to mechanical valves for older patients with a life expectancy of < 10 years and for those who are unable to take long-term anticoagulants.

KEY FACT

Valves should be chosen on the basis of life expectancy and suitability for long-term anticoagulation.

TABLE 3.12. Valvular Heart Disease

	Aortic Stenosis	Aortic Insufficiency	Mitral Stenosis	Mitral Valve Prolapse	Mitral Insufficiency
Cause	Rheumatic (world), bicuspid valve, senile calcific stenosis.	Valve leaflet destruction (endocarditis, rheumatic, aortic stenosis), acute aortic dissection (Marfan).	Rheumatic (most), occasionally endocarditis, calcification of mitral annulus.	Idiopathic, familial, Marfan, Ehlers-Danlos, post-MI, reduced LV size, flail leaflet.	Endocarditis, MI, trauma to valve, MVP, rheumatic.
Symptoms	**Angina, syncope, heart failure,** dyspnea, ↓ exercise tolerance.	Often asymptomatic until heart failure develops.	Dyspnea, hemoptysis, symptoms from pulmonary HTN, right heart failure, or PE.	Often asymptomatic. MVP syndrome = atypical CP, palpitations, dizziness **not** related to valve dysfunction.	Acute: Cardiogenic shock. Chronic: ↓ exercise tolerance, fatigue, dyspnea.
Murmur	Systolic crescendo-descrescendo, radiates to carotids.	Diastolic decrescendo blowing at base (in severe cases, apical diastolic rumble is heard, as in MS).	Diastolic apical rumble after an opening snap.	Midsystolic click and murmur at the apex.	Holosystolic, high pitched, best at apex in left lateral decubitus position with diaphragm of stethoscope.
Exam findings	Sustained PMD, ↓ S2, systolic click if bicuspid.	↓ S1, wide pulse pressure, water-hammer pulses.	↓ pulses, ↑ S1, signs of right heart failure (↑ JVP, edema).		↓ S1, ⊕ S3, if acute signs of left heart failure.
Diagnosis	Echo (asymptomatic until valve area < 1 cm³, pressure gradient > 40 mmHg).	Echo (if acute, may need TEE to r/o endocarditis).	Echo (evaluate valve area, pressure gradient, morphology).	Echo (assess if regurgitation or ↓ LV function).	Echo.
Treatment	Valve replacement once symptomatic. Survival is 2–5 years without treatment once symptoms develop.	Afterload reduction (ACEI). Valve replacement if symptoms or worsening LV dilation/function.	Percutaneous balloon valvotomy if no regurg or thrombus; valve replacement.	Usually not necessary.	Acute: Surgery. Chronic: Valve repair/replacement if new AF and decreased LV systolic function.
Complications	LV systolic dysfunction.	Left atrial enlargement, pulmonary HTN, right heart failure, AF.	AF, pulmonary HTN, PE, right heart failure.		Heart failure, infectious endocarditis, AF.

TABLE 3.13.　Anticoagulation in Heart Disease

	CONDITION	PRIMARY RECOMMENDATION	SECONDARY RECOMMENDATION
Cardiovascular disease	CAD.	ASA.	Clopidogrel if cannot take ASA.
	Acute ACS.	ASA + heparin + clopidogrel.	
	After ACS.	ASA, continue clopidogrel at least × 1 mo for patients managed medically without stent.	
	After bare metal stent.	ASA, clopidogrel at least × 1 mo.	
	After drug eluting stent.	ASA, clopidogrel at least × 1 yr.	
Arrhythmia	AF/atrial flutter.	Warfarin; see section on AF/atrial flutter for details.	
	Postcardioversion.	Warfarin for 4 weeks if maintains NSR.	
CHF		**Not routine;** some consider warfarin if LVEF < 30 or LV thrombus.	**Warfarin** if AF or history of systemic embolism also present.
Valvular disease	Mitral valve disease.	**Not routine.**	**Warfarin** if AF or history of systemic embolism also present.
	Aortic valve disease.	**Not routine.**	**Warfarin + ASA** if repeated systemic embolism.
Prosthetic heart valves	Mechanical.	**Warfarin** for lifetime.	**Warfarin + ASA** if other thrombolic risk factors.
	Bioprosthetic.	**Warfarin** for first 3 months, **ASA** for lifetime.	**Warfarin + ASA** if other thrombotic risk factors.
Cerebrovascular disease	Ischemic embolic stroke.	Depends on source of emboli (AF, carotid, endocarditis, etc).	
	Ischemic thrombotic stroke.	ASA.	If stroke while on ASA, clopidogrel or GIIb–IIIa antagonist.
	Hemorrhagic stroke.	Avoid.	

*Other thrombotic risk factors: AF, prior thromboembolism, hypercoagulable state, ↓ LVEF < 30.

ENDOCARDITIS PROPHYLAXIS

Antibiotics to prevent endocarditis during procedures should be limited to patients with cardiac conditions with very high risk of adverse outcomes from endocarditis.

■ The American Heart Association recommends prophylactic antibiotics for **prosthetic heart valves, prosthetic material** used in valve repair or repair of congenital heart disease, unrepaired **cyanotic congenital heart disease** (or partially repaired with residual defects), valve pathology in a **transplanted heart,** and **prior history** of endocarditis.
■ Prophylactic antibiotics are no longer recommended for aortic stenosis, bicuspid aortic valve, aortic regurgitation, mitral stenosis, mitral valve prolapse, mitral regurgitation, and hypertrophic cardiomyopathy.
■ Procedures that need prophylaxis include dental procedures and respiratory procedures **if** they involve biopsy or incision of mucosa (eg, tonsillectomy, bronchoscopy).
■ Procedures that do not need prophylaxis include GI or GU procedures (unless patient has known active infection), C-section, or vaginal delivery.

 MNEMONIC

Prophylaxis for endocarditis in HEaRT:

Hole (unrepaired or partially repaired congenital lesion)
Endocarditis previously
Repair with prosthetic material (of valve or congenital lesion)
Transplanted heart with valve pathology

- **Antibiotic regimen:** Amoxicillin. If patient is allergic, can use cephalexin, clindamycin, azithromycin.

Anticoagulation in Heart Disease

Table 3.13 reviews the medications and indications for anticoagulation in various cardiovascular diseases.

Cardiomyopathies

Diseases of the heart muscle that have a variety of causes. The clinical presentation is variable and related to the underlying etiology.

- **Hypertrophic:** A genetic disorder with autosomal-dominant inheritance but variable penetrance. First-degree family members of affected individuals should be screened q1 year between ages 12–18, then q5 years with an ECG, possibly an echocardiogram.
- **Restrictive:** Impaired diastolic filling with preserved systolic functioning.
  - Infiltrative (amyloid, sarcoid).
  - Noninfiltrative (familial, idiopathic).
  - Storage (hemochromatosis, Fabry).
  - Endomyocardial fibrosis (endemic in certain areas of the world, radiation treatment).
- **Dilated:** Dilation and impaired contraction of one or both ventricles.
  - Ischemic.
  - Valvular.
  - Infectious (viral, Chagas, HIV, Lyme).
  - Toxic (alcohol, cocaine, methamphetamine, some chemotherapeutic agents).
  - Genetic.
  - Idiopathic.

SYMPTOMS/EXAM

- **Hypertrophic:** Often asymptomatic and found on routine family screening. Can present with symptoms of heart failure, sudden cardiac death, syncope, or arrhythmias.
- **Restrictive:** Presents with symptoms of heart failure.
- **Dilated:** Can present with arrhythmias, heart failure, or sudden death.

DIAGNOSIS

- **Hypertrophic:**
  - Echo: LV thickening, may be asymmetric around the septum → systolic pressure gradient.
  - ECG: LVH; prominent Q in II, III, aVF; P wave ↑ (LA enlargement).
  - Murmur: Systolic crescendo-decrescendo, radiating to axilla/base. ↑ with Valsava or standing (decreased blood return → less ventricular filling → increased obstruction). ↓ with squatting.
- **Restrictive:** Ventricles have normal size and wall thickness but rigid walls on echocardiogram. Can have similar findings as constrictive pericarditis (see section on constrictive pericarditis). Chest CT, cardiac MRI, or cardiac catheterization may assist in differentiating from constrictive pericarditis.
- **Dilated:** On echocardiogram: ↓ wall thickness, ↓ EF, ↑ LV volume.

TREATMENT

- **Hypertrophic:** Treatment with negative inotropes such as β-blockers or verapamil is directed toward improving diastolic filling in patients who are symptomatic. Avoid volume depletion, avoid vasodilators, and start activity restriction.
- **Restrictive:** Treatment aims to ↓ elevated filling pressures and treat symptoms of heart failure. Diuretics may relieve symptoms; CCBs may improve diastolic relaxation. Consider amiodarone or a defibrillator for high-risk patients with previous dysrhythmias, LVH, syncope, or specific genetic mutations.
- **Dilated:** Treatment is influenced by the development of heart failure.

Pericardial Disease

Pericardial disease often results from systemic disease. Often presents with both pericarditis and an effusion.

ACUTE PERICARDITIS

Etiologies of acute pericarditis are as follows:

- **Idiopathic:** The most common cause.
- **Infectious:** Usually viral (including HIV, coxsackie, Epstein-Barr virus [EBV], cytomegalovirus [CMV]) but may also be caused by TB, other bacteria, or parasites.
- **Metabolic disorders:** Most commonly uremia, also hypothyroidism.
- **Other:** **Previous radiation, postinfarction** (Dressler syndrome), **inflammatory/autoimmune** (lupus, RA, scleroderma), **neoplastic** (often lung or breast cancer), **degenerative, traumatic, medications** (INH, hydralazine).

SYMPTOMS/EXAM

- Presents with sudden onset, sharp, pleuritic chest pain that ↑ when the patient is supine and ↓ when the patient leans forward. Can be angina-like.
- **Pericardial friction rub.**
- **Diffuse ST elevations** are found on ECG, as seen in Figure 3.12. Sometimes ↑ cardiac markers. Echo is often normal unless associated effusion present.
- **High-risk features** include high fever, gradual onset, evidence of tamponade or large effusion, acute trauma, leukocytosis, and failure to respond to medical therapy within 7 days.

DIAGNOSIS

Diagnosed clinically based on the findings above. Usually benign course.

TREATMENT

NSAIDs. Colchicine and steroids can also be used.

PERICARDIAL EFFUSION

Often accompanies acute pericarditis. Causes are similar to those of acute pericarditis, with the most common being idiopathic, infectious, malignancy, trauma, and post-MI.

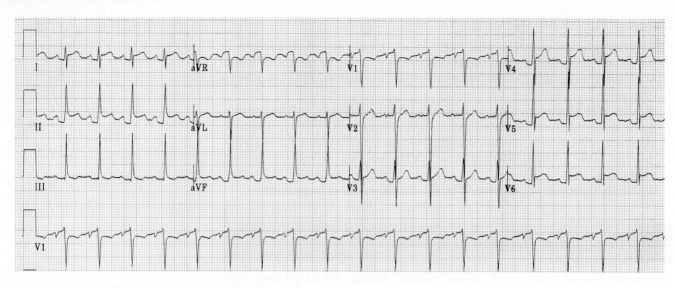

FIGURE 3.12. **Diffuse ST elevations in pericarditis.** (Reproduced, with permission, from Knoop KJ, Stack LB, Storrow AB, Thurman RJ. *The Atlas of Emergency Medicine,* 3rd ed. http://www.accessmedicine.com. Copyright © The McGraw-Hill Companies, Inc. All rights reserved.)

SYMPTOMS/EXAM

Similar to acute pericarditis; sometimes persistent fever, L > R pleural effusion, cardiomegaly.

DIAGNOSIS

- **ECG:** May show associated pericarditis; if large enough, effusion can look like tamponade (see tamponade information below—low voltage, electrical alternans).
- **CXR:** May show enlarged cardiac silhouette with a "water-bottle configuration" (see Figure 3.13A).
- **Echocardiography:** Confirms the presence of effusion and determines the hemodynamic impact (impaired ventricular filling).
- **Pericardiocentesis:** Most useful for cytology and cultures. Not always indicated, depending on cause/size of effusion.

TREATMENT

Treatment is specific to the cause.

KEY FACT

Pericardial effusion may accompany acute pericarditis.

TAMPONADE

Caused by an effusion under pressure → impaired ventricular filling. May be acute or subacute. Etiologies are:

- **Acute:** Usually traumatic (penetrating trauma, aortic rupture, procedures such as pacer placement).
- **Subacute:** Neoplasm, pericarditis.

SYMPTOMS/EXAM

- **Acute:** Presents with chest pain and dyspnea. Classic exam findings include **elevated JVP, muted heart sounds, and hypotension.** Potentially life-threatening.
- **Subacute:** Presents with chest pain. On exam, hypotension, tachycardia, and a narrowed pulse pressure may be seen.

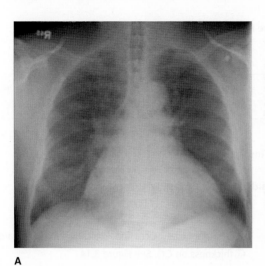
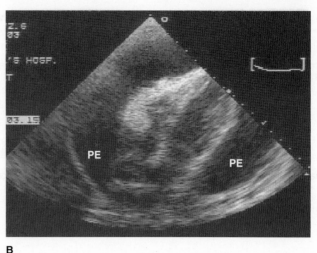

A

B

FIGURE 3.13.   Pericardial effusion and tamponade. (A) CXR with enlargement of the cardiac silhouette ("water-bottle heart") in a patient with pericardial effusion. **(B)** Apical 4-chamber transthoracic echocardiogram with large pericardial effusion (PE) and collapse of the right atrium/ventricle during diastole in a patient with cardiac tamponade. (Image A reproduced, with permission, from USMLERx.com. Image B reproduced, with permission, from Hall JB, et al. *Principles of Critical Care*, 3rd ed. New York: McGraw-Hill, 2005: Fig. 28-7A.)

DIAGNOSIS

- **ECG:** Low voltage, sinus tachycardia; "electrical alternans"—QRS shifts from beat to beat due to swinging of heart in large effusion.
- **Pulsus paradoxus:** An SBP ↓ of > 10 mmHg during inspiration. Occurs with tamponade, constrictive pericarditis, asthma, and COPD.
- **Echocardiography:** Shows right atrial collapse during diastole and equalization of RV and LV pressures (see Figure 3.13B).

> **KEY FACT**
>
> Cardiac tamponade is an effusion under pressure → impaired ventricular filling. Classic exam findings include elevated JVP, distant heart sounds, and hypotension.

TREATMENT

Drainage via either pericardiocentesis or an open procedure is required. Pericardiectomy may also be necessary.

CONSTRICTIVE PERICARDITIS

Constrictive pericarditis results from subacute or chronic scarring and loss of elasticity of the pericardial sac, so cardiac filling is impeded by external force. Because of less stretch, LV and RV are more interdependent. Many findings are similar to restrictive cardiomyopathy (see Table 3.14 and Figure 3.14).

Peripheral Vascular Disease

Almost always due to peripheral atherosclerosis; therefore, risk factors are the same as those in coronary atherosclerosis (tobacco use, hypertension, hyperlipidemia, diabetes).

SYMPTOMS/EXAM

- Often asymptomatic. **The classic symptom is claudication,** or pain in a muscle group that is reproduced with exercise and relieved by rest. Severity varies and symptoms do not always correlate with degree of vessel stenosis.
- The calf is the most frequently affected area, but the buttocks, thighs, and feet may also be affected.
- Poor wound healing.

TABLE 3.14. Comparison of Restrictive Cardiomyopathy and Constrictive Pericarditis

	RESTRICTIVE CARDIOMYOPATHY	CONSTRICTIVE PERICARDITIS
Causes	Infiltrative (amyloid sarcoid), storage (hemochromatosis, Fabry), idiopathic, familial, hypereosinophillic syndromes.	Scarring from previous pericardial disease (idiopathic, viral, radiation, postsurgical, connective tissue disease).
Exam	↑ JVP. Kussmaul sign (lack of JVP decline during inspiration).	
ECG changes	Low voltage (more with constrictive pericarditis or amyloidosis), LVH, Q waves, impaired AV conduction, nonspecific ST changes.	
CXR	Mild cardiomegaly.	Mild cardiomegaly. Occasional calcification of pericardium (↑ thickness on CT). See Figure 3.14.
BNP	↑ (wall stretches).	Normal (wall can't stretch).

■ Rest pain is a late finding that often occurs at night.
■ Exam findings include ↓ pulses, peripheral bruits, and cool, shiny extremities with ↓ hair.

DIAGNOSIS

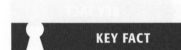

Ankle-brachial index (ABI) < 0.9 (indicates > 50% stenosis of one or more vessels). Highest systolic ankle pressure/systolic brachial pressure by Doppler. Performed at rest and after exercise. Calcified vessels can cause an abnormally high ABI (> 1.3). ABI of < 0.4 indicates ischemia.

■ **Segmental limb pressures** are used to evaluate the extent of disease.
■ Other modalities: Ultrasound with duplex, MRI, CT.

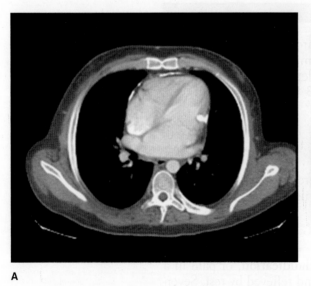

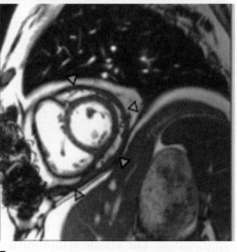

A   B

FIGURE 3.14. Constrictive pericarditis. (Image A reproduced, with permission, from Fuster V, O'Rourke RA, Walsh RA, Poole-Wilson P. *Hurst's The Heart*, 12th ed., Fig. 21-25. http://www.accessmedicine.com. Copyright © The McGraw-Hill Companies, Inc. All rights reserved. Image B reproduced, with permission, from Fauci AS, Kasper DL, Braunwald E, et al. *Harrison's Principles of Internal Medicine*, 17th ed. New York: McGraw-Hill, 2008, Fig. 222-9.)

TREATMENT

- **Risk factor reduction:** Tobacco cessation; treatment of hyperlipidemia; glucose and BP control. Rehabilitation and structured exercise programs.
- **Pharmacologic:**
  - **Aspirin:** Has only modest benefit. Ticlopidine and clopidogrel can also be used.
  - **Cilostazol:** Inhibits platelet aggregation and ↑ vasodilation.
  - **Pentoxifylline:** ↑ RBC deformity and ↓ serum viscosity.
  - **Ginkgo biloba:** Has been shown to be somewhat effective, although the mechanism is unclear.
- **Interventional procedures:**
  - Indicated for symptoms that limit activity as well as with rest pain or tissue loss (ischemic ulcers or gangrene).
  - Include percutaneous revascularization with percutaneous angioplasty or stents, generally for more focal lesions.
  - Surgical revascularization (endarterectomy or bypass grafting) if cannot be done percutaneously.

CHAPTER 4

Endocrinology

Kelly Eagen, MD

Diabetes Mellitus (DM)

 An 81-year-old man comes to your clinic concerned that he has diabetes. He recently had his blood sugar checked at a health fair and was told that it was around 200 mg/dL. He denies any symptoms of diabetes. You order a fasting blood glucose test, which reveals his level to be 150 mg/dL. Further labs reveal an HbA$_{1c}$ of 8.2% and a creatinine level of 1.3 mg/dL. What further testing should you do before starting the patient on metformin?

A second fasting blood glucose test to confirm the diagnosis and tests to determine creatinine clearance since serum creatinine can be misleading in elderly individuals with low muscle mass.

DM is an impairment in carbohydrate metabolism leading to hyperglycemia. There are 2 main types of DM:

- **Type 1:** Due to absolute insulin insufficiency caused by destruction of pancreatic islet cells. Type 1 DM is typically autoimmune but can be idiopathic.
- **Type 2:** Due to insulin resistance and variable degrees of relative insulin deficiency. Type 2 DM accounts for approximately 90% of DM cases in the United States. Although type 1 DM was formerly known as juvenile diabetes, more children are currently being diagnosed with type 2 than with type 1 DM.
- A third type of diabetes is gestational diabetes, a complication of pregnancy (see the Reproductive Health chapter).

SYMPTOMS/EXAM

- **May be asymptomatic (common in type 2 DM).**
- Presents with the 3 P's: **polyuria, polydipsia,** and **polyphagia.**
- Weight loss, blurry vision, acanthosis nigricans (a sign of insulin resistance; see Figure 4.1), dehydration, and neuropathy may also be seen.
- **Diabetic ketoacidosis (DKA)** and **hyperosmolar nonketotic coma (HONKC)** are acute complications (see below).

DIAGNOSIS

The American Diabetes Association (ADA) diagnostic criteria for DM are as follows:

- Symptoms of diabetes plus a **random** plasma glucose concentration of **≥ 200 mg/dL.**
- A **fasting** plasma glucose of **≥ 126 mg/dL** on **2** separate occasions.
- A plasma glucose of ≥ 200 mg/dL 2 hours after a 75-g glucose load during an oral glucose tolerance test.

SCREENING

- The U.S. Preventive Services Task Force (USPSTF) recommends screening for asymptomatic adults with sustained blood pressure (treated or untreated) > 135/80 mmHg.
- Symptomatic individuals should be screened.

KEY FACT

Type 1 DM used to be called juvenile diabetes, but now more children are being diagnosed with type 2 DM than with type 1.

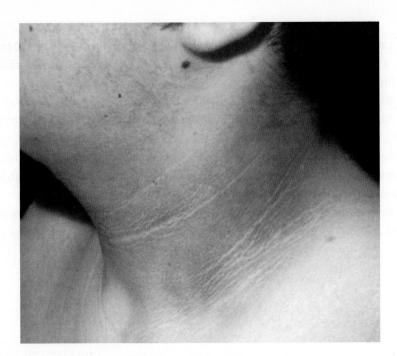

FIGURE 4.1. **Acanthosis nigricans.** (Reproduced, with permission, from Wolff K, Johnson RA. *Fitzpatrick's Color Atlas & Synopsis of Clinical Dermatology,* 6th ed. New York: McGraw-Hill, 2009, Fig. 5e-AN-1.)

TREATMENT

- **Routine diabetic care:** Table 4.1 outlines the routine management of diabetes.
- **Glycemic control:** Nonpharmacologic modalities are typically the first approach to glycemic control but the addition of pharmacologic agents is often necessary for tight control.
- **Nonpharmacologic:** Diet, exercise, weight loss, and stress management can all help control glucose levels and ↓ the need for other medications in type 2 DM.
- **Pharmacologic:**
  - Table 4.2 outlines medications for the treatment of type 2 DM. Metformin and/or sulfonylureas are first-line agents.
  - **Insulin** is appropriate for type 1 and type 2 DM (see Table 4.3). Options include a "basal-bolus" regimen (basal coverage with intermediate- to long-acting insulin plus a short-acting bolus insulin before meals), insulin in combination with other agents, or continuous insulin infusion via an SQ catheter.
  - **Experimental treatment:** Immunosuppression in type 1 DM; pancreatic/islet cell transplantation.

KEY FACT

Metformin is the first-line agent in obese patients with a creatinine level < 1.5 mg/dL in men and < 1.4 mg/dL in women because it promotes weight loss.

KEY FACT

Hold metformin in surgery patients until renal function has normalized after surgery because of the ↑ risk of lactic acidosis. Metformin may also cause GI upset, and providers should counsel patients to take it with meals and titrate up slowly to minimize side effects.

ACUTE COMPLICATIONS

 A 10-year-old boy presents to the ER with lethargy, nausea, and vomiting. Exam reveals that he is tachypneic and has a fruity odor to his breath. His urine shows 4+ glucose and ketones, and his bedside blood glucose level is > 500 mg/dL. Even before labs are obtained, what therapy can be initiated in this patient?

NS and IV insulin.

Labs are obtained and show a K+ level of 4.0, a blood glucose level of 550 mg/dL, a serum HCO_3 level of 15 mEq/L, and a pH of 7.29. What can now be added to his fluids?

K+ supplementation. Should bicarbonate be given?

No; bicarbonate is indicated only with severe acidosis (pH < 7.2 or HCO_3 < 15 mEq/L).

Several hours later, the boy's labs show a blood glucose level of 210 mg/dL, a K+ level of 4.2, and a serum HCO_3 level of 15 mEq/L. Should you switch to an SQ insulin regimen?

Not yet; instead, add 5% dextrose to the boy's fluids and continue IV insulin until acidosis resolves.

TABLE 4.1.   Routine Management of Diabetes

Glucose control	Goal HbA_{1c} is < 6.5%–7.0%. HbA_{1c} reflects glucose levels over the past 3 months. Check at least biannually in stable patients.
BP control	Goal BP is < 130/80 mmHg.
Lipid control	Goal LDL is < 100 mg/dL and < 70 mg/dL in high-risk patients.
Aspirin therapy	Daily aspirin therapy is recommended as followed: 1. 2° prevention in high-risk groups such as those with a history of MI, CAD, and PVD. 2. 1° prevention in diabetic patients with ↑ cardiovascular risk (10-year risk > 10%).
Smoking cessation	Advise all patients to stop smoking.
Nephropathy screening	Screen annually for microalbuminuria with spot urine protein/creatinine or albumin/creatinine ratio as follows: 1. Type 2 DM patients: screen immediately after diagnosis. 2. Type 1 DM patients: screen 5 years after diagnosis. Treat with ACEIs or ARBs. Tolerate up to a 15%–20% ↑ in serum creatinine with the initiation of ACEIs/ARBs. Tight BP and glucose control also delays development.
Retinopathy screening	Schedule an annual ophthalmology exam as follows: 1. Type 2 DM patients: immediately after diagnosis. 2. Type 1 DM patients: 5 years after diagnosis. Maintain tight glucose and BP control for prevention. Laser therapy can slow diabetic retinopathy and ↓ the risk of vision loss.
Foot care	Perform an annual complete foot exam with monofilament testing, visual inspection on each visit, and prophylactic foot care education for all diabetic patients.
Immunizations	Vaccinate adults with the pneumococcal vaccine and the annual influenza vaccine.
Tuberculosis testing	High-risk populations should be tested because of ↑ reactivation rates.

TABLE 4.2.   Medications Used in Type 2 DM

CLASS	DRUGS	ADVERSE EFFECTS	COMMENTS
Sulfonylureas	Glipizide, glyburide, glimepiride, tolazamide, tolbutamide.	Hypoglycemia.	Often first-line treatment; can cause weight gain.
Biguanides	Metformin.	GI side effects (nausea, diarrhea), lactic acidosis ($\uparrow$ risk in renal disease [Cr > 1.5]), CHF, respiratory disease, liver disease in the elderly.	Often first-line treatment. Promote weight loss; hypoglycemia is rare.
Meglitinides	Repaglinide, nateglinide.	Hypoglycemia.	Short acting; use for postprandial hyperglycemia.
Thiazolidinediones	Rosiglitazone, pioglitazone.	Rare hypoglycemia; fluid retention, liver disease. $\uparrow$ rates of cardiovascular death in patients on rosiglitazone.	Monitor LFTs; do not use in patients with CHF. Last-choice oral agent.
α-glucosidase inhibitors	Miglitol, acarbose.	Gas, bloating, diarrhea.	Start low and gradually $\uparrow$ dosage.
Amylin replacement	Pramlintide.	Nausea.	Given SQ with meals in patients on basal-bolus insulin.
GLP-1 agents	Exenatide.	Nausea, vomiting, diarrhea.	SQ; promote weight loss.
DPP-4 inhibitors	Sitagliptin, vildagliptin.	GI upset.	Oral agents, weight neutral.

Acute complications of DM include the following:

- **DKA:** Much more common in type 1 than in type 2 DM. Can be the initial manifestation of type 1 or may occur later in either type 1 or type 2. Look for a stressor (eg, infection, surgery, infarction, medical noncompliance) that may have precipitated DKA.
  - **Sx/Exam:** Abdominal pain, vomiting, Kussmaul respirations (rapid deep breaths), a fruity breath odor (from acetone), and lethargy. Can progress to coma.
  - **Dx:** Lab findings include hyperglycemia, hyperosmolality, and a high anion-gap metabolic acidosis (serum $HCO_3 < 15$ mEq/L; pH < 7.3; serum ketones > 5 mmol/L) (see Table 4.4).
  - **Tx:**
    - **Insulin drip:** To close the anion gap and $\downarrow$ plasma glucose. Switch to SQ insulin only when the anion gap has closed.

TABLE 4.3.   Insulin Types

	INSULIN TYPE	ONSET	PEAK ACTION	DURATION
Ultra-short-acting	Lispro, insulin aspart, glulisine.	5–15 minutes.	1.0–1.5 hours.	3–4 hours.
Short-acting	Regular.	15–30 minutes.	1–3 hours.	5–7 hours.
Intermediate-acting	Lente, NPH.	2–4 hours.	8–10 hours.	18–24 hours.
Long-acting	Ultralente, glargine, detemir.	4–5 hours.	8–14 hours (glargine has virtually no peak).	25–36 hours.

TABLE 4.4. Diabetic Ketoacidosis vs. Hyperosmolar Nonketotic Coma

	DKA	HONKC
Onset	Short (hours to days).	Insidious (days to weeks).
Blood glucose	> 250 mg/dL.	> 600 mg/dL.
pH	> 7.3.	< 7.3.
HCO_3	< 320 mEq/L.	> 330 mEq/L.
TBW deficit	5–7 L.	8–10 L.
Fluid repletion	Initial goal is to correct intravascular volume, then correct TBW deficit in the following 24–48 hours.	Goal is to replace one-half of TBW deficit over the first 12 hours and remainder in the next 24 hours.

TBW = total body water.

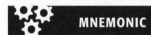

- **Fluids:** Glucose-induced osmotic diuresis causes a fluid loss of approximately 3–6 L. Start with NS and then switch to 1/2 NS. Add D5 when glucose is < 250 mg/dL.
  - **Electrolytes: Potassium** is usually falsely elevated initially because of acidosis and will ↓ with treatment. Start potassium replacement with plasma levels in the 4.0–4.5 range.
  - **Bicarbonate therapy is not usually indicated** unless there is severe acidosis (pH < 7.2 or HCO_3 < 10 mEq/L).
- **HONKC:** Defined as significant hyperglycemia, hyperosmolality, and dehydration without ketosis. Look for a stressor (eg, infection, infarction, intoxication, medical noncompliance) that may have precipitated HONKC.
  - **Sx/Exam:** Presents with **polyuria, polydipsia, polyphagia,** weakness, lethargy, confusion, and coma.
  - **Dx:** Serum glucose is often > 800 mg/dL. Serum HCO_3 is normal to slightly low; pH is > 7.3 (see Table 4.4).
  - **Tx: Treat the underlying stressor;** give fluids, insulin drip, and electrolyte replacement. Similar to treatment for DKA. Often need 6–10 L of fluids in these patients. Watch for pulmonary edema and volume overload in elderly patients.
  - **Cx:** Mortality may be as high as 50%, likely due to the comorbidities of the population affected.
- **Hypoglycemia:** A common occurrence in diabetic patients on insulin therapy. Can also occur with use of oral hypoglycemics, especially sulfonylureas.
  - **Sx/Exam:**
    - **Neuroglycopenic symptoms:** Include confusion, stupor, coma, and focal neurologic findings. Result from low glucose delivery to the brain.
    - **Autonomic symptoms:** Tachycardia, palpitations, sweating, tremulousness, nausea, hunger.
  - **Tx:**
    - **Conscious patients:** Give glucose tablets, juice, and other high-glucose drinks or snacks.
    - **Unconscious patients:** Administer glucagon 1 mg IM or 50% glucose IV.

CHRONIC COMPLICATIONS

Most of the **chronic complications** of DM begin about 5 years after disease onset. Screening of type 1 patients begins 5 years after diagnosis, but screening of type 2 patients begins immediately after diagnosis, since type 2 patients usually have had the disease for years before diagnosis. **Tight glycemic control** can ↓ the incidence of chronic complications, especially microvascular disease.

- Microvascular:
    - **Retinopathy:** Schedule an annual eye exam by an ophthalmologist. Retinal neovascularization can be treated with photocoagulation therapy (see Figure 4.2).
    - **Nephropathy:** Screen annually for microalbuminuria. ACEIs or ARBs can slow progression of renal disease in patients with microalbuminuria.
    - **Neuropathy:** Peripheral neuropathy initially involves the distal feet and later the hands. Stress the importance of foot care and annual foot exams to prevent complications. Autonomic neuropathy may cause orthostatic hypotension, gastroparesis, neurogenic bladder, and impotence. Manage with improved glycemic control and pain management strategies.
    - **Diabetic ulcers and osteomyelitis:** Neuropathy and trauma may result in bony deformations, including those of the foot, such as a Charcot joint. People with diabetes are also at higher risk for infections of the soft tissue (cellulitis) and bones (osteomyelitis) (see Figure 4.3).

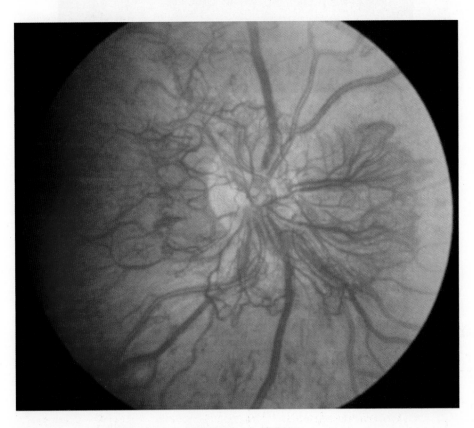

FIGURE 4.2.   Florid optic neovascularization in diabetes. (Reproduced, with permission, from McPhee SJ, Papadakis MA. *Current Medical Diagnosis and Treatment,* 49th ed. New York: McGraw-Hill, 2009.)

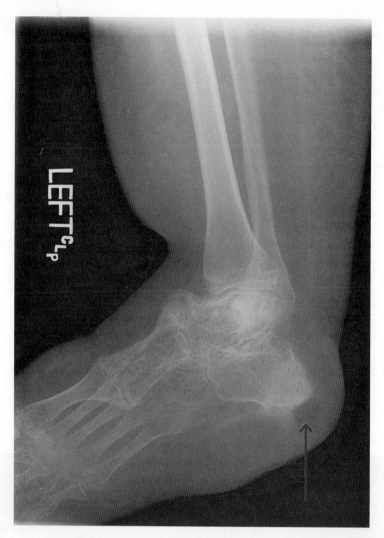

FIGURE 4.3.   Diabetic foot. Osteopenia and destruction of the ankle and tarsal joints (Charcot joints). Also, note the soft-tissue ulcer at the heel (*arrow*) with sclerosis of the underlying calcaneus that likely represents chronic osteomyelitis. (Reproduced, with permission, from USMLERx. com.)

- **Macrovascular complications:** Associated with an ↑ risk of MI and stroke. Control risk factors by instituting the following measures:
    - **Daily aspirin** (see Table 4.1); **smoking cessation.**
    - **BP control:** Goal BP is < 130/80 mmHg.
    - **Lipids:** Goal LDL is < 100 mg/dL, or < 70 mg/dL in high-risk patients.
    - Diet and exercise.

METABOLIC SYNDROME

Also known as insulin resistance syndrome or "Syndrome X." Represents a combination of traits associated with insulin resistance and an ↑ risk of type 2 DM.

DIAGNOSIS

Diagnosis is based on any **3** of the following Adult Treatment Panel III criteria:

- Abdominal obesity (waist circumference > 40 inches in men, > 35 inches in women).
- TG ≥ 150 mg/dL.
- HDL < 40 mg/dL in men and < 50 mg/dL in women.
- BP ≥ 130/85 mmHg.
- Fasting glucose ≥ 110 mg/dL.

TREATMENT

Directed toward preventing the development of type 2 DM and coronary vascular disease. Focus on lifestyle modifications (diet, weight loss, exercise) and, if needed, medication for treatment of insulin resistance.

Pituitary Disorders

The pituitary gland releases 8 hormones that regulate the body's endocrine functions. The hypothalamus produces oxytocin and ADH, which are then stored and released by the posterior pituitary. The anterior pituitary produces 6 hormones: ACTH, TSH, FSH, LH, GH, and prolactin (see Figure 4.4 and Table 4.5).

PITUITARY TUMORS

Pituitary tumors may arise from any cell. They are classified as **microadenomas** (< 1 cm) and **macroadenomas** (> 1 cm). They may ↑ or ↓ hormones produced by the cells of origin by mass effect. Subtypes include the following:

- **Pituitary adenomas:**
  - Prolactinomas (the most common pituitary microadenoma).
  - GH-secreting.
  - Nonfunctioning (account for one-third of all pituitary tumors; the most common macroadenoma).
  - ACTH-secreting.
  - TSH-secreting (rare).
- **Pituitary carcinomas.**

SYMPTOMS/EXAM

- Incidental discovery on MRI is very common; up to 10% of the general population has asymptomatic pituitary adenomas.
- Symptomatic cases may present as follows:
  - **Neurologic:** Headaches; visual field deficits (bitemporal hemianopia due to mass effect on the optic chiasm).
  - **Hormonal excess/deficiency:** Hypothyroidism, hypogonadism, hyperprolactinemia (see specific sections for symptomatology).

DIFFERENTIAL

The differential for sellar masses includes other benign masses (craniopharyngioma, meningioma), malignancies (1°—germ cell tumors and lymphomas; me-

KEY FACT

Prolactinomas are usually associated with a prolactin level > 200 ng/dL.

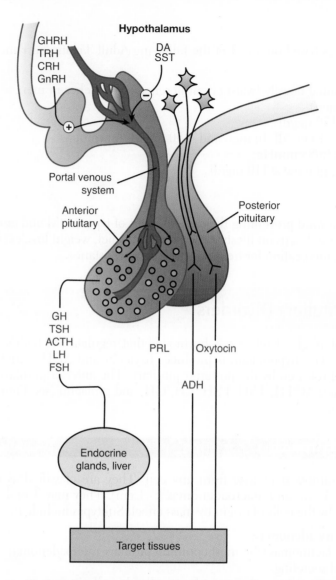

FIGURE 4.4. **The hypothalamic-pituitary endocrine system.** Except for prolactin, hormones released from the anterior pituitary stimulate the production of hormones by a peripheral endocrine gland or the liver. Prolactin and the hormones released from the posterior pituitary (vasopressin and oxytocin) act directly on target tissues. Hypothalamic factors regulate the release of anterior pituitary hormones. (Reproduced, with permission, from Katzung BG, et al. *Basic and Clinical Pharmacology,* 11th ed. New York: McGraw-Hill, 2009, Fig. 37-1.)

tastases—especially breast and lung cancer), cysts (Rathke cleft, arachnoid, and dermoid cysts can cause sellar enlargement), and infections (abscesses, TB).

DIAGNOSIS

- **Labs:** Check prolactin, insulin-like growth factor-1 (IGF-1), 24-hour urine for cortisol, ACTH, TSH, LH, FSH, and testosterone levels.
- **Imaging:** MRI of the pituitary/sella (see Figure 4.5).

TREATMENT

- Observation may suffice if the tumor is < 20 mm and is not causing signs or symptoms.

TABLE 4.5.   Pituitary Hormones and Their Function

HORMONE	INCREASED BY	DECREASED BY	EXCESS	DEFICIENCY	NOTES
ADH	Thirst, high serum osmolality.	Low serum osmolality, low serum K^+.	SIADH.	DI.	
ACTH	CRH, stress.	High cortisol.	Cushing syndrome.	Adrenal insufficiency.	Diurnal variation (peak at 3–4 A.M.).
TSH	TRH.	High T_4 and/or T_3.	Hyperthyroidism.	Hypothyroidism.	
LH/FSH	GnRH.	Gonadal sex steroids.		Hypogonadism.	In men, inhibin inhibits FSH.
GH	GHRH, hypoglycemia, dopamine.	Somatostatin.	**Childhood:** gigantism. **Adulthood:** acromegaly.	**Childhood:** short stature. **Adulthood:** poor sense of well-being.	
Prolactin	Pregnancy, nursing, TRH, stress.	Dopamine.	Galactorrhea, hypogonadism.	Inability to lactate.	Under tonic inhibition by hypothalamic dopamine.

(Reproduced, with permission, from Le T, et al. *First Aid for the Internal Medicine Boards,* 1st ed. New York: McGraw-Hill, 2006: 177.)

- Treatment for symptomatic disease is as follows:
    - **Medical:** Treat hormone deficiency or excess as appropriate (discussed in following sections).
    - **Surgical:** The transsphenoidal approach is successful in approximately 90% of microadenomas.
    - **Radiation:** Conventional or stereotactic radiation. Side effects include panhypopituitarism (seen in up to 90% of cases) requiring lifelong hormonal supplementation.

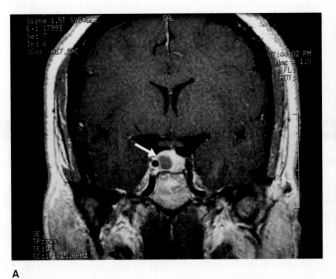

A

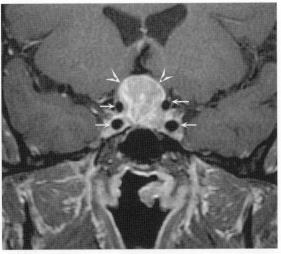

B

FIGURE 4.5.   Pituitary adenomas. Coronal gadolinium-enhanced MR images demonstrating (**A**) a microadenoma (*arrow*), which enhances less than the adjacent pituitary tissue, and (**B**) a pituitary macroadenoma (*arrowheads*) extending superiorly from the sella turcica to the suprasellar region. Arrows denote the internal carotid arteries. (Image A reproduced, with permission, from Schorge JO, et al. *Williams Gynecology.* New York: McGraw-Hill, 2008, Fig. 15-8A. Image B reproduced, with permission, from Fauci AS, et al. *Harrison's Principles of Internal Medicine,* 17th ed. New York: McGraw-Hill, 2008, Fig. 333-4.)

DIABETES INSIPIDUS (DI)

DI causes polyuria and an inability to concentrate urine because of a deficiency of ADH (also known as vasopressin) action. Central and nephrogenic types are distinguished as follows:

- **Central DI:** ↓ release of ADH. Causes include neurosurgery, trauma, tumors, ischemia, infiltrative diseases, or idiopathic DI.
- **Nephrogenic DI:** Resistance to ADH at the level of the kidneys. Causes include chronic renal disease, hereditary factors, hypercalcemia, hypokalemia, and **lithium toxicity.**

SYMPTOMS/EXAM

- Presents with inappropriately **dilute** urine (low urine osmolality) in the setting of ↑ **serum osmolality.**
- **Polyuria** and polydipsia are also seen.
- There is no component of glucose dysregulation with DI.

DIFFERENTIAL

Osmotic diuresis (eg, elevated serum and urine osmolality); **psychogenic polydipsia** (low serum and urine osmolality).

DIAGNOSIS

- **High plasma and low urine osmolality.**
- **Water deprivation test** to confirm DI.
- **Desmopressin (DDAVP) test** (synthetic vasopressin [ADH]) to differentiate between central and nephrogenic DI.
- If tests confirm central DI, perform MRI of the sella turcica to evaluate for an underlying cause.

TREATMENT

- **Central DI: Treat any underlying lesion if present.** Administer intranasal DDAVP.
- **Nephrogenic DI:** Treat the underlying disorder. Thiazide diuretics and amiloride may help (presumably by inducing mild hypovolemia, thus increasing proximal reabsorption of sodium and water and decreasing overall urine output).

COMPLICATIONS

Dehydration, hydronephrosis.

SYNDROME OF INAPPROPRIATE SECRETION OF ADH (SIADH)

An excessive secretion of ADH that may be idiopathic or caused by the following factors:

- **CNS disturbances:** CNS pathology, including hemorrhage, stroke, or infection, can enhance ADH secretion.
- **Tumors:** Tumors (the most common being small-cell lung carcinoma) may cause ectopic production of ADH.
- **Drugs:** Many drugs can ↑ the release of ADH or enhance its effects. These include carbamazepine, SSRIs, vincristine, haloperidol, amitriptyline, and amiodarone.

KEY FACT

If a patient is volume depleted with SIADH, he or she will have low urine sodium. These patients will respond to a saline load with an ↑ in urine sodium, and urine osmolality will remain high.

SYMPTOMS/EXAM

Initially, mild SIADH may be asymptomatic. Later symptoms of **hypona-tremia**, with nausea and malaise progressing to headaches, lethargy, and eventually seizures and coma, may develop.

DIAGNOSIS

SIADH should be suspected in anyone with **hyponatremia, low plasma osmolality, a urine osmolality > 100 mOsm/kg, a urine sodium concentration** normally > **40 mEq/L**, normal acid-base and potassium balance, and frequently a low plasma uric acid concentration. SIADH is a diagnosis of exclusion after ruling out other causes of hyponatremia.

TREATMENT

- **Water restriction:** The mainstay of treatment. Avoid in SAH, as it may precipitate cerebral vasospasm or infarction.
- **Salt administration:** IV saline or hypertonic saline may be needed if hyponatremia is severe or symptomatic.
- **Loop diuretics:** Can enhance the effect of hypertonic saline.
- **Lithium and demeclocycline:** Act on collecting tubules to ↓ their response to ADH. Reserved for very severe cases.

KEY FACT

Be aware of causing central pontine myelinolysis by correcting hyponatremia too rapidly.

HYPOPITUITARISM

↓ secretion of 1 or more pituitary hormones. May be idiopathic or caused by the following factors:

- **Invasive causes:** Pituitary adenomas, craniopharyngiomas, sinus tumors.
- **Infiltrative causes:** Sarcoidosis, hemochromatosis, histiocytosis X.
- **Infarction:**
  - **Sheehan syndrome:** Infarction of the pituitary occurring postpartum following substantial blood loss in childbirth. Presents with the inability to lactate, lethargy, and amenorrhea.
  - **Pituitary apoplexy:** Sudden hemorrhage, often into a pituitary adenoma. Presents with severe headache, visual field defects, and hypotension. May resolve spontaneously or require high-dose steroids +/- decompression.
- **Injury:** Head trauma can cause anterior pituitary dysfunction and vasopressin deficiency.
- **Immunologic causes:** Lymphocytic hypophysitis leading to lymphocytic infiltration. Can occur late in pregnancy or postpartum.
- **Iatrogenic:** Post–radiation therapy.
- **Infectious:** Rare. Etiologic agents include TB, syphilis, and fungi.
- **Empty sella syndrome:** Enlarged sella turcica not entirely filled with pituitary. May be 1° or 2°.
  - **1°:** A defect in the diaphragm sella leading to infiltration with CSF fluid.
  - **2°:** Enlargement of the sella by a mass that is then removed by surgery, radiation, or infarction.

KEY FACT

Remember the **8 I's** of hypopituitarism: **I**nvasion, **I**nfiltrative, **I**nfarction, **I**njury, **I**mmunologic, **I**atrogenic, **I**nfectious, **I**diopathic.

SYMPTOMS/EXAM

May be asymptomatic or may present with symptoms 2° to mass effect and/or signs of hormone deficiency:

- **ACTH deficiency:** ↓ cortisol secretion (hypotension, tachycardia, weakness, anorexia).
- **TSH deficiency:** Hypothyroidism.

- **LH/FSH deficiency:** Hypogonadism. In women, presents with anovulation, infertility, and ↓ estrogen secretion. In men, infertility and ↓ testosterone are seen.
- **GH deficiency:** Presents as short stature in children. May cause a variety of subtle effects in adults, including ↓ muscle mass, ↓ bone mineral density (BMD), and ↑ cardiovascular risk.
- **Prolactin deficiency:** Inability to lactate postpartum.

DIAGNOSIS

Diagnosed by hormonal testing:

- **ACTH:** Abnormal ACTH and cortisol levels with failure of synthetic corticotropin stimulation test.
- **Thyroid:** Low free T_4 (TSH may be low or normal).
- **Gonadotropins:** Low FSH/LH.
- **GH:** Low IGF-1.
- **Prolactin:** Low.

TREATMENT

Treat the underlying cause. Correct hormone deficiencies as follows:

- **ACTH:** Steroids.
- **TSH:** Levothyroxine.
- **GnRH:** In men, treat with testosterone replacement. In women, initiate estrogen replacement but keep in mind ↑ cardiovascular risk and ↑ estrogen-dependent cancers with unopposed estrogen.
- **GH:** Human GH. Replacement of GH in adults is controversial.
- **ADH:** Intranasal DDAVP.
- **Prolactin:** No treatment.

GROWTH HORMONE (GH) EXCESS

Etiologies are as follows:

- **Pituitary adenoma:** Accounts for > 99% of cases. Often has an insidious onset, causing the diagnosis to be delayed for > 10 years. Accounts for approximately one-third of all hormone-secreting tumors.
- **Iatrogenic:** Exogenous GH.
- **Ectopic GH or GHRH:** Very rare; can be seen with lung carcinoma, carcinoid, and pancreatic islet cell tumors.

SYMPTOMS/EXAM

- **Childhood: Gigantism** from delayed epiphyseal closure, leading to extremely tall stature.
- **Adulthood:**
    - Presents with **acromegaly.** Usually has an insidious onset.
    - Affects many different tissues and organs, with symptoms that may include **enlargement of the hands and feet,** glucose intolerance, hypertension, heat intolerance, weight gain, and fatigue.
    - May affect the heart by causing hypertrophic cardiomyopathy.

DIAGNOSIS

- **Labs:** IGF-1 levels must be assessed. Random GH is not helpful.
- **Imaging: MRI** of the pituitary.

TREATMENT

- **Surgery:** Transsphenoidal resection is curative in 60%–80% of cases but carries a risk of hypopituitarism or DI.
- **Medical:** Bromocriptine, octreotide, lanreotide, pegvisomant.

HYPERPROLACTINEMIA

A 31-year-old woman who is on OCPs presents to your office with bilateral galactorrhea of 4 months' duration and absent menses for the last year. Physical exam reveals a milky breast discharge and an otherwise normal breast exam. Her serum prolactin level, confirmed on 2 occasions, is > 200 ng/dL. What is the most likely diagnosis?

With a prolactin level of > 200 ng/dL, a prolactinoma is the most likely etiology. Although many drugs, including OCPs and antipsychotics, can ↑ prolactin levels, they would not do so to this level.

Which diagnostic studies should you order?

MRI of the pituitary with gadolinium enhancement.

What treatment should you initiate?

If a prolactinoma is found, start the woman on a dopamine agonist such as bromocriptine or cabergoline.

Elevated serum prolactin can be caused by a variety of physiologic conditions. **Prolactinomas,** the most common type of pituitary tumor, account for the majority of pathologic cases. Most are microadenomas (< 1 cm). Other etiologies are as follows:

- **Drugs:** Medications associated with hyperprolactinemia include dopaminergic drugs (eg, antipsychotics, antihypertensives) as well as estrogen and SSRIs (although not typically clinically significant).
- ↓ **dopaminergic inhibition of prolactin.**
- **Pregnancy:** Prolactin can reach 200 ng/mL in the second trimester.
- **Hypothalamic lesions:** May cause pituitary stalk compression or damage.
- **Hypothyroidism:** TRH stimulates prolactin secretion.

SYMPTOMS/EXAM

↑ prolactin inhibits GnRH, leading to ↓ FSH/LH, in turn leading to ↓ estrogen and testosterone, with the following clinical features:

- **Women:** Galactorrhea; anovulatory cycles with amenorrhea or oligomenorrhea.
- **Men:** Impotence, ↓ libido, galactorrhea (very rare).
- **Both:** Mass effect from large tumor (headache, visual field cuts, and hypopituitarism).

DIAGNOSIS

- **Labs:** Show ↑ prolactin (typically > 200 ng/mL) with normal TSH; ⊖ pregnancy test.
- **Imaging:** Obtain an MRI in anyone with hyperprolactinemia in the absence of pregnancy or drugs known to cause elevation.

KEY FACT

The most common cause of amenorrhea and galactorrhea in a premenopausal woman is pregnancy!

TREATMENT

- **Pharmacologic:** Treat with a dopamine agonist such as **bromocriptine** or **cabergoline.**
- **Surgical:** Transsphenoidal resection is sometimes necessary if medical therapy is ineffective or if the tumor is causing a mass effect.

MULTIPLE ENDOCRINE NEOPLASIA (MEN) SYNDROME

Inherited in an autosomal-dominant pattern.

- Type I: Pancreatic, parathyroid, pituitary tumors.
- Type II: Medullary thyroid carcinoma, pheochromocytoma, parathyroid hyperplasia.
- Type III (IIb): Medullary thyroid carcinoma, pheochromocytoma, mucosal and gastrointestinal neuromas.

Thyroid Disorders

HYPERTHYROIDISM

Etiologies, classified by nuclear imaging findings of radioactive iodine (RAI) uptake by the thyroid, are as follows (see also Table 4.6):

- ↑ RAI uptake:
  - **Graves disease:** An autoimmune disorder in which **TSH receptor antibodies**—also known as **thyroid-stimulating immunoglobulin (TSI)**—stimulate the receptor to produce excess thyroid hormone. The most common cause of hyperthyroidism (60%–90% of cases). Females are affected more often than males (5:1).
  - **Solitary toxic hyperactive nodule.**
  - **Toxic multinodular goiter (Plummer disease).**
- ↓ RAI uptake: Thyroiditis; exogenous thyroid hormone.

TABLE 4.6. Causes and Treatment of Hyperthyroidism

DISORDER	CLINICAL FINDINGS	LAB FINDINGS	RAI UPTAKE AND SCAN	TREATMENT
Graves disease	Diffusely enlarged thyroid; possibly bruit.	TSH receptor antibody (80%–95% sensitive); TPO (50%–85% sensitive; low specificity).	Diffusely ↑ uptake.	MMI, PTU; β-blockers; RAI.
Solitary toxic nodule	Single palpable nodule.		Single-focus ↑ uptake.	Medications or RAI.
Multinodular goiter	"Lumpy-bumpy," enlarged thyroid.		Multiple hot and/or cold nodules.	Medications or RAI.
Subacute thyroiditis (eg, de Quervain)	Tender, enlarged thyroid/painless.	Often postviral. ↑ ESR.	Diffusely ↓ uptake.	NSAIDs +/− steroids.
Exogenous hyperthyroidism	Normal.	Thyroglobulin levels are low.	Diffusely ↓ uptake.	Discontinue or ↓ thyroid hormone.

SYMPTOMS/EXAM

- Presents with anxiety, weakness, palpitations, heat intolerance, diaphoresis, weight loss, and oligo- or amenorrhea.
- Exam reveals tachycardia, hyperreflexia, thin hair, lid lag, exophthalmos, and pretibial myxedema. Goiter may be present.

DIAGNOSIS

- **Labs:** TSH, free T_4, free T_3, thyroid antibodies in Graves disease (thyroglobulin and TPO are present in 50%–80% of patients; TSH receptor antibodies are found in 80%–95%).
- **Imaging:** RAI uptake and nuclear scan.

TREATMENT

- **Medications:**
    - **Antithyroid medications:** Block thyroid hormone production; can induce remission in 50% of patients with Graves disease. Check periodic leukocyte counts as antithyroid medications can cause the rare but serious side effect of agranulocytosis.
    - **Propylthiouracil (PTU):** Blocks peripheral conversion of T_4 to T_3 at high doses; first choice during pregnancy.
    - **Methimazole (MMI):** Has a longer half-life, so can be used once per day.
    - **β-blockers:** For symptomatic treatment.
- **RAI:** Works by destroying thyroid follicular cells. Highly effective in toxic nodules and multinodular goiters; 90% effective in Graves disease. May result in hypothyroidism requiring lifelong levothyroxine supplementation.
- **Surgery:** Subtotal thyroidectomy is used only in rare cases (eg, for uncontrolled disease in pregnancy, very large goiters, goiters obstructing the airway, or patient preference). Side effects include hypothyroidism, hypoparathyroidism, or recurrent laryngeal nerve damage.

COMPLICATIONS

- **Cardiac:** Tachycardia, ↑ contractility, CHF, arrhythmias (of which **atrial fibrillation** is most common and occurs in 5%–15% of patients), atrial flutter, paroxysmal atrial tachycardia.
- **Graves ophthalmopathy:** Occurs in approximately 20% of patients. More common in **smokers.** Caused by accumulation of hydrophilic glycosaminoglycans, principally hyaluronic acid, in tissues. Can be worsened by RAI therapy. Treatment includes steroids and eye surgery. Treatment of hyperthyroidism does not cure exophthalmos, only stops progression of eye disease.
- **Thyroid storm:** Presents with fever, tachycardia, delirium, diarrhea, vomiting, and CHF. Treat with high-dose propranolol, PTU, steroids, and iodide. This is a **life-threatening** medical emergency. Look for an underlying stressor that may have triggered the storm.

HYPOTHYROIDISM

May be caused by a variety of conditions, including the following:

- **Hashimoto thyroiditis:** An autoimmune thyroiditis that commonly leads to hypothyroidism but may initially present as hyperthyroidism. The most common cause of hypothyroidism in the United States.
- **Iodine deficiency:** Rare in developed countries, but the most common cause of hypothyroidism worldwide.

- **Drugs:** Amiodarone, lithium, interferon, and drugs used to treat hyperthyroidism (iodide, PTU, MMI).
- **Iatrogenic:** Neck irradiation, thyroidectomy, RAI.
- **Subacute thyroiditis:** Typically transient.
- **Other:** 2° hypothyroidism (hypopituitarism); 3° hypothyroidism (hypothalamic dysfunction); peripheral resistance to thyroid hormone.

SYMPTOMS/EXAM

- Causes a generalized slowing of metabolic processes, leading to a vague, nonspecific constellation of symptoms that includes **fatigue, weight gain, cold intolerance, dry skin, constipation, menstrual irregularities,** and **depression.**
- Look for exam findings, including bradycardia and delayed relaxation phase of DTRs. Accumulation of matrix glycosaminoglycans in many tissues can also cause symptoms of coarse hair, enlargement of the tongue, hoarseness, and periorbital edema.
- Be aware that hypothyroidism may have an atypical presentation in the elderly.

DIAGNOSIS

- **Labs:** Generally show ↑ **TSH** and ↓ **free T_4**. ↑ TSH in the presence of a normal T_4 is considered subclinical hypothyroidism. Do not treat subclinical hypothyroidism unless symptomatic. If both TSH and free T_4 are low, think 2° or 3° hypothyroidism (occasionally can see mild depression of both TSH and T_4 with euthyroid sick syndrome). Check for ⊕ antibodies (TPO, which is most sensitive, is found in 90%–100% of patients with Hashimoto thyroiditis).
- **Imaging:** Not generally indicated.

TREATMENT

- **Thyroid hormone replacement:** Synthetic thyroxine (T_4). Titrate to normalize TSH.
- Pregnancy as well as some drugs (eg, OCPs and other hormones) can affect the amount of thyroid-binding globulin (TBG) and may therefore ↑ the need for T_4.

COMPLICATIONS

- Hypothyroidism may precipitate depression and hyperlipidemia and may cause modest weight gain. Consider checking TSH in patients presenting with these symptoms.
- **Myxedema coma:** Severe hypothyroidism constituting a medical emergency. Characterized by ↓ mental status and hypothermia. Can progress to shock and death. Treatment is IV T_3 and/or T_4 along with supportive therapy, especially rewarming.

THYROIDITIS

Inflammation of the thyroid may present with hyper-, hypo-, or euthyroid states. Table 4.7 outlines the causes, presentation, and treatment of thyroiditis.

KEY FACT

Hypothyroidism may cause galactorrhea because of the effect of TSH on prolactin secretion.

KEY FACT

Excess thyroid hormone replacement can cause ↓ bone density.

TABLE 4.7. **Clinical Features and Differential Diagnosis of Thyroiditis**

Disorder	Etiology	Clinical Findings	Lab Findings	Treatment
Subacute granulomatous thyroiditis (de Quervain)	Viral.	Hyperthyroid early; then hypothyroid. Presents with a tender, enlarged thyroid and with fever.	↑ ESR; ↓ RAI uptake.	NSAIDs; acetaminophen +/− steroids.
Hashimoto thyroiditis	Autoimmune.	Usually hypothyroid; painless, +/− goiter.	Some 95% have ⊕ antibodies; anti-TPO antibodies are most sensitive.	Thyroid hormone.
Suppurative thyroiditis	Bacteria are more commonly implicated than other infectious agents.	Fever, neck pain, tender thyroid.	TFTs are normal. No uptake on RAI scan; ⊕ cultures.	Antibiotics and drainage.
Amiodarone use	Am**IOD**arone contains **IOD**ine.	1. Asymptomatic TFT changes. 2. Hypothyroidism. 3. Hyperthyroidism.	1. ↑ free T_4 and total T_4; then low T_3 and high TSH. 2. High TSH; low T_4 and T_3. 3. Low TSH; high T_4 and T_3.	1. Usually not necessary to stop medications; will normalize over time. 2. As for other hypothyroidism. 3. As for other and T_3. Hyperthyroidism +/− steroids.
Other medications	**Lithium,** α-interferon, interleukin-2.		Lithium usually causes hypothyroidism.	Stop medication if possible.
Postpartum thyroiditis	Lymphocytic infiltration; seen after up to 10% of pregnancies.	Small, nontender thyroid. Mild symptoms.	May see hyper- or hypothyroidism. Antibodies are often ⊕; RAI uptake is ↓.	β-blockers if needed. Otherwise, no treatment is necessary.

THYROID NODULES AND CANCER

A 62-year-old woman comes to your office for a routine visit. Exam reveals a 2-cm thyroid nodule. The exam is otherwise normal. What tests do you order?
You order TSH, which is found to be within normal limits.
What further workup is indicated?
Fine-needle aspiration (FNA).

The "90%" mnemonic applies to thyroid nodules: 90% of nodules are benign; 90% are cold on RAI uptake scan, with 5%–10% of these malignant (hot nodules are rarely malignant); **90%** of thyroid malignancies present as a thyroid nodule or lump. Etiologies include the following:

- **Benign lesions:** Often regress spontaneously or with T_4 therapy.
- **1° thyroid cancer:**
  - **Papillary:** The **most common type.** Carries an excellent prognosis, with a 98% survival rate for stage I or II disease. Many tumors secrete thyroglobulin.
  - **Follicular:** A more aggressive form associated with metastasis to bone, lungs, and brain. Often retains the ability to form thyroglobulin and occasionally thyroid hormone (ie, "functioning thyroid cancer").
  - **Medullary:** May secrete **calcitonin** and can be associated with MEN 2A and 2B.
  - **Anaplastic:** Undifferentiated thyroid gland tumors. Very aggressive.
  - **Other:** Lymphoma, metastasis to thyroid (breast, kidney, melanoma, lung).

SYMPTOMS/EXAM

- Typically presents with a single, firm, palpable nodule. Otherwise, often asymptomatic unless associated with thyroid hormone abnormalities or advanced carcinoma.
- **Red flags** for thyroid carcinoma are **male** gender; age < 20 or > 65 years; a ⊕ history of head/neck irradiation; a ⊕ family history of thyroid cancer; a **hard, fixed nodule > 4 cm;** rapid growth of the nodule; and symptoms related to local invasion (**dysphagia, hoarseness**).

DIAGNOSIS

Start the evaluation by checking TFTs. In a patient with a **low TSH,** the next step is RAI **uptake and scan.** If the nodule is hot, the evaluation ends there. If

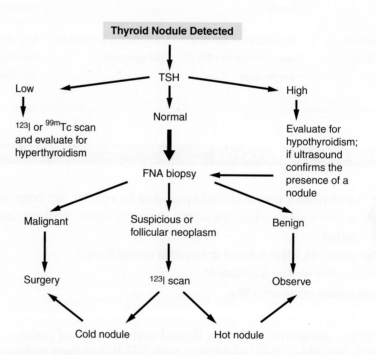

FIGURE 4.6.   Decision matrix for workup of a thyroid nodule. (Reproduced, with permission, from Gardner DG, Shoback D. *Greenspan's Basic & Clinical Endocrinology,* 8th ed. New York: McGraw-Hill, 2008: Fig. 8-45.)

the nodule is cold or if TSH is normal or ↑, perform an ultrasound. Nodules > 1–1.5 cm with suspicious characteristics should be biopsied with **FNA** (see Figure 4.6). FNA is the most reliable test for determining if a mass is malignant.

TREATMENT

- **Benign nodules:** Observe if asymptomatic and confirmed to be benign. T₄ suppression therapy is only 50% effective. Surgical excision can be considered.
- **Malignancies:** Total thyroidectomy followed by **RAI ablation.** Markers such as thyroglobulin and calcitonin (medullary carcinoma only) can be used to monitor for recurrence. For low-risk cases with very small nodules (< 1 cm), lobectomy can be considered.

Calcium and Bone Disorders

CALCIUM METABOLISM

Figure 4.7 illustrates the hormonal control loop that governs vitamin D and calcium metabolism and function.

KEY FACT

Concerning characteristics of thyroid nodules:
- Fixed
- Irregular texture
- History of radiation to the neck
- Rapid growth
- Vocal changes
- Cervical lymphadenopathy

KEY FACT

Thyroid nodules on nuclear imaging:
- **Hot nodules:** Hyperfunctioning. Low likelihood of malignancy.
- **Cold nodules:** Hypofunctioning. Approximately 20% malignant.

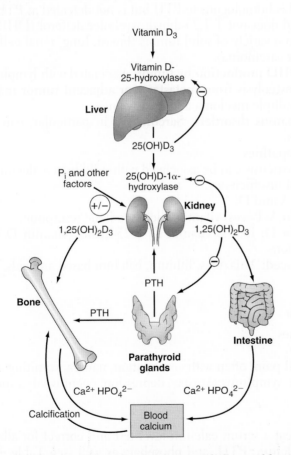

FIGURE 4.7.   Hormonal control loop for vitamin D metabolism and function. (Reproduced, with permission, from Kasper DL, et al. *Harrison's Principles of Internal Medicine,* 16th ed. New York: McGraw Hill, 2005: 2246.)

HYPERCALCEMIA

A 52-year-old man presents with nausea, constipation, lethargy, and impaired concentration and memory. His physical exam is essentially normal. His CBC and chemistry reveal ↑ calcium levels. What medications can cause hypercalcemia?
Vitamins A and D, thiazide diuretics, calcium-containing antacids, and lithium.
His PTH is low. What is the likely etiology of this patient's hypercalcemia?
Malignancy.
How should you treat him?
Institute aggressive fluids, loop diuretics, calcitonin, and bisphosphonate.

High levels of calcium in the blood can stem from a variety of causes, but **1° hyperparathyroidism** and **malignancy** account for 80%–90% of cases. Pathophysiologic mechanisms are as follows:

- **1° hyperparathyroidism:** See section below.
- **Malignancy-associated hypercalcemia:** Can occur in up to 10%–15% of malignancies via several mechanisms:
  - **Tumor release of PTH-related peptide (PTHrP): Most common.** PTHrP is homologous to PTH but is not detected as PTH by serum assays and does not ↑ 1,25-dihydroxycholecalciferol (DHD) production. Seen in a variety of solid tumors (breast, lung, renal cell, ovarian, and bladder carcinoma).
  - **1,25-DHD production by tumor:** Associated with lymphomas.
  - **Local osteolysis from metastases or adjacent tumor mass:** Associated with multiple myeloma and breast cancer.
- **Granulomatous disorders: Sarcoidosis,** in particular, can ↑ vitamin D production.
- **Endocrinopathies:**
  - **Thyrotoxicosis** can be associated with mild hypercalcemia.
  - Adrenal insufficiency.
- **↑ vitamin A and D:**
  - **Vitamin A:** Excess vitamin A leads to bone resorption.
  - **Vitamin D:** Excess vitamin D ↑ 25-hydroxyvitamin D (25-HD) concentrations.
- **Drug induced:** Thiazides, lithium, calcium-based antacids, estrogens, androgens.

KEY FACT

Hallmarks of hypercalcemia: Stones, bones, groans, and psychiatric overtones.

SYMPTOMS/EXAM

- Renal **stones.**
- Bone pain.
- **Abdominal pain,** often with constipation, nausea, vomiting, and anorexia.
- **Psychiatric symptoms:** Anxiety, depression, cognitive dysfunction.

DIAGNOSIS

- **Labs:** Repeat a serum calcium level test and correct for albumin. Check ionized calcium, **PTH,** and phosphate as well (see Table 4.8). Consider protein electrophoresis to rule out multiple myeloma.
- **Imaging:** In a patient with normal PTH, perform CXR to look for sarcoidosis or malignancy.

TABLE 4.8. Laboratory Findings Associated with Hypercalcemia

	CALCIUM	PHOSPHORUS	PTH	PTHrP	OTHER
PTH mediated	↑	↓	↑	↓	
PTHrP mediated	↑	↓	↓	↑	
1,25-DHD mediated	↑	↑	↓	↓	↑ 1,25-DHD
Vitamin D intoxication	↑	↑	↓	↓	↑ 25-HD

TREATMENT

Treatment should be aimed at lowering the calcium level, especially if the patient is symptomatic, and treating the underlying cause.

- ↑ **urinary excretion:**
  - **Fluids:** Begin with isotonic saline to expand volume and ↑ urinary excretion. Hydration with normal saline is the essential element in treating acute hypercalcemia.
  - Loop diuretics.
- **Inhibit bone reabsorption:**
  - **Calcitonin (SQ):** ↓ bony reabsorption by interfering with osteoclast function; also ↑ renal excretion. However, efficacy is lost after 3 days because tachyphylaxis develops. Also helpful in treating bone pain.
  - **Bisphosphonates (IV):** Toxic to osteoclasts; more potent than calcitonin. Effects on serum calcium are seen 48–72 hours after initiation of therapy.
- ↓ **intestinal absorption:**
  - **Glucocorticoids:** First-line treatment in patients with vitamin A- or D-mediated hypercalcemia.
  - **Phosphate:** Oral administration to bind calcium in the gut. Minimal effect on hypercalcemia.
- Chelation of ionized calcium with sodium EDTA or IV phosphate works quickly but is potentially toxic.
- Dialysis is used as a last resort.

COMPLICATIONS

Long-standing or very high levels of hypercalcemia can cause deposition of calcium in heart valves, coronary arteries, and myocardial fibers and can also cause severe renal disease and neurologic deficits.

1° HYPERPARATHYROIDISM

A 50-year-old man comes to your office for a routine screening. Lab studies indicate that he has elevated serum calcium. What lab value do you check next?

In addition to rechecking serum calcium with an albumin and an ionized calcium, check PTH.

If the PTH is elevated, what are the indications for parathyroidectomy?

Age < 50 years, serum calcium > 1 mg/dL above normal, osteoporosis, unexplained ↓ creatinine clearance, and hypercalciuria (> 400 mg/dL).

Approximately 80% of cases of 1° hyperparathyroidism are due to a single parathyroid adenoma; the remainder are due to gland hyperplasia and cancer.

SYMPTOMS/EXAM

- Approximately **85% of cases are asymptomatic** and are diagnosed on screening labs.
- Hypercalcemia causes **"stones, bones, groans, and psychiatric overtones"** (see Figure 4.7).
- Osteoporosis is commonly seen.

DIFFERENTIAL

- **Familial benign hypocalciuric hypercalcemia:** A hereditary, autosomal-dominant disorder causing lifelong asymptomatic mild hypercalcemia. Differentiated from 1° hyperparathyroidism by marked hypocalciuria. PTH can be normal or mildly elevated. No therapy is required.
- **MEN syndromes.**
- **Lithium therapy:** Lithium shifts the set point for PTH secretion, causing hypercalcemia.

DIAGNOSIS

- Labs reveal ↑ PTH, ↑ Ca^{++}, and ↓ phosphorus.
- To investigate possible complications of 1° hyperparathyroidism, also check 24-hour urine calcium/creatinine, renal function, and BMD.
- Preoperative imaging with sestamibi scanning can help determine the surgical technique (ie, minimally invasive vs. bilateral neck exploration) for a parathyroidectomy.

TREATMENT

- **Indications for surgery include:**
  - Age < 50 years.
  - Serum calcium > 1 mg/dL above normal.
  - Osteoporosis. Treat osteoporosis with estrogen therapy or bisphosphonates.
  - Hypercalciuria (calcium > 400 mg/day).
  - Unexplained worsening in renal function.
- **If surgery is not indicated, observe.**
- **Parathyroidectomy** is the only curative treatment. The cure rate is 95%, and the complication rate is low.

COMPLICATIONS

Nephrolithiasis, nephrocalcinosis with renal insufficiency, osteopenia, osteoporosis.

HYPOCALCEMIA

Serum calcium concentrations are regulated by DHD and PTH. Hypocalcemia can be caused by abnormalities in these regulatory mechanisms:

- **Hypoparathyroidism:** Most often follows thyroid or parathyroid surgery. Can also be autoimmune, familial, infiltrative, or idiopathic. Treat with chronic oral calcitriol (DHD) and calcium.
- **Pseudohypoparathyroidism:** Results from target organ resistance to PTH. Can be isolated or associated with Albright hereditary osteodystrophy

(short stature, round face, short neck, brachydactyly). Treat the same as hypoparathyroidism.

- **Vitamin D deficiency:**
  - Caused by malabsorptive states (eg, IBD, celiac sprue), lack of sun exposure, and dark skin.
  - In children: **Rickets** (bony deformities with rachitic rosary, bowing of the lower extremities, and frontal bossing).
  - In adults: **Osteomalacia** with myopathy and poor bone mineralization.
  - Diagnose with a **low 25-HD level** (< 20 ng/mL), hypocalcemia, hypophosphatemia, and 2° hyperparathyroidism.
  - Treatment is high-dose oral vitamin D replacement and calcium.
- **Acute deposition or complex formation of calcium:** Acute hyperphosphatemia (tumor lysis, excessive phosphate administration); acute pancreatitis; blood transfusion (citrate buffer in packed RBCs precipitates with calcium); hungry bone syndrome (relative hypoparathyroidism following parathyroidectomy or thyroidectomy).

Symptoms/Exam

- **Neuromuscular manifestations:**
  - **Tetany:** Neuromuscular irritability, leading to a mixture of spontaneous muscular and sensory nerve dysfunctions.
  - **Chvostek sign: Contraction of the facial muscles** in response to tapping of the facial nerve. Approximately 25% of normal individuals have a ⊕ Chvostek sign.
  - **Trousseau sign:** Induction of carpal spasm by inflation of a BP cuff to 20 mmHg above SBP for 3 minutes. ⊕ in 1%–4% of normal individuals.
  - **Paresthesias, especially of the fingertips and perioral area.**
  - **Other:** Seizures, psychiatric symptoms.
- **Cardiac:** The hallmark is a **prolonged QT interval.**
- **Other:** Cataracts, skeletal abnormalities.

Diagnosis

Lab studies reveal a ↓ calcium level when corrected for albumin; low-normal phosphorus; normal magnesium; and ↓ PTH. If PTH is ↑ or normal, check 25-HD and renal function (see Table 4.9).

Treatment

- **Acute:** In the presence of tetany, give a continuous IV calcium drip, start oral calcium, and add calcitriol if needed.
- **Chronic:** Oral calcium and calcitriol if needed.

TABLE 4.9. Laboratory Findings Associated with Hypocalcemia

	CALCIUM	PHOSPHORUS	PTH	OTHER
Hypoparathyroidism	↓	↑	↓	
PTH resistance	↓	↑	↑	
Vitamin D deficiency	↓	↓	↑	↓ 25-HD
1,25-DHD resistance	↓	↓	↑	↑ 1,25-DHD

KEY FACT

The most common fractures in Paget disease are vertebral crush fractures.

PAGET DISEASE

A skeletal disease with **accelerated bone turnover** as its hallmark. Incidence is approximately 3%–4% in patients > 40 years of age. More common among whites.

SYMPTOMS/EXAM

- **Two-thirds of patients are asymptomatic.** Symptoms can include **pain** (worsens with weight bearing and often occurs at night), **fractures,** and bony **deformity** most commonly affecting the sacrum, spine, femur, skull, and pelvis.
- Look for signs, including skull enlargement, frontal bossing, bowed legs, and often skin changes of the affected areas (erythema, warmth, tenderness).

DIFFERENTIAL

Bony tumors, including malignancies.

DIAGNOSIS

- **Labs:** ↑ **alkaline phosphatase** and markers of bone turnover (osteocalcin, urinary hydroxyproline, N-telopeptide). Ca^{++} and phosphorus are usually normal.
- **Imaging:** Plain films of involved bones show ↑ density and size; erosions can be seen in the skull. Bone scan shows ↑ uptake in affected areas (see Figure 4.8).

TREATMENT

Bisphosphonates are the treatment of choice and often → remission.

COMPLICATIONS

↑ risk of bone tumors. Immobilizing a patient with active Paget disease can cause hypercalcemia.

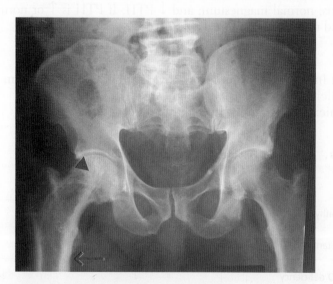

FIGURE 4.8. Paget disease, right femur. Note the thickened cortex *(arrow)*, thickened trabeculae *(arrowhead)*, and expansion of the right femoral head and neck compared with the left femur. (Reproduced, with permission, from Fauci AS, et al. *Harrison's Principles of Internal Medicine,* 17th ed. New York: McGraw Hill, 2008, Fig. 349-3.)

OSTEOPOROSIS

Low BMD is associated with ↑ risk of skeletal fragility and fracture. Osteoporosis often presents with pathologic fractures, particularly of the vertebrae, hip, or wrist (see Figure 4.9).

DIAGNOSIS

- T-score is the number of standard deviations the BMD is above or below the average BMD of a young, healthy control of the same sex. T-score < –2.5 establishes osteoporosis. A t-score between –1 and –2.5 establishes osteopenia.
- DEXA scan is the standard imaging modality to determine t-score.

SCREENING

The USPSTF recommends universal screening for women ≥ 65 years of age and for at-risk women 60–65 years of age. There is no evidence for screening

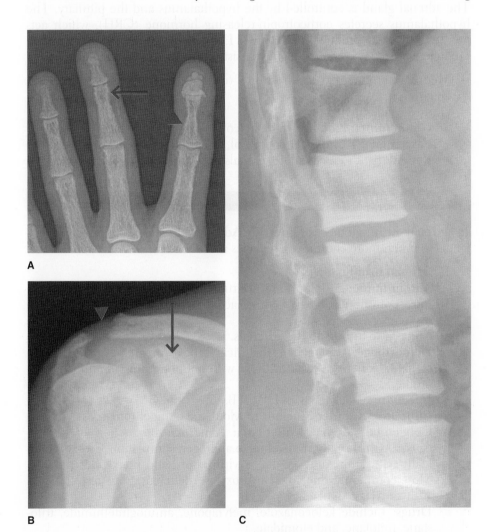

FIGURE 4.9. Skeletal changes of hyperparathyroidism. (A) Subperiosteal resorption of the phalanges *(arrow)* and digital artery calcifications *(arrowhead)*. **(B)** Restoration of the distal clavicle *(arrowhead)* and soft-tissue calcifications *(arrow)*. **(C)** "Rugger jersey" appearance of the spine (bands of osteosclerosis alternating with normal bone). (Reproduced, with permission, from Imboden J, et al. *Current Rheumatology Diagnosis & Treatment,* 2nd ed. New York: McGraw Hill, 2007, Fig. 54-5.)

men not at ↑ risk. Screening allows asymptomatic patients with osteoporosis to be identified and treated.

TREATMENT

- Prevention should begin with lifestyle changes including ↑ weight-bearing exercise, modification of risk factors, smoking cessation, avoidance of excessive alcohol intake, and ↑ dietary intake of calcium and vitamin D.
- Pharmacologic treatment of osteoporosis includes bisphosphonates (eg, alendronate), selective estrogen receptor modulators (eg, raloxifene), and calcitonin. Bisphosphonates are first-line agents, may be dosed weekly, and ↓ fracture risk by as much as 50% in the first year. Side effects include erosive esophagitis and jaw necrosis.

Adrenal Disorders

The adrenal gland is controlled by the hypothalamus and the pituitary. The hypothalamus secretes corticotropin-releasing hormone (CRH), which acts on the pituitary to produce ACTH. ACTH then acts on the adrenal gland to produce cortisol. The adrenal gland consists of the medulla and the cortex.

- **Medulla:** Produces catecholamines (epinephrine, norepinephrine, and dopamine).
- **Cortex:** Made up of 3 layers:
  - **Glomerulosa:** Produces mineralocorticoids (aldosterone).
  - **Fasciculata:** 1° producer of cortisol, also produces some androgens.
  - **Reticularis:** Produces androgens, also produces some cortisol.

ADRENAL INSUFFICIENCY

1° adrenal insufficiency is known as **Addison disease.** 2° adrenal insufficiency is much more common. Etiologies are as follows:

- 1° adrenal insufficiency:
  - **Autoimmune:** Autoimmune destruction of the adrenal gland is the **most common** etiology. Can be accompanied by other autoimmune disorders.
  - **Metastatic tumors to the adrenals.**
  - **Hemorrhage:** Can occur in critical illness, pregnancy, and anticoagulated patients as well as those with antiphospholipid antibody syndrome.
  - **Infection:** Associated with **HIV**, TB, fungi, and CMV.
  - **Infiltrative disorders:** Include amyloid and hemochromatosis.
  - **Congenital adrenal hyperplasia:** Abnormal production of cortisol causes ACTH synthesis, leading to androgen stimulation. Presents clinically with ambiguous genitalia, virilization, and precocious puberty. Most commonly due to 21-hydroxylase deficiency but also 11- and 17-hydroxylase deficiency.
  - **Drugs:** Include ketoconazole, metyrapone, aminoglutethimide, trilostane, mitotane, and etomidate.
- 2° adrenal insufficiency:
  - **Iatrogenic:** 2° to glucocorticoid and anabolic steroid administration.
  - Pituitary or hypothalamic tumors.

Symptoms/Exam

- Presents with weakness, fatigue, anorexia, weight loss, nausea, vomiting, diarrhea, abdominal pain, and orthostatic hypotension, coma, and death.
- **Hyperpigmentation** of the oral mucosa and palmar creases is found in 1° disease.

Diagnosis

- Labs: Hyponatremia and hyperkalemia (in 1° disease).
- Confirm the diagnosis as follows:
  - **Random cortisol test:** A random level ≥ 18 µg/dL rules out adrenal insufficiency. **Early-morning cortisol < 5 µg/dL strongly suggests adrenal insufficiency.**
  - **Cosyntropin stimulation test:**
    - Obtain baseline ACTH and cortisol levels.
    - Inject cosyntropin (synthetic ACTH) 250 µg IM or IV.
    - Check cortisol level 45–60 minutes later.
    - A peak ≥ 18–20 µg/dL excludes adrenal insufficiency. Can be falsely ⊖ in acute 2° adrenal insufficiency.
- **Distinguish 1° from 2° adrenal insufficiency:** An ↑ ACTH level in a patient with adrenal insufficiency is consistent with 1° adrenal insufficiency. In 2° disease, ACTH is low because of the presence of ACTH-like hormones.
- **Evaluate the cause:** Exclude exogenous or iatrogenic steroids. In 1° adrenal insufficiency, obtain a CT of the adrenal gland. In 2° disease, obtain a pituitary MRI.

Treatment

- **Hydrocortisone** two-thirds in the morning and one-third in the evening, or **prednisone** daily. Administer "stress-dose" steroids during illness or surgery.
- In 1° adrenal insufficiency, use **fludrocortisone** to replace mineralocorticoid deficiency.

Complications

Adrenal crisis, an acute deficiency of cortisol, usually occurs 2° to abrupt discontinuation of exogenous steroids or major stress in the setting of adrenal insufficiency. Presents with headache, nausea, vomiting, confusion, fever, hypotension, and coma. Treat immediately with steroids as complications include death.

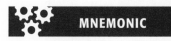

MNEMONIC

4 S's of adrenal management:

Salt—0.9% saline
Steroids—IV
Supportive care
Search for underlying disease

CUSHING SYNDROME

A syndrome due to excess exogenous or endogenous cortisol.

- **Exogenous corticosteroids:** The **most common** cause.
- **Cushing disease:** Caused by ACTH hypersecretion from a **pituitary** microadenoma. Female-to-male ratio is 8:1.
- **Ectopic ACTH:** ACTH secretion from a nonpituitary neoplasm (**small-cell lung carcinoma,** bronchial carcinoids).
- **Adrenal disease:** Adenoma, carcinoma, or nodular adrenal hyperplasia.

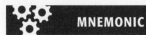

MNEMONIC

Features of Cushing syndrome:

MR. CUSHING

Menstrual irregularities

Rounded facies

Central obesity/**C**ervical fat pad (buffalo hump)

Urinary glucose and cortisol ↑

Striae/**S**uppressed immune system

Hirsutism/HTN/hyperglycemia/ hypercortisol

Iatrogenic excess corticosteroid intake (most common cause)

Neoplasm of the pituitary (second most common cause)

Glucose intolerance

SYMPTOMS/EXAM

Presents with centripetal obesity (with moon facies and buffalo hump), menstrual irregularities, hypertension, emotional lability, dermatologic manifestations (eg, plethora, hirsutism, striae), and glucose intolerance. Excess ACTH may also cause hyperpigmentation.

DIAGNOSIS

- Confirm excess cortisol production with an overnight dexamethasone suppression test.
- A.M. cortisol < 1.8 µg/dL is a ⊖ test result and rules out excess cortisol.
- If ↑, check 24-hour urinary free cortisol.
- Check ACTH:
  - If < 5 pg/mL, the source is likely adrenal, warranting CT of the adrenal glands.
  - If > 10 pg/mL, the source is either pituitary or ectopic, warranting:
    - **MRI of the pituitary.**
    - **If MRI is ⊖, inferior petrosal sinus sampling (IPSS):** Measures levels of ACTH draining from the pituitary and periphery before and after CRH stimulation to see if the gradient is greater from the pituitary or the periphery.

TREATMENT

- **Adrenal tumors:** Adrenalectomy.
- **Cushing disease:** Transsphenoidal pituitary adenoma resection.
- **Ectopic ACTH:**
  - Treat the underlying neoplasm.
  - Blockade of steroid synthesis (ketoconazole, metyrapone, aminoglutethimide).
  - Potassium replacement (spironolactone can be helpful).
  - Bilateral adrenalectomy if needed.

COMPLICATIONS

Complications may arise from long-term excess glucocorticoids (diabetes, hypertension, cardiovascular disease, obesity, osteoporosis). May also ↑ susceptibility to infections.

HYPERALDOSTERONISM

Excess aldosterone can stem from a variety of sources and can be a cause of 2° hypertension. Common etiologies include the following:

- **Aldosterone-producing adenoma (Conn disease):** More common in women than in men. Accounts for over one-half of 1° aldosteronism.
- **Idiopathic hyperaldosteronism:** Accounts for approximately one-third of cases.
- **Glucocorticoid-suppressible aldosteronism:** A rare autosomal-dominant disorder.
- **Angiotensin II–responsive adenoma.**
- **Aldosterone-producing adrenocortical carcinoma:** Rare. Hyperandrogenism occurs as well.

SYMPTOMS/EXAM

Most patients are asymptomatic. **Hypertension** and **hypokalemia** are classic, but potassium can be normal.

DIAGNOSIS

- Check **plasma aldosterone concentration and plasma renin activity.** Measure after a high-salt diet or salt supplementation for a week.
- Review 24-hour urine **aldosterone level.**
- In patients with primary hyperaldosteronism, CT or MRI should be performed to search for an adrenal adenoma.

TREATMENT

- **Spironolactone:** Give high-dose **spironolactone** or **eplerenone** mineralo-corticoid receptor to normalize potassium levels. Side effects include gynecomastia in men, rash, impotence, and epigastric discomfort.
- **Unilateral adrenalectomy** in patients with a single adenoma.

COMPLICATIONS

Complications may arise 2° to hypertension or hypokalemia.

PHEOCHROMOCYTOMA

A rare tumor of the cells from the adrenal medulla of the adrenal glands that produce **epinephrine and/or norepinephrine.** Approximately 90% arise in the adrenal gland itself and others occur extra-adrenally.

SYMPTOMS/EXAM

- Patients most commonly present with episodic attacks of throbbing **headaches,** diaphoresis, and palpitations but pheochromocytoma may also be associated with tremor, anxiety, nausea, vomiting, fatigue, weight loss, chest pain, and abdominal pain.
- The majority of patients have hypertension, which may only be episodic. Check **orthostatics** as well because orthostasis is commonly present.

DIAGNOSIS

Pheochromocytoma is usually suggested by the history of a symptomatic patient, particularly those with a history of familial disease. Diagnose as follows:

- Establish biochemistry: The finding of markedly elevated urinary metanephrines and catecholamines in a 24-hour urine collection or plasma metanephrines confirms a biochemical diagnosis.
- Next, localize the lesion with **MRI/CT imaging** of the adrenal glands (see Figure 4.10). If the adrenals appear normal, ^{123}I-MIBG scan can be used to localize extra-adrenal pheochromocytomas and metastases.

TREATMENT

- **Adrenergic blockade:** Phenoxybenzamine is the key first step.
- **β-blockers:** Used to control heart rate, but only after adrenergic blockade.
- **Surgical resection:** Has a 90% cure rate. It is important to hydrate patients and control symptoms before surgery.

MNEMONIC

Pheochromocytoma rule of 10's:

10% are normotensive
10% occur in children
10% are familial
10% are bilateral
10% are malignant
10% are extra-adrenal

KEY FACT

Do not use β-blockers in patients with pheochromocytoma before adequate adrenergic blockade is achieved as this can worsen hypertension and precipitate a hypertensive crisis.

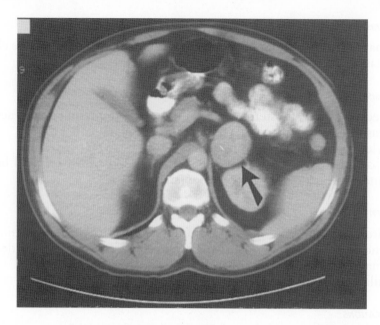

FIGURE 4.10. Left adrenal pheochromocytoma. Large heterogeneously enhancing mass with a thin area of calcification in the left adrenal gland *(arrow)* on transaxial image from a contrast-enhanced CT scan. (Reproduced, with permission, from Brunicardi FC, et al. *Schwartz's Principles of Surgery,* 9th ed. New York: McGraw-Hill, 2010, Fig. 38-46.)

COMPLICATIONS

Hypertensive crises, MI, CVAs, arrhythmias, renal failure, dissecting aortic aneurysm.

ADRENAL INCIDENTALOMAS

Adrenal lesions are found incidentally in approximately 2% of patients undergoing abdominal CT scans for unrelated reasons. Autopsies indicate a prevalence of approximately 10%. Subtypes are as follows:

- **Functioning adenoma:** Cushing syndrome, pheochromocytoma, Conn disease.
- **Nonfunctioning adenoma:** Carcinoma, benign adenoma, metastatic lesion.

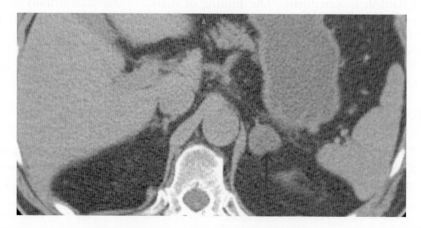

FIGURE 4.11. Adrenal adenoma. Cropped transaxial image from a noncontrast CT scan showing a small, low-density mass in the left adrenal gland *(arrow)*. (Reproduced, with permission, from USMLERx.com.)

In patients with a history of malignancy, the probability that an adrenal lesion is metastatic is > 25%. CT and/or MRI can often determine if a mass is an incidental adrenal adenoma or a metastasis. In equivocal or suspicious cases, biopsy may be indicated.

SYMPTOMS/EXAM

Many are nonfunctioning. See above for functioning lesions.

DIAGNOSIS

- **Rule out functioning tumor:**
    - Plasma metanephrines or 24-hour urine for catecholamine and metanephrines to rule out pheochromocytoma.
    - Dexamethasone suppression test to rule out Cushing disease.
    - If the patient is hypertensive, check plasma renin activity and aldosterone level to rule out aldosteronoma.
- **CT/MRI:** Characteristics of a CT or MRI can help define whether a lesion is likely benign or malignant (see Figure 4.11).

TREATMENT

Treat based on the size and functional status of the lesion:

- **Lesions < 4 cm and nonfunctioning:** Repeat imaging in 3–6 months.
- **Lesions > 4 cm and nonfunctioning:** Resect.
- **Functioning lesions:** Treat as appropriate for the disorder (see previous sections).

NOTES

CHAPTER 5

Gastroenterology

Brett Spitnale, MD

Esophageal Disorders

ESOPHAGEAL DYSPHAGIA

Defined as a sensation of food sticking or obstruction of the esophagus (vs. **odynophagia,** which is pain on swallowing). Due to disease in the body of the esophagus, the lower esophageal sphincter (LES), the cardia, or nearby structures. Patients typically complain of symptoms **seconds after swallowing** and identify the **suprasternal notch** or **retrosternal area** as the source of their discomfort. Etiologies include the following:

- **Gastroesophageal reflux.**
- **Anatomic abnormalities of the esophagus:** Zenker diverticulum, cricopharyngeal bars, peptic strictures, radiation injury, esophageal webs/rings, and esophageal carcinoma.
- **Esophageal motility disorders:**
    - **Achalasia:** Failure of the LES due to idiopathic degeneration of neurons in the esophageal wall leading to failure of relaxation and distal peristalsis. Cases are largely 1° in the United States but can also be 2° to other conditions (eg, Chagas disease). Symptoms are progressive, worsen at night, and usually occur without heartburn (see Figure 5.1).

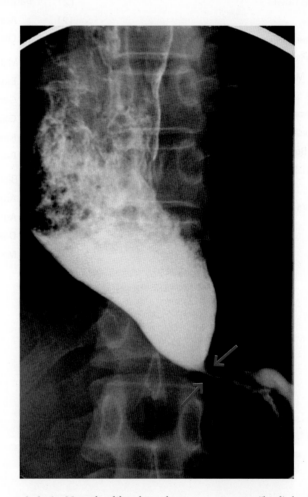

FIGURE 5.1.   Achalasia. Note the dilated esophagus tapering to a "bird's-beak" narrowing at the LES. (Reproduced, with permission, from Doherty GM. *Current Diagnosis & Treatment: Surgery,* 13th ed. New York: McGraw-Hill, 2010, Fig. 20-5.)

- **1° motility disorders:** A group of disorders with an unclear pathologic or pathophysiologic basis, each characterized by specific manometric findings. Features include diffuse esophageal spasm, nutcracker esophagus, and hypertensive LES. Chest pain is common.
- **Globus sensation:** A persistent or intermittent sensation of a lump or foreign body in the throat for > 12 weeks that is present **even when the patient is not swallowing.** More common in women and usually worsens with emotional stress. An association with GERD has not been substantiated.
- **Autoimmune disorders:** Scleroderma; Sjögren syndrome (dysphagia is independent of xerostomia but is worsened by it).
- **Cardiovascular abnormalities:** Can lead to dysphagia via compression of the esophagus (eg, vascular rings, aneurysms, left atrial enlargement).
- **Xerostomia** (eg, anticholinergics).
- **Functional dysphagia:** Dysphagia for > 12 weeks over 1 year with no identifiable cause.
- **Esophageal cancer:** Progressive dysphagia, weight loss, anemia/heme-⊕ stools.

KEY FACT

Dysphagia only for solids suggests a mechanical obstruction (but often progresses to include liquids with severe obstruction). Dysphagia for solids and liquids equally suggests a motility disorder.

DIFFERENTIAL

Oropharyngeal dysphagia, in which patients complain of food getting stuck **immediately upon swallowing (which is frequently followed by coughing and choking)** and identify the **cervical region** as the source of discomfort. Caused by a variety of neuromuscular disorders (eg, CVA).

DIAGNOSIS

- **EGD:** Most commonly used for the diagnosis of esophageal dysphagia.
- **Barium swallow:** Less diagnostic but safer than EGD; the initial test of choice for suspected achalasia, revealing classic "bird's beak" narrowing (see Figure 5.1).
- **Esophageal manometry:** Usually performed if the aforementioned studies are ⊖ to evaluate for a 1° esophageal dysmotility disorder. Also confirmatory for achalasia.
- **Videofluoroscopic swallow study:** Useful in the evaluation of oropharyngeal dysphagia.
- **Laryngoscopy:** Should be considered in patients with globus sensation to rule out malignancy.

KEY FACT

It is essential to rule out cardiac chest pain in a patient suspected of having a 1° esophageal dysmotility disorder.

TREATMENT

Directed at the underlying cause.

ESOPHAGITIS

Inflammation of the esophagus with variable etiologies (see Table 5.1). Can be asymptomatic or can present with symptoms such as odynophagia, dysphagia, heartburn, retrosternal chest pain, or gastrointestinal bleeding.

TABLE 5.1. **Etiologies and Presentation of Esophagitis**

SUBTYPE	CHARACTERISTICS	DIAGNOSIS	TREATMENT
HSV	Usually found in immunocompromised patients. Has an acute onset, and exam may reveal concomitant vesicles on the nose and lips.	EGD, biopsy, culture.	Acyclovir.
CMV	Usually found in immunocompromised patients. Presents with odynophagia, chest pain, hematemesis, nausea, and vomiting.	EGD, biopsy, culture.	Ganciclovir.
HIV	May present in 1° infection.	HIV testing.	Usually self-limited.
Candida	Often found in immunocompromised patients. Exam may reveal thrush, but **the absence of thrush does not preclude the diagnosis.**	EGD, biopsy; alternatively, therapeutic trial.	Fluconazole.
Radiation	A complication of therapy for head and neck tumors. May present as acute or chronic (from fibrosis and ischemia).	Usually clinical, EGD	Acutely, viscous lidocaine; indomethacin may ↓ chronic damage.
Corrosive	Caustic ingestion.	Usually clinical, EGD	Acutely, prednisone; strictures formed later require balloon dilation.
Pill	Relatively sudden onset; classically caused by taking an offending medication without water before sleep. Commonly implicated drugs include antibiotics (tetracycline, doxycycline, clindamycin), vitamin C, $FeSO_4$, KCl, NSAIDs, and bisphosphonates.	Usually clinical.	Prevention. The role of acid suppression is unsubstantiated in the absence of GERD.
Eosinophilic	Causes are idiopathic or allergic; usually leads to dysphagia and food impaction due to stricture and ring formation.	EGD, biopsy.	PPI, esophageal dilation, swallowed aerosolized fluticasone, systemic steroids, elimination diet trial.
Reflux	See section on GERD.		

GASTROESOPHAGEAL REFLUX DISEASE (GERD)

Caused by **failure of antireflux mechanisms,** which consist of the LES, the crural diaphragm, and the portion of the gastroesophageal junction below the hiatus. Its prevalence is high: 15% of affected patients experience symptoms at least once a week and 7% have daily symptoms.

SYMPTOMS/EXAM

- Presents with regurgitation of sour material in the mouth along with heartburn (usually postprandial), dysphagia, chest pain, and water brash (hypersalivation).
- In severe cases, laryngitis, chronic coughing, morning hoarseness, and pulmonary aspiration may be seen.
- Exam is usually normal.

KEY FACT

Asthma unresponsive to conventional therapy is highly suspicious for GERD.

DIFFERENTIAL

Infectious esophagitis, pill esophagitis, gastritis, peptic ulcer disease (PUD), functional dyspepsia, biliary tract disease, CAD, esophageal motility disorders.

DIAGNOSIS

- Mild, low-risk cases (ie, those with no dysphagia, odynophagia, anemia, or weight loss) are usually diagnosed clinically and supported by patients' response to empiric treatment.
- **EGD:** Can be used to evaluate for Barrett esophagus, erosions, strictures, or ulcers. Barium swallow is less popular because of its lower sensitivity in milder cases of GERD.
- **Wireless capsule endoscopy:** Has been approved by the FDA for evaluation of the esophagus in patients with heartburn. Sensitivities are nearly equal to those of EGD.
- **A 24-hour pH probe monitoring:** Can be useful for confirming the disease in patients with persistent symptoms, especially if a trial of acid suppression has failed and/or EGD is ⊖.

TREATMENT

- **Lifestyle modifications:**
  - **Elevation of the head of the bed:** Especially beneficial for nocturnal or laryngeal symptoms. Elevation should be approximately 6 inches.
  - **Dietary modifications:** Avoidance of **reflux-inducing foods** (chocolate, peppermint, alcohol, fatty foods); avoidance of **acidic foods** (orange juice, coffee, colas, red wine); consumption of **smaller, more frequent meals;** and use of lozenges or chewing gum (to promote salivation, which neutralizes gastric contents).
  - **Other:** Avoidance of tight-fitting garments; smoking and alcohol cessation.
- **Antacids:**
  - **H$_2$ blockers:** Good for mild cases, but not effective for more severe disease.
  - **PPIs:** More effective than H$_2$ blockers in healing and providing symptomatic relief.
  - Intermittent therapy with 2–4 weeks of H$_2$ blockers or PPIs is a reasonable approach for mild GERD.
  - Maintenance therapy is usually required, with doses titrated to the minimum needed to prevent recurrence.
- **Prokinetics:** Metoclopramide, bethanechol. Useful adjuncts, but not appropriate as monotherapy. Side effects limit their use.
- **Surgery:**
  - Generally reserved for patients whose symptoms persist despite optimal medical therapy; those who are unable to tolerate or comply with medical management; and those with severe esophagitis, stricture, Barrett metaplasia, or pulmonary complications.
- The most common techniques (**Nissen fundoplication, Hill repair, Belsey Mark IV**) improve symptoms and heal the disease in approximately 85% of cases.

COMPLICATIONS

Complications of GERD include the following:

- **Complications of prolonged acid suppression:** Include pneumonia and enteric infections (due to easier colonization of pathogens in the upper GI tract) as well as vitamin B$_{12}$ malabsorption (associated with prolonged omeprazole use).

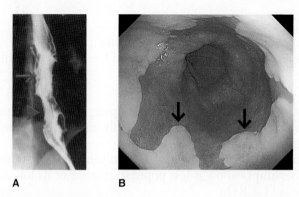

FIGURE 5.2. **Barrett esophagus.** **(A)** Barrett esophagus with adenocarcinoma on barium esophagram. Note the nodular mucosa *(arrow)* and the raised filling defect *(arrowhead)*, representing adenocarcinoma. **(B)** Endoscopic image showing the pink tongues of Barrett esophagus *(arrows indicate normal esophagus)*. (Image A reproduced, with permission, from Chen MY, et al. *Basic Radiology.* New York: McGraw-Hill, 2004, Fig. 10-19. Image B reproduced, with permission, from Fauci AS, et al. *Harrison's Principles of Internal Medicine,* 17th ed. New York: McGraw-Hill, 2008, Fig. 285-3A.)

- **Barrett esophagus:**
  - Metaplastic process in which stratified squamous epithelium is replaced by **intestinal-type (columnar) epithelium** during the healing phases of esophagitis (see Figure 5.2). Occurs in 4%–10% of patients with significant heartburn.
  - The presence of Barrett esophagus ↑ the risk of esophageal adenocarcinoma, with an annual cancer incidence of 0.2%–2.0%. Treatment includes aggressive antireflux therapy.
  - There are no well-established guidelines for cancer surveillance; however, patients ≥ 50 years of age with persistent GERD symptoms are sometimes screened with EGD and biopsy.
- **Peptic stricture:** Suggested by progressive dysphagia and episodic obstruction. Barium swallows are helpful in diagnosis. The treatment of choice is endoscopic balloon dilation along with high-dose acid suppression.
- **Asthma:** Caused by microaspiration and ↑ vagal tone from acid stimulation of the esophagus. Can occur in the absence of other reflux symptoms. Consider in asthmatic patients who fail to respond to conventional asthma therapy.
- **Others: Chronic cough,** periodontal disease, chronic sinusitis, recurrent pneumonitis, nocturnal choking, chronic hoarseness, pharyngitis, subglottic stenosis, laryngeal/tracheal stenosis.

Disorders of the Stomach

GASTROPATHY

Defined as injury to the mucosa of the stomach, with epithelial cell damage and regeneration. **Injury is unrelated to inflammation.** The etiologies of gastropathy include drugs **(NSAIDs),** alcohol, bile reflux, severe illness, and portal hypertension.

GASTRITIS

Defined as injury to the mucosa of the stomach, with epithelial cell damage and regeneration, 2° **to inflammatory response.** Etiologies include the following:

- **Acute gastritis:** Typically caused by an acute *Helicobacter pylori* **infection,** although etiologic agents such as CMV have been implicated in immunocompromised and iatrogenic cases. Can progress to chronic gastritis if not treated.
- **Chronic (metaplastic) gastritis:** Categorized according to the site affected.
    - **Type A:** Primarily affects the fundus and body, with antral sparing. Includes **autoimmune gastritis,** in which antibodies against parietal cells and intrinsic factor (IF) lead to pernicious anemia (cobalamin deficiency, megaloblastic anemia, subacute combined degeneration) and achlorhydria.
    - **Type B:** Predominantly affects the antrum, progressing to the fundus. Caused by *H pylori.* Can lead to multifocal atrophic gastritis, gastric atrophy, and metaplasia, increasing the risk of developing gastric adenocarcinoma.

SYMPTOMS OF GASTROPATHY AND GASTRITIS

There is a **poor correlation** between symptoms (eg, pain and dyspepsia) and endoscopic findings. However, acute *H pylori* gastritis can cause **sudden onset of epigastric pain, nausea, and vomiting,** while gastropathy caused by NSAID use, alcohol, or portal hypertension can present with **GI bleeding.**

EXAM

- Exam is usually unremarkable, but abdominal tenderness may be seen.
- Signs of vitamin B_{12} deficiency (anemia, neurologic signs) may also be noted.

DIFFERENTIAL

See the differential for PUD, below. Rarer causes include granulomatous disease (TB, fungal, sarcoid, Crohn disease) and Ménétrier disease (characterized by giant thickened folds of mucosa).

DIAGNOSIS

- Diagnosis is largely clinical but can include noninvasive *H pylori* testing (see Table 5.2), evaluation for suspected autoimmune gastritis via anti–parietal cell and IF antibodies, and analysis of the serum pepsinogen I-to-II ratio.
- **EGD** with biopsy can provide a pathologic diagnosis.

TREATMENT

- Treatment generally consists of avoidance of causative factors (eg, NSAIDs, alcohol) along with **prophylaxis** (PPIs; nonselective β-blockers for varices).
- *H pylori* eradication; parenteral vitamin B_{12} for pernicious anemia.

KEY FACT

Indications for prophylactic PPI use in hospitalized patients include coagulopathy (platelets < 50,000 μL, INR > 1.5); intubated > 48 hours; history of GI bleed or ulcer in the past year; 2 or more of the following criteria: sepsis, ICU admission > 1 week, occult GI bleed > 6 days, glucocorticoid treatment (> 250 mg hydrocortisone or equivalent).

TABLE 5.2.   Testing Methods for *H pylori*

TYPE	ADVANTAGES	DISADVANTAGES
Invasive		
Biopsy urease test	The test of choice; sensitivity is 90%–95% and specificity 95%–100%.	False ⊖s occur with use of PPIs and H_2 blockers as well as with GI bleeding, antibiotics, and bismuth.
Histology	Useful in excluding gastritis, intestinal metaplasia, and MALT lymphoma.	Prone to sampling error and interobserver variability; has ↓ sensitivity if the patient is taking antisecretory therapy.
Brush cytology	Sensitivity and specificity are similar to those of the biopsy urease test.	Not commonly done unless the patient has a bleeding disorder.
Culture for *H pylori*		Not done routinely; mostly for suspected antibiotic resistance if sensitivities are needed.
Noninvasive		
Urea breath test	The best nonendoscopic test. Uses urea with radiolabeled carbon, allowing liberated CO_2 to be detected. Has 88%–95% sensitivity and 95%–100% specificity.	The same factors causing false ⊖s with the biopsy urease test apply.
Stool antigen testing	As good as the urea breath test.	Less accurate if the patient is on PPIs or bismuth.
H pylori serology (IgG, IgA)	Inexpensive and has good sensitivity (90%–100%).	Specificity is 76%–96%; reliable if consistent with pretest probability. Not useful to confirm eradication, as it takes several months for patients to seroconvert. Cannot differentiate from old infection.

PEPTIC ULCER DISEASE (PUD)

A 50-year-old man presents with 1 month of epigastric pain that seems to improve with meals and calcium carbonate. He has no family history of upper GI malignancies, weight loss, early satiety, vomiting, or dysphagia, and he has no signs of anemia. His only medication is naproxen, which he takes for low back pain. He does not smoke but enjoys having a glass of wine with each dinner. What do you tell the patient?

You tell the patient that something may be wrong in his upper GI tract, and you recommend an EGD. He should stop taking naproxen and stop drinking wine. The patient's EGD demonstrates a duodenal ulcer, and his biopsy urease test is ⊕ for *H pylori*.

How will you treat him?

You prescribe him triple therapy. Two months later, he reports some improvement but continues to have symptoms and remains on his PPI.

Should you order a stool *H pylori* antigen test to check for eradication?

You defer this, as you know it will not be accurate while he is on a PPI. On closer questioning, you find that he actually never filled his prescription for the antibiotics because he felt that the drugs were "too expensive."

The principal cause of PUD is ***H pylori* infection,** which causes 70%–80% of duodenal and 60%–70% of gastric ulcers. Most cases that are not associated with *H pylori* are related to **NSAID** use. Zollinger-Ellison syndrome is another significant cause. Additional risk factors include tobacco, medications (eg, aspirin, KCl, mycophenolate), physiologic stress (ie, ICU), and, less often, CMV, HSV-1, and chemoradiation. **Psychological stress is not a cause, and corticosteroids are not a contributing factor unless they are used in association with NSAIDs.**

SYMPTOMS

- May be asymptomatic ("silent disease"; more common in the elderly and in NSAID users), or may present with dyspepsia or with severe, hunger-like epigastric pain accompanied by burning and gnawing.
- Symptoms are further distinguished as follows:
  - **Gastric ulcers:** Classically present with **severe pain soon after meals. Relief with antacid intake or food consumption is less frequent than with duodenal ulcers.**
  - **Duodenal ulcers:** Classically present as **pain 2–5 hours after meals** along with night symptoms occurring from 11 PM to 2 AM Food and antacids tend to relieve symptoms.

EXAM

Exam may reveal epigastric tenderness.

DIFFERENTIAL

Functional dyspepsia, gastric cancer, drug-induced dyspepsia (NSAIDs), sarcoidosis, Crohn disease, infections (TB, strongyloidiasis, giardiasis), GERD, biliary tract disease, gastroparesis, pancreatitis, malabsorption.

DIAGNOSIS

- **EGD:** The diagnostic **gold standard,** allowing for the **differentiation of benign ulcers from cancer.** Indicated to rule out malignancy if any **alarm signs** are present (eg, if patients are > 45 years of age and have weight loss, anemia, bleeding, vomiting, dysphagia, a family history of gastric cancer, or previous gastric surgery) (see Figure 5.3).
- **Upper GI series:** Less favored because of its variable sensitivity (50%–90%).
- *H pylori* **testing** (see Table 5.2).

TREATMENT

- **Lifestyle modifications: Smoking cessation;** alcohol avoidance; caffeine avoidance; and avoidance of NSAIDs or aspirin.

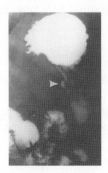
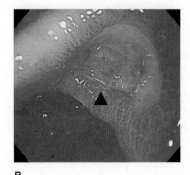

A   **B**

FIGURE 5.3. **Gastric ulcer.** (**A**) Barium upper GI study shows a benign gastric ulcer as pooling of contrast (*arrowhead*) extending beyond the adjacent gastric wall. (**B**) Benign gastric ulcer (*arrowhead*) at endoscopy. (Image A reproduced, with permission, from Chen MY, et al. *Basic Radiology.* New York: McGraw-Hill, 2004, Fig. 10-21. Image B reproduced, with permission, from Fauci AS, et al. *Harrison's Principles of Internal Medicine,* 17th ed. New York: McGraw-Hill, 2008, Fig. 285-2A.)

- **Acid suppressors:** Include H_2 blockers, PPIs, and sucralfate. Maintenance acid suppression may be required to prevent recurrence or to treat complications.
- ***H pylori* infection:** Eradicate *H pylori* if indicated. Continued acid suppression is necessary to allow the ulcer to heal. In complex cases, *H pylori* testing should be repeated approximately 4 weeks after healing to confirm disease resolution. Treatment regimen includes PPI BID, clarithromycin 500 mg BID, amoxicillin 1 g BID for 10–14 days. Metronidazole may be substituted for amoxicillin if patient is PCN allergic, but resistance is common.
- **Surgical intervention:** Indications include failure of medical management; suspicion of cancer (eg, a gastric ulcer that fails to heal after 12 weeks); perforation; outlet obstruction (failing to resolve after > 72 hours); and failure to arrest bleeding. Duodenal ulcers are typically treated with a highly selective vagotomy, with either pyloroplasty or antrectomy (with a Billroth I or II anastomosis); gastric ulcers are treated with distal gastrectomy/antrectomy with a Billroth anastomosis, but vagotomies are not performed unless there is a coexisting duodenal ulcer.

COMPLICATIONS

- **Lack of response:** Causes of treatment failure include *H pylori* resistance, noncompliance with medical therapy/supportive measures, giant ulcers (those > 2 cm have a lesser chance of healing), H_2 blocker/PPI resistance or tolerance, cancer, Crohn disease, infection, and **Zollinger-Ellison syndrome** (pancreatic gastrinoma; ↑ **fasting serum gastrin**).
- Fibrotic scar, penetrating ulcers (more localized and intense pain radiating to the back), perforation (sudden diffuse abdominal pain and peritonitis), pyloric channel obstruction (early satiety, vomiting, nausea, weight loss, pain, and bloating), hemorrhage (nausea, hematemesis, melena, and dizziness).
- **Complications of surgery:** Ulcer recurrence, afferent loop syndrome (due to bacterial overgrowth or partial obstruction of loop), dumping syndrome (due to ↑ hyperosmolar loads to the small bowel), postvagotomy diarrhea, bile reflux gastropathy, maldigestion, malabsorption, and gastric cancer.

GASTROPARESIS

Obstructive symptoms in the stomach/bowel in the **absence of an anatomic lesion.** May be idiopathic or 2° to diabetes, hypothyroidism, neurologic disorders, rheumatologic disease (scleroderma), amyloidosis, paraneoplastic disease, or drugs (eg, anticholinergics, calcium channel blockers, α_2-adrenergic agonists).

SYMPTOMS/EXAM

- Presents with early satiety, nausea, bloating/distension, and vomiting soon after meals.
- Exam may reveal abdominal distention and/or succussion splash (heard when shaking the abdomen by holding the pelvis, indicating free fluid).

DIAGNOSIS

- **Plain films:** Occasionally show gaseous distention of the stomach or the bowel.
- **Upper GI series with small bowel follow-through:** Used to rule out mechanical obstruction.
- **Gastric scintigraphy:** Establishes delayed gastric emptying.

TREATMENT

- **Acute episodes:** Treat with NPO, NG suction, and IV fluids.
- **Nutritional support:** Small, frequent meals with fewer fatty or gas-forming foods. Parenteral nutrition if necessary.
- **Prokinetics: Metoclopramide,** cisapride (has limited use in the United States because drug interactions ↑ the risk of fatal arrhythmias). **IV erythromycin** for acute episodes.
- **Strict glycemic control** in diabetic gastroparesis is recommended.
- Discontinue drugs that slow intestinal motility (eg, anticholinergics, opioids).

Disorders of the Bowel

ACUTE DIARRHEA

Defined as diarrhea lasting ≤ **2 weeks.** One of 5 leading causes of death worldwide. **Ninety percent** of cases are caused by **infectious agents.** Most are viral, but severe cases are more frequently caused by bacteria (1.5%–5.6% of mild cases are due to bacterial infection, vs. 87% of severe cases). The remaining 10% are from **medications, toxin ingestion, and ischemia.** Some chronic cases present acutely, as in **IBD** or **diverticulitis.** Risk factors for acute infection are as follows:

- **Travel:** Approximately 40% of travelers to Asia, Latin America, or Africa get "traveler's diarrhea." The most common infectious agents are enterotoxigenic *Escherichia coli*, *Campylobacter*, *Shigella*, and *Salmonella*. Campers, backpackers, and travelers to Russia are susceptible to *Giardia*.
- **Contaminated food ingestion:** Usually associated with food consumption at picnics, banquets, or restaurants. Commonly implicated foods include chicken, hamburger (enterohemorrhagic *E coli*), fried rice, mayonnaise, eggs, and raw seafood.
- **High-risk populations:** Include immunocompromised patients, day care workers and their contacts, and health care workers.
- **Recent antibiotic use:** Can be related or unrelated to *Clostridium difficile* infection.
- **Viral gastroenteritis:** Etiology includes rotavirus, norovirus, enteric adenovirus, and astrovirus. Usually has rapid onset (24–48 hours incubation period) and is short lasting (12–60 hours). Symptoms often include vomiting. Most outbreaks (cruise ships, nursing homes, military environments, etc) are caused by norovirus.

DIAGNOSIS

- Indications for evaluation include profuse diarrhea with dehydration, grossly bloody stools, fever ≥ 38.5°C (101.3°F), illness lasting > 48 hours without improvement, advanced age, severe abdominal pain in patients > 50 years of age, community outbreaks, > 6 stools in 24 hours, recent use of antibiotics, and hospitalization.
- Diagnostic modalities include the following:
    - **Fecal leukocytes:** Sensitivity and specificity for inflammation vary from 20%–90%. Useful if preclinical suspicion for an inflammatory etiology is high.
    - **Bacterial stool culture:** Controversial because acute infectious diarrhea is often viral and bacterial cases are usually self-limited. However,

KEY FACT

Etiologies of bloody diarrhea include *E coli* O157:H7, *Shigella*, *Campylobacter*, and *Salmonella*.

KEY FACT

Do not give antibiotics to patients with suspected enterohemorrhagic *E coli* infection (bloody stools, abdominal pain/tenderness, little or no fever), as there is no evidence that antibiotics are of benefit, and there is a theoretical risk of causing hemolytic-uremic syndrome.

stool cultures should be obtained in immunocompromised patients, those with significant comorbidities, and those with IBD (to differentiate flare from infection). Routine cultures will identify *Salmonella, Shigella,* and *Campylobacter* but not *Yersinia* or *Aeromonas.* The **false-⊖ rate is low** (ie, repeat testing is not necessary).

- **Viral stool culture and antigens.**
- **Stool ova and parasites (O&P):** Usually obtained if diarrhea is persistent (> 2 weeks) or for patients who have traveled to developing countries, men who have sex with men (MSM), AIDS patients, those involved in waterborne outbreaks, and those with bloody diarrhea with few or no fecal leukocytes (suggestive of amebiasis). Send O&P on 3 consecutive days, each spaced > 24 hours apart.
- **Endoscopy/colonoscopy:** Appropriate if IBD or pseudomembranous/ischemic colitis is suspected.
- **Other:** Toxin assays (eg, *C difficile*); stool *Giardia* antigen; *Entamoeba histolytica* antigen.

TREATMENT

- **Fluid and electrolyte replacement:** Consists of ½ teaspoon of salt, ½ teaspoon of baking soda, and 4 tablespoons of sugar in 1 L of water for oral rehydration. IV fluids may be needed.
- **Loperamide and diphenoxylate:** Generally safe for the alleviation of symptoms in afebrile and nonbloody cases, but may prolong disease in patients who are febrile. Avoid in suspected *C difficile* infection, as this can lead to toxic megacolon.
- **Bismuth subsalicylate:** Can ↓ nausea and vomiting, but avoid in immunocompromised patients because of the risk of bismuth encephalopathy.
- **Antibiotics** if indicated:
  - **Fluoroquinolones:** For suspected bacterial infection; give for 3–5 days. Administer a **macrolide** if resistance is suspected, especially in traveler's diarrhea.
  - **Metronidazole:** For cases suspected to be related to *Giardia* or *C difficile.*
  - Always give antibiotics to elderly patients, immunocompromised patients, and those with heart or vascular grafts.
- **Probiotics:** Proven to aid recolonization in pediatric patients, but their efficacy has not been established in adults. Examples include *Saccharomyces, Lactobacillus, Bifidobacterium.*

CHRONIC DIARRHEA

Defined as diarrhea **lasting > 4 weeks.** In developing countries, it is most often due to chronic infections, whereas in developed countries it is primarily caused by IBS, IBD, and malabsorption syndromes. Subtypes are as follows:

- **Secretory:** Deranged transport of fluid and electrolytes across the mucosa. Usually presents with watery, large-volume diarrhea that persists with fasting. Causes include medications, laxatives, chronic alcohol consumption (enterocyte injury), toxins, cholerrheic diarrhea, partial obstruction/strictures/fecal impaction (leading to paradoxical hypersecretion), carcinoid, and VIPoma.
- **Osmotic:** Due to a poorly absorbed osmotically active substance. Diarrhea is usually watery and ↑ with increasing solute load. Characterized by ↑ **stool osmotic gap, calculated as 290 − [2 (Na + K)].** Causes include carbohydrate malabsorption (leading to watery diarrhea) and fat malabsorption (leading to greasy diarrhea).

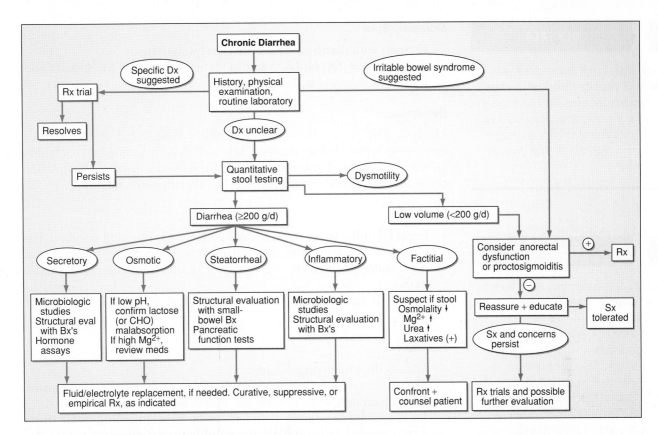

FIGURE 5.4. Diagnosis of chronic diarrhea. (Reproduced, with permission, from Kasper DL, et al. *Harrison's Principles of Internal Medicine,* 16th ed. New York: McGraw-Hill, 2005: 230.)

- **Inflammatory:** Due to mucosal inflammation. Diarrhea is generally bloody and accompanied by fever and abdominal pain. Causes include infections, IBD, radiation enterocolitis, and eosinophilic gastroenteritis.
- **Dysmotile:** Associated with hyperthyroidism, diabetes, carcinoid, drugs, and IBS.
- **Factitious:** Associated with Munchausen syndrome and bulimia.

DIAGNOSIS

Figure 5.4 shows an algorithm to guide the diagnosis of chronic diarrhea.

TREATMENT

- Treat the underlying cause.
- **Pharmacotherapy:**
  - **Loperamide and diphenoxylate:** Can be used for mild or moderate watery diarrhea.
  - **Codeine, octeotride, and tincture of opium:** Can be used for more severe diarrhea, but avoid in inflammatory diarrhea (can precipitate toxic megacolon in IBD).
- Fluid, electrolyte, and vitamin replacement as needed.

FAT MALABSORPTION

Results from failure to digest, absorb, or transport fat or from a deficiency of bile with failed compensatory hepatic synthesis.

> **KEY FACT**
>
> Nocturnal diarrhea is not characteristic of IBS and must be evaluated for another cause.

SYMPTOMS/EXAM

■ Presents with diarrhea, steatorrhea, and weight loss.
■ Symptoms of fat-soluble vitamin deficiencies may be seen (associated blindness, osteopenia, and bleeding).

DIFFERENTIAL

Lipolysis defects (ie, chronic pancreatitis); ↓ bile acid synthesis (liver disease) or secretion (biliary disease); bile acid deconjugation (ie, bacterial overgrowth) or loss (ie, Crohn disease, ileal resection); mucosal dysfunction (ie, celiac disease); postabsorption defects (ie, abetalipoproteinemia).

DIAGNOSIS

■ **Fecal fat collection** (72-hour stool collection): The gold standard. Fat malabsorption is defined as stool fat excretion > 6 g/day; however, patients with steatorrhea excrete > 20 g/day. The inconvenience of the test limits its use.
■ **Sudan III stain for fecal fat/stool acid steatocrit:** Alternative, qualitative tests.

TREATMENT

■ Address the underlying disorder.
■ Restrict long-chain fatty acids to 40 g/day, with supplementation of medium-chain fatty acids to maintain nutritional balance.
■ Treat fat-soluble vitamin deficiencies by supplementing **5–10 times** the recommended daily value. **Water-soluble preparations** are necessary.
■ Calcium and magnesium bind fatty acids in severe fat malabsorption, requiring supplementation.

CARBOHYDRATE METABOLISM

Lactose Intolerance

A prototypical carbohydrate malabsorption disorder. Has a high prevalence in East Asians and Native Americans and a moderate prevalence in blacks. Least common in whites (but still has up to 20% prevalence).

SYMPTOMS/EXAM

■ Presents with diarrhea, cramps, abdominal pain, and/or flatus following the ingestion of milk products. Symptom severity depends on the amount of lactose ingested and the fat content of the product (skim milk empties from the stomach faster, causing more symptoms).
■ Exam may reveal abdominal distention and hyperactive bowel sounds.

DIFFERENTIAL

See the differential for chronic diarrhea.

DIAGNOSIS

Usually clinical, with trial of empiric restriction of lactose intake.

■ **Lactose tolerance test:** Measures serum glucose in blood 0, 60, and 120 minutes after the ingestion of 50 g of lactose. An ↑ in glucose of > 20 mg/dL in conjunction with symptoms is diagnostic.

- **Lactose breath hydrogen test:** Measures H_2 in the breath at 30-minute intervals following an oral challenge of 2 g/kg. An ↑ in breath hydrogen of > 20 ppm is diagnostic (the ↑ is due to bacterial fermentation of nonabsorbed lactose).
- **Other:** Nonspecific tests such as stool pH, stool-reducing substances, and stool osmotic gap (osmotic diarrhea) can aid in diagnosis.

TREATMENT

- Lactose restriction (milk and ice cream have more lactose than cheese).
- Lactase preparations can ↓ symptoms.
- Calcium and vitamin D supplementation needed because of decreased intake of milk products.

CELIAC DISEASE

An immune disorder that is triggered by the **gliadin component of gluten** and can affect any part of the intestine. Once considered a disease of infancy, it now presents more often at 10–40 years of age, presumably because of longer breast-feeding periods and later introduction of gluten into the diet. **Spontaneous remissions and exacerbations** are common. Associated with autoimmune disorders (type 1 DM, autoimmune thyroiditis, autoimmune hepatitis) as well as with dermatitis herpetiformis and IgA deficiency. More common among whites.

SYMPTOMS/EXAM

- Can range from significant disease causing diarrhea, steatorrhea, and weight loss to the absence of symptoms except those of a single nutrient deficiency (eg, anemia, metabolic bone disease).
- Exam may reveal no abnormalities or only those due to a particular nutrient deficiency.

DIAGNOSIS

- **Small intestinal biopsy:** The gold standard. Reveals suggestive (not diagnostic) changes that are confirmed by reversion to normal histology following initiation of a gluten-free diet.
- **Antiendomysial IgA** and **anti–tissue transglutaminase (anti-TTG) IgA:**
  - Excellent screening tests, with 95% and 100% sensitivities, respectively. Can also be used to follow titers in order to gauge clinical improvement.
  - Screens should be followed by endoscopy with biopsy.
  - Antigliadin IgA is no longer favored because of its lower sensitivity and specificity.
  - Transaminases may be elevated.

TREATMENT

- **Dietary modifications:**
  - Institute a **gluten-free diet** (avoidance of wheat, rye, and barley products), supplemented by nutritional counseling.
  - Avoid lactose, as 2° intolerance is common.
  - Specific dietary deficiencies, such as deficiencies of iron, folic acid, calcium, vitamin D, and, rarely, vitamin B_{12}, should be corrected.

- Educate patients about the relapsing and remitting nature of the disease.
- Consider pneumococcal vaccination, as celiac disease is associated with hyposplenism.

COMPLICATIONS

Refractory sprue. May be due to other dietary agents. Associated with ↑ risk of progressive malabsorption and death. Treatment consists largely of immunosuppression (steroids) and, increasingly, immunomodulator therapy.

SHORT GUT SYNDROME

A malabsorptive state following massive small bowel resection, usually for Crohn disease, malignancy, mesenteric ischemia, or radiation.

SYMPTOMS/EXAM

Presents with diarrhea and symptoms or signs of specific nutrient or vitamin deficiencies, depending on the nature of the resection. Common examples: resection of > 60 cm of terminal ileum leads to malabsorpion of IF-bound vitamin B_{12}; resection of > 100 cm of ileum leads to bile salt and, therefore, fat malabsorption; loss of ileocecal valve leads to bacterial overgrowth and ↓ intestinal transit time.

DIAGNOSIS

Usually clinical and suggested by the surgical history.

TREATMENT

- Treat with dietary adjustment to maximize nutrition while avoiding steatorrhea or osmotic diarrhea. Fiber can help absorb water and also ↑ bacterial production of short-chain fatty acids to provide additional calories.
- Moderate use of **opiates** can ↑ transit time.
- **Cholestyramine** for choleraic diarrhea; **calcium supplementation** for hyperoxaluria.
- Monitor and replace vitamins and minerals (eg, monthly vitamin B_{12} IM).
- TPN may be necessary if alimentary feeds are insufficient.
- Intestinal transplantation if extensive resection has occurred and medical therapy fails.

BACTERIAL OVERGROWTH

There are relatively fewer bacteria in the upper GI tract than in the lower GI tract (especially the colon). In bacterial overgrowth, there is an ↑ in the number of bacteria in the more proximal GI tract. This can result from anything causing abnormal stasis (eg, stricture, blind loops), ↓ motility, or abnormal communications between the proximal and distal GI tract (eg, fistula, ileocecal valve resection). Bacterial overgrowth leads to **carbohydrate malabsorption** (due to bacterial consumption), **fat malabsorption** (through deconjugation of bile, which also has a direct toxic effect on the mucosa, aggravating carbohydrate malabsorption), and vitamin B_{12} **deficiency** (as bacteria compete with the host for vitamin B_{12}). **Altered intestinal motility** is also seen.

KEY FACT

Bacterial overgrowth should be suspected in any patient with a predisposing condition who presents with malabsorptive symptoms.

SYMPTOMS/EXAM

- Presents with diarrhea, steatorrhea, bloating, flatulence, anemia, sub-acute combined degeneration, weight loss, and associated calcium and fat-soluble vitamin deficiencies.
- Exam may reveal a succussion splash or distention.

DIAGNOSIS

The gold standard is a **jejunal aspirate** showing a bacterial count of $> 10^5$; breath hydrogen testing can also be done. Alternatively, an empiric trial of antibiotics can be attempted.

TREATMENT

- Treat the disorder predisposing to overgrowth.
- Correct vitamin deficiencies if present.
- **Antibiotics** to alter (not eliminate) flora include amoxicillin-clavulanate, cephalexin plus metronidazole, TMP-SMX plus metronidazole, norfloxacin, and oral gentamicin plus metronidazole. Usually given for 7–10 days, but it may be necessary to prolong treatment, offer repeat courses, and rotate antibiotics to prevent resistance.
- ↓ drugs that slow motility or gastric acidity.
- Periodic polyethylene glycol can help with overgrowth by transient reduction.
- A high-fat, low-carbohydrate diet is of benefit, as bacteria rely more on carbohydrates.
- Probiotics may be tried, but their efficacy is unclear.

INFLAMMATORY BOWEL DISEASE (IBD)

Chronic inflammatory disease of the GI tract. The 2 main subtypes are **Crohn disease** (see Figure 5.5) and **ulcerative colitis** (see Figure 5.6). Table 5.3 outlines symptoms and disease characteristics of these 2 subtypes.

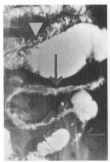 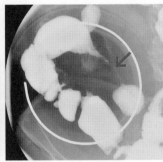 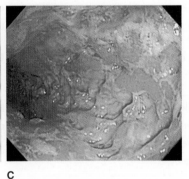

A   B   C

FIGURE 5.5.   Crohn disease. (A) Small bowel follow-through (SBFT) barium study shows skip areas of narrowed small bowel with nodular mucosa (*arrows*) and ulceration. Compare with normal bowel (*arrowhead*). (B) Spot compression image from SBFT shows "string sign" narrowing (*arrow*) due to stricture. (C) Deep ulcers in the colon of a patient with Crohn disease, seen at colonoscopy. (Image A reproduced, with permission, from Chen MY, et al. *Basic Radiology.* New York: McGraw-Hill, 2004, Fig. 10-30. Image B reproduced, with permission, from USMLERx.com. Image C reproduced, with permission, from Fauci AS, et al. *Harrison's Principles of Internal Medicine,* 17th ed. New York: McGraw-Hill, 2008, Fig. 285-4B.)

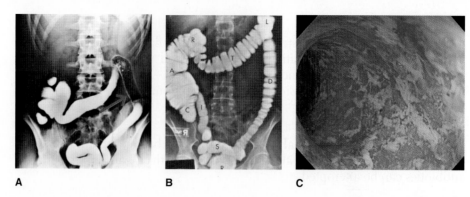

A   B   C

FIGURE 5.6. **Ulcerative colitis.** (A) Radiograph from a barium enema showing a feature-less ("lead pipe") colon with small mucosal ulcerations (*arrow*). Compare with normal haustral markings in (**B**). (**C**) Diffuse mucosal ulcerations and exudates at colonoscopy in chronic ulcerative colitis. (Image A reproduced, with permission, from Doherty GM. *Current Diagnosis & Treatment: Surgery,* 13th ed. New York: McGraw-Hill, 2010, Fig. 30-17. Image B reproduced, with permission, from Chen MY, et al. *Basic Radiology.* New York: McGraw-Hill, 2004, Fig. 10-10A. Image C reproduced, with permission, from Fauci AS, et al. *Harrison's Principles of Internal Medicine,* 17th ed. New York: McGraw-Hill, 2008, Fig. 285-4A.)

TABLE 5.3. **Crohn Disease vs. Ulcerative Colitis**

	CROHN DISEASE	ULCERATIVE COLITIS
Symptoms	Chronic diarrhea, crampy abdominal pain, fever, weight loss, and fatigue. Strictures leading to obstructive symptoms. Fistulization causing recurrent UTIs/pneumoturia, gas/feces from vagina, psoas abscesses, and ureteral obstruction.	Chronic bloody diarrhea, abdominal pain, cramps, tenesmus, and fecal urgency.
GI tract involvement	**Transmucosal inflammation** leading to ulceration, strictures, fistulas, and abscesses. May affect any part of the GI tract, from the mouth to the anus, but typically affects the **small bowel and colon.** 30% of disease occurs in the ileum; 20% occurs in the colon; and 50% occurs in both.	**Mucosal inflammation** leading to friability, erosions, and bleeding. The **rectum** is invariably involved. Extends **proximally** in a **continuous** fashion to involve the colon. 50% of cases involve the rectosigmoid colon; 30% extend to the splenic flexure; and 20% extend proximal to the splenic flexure.
GI bleeding manifestations	Guaiac-⊕ stools are common; **grossly bloody stools are uncommon.**	**Bloody stools are common.**
Exam	Exam may reveal pallor, weight loss, a palpable mass (in some cases of perforation and localized peritonitis), **aphthous ulcers, anal fissures, perirectal abscesses,** and **anorectal fistulas.**	Exam reveals abdominal tenderness and **gross blood on DRE.**
Extraintestinal manifestations	Uncommon, but those seen in ulcerative colitis may also be seen in Crohn disease.	Uveitis, episcleritis, erythema nodosum, pyoderma gangrenosum (see Figure 5.7), arthritis, ankylosing spondylitis, venous/arterial thromboembolism, sclerosing cholangitis.

TABLE 5.3. Crohn Disease vs. Ulcerative Colitis (continued)

	CROHN DISEASE	ULCERATIVE COLITIS
Differential	Ulcerative colitis, acute infectious diarrhea (*Shigella, Salmonella, Campylobacter, E coli* O157:H7), acute ileitis (*Yersinia* spp.), TB of the bowel, amebiasis, pseudomembranous colitis, CMV colitis (in the immunosuppressed), appendicitis, diverticulitis, ischemic colitis, lymphoma, carcinoma.	Crohn disease, radiation proctitis, ischemic/pseudomembranous/infectious colitis, infectious proctitis (gonorrhea, chlamydia, herpes, syphilis), amebiasis, CMV/Kaposi sarcoma in the immunosuppressed.
Endoscopic evaluation	**Colonoscopy** with intubation of the terminal ileum (reveals skip lesions, linear ulcers, and cobblestone mucosa) with biopsy. An upper GI series with small bowel follow-through or barium enema may also be needed to identify disease in the small bowel.	**Flexible sigmoidoscopy** is usually adequate (shows pseudopolyps, bleeding, petechiae, ulcers, and exudates) with biopsy. Colonoscopy may cause perforation in severe disease but may be used to evaluate the extent of disease.
Autoantibodies (sent if diagnosis after endoscopy remains uncertain)	**ASCA** is present in 60%–70% of cases; **p-ANCA** is present in 5%–10%. **ASCA**-⊕/p-ANCA-⊖ findings are 90% specific for Crohn disease.	**p-ANCA** is present in 50%–70% of cases; **ASCA** is present in 10%–15%. **p-ANCA**-⊕/ASCA-⊖ findings are 98% specific for ulcerative colitis.
Labs	Micro- or macrocytic anemia, leukocytosis, hypoalbuminemia. Stool studies are ⊖ for an infectious cause.	Same (but macrocytic anemia is less likely).
Suggested diet	High-fiber diet with colonic involvement; conversely, low roughage if obstructive symptoms are present. A trial of lactose elimination may benefit those with 2° intolerance.	High-fiber diet; limit caffeine and gas-producing foods. A trial of lactose elimination may be beneficial.
Medical therapy	**Ileitis:** Mesalamine (sulfasalazine is activated in the colon, so it should not be used). **Ileocolitis/colitis:** Mesalamine or sulfasalazine. Steroids or antibiotics (ciprofloxacin for ileitis; metronidazole for ileocolitis/colitis) may be required. Refractory cases require azathioprine, 6-MP, or infliximab. **Surgery is not curative.**	**Proctitis:** 5-ASA suppositories (or steroid suppositories/foams); 5-ASA enemas (or steroid enemas) for left-sided colitis. **Extensive/pancolitis:** Combined oral/rectal ASA agents and/or steroid enemas, with oral corticosteroids for refractory cases (cyclosporine if steroid refractory). Treat severe/fulminant cases with bowel rest, IV steroids, and antibiotics if the patient appears septic. **Colectomy is curative.**
Complications	Localized perforation/peritonitis, abscess, fistulas, bowel obstruction, massive hemorrhage, toxic megacolon, colon cancer, short gut syndrome (after resection).	Massive hemorrhage, fulminant colitis, toxic megacolon, perforation, stricture, colon cancer.

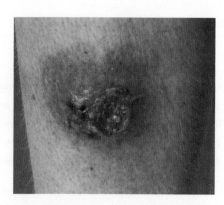

FIGURE 5.7. **Pyoderma gangrenosum.** (Reproduced, with permission, from Wolff K, et al. *Fitzpatrick's Dermatology in General Medicine,* 7th ed. New York: McGraw-Hill, 2008, Fig. 32-6.)

IRRITABLE BOWEL SYNDROME (IBS)

A 35-year-old female human resource manager returns for her follow-up visit for 6 months of intermittent lower abdominal discomfort and bloating. She also has frequent diarrhea, which alleviates her discomfort to some degree. She is able to sleep well at night and has had no fever, weight loss, or bloody stools. She denies a family history of colorectal cancer. Initial tests, including a complete metabolic panel, CBC, TSH, fecal occult blood test (FOBT), and stool O&P, have all been ⊖, and 2 weeks of a food journal have revealed no dietary triggers. What is the most likely diagnosis?

Irritable bowel syndrome.

What treatments would you offer?

Low-dose TCAs and loperamide as well as elimination trials of dairy, caffeine, and gas-causing foods.

A functional disorder characterized by **abdominal pain and discomfort**, with associated **disturbed defecation**. Its etiology is believed to be multifactorial, involving altered gut motility/secretion, visceral hypersensitivity, and brain–gut axis dysregulation. IBS is the most commonly diagnosed GI condition and the second most common cause of work absenteeism, exceeded only by the common cold. It is more prevalent in women and generally presents at 30–50 years of age.

SYMPTOMS/EXAM

- **1° symptoms:** Abdominal discomfort, relief of discomfort with defecation, a change in frequency and/or form of stool (may be diarrhea- or constipation-predominant).
- **Other symptoms:** Straining, urgency, or a feeling of incomplete evacuation; passage of mucus; bloating.
- Exam typically yields no physical findings, but mild lower abdominal tenderness may be seen.

DIFFERENTIAL

IBD, colon cancer, hyperthyroidism, hypothyroidism, chronic diarrhea (infectious, malabsorption), chronic constipation, celiac sprue.

DIAGNOSIS

- Presumes the absence of a structural or biochemical explanation for the symptoms.
- The absence of alarm signs (eg, fever, weight loss, blood in the stool, anemia, a family history of IBD or colon cancer, progressive symptoms, pain preventing sleeping or awakening the patient from sleep) is essential to diagnosis.
- Diagnostic tests may be used on a limited basis to exclude organic disease and include stool hemoccult, CBC, ESR (especially in younger patients), serum chemistry, albumin, stool O&P × 3, TSH, and antiendomysial/anti-TTG antibodies.

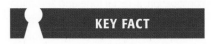

KEY FACT

IBS is a clinical diagnosis, so diagnostic testing should be limited.

TREATMENT

- **Establishment of a therapeutic alliance:** It is important to remain nonjudgmental, to provide reassurance that the disease is benign, and to promote patient involvement in treatment decisions.
- **Dietary modification:** Limitation of dairy products, caffeine, and gas-producing foods (eg, beans, onions) may be of benefit. A symptom diary to identify possible triggers may be useful as well.
- **Pain medications:**
  - **Antispasmodics:** Dicyclomine or hyoscyamine.
  - **Antidepressants:** Low-dose TCAs or occasionally SSRIs, especially with comorbid depression, may be of use.
  - For **constipation:** Lubiprostone, ↑ dietary fiber unless bloating is a major factor.
  - For **diarrhea:** Loperamide, diphenoxylate, atropine, alosetron.

CONSTIPATION

Has variable causes, including IBS, medication side effects, and metabolic, neurologic, or obstructive intestinal disease (see Table 5.4). Chronic constipation is more common in women, nonwhites, and those > 60 years of age.

TABLE 5.4.   Causes of Constipation in Adults

TYPE OF CONSTIPATION	EXAMPLES
Recent onset	
Colonic obstruction	Neoplasm, stricture (ischemic, diverticular, inflammatory).
Anal sphincter spasm	Anal fissure, painful hemorrhoids.
Medications	Narcotics.
Chronic	
IBS	Constipation-predominant, alternating.
Medications	Narcotics, Ca^{2+} blockers, antidepressants.
Colonic pseudo-obstruction	Slow-transit constipation, megacolon (rarely, Hirschsprung and Chagas disease).
Disorders of rectal evacuation	Pelvic floor dysfunction, anismus, descending perineum syndrome, rectal mucosal prolapse, rectocele.
Endocrinopathies	Hypothyroidism, hypercalcemia, pregnancy.
Psychiatric disorders	Depression, eating disorders, drugs.
Neurologic disease	Parkinsonism, MS, spinal cord injury.
Generalized muscle disease	Progressive systemic sclerosis.

Reproduced, with permission, from Fauci AS, et al. *Harrison's Principles of Internal Medicine,* 17th ed. New York: McGraw-Hill, 2008, Table 40-5.

Constipation can also be idiopathic, characterized by patterns seen on bowel function studies. For example, in **slow-transit constipation,** there is normal resting colonic motility but little or no ↑ after meals or with stimulants. With **dyssynergic defecation,** the pelvic floor muscles and external anal sphincter fail to relax during defecation, making evacuation difficult.

DIAGNOSIS

- Diagnosis is largely clinical. IBS should be excluded. Drugs should be reviewed for possible temporal relationships.
- Alarm signs for obstruction 2° to malignancy include weight loss, a family history of colon cancer or IBD, anemia, hematochezia, a ⊕ FOBT, or acute onset of symptoms. The presence of an alarm sign should prompt endoscopic evaluation.
- Laboratory tests include serum calcium for hypercalcemia and TSH for hypothyroidism.
- Barium enemas can detect structural changes, megacolon, and megarectum.
- If idiopathic constipation is suspected, workup with marker studies, defecography, or anorectal manometry may prove useful.

TREATMENT

- **Patient education:** Recommend that patients ↑ fluid and fiber intake, take advantage of ↑ colonic transit after meals (go to the bathroom after eating), and participate in regular physical activity (immobility worsens the condition).
- **Pharmacotherapy:** Fiber, stool surfactants (eg, docusate), stimulant laxatives (eg, bisacodyl, senna), osmotic laxatives (eg, lactulose, polyethylene glycol).
- **Others:**
  - Enemas, biofeedback, digital rectal stimulation.
  - Slow-transit constipation requires aggressive medical treatment. Treatment failure or the presence of a megarectum or megacolon may suggest the need for surgery.

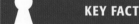

FECAL INCONTINENCE

Affects men and women equally (about 0.5%–2.0% of the population), but tends to be more severe in women and the elderly. Usually multifactorial, but generally due to sphincter dysfunction, abnormal rectal compliance, ↓ rectal sensation, or abnormal puborectalis muscle function. Specific etiologies include anal sphincter tears or pudendal nerve trauma during vaginal childbirth, surgical trauma (during fistula or hemorrhoid repairs), ulcerative/radiation proctitis, impaired rectal sensation (eg, neurologic disease, dementia), fecal impaction, or a cancer/obstructing mass.

EXAM

- Anal wink reflex should be elicited bilaterally; its absence suggests nerve damage.
- DRE may show a mass or fecal impaction or reveal weakened anal tone.

DIFFERENTIAL

Incontinence must be distinguished from bowel urgency and frequency **without loss of bowel contents,** which suggests etiologies such as IBD or IBS.

DIAGNOSIS

- Mostly **clinical,** based on the history and physical exam.
- **Sigmoidoscopy** to evaluate for inflammatory causes or a mass.
- Anorectal manometry, pudendal nerve terminal latency, endorectal ultrasound, defecography, and EMG of the anal sphincter can be done if further evaluation is required.

TREATMENT

- If present, diarrhea should be further evaluated and treated.
- **Stool disimpaction and bowel regimen:** If fecal impaction is the cause.
- **Regular defecation program:** Appropriate if the disorder is related to mental dysfunction or physical disability.
- **Biofeedback programs.**
- **Pharmacotherapy:**
  - **Bulk-forming laxatives:** Indicated with low-volume, loose stools.
  - **Loperamide:** ↓ stool frequency and ↑ internal anal sphincter tone.
  - **Anticholinergics** (hyoscyamine) may be helpful.
  - **Topical phenylephrine gel:** ↑ anal sphincter tone (α_1-agonist).
- **Surgical repair:** Usually successful in patients with single anal sphincter tears following vaginal delivery or fistula surgery. Additional surgical options include plication of the posterior part of the sphincter, anal encirclement, and muscle transfer procedures.
- **Other modalities:** Novel treatments include implantable incontinence devices, silicone biomaterial injections (augmenting the internal anal sphincter), and sacral nerve stimulation.

Liver Disease

Table 5.5 outlines the differential diagnosis and treatment of common liver diseases. Viral hepatitis (HAV, HBV, and HCV) is not included in this table, as it is covered in detail in the Infectious Diseases chapter. The subtopics that follow discuss cirrhosis and related complications.

A 50-year-old woman presents to your office with fatigue, pruritus, and mild jaundice. Her electrolytes and CBC are normal, but a liver panel reveals an alkaline phosphatase level twice that of normal in the setting of a mildly elevated bilirubin and normal AST/ALT. What do you recommend?

The setting is suspicious for 1° biliary cirrhosis, so you check for antimitochondrial antibodies and order an ultrasound. The patient's liver ultrasound is normal, and her antimitochondrial antibodies are ⊕. How should you proceed?

Given the high specificity and sensitivity of the antimitochondrial antibody test and the patient's normal ultrasound, the diagnosis of 1° biliary cirrhosis is likely but must be confirmed and staged by percutaneous liver biopsy.

These confirm the diagnosis. What further procedures are necessary, and how should the patient be treated?

The woman should have a DEXA scan to screen for osteoporosis. She can then be started on ursodeoxycholic acid to delay disease progression along with cholestyramine to relieve her itching.

TABLE 5.5.   Common Liver Diseases

Disease	Clinical Caveats	Symptoms/Exam
Drug/toxin-induced liver disease (always review meds in patients with liver disease)	Common offenders include **acetaminophen, INH, tetracyclines,** and some antiepileptics.	Variable.
Alcoholic liver disease	Includes (1) alcoholic fatty liver (develops in 90% of alcoholics), (2) alcoholic hepatitis (develops in 10%–20%), and (3) alcoholic cirrhosis. Women are affected more than men; concomitant HCV is a risk factor.	**Fatty liver:** May be asymptomatic or present with hepatomegaly. **Alcoholic hepatitis:** Begins after a recent period of heavy drinking and presents with anorexia, nausea, hepatomegaly, and jaundice.
Nonalcoholic steatohepatitis	A condition in which **biopsy findings are indistinguishable from alcoholic hepatitis** in patients without significant alcohol consumption. Most commonly found in patients 40–60 years of age; affects women more than men. Metabolic syndrome is a risk factor.	Usually asymptomatic, but may present with fatigue, malaise, RUQ discomfort, and hepatomegaly.
Ischemic hepatopathy (shock liver)	Liver disease due to an acute ↓ in cardiac output (eg, MI, arrhythmia).	Variable; signs of fulminant failure may be present (eg, encephalopathy, jaundice, coagulopathy).
Hemochromatosis	The **most common genetic disorder in whites.** Characterized by inappropriately ↑ absorption of dietary iron, causing deposition in the liver, heart, pancreas, and pituitary (leading to end-stage liver disease, hepatocellular carcinoma, dilated cardiomyopathy, DM, and hypogonadism). Associated with mutations of the **HFE gene on chromosome 6.**	Presents with weakness, fatigue, malaise, hepatomegaly, RUQ pain, arthralgias, impotence, amenorrhea, and slate-gray pigmentation of the skin (due to iron and melanin deposition; also known as "bronze diabetes").
Wilson disease	An **autosomal-recessive** disease (involving the **ATP7B gene**) causing ↓ transmembrane transport (excretion) of copper in hepatocytes, leading to copper accumulation in organs (liver, brain, kidneys, cornea).	Presents with symptoms of liver failure. Coombs-⊖ hemolytic anemia, ARF, **Kayser-Fleischer rings,** behavior change, cognitive decline, tremor, lack of motor coordination, drooling, dysarthria, dysphonia, spasticity, oropharyngeal dysphagia, depression, anxiety, and psychosis.

LFT Pattern	Other Findings	Treatment
Variable.		**Stop the offending medication.** For acetaminophen toxicity, give *N*-acetylcysteine if **toxicity is likely** based on nomogram (> 200 µg/mL at 4 hours).
Fatty liver: Modest elevation of aminotransferases (100–200s). **Alcoholic hepatitis:** AST usually < 300–400 and 2 × ALT, alkaline phosphatase and bilirubin are generally ↑.	Fatty liver on ultrasound, CT, or MRI; biopsy shows **macrovesicular** fatty change; PMNs and Mallory bodies are seen.	**Abstinence;** alcohol rehabilitation (AA, family therapy); aggressive nutritional support **(thiamine, folate); prednisolone if encephalopathic** or **discriminant function > 32** (PT – control × 4.6 + total bilirubin). **Liver transplantation** can be considered with abstinence > **6 months.**
↑ ALT and AST are seen in 90% of patients; unlike alcoholic hepatitis, the **ALT-to-AST ratio is** > 1.	Indistinguishable from that in alcoholic hepatitis (above).	**Gradual weight loss** (rapid loss can exacerbate NASH), dietary **fat restriction, exercise.** Can recur following liver transplantation.
A **striking ↑ of transaminases** (often > **5000**); corrects quickly if reversed, ↑ PT may occur.		Restore perfusion; aminotransferases usually correct quickly **(within 1 week).**
Variable (usually mild) elevation of AST and alkaline phosphatase is seen, depending on the stage of the disease.	Fasting **transferrin saturation > 45%;** ↑ **ferritin; genotype testing** (performed if iron studies are ⊕ or there is a history of the disease in first-degree relatives). Liver biopsy should be offered to document the degree of fibrosis in homozygotes > 40 years of age with ↑ AST and ferritin > 1000 ng/mL. **Hepatic iron index** has **fallen out of favor** for diagnosis with genetic testing.	**Phlebotomy therapy** (remove 1 unit of blood 1–2 times per week). **Deferoxamine** is **rarely needed.** A normal diet is acceptable, but avoid iron supplements, vitamin C, **shellfish** (↑ susceptibility to *Vibrio vulnificus* and others). Liver transplant has relatively low survival because of concurrent cardiac disease and ↑ infection risk.
↑ **aminotransferases** are seen. Alkaline phosphatase is usually low.	**Low copper** and serum **ceruloplasmin** (< 5 mg/dL is strongly suggestive; low because of ↓ incorporation causing ↓ half-life); ↑ **24-hour urinary copper excretion** (> 40 µg is suggestive); **hepatic copper content on biopsy** (> 250 µg/g is the best biochemical evidence of disease; < 40–50 µg/g excludes the diagnosis); **slit-lamp exam** for Kayser-Fleischer rings (diagnostic with ceruloplasmin < 20 mg/dL); brain MRI to evaluate for neurologic complications.	**D-penicillamine** (binds copper and enhances urinary excretion); trientene is an alternative for patients who cannot tolerate D-penicillamine. **Oral zinc** interferes with the absorption of copper in the GI tract. Reduction of copper-containing foods (shellfish, organs, legumes) is essential. Liver transplant for end-stage liver disease and fulminant failure.

(continues)

TABLE 5.5.　**Common Liver Diseases** *(continued)*

Disease	Clinical Caveats	Symptoms/Exam
Autoimmune hepatitis	Unknown etiology; likely a heterogeneous group of liver disorders characterized by (1) **autoantibodies** and (2) **high serum globulins.** Can be seen with other autoimmune diseases (hemolytic anemia, ITP, DM, ulcerative colitis, celiac disease, thyroiditis). Female predominance.	May be asymptomatic or fulminant (20%–25%, with jaundice and coagulopathy). A subset of patients are **young, otherwise healthy women** with fatigue, malaise, spider nevi, anorexia, amenorrhea, acne, arthralgias, and jaundice.
1° biliary cirrhosis	An **autoimmune disorder** causing granulomatous destruction of the intrahepatic bile ducts and cholestasis. Ninety-five percent of patients are women, and onset is at 40–60 years of age. Osteopenia/osteoporosis develops in 25% of patients because of osteoblast dysfunction. Frequently associated with other autoimmune disorders such as Sjögren and CREST.	**Usually asymptomatic** (60% are asymptomatic at the time of diagnosis), but fatigue and pruritus are common presenting symptoms. Jaundice, skin hyperpigmentation, xanthomas, hepatosplenomegaly, and other findings of end-stage liver disease may be present. **Osteoporosis** is seen.
1° sclerosing cholangitis	An uncommon disease characterized by diffuse inflammation, fibrosis, and stricturing of the biliary tract as well as an ↑ risk of cholangiocarcinoma (associated with a 10%–15% lifetime risk). **Two-thirds** of patients have **ulcerative colitis** (but only 5% of ulcerative colitis patients have 1° sclerosing cholangitis). Affects males more than females.	Presents with **progressive jaundice,** with associated malaise, pruritus, anorexia, and indigestion. May have occasional bouts of acute cholangitis. Steatorrhea, fat-soluble vitamin deficiency, and osteopenia develop.

CIRRHOSIS

Generally irreversible scarring of the liver, with fibrosis and nodular regeneration. Represents the tenth leading cause of death in the United States.

The fibrosis and resulting distorted vasculature lead to portal hypertension, causing ascites, esophageal and rectal varices, and splenomegaly (see Figure 5.8).

SYMPTOMS

- Weakness, fatigability, disturbed sleep, muscle cramps, and weight loss are common.
- Anorexia, nausea, vomiting, and abdominal pain may be seen.
- Men may develop impotence, loss of libido, sterility, and gynecomastia; women may develop amenorrhea.

EXAM

- The liver can be enlarged, normal, or shrunken, and usually is firm. Splenomegaly, spider nevi, palmar erythema, Dupuytren contractures, gynecomastia, caput medusa, weight loss, and wasting may be seen.

LFT Pattern	Other Findings	Treatment
Aminotransferases are ↑ (100–1000s).	↑ **gamma globulin** (SPEP). Autoantibodies include **ANA, ASMA (type 1)**, and **ALKM (type 11).** Liver biopsy may be nonspecific but aids in diagnosis, prognosis, and response to therapy.	Treatment is indicated if (1) aminotransferases are elevated tenfold, (2) aminotransferases are elevated fivefold AND serum globulin is elevated twofold, or (3) bridging or multiacinar necrosis is found on biopsy. Treat with **prednisone with azathioprine** or **6-MP.** Disease can recur after liver transplantation (especially as immunosuppression is ↓).
Usually diagnosed in the presymptomatic phase, with **alkaline phosphatase** often more than **twice normal** (with elevations of GGT and 5-NT). **Bilirubin** ↑ with disease progression. AST and ALT may be normal.	**Antimitochondrial antibodies** are 95% sensitive and 98% specific for the disease. **Liver biopsy** is confirmatory. Other causes of cholestasis should be excluded (eg, by ultrasound or cholangiography). **DEXA scans** to evaluate for concurrent osteoporosis.	**Ursodeoxycholic acid** delays progression, enhances survival, and is well tolerated. **Cholestyramine** improves pruritus (rifampin is second line). **Liver transplantation** is appropriate for treatment failure or severe osteoporosis.
Usually diagnosed in the presymptomatic phase with **alkaline phosphatase elevation;** aminotransferases may be ↑ to the 300s.	Diagnosis is established by **ERCP** (or MRCP) unless the disease is **confined to small intrahepatic ducts,** in which case a **liver biopsy** is needed to establish the diagnosis and staging. ANCA, ANA, anticardiolipin antibodies, anti-TPO antibodies, and RF may be ⊕.	Medical therapy has failed to show consistent benefit in survival. However, **ursodeoxycholic acid** relieves pruritus, improves biochemical abnormalities, and stabilizes hepatic inflammation. Dominant biliary strictures should be **biopsied to rule out carcinoma, with balloon dilation or stent placement** to relieve obstruction. **Liver transplantation** significantly improves survival.

- Late signs include jaundice, ascites, pleural effusions, ecchymoses, encephalopathy, asterixis, tremor, and GI bleeding.

DIAGNOSIS

- **Liver biopsy:** The gold standard, but diagnosis is usually made with clinical, lab, and radiologic findings.
- **Labs:** Anemia, leukopenia, and thrombocytopenia may be seen. AST and alkaline phosphatase are mildly ↑, and albumin is low. Rising total bilirubin, INR, and creatine indicate worsening liver function.
- **Imaging: Ultrasound** to assess the extent of disease and to detect nodules (which can be further evaluated by CT/MRI if suspicious for HCC); Doppler studies (to assess flow patterns in vasculature). Figure 5.9 shows a CT scan in a cirrhotic patient, with subsequent portal hypertension.

TREATMENT

Rule out reversible causes (eg, autoimmune hepatitis); stop alcohol; treat HBV and HCV if possible. Immunize against HAV and HBV; limit hepatotoxic drugs (eg, acetaminophen < 2 g/day), manage complications, and consider transplantation referral.

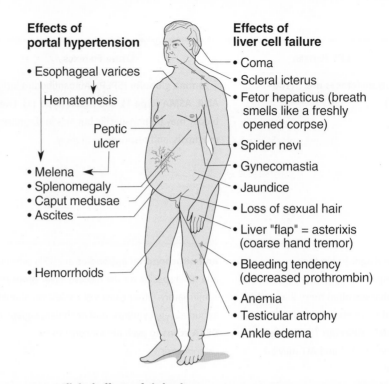

FIGURE 5.8.   Clinical effects of cirrhosis. (Reproduced, with permission, from Chandrasoma P, Taylor CR. *Concise Pathology*, 3rd ed. Originally published by Appleton & Lange. Copyright © 1998 by The McGraw-Hill Companies, Inc.)

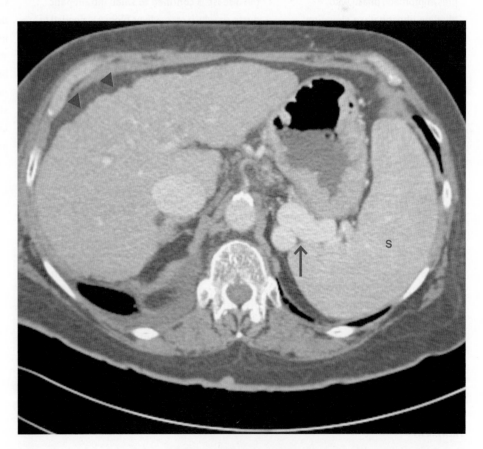

FIGURE 5.9.   Cirrhosis. Transaxial image from contrast-enhanced CT shows a nodular liver contour *(arrowheads)* and the stigmata of portal hypertension, including splenomegaly (S) and perisplenic varices *(arrow)*. (Reproduced, with permission, from USMLERx.com.)

TABLE 5.6.   Causes of Ascites

High Albumin Gradient (SAAG > 1.1 g/dL)	Low Albumin Gradient (SAAG < 1.1 g/dL)
Cirrhosis	Peritoneal carcinomatosis
Portal hypertension	Peritoneal tuberculosis
Alcoholic hepatitis	Pancreatitis
Nonalcoholic steatohepatitis (NASH)	Serositis
Chronic hepatitis C	Nephrotic syndrome
Congestive heart failure	Dialysis
Massive hepatic metastases	Chlamydial peritonitis
Hypothyroidism	
Budd-Chiari syndrome	

ASCITES

Intra-abdominal fluid accumulation caused by transudative movement of fluid into the abdominal cavity as a result of portal hypertension and decreased serum oncotic pressure. Table 5.6 lists causes of ascites.

SYMPTOMS/EXAM

Presents with abdominal distention; exam may reveal flank dullness (eg, shifting dullness), indicating at least 1500 cc of ascitic fluid.

DIAGNOSIS

- Diagnosis is usually clinical but can be difficult in obese patients (for whom ultrasound can be useful).
- Usually occurs in the presence of portal hypertension (**serum-ascites albumin gradient [SAAG] > 1.1**).

TREATMENT

- **Sodium restriction:** Restrict patients to 2 g (88 mmol) per day. Fluid restriction should be reserved for patients with Na < 120.
- **Spironolactone and furosemide:** If sodium restriction is inadequate, 90% of patients will respond to sodium restriction and spironolactone/furosemide starting at 100 mg/40 mg, respectively (ratio ensures normokalemia with normal renal function).
- **Repeated large-volume paracentesis:** Albumin replacement should be considered if > 4–5 L is removed.
- **Transjugular intrahepatic portosystemic shunt (TIPS):** Controversial. Improves ascites (and a last resort for variceal hemorrhage), but can ↑ encephalopathy and has a high occlusion rate.
- **Liver transplantation:** For refractory cases.

SPONTANEOUS BACTERIAL PERITONITIS (SBP)

 A 57-year-old woman with a history of IV drug use is admitted to the inpatient service with a diagnosis of SBP. The admitting intern reports that he performed a diagnostic paracentesis in the ER and sent it for a cell count and culture before starting cefotaxime. What else would you recommend?

KEY FACT

New-onset ascites should have diagnostic paracentesis; fluid should be sent for albumin, total protein, cell count, Gram stain, and culture.

KEY FACT

Albumin replacement: On Day 1, give 1.5 g/kg of 25% albumin; on Day 3, give 1.0 g/kg of 25% albumin.

> You add an order to start an albumin infusion to prevent hepatorenal syndrome. In addition, you call the lab to add a total protein, glucose, and LDH to rule out 2° peritonitis. The patient's ascitic fluid glucose level is 30; her ascitic fluid LDH is twice the level of serum; and her total protein level is 2 g/dL. What should you do next?
>
> You order stat supine and upright films of the abdomen, which reveal free air. General surgery is called, and the patient is immediately taken to the operating room for bowel perforation. The ascites culture eventually grows multiple organisms.

Defined as infection of ascitic fluid caused by translocation of enteric bacteria across the gut wall or mesenteric lymphatics. Virtually all cases are monomicrobial, with *E coli*, *Klebsiella*, *Enterococcus*, and *Pneumococcus* most frequently implicated.

Symptoms/Exam

Patients present with fever, ascites, and abdominal pain.

Differential

- **Culture-⊖ neutrocytic ascites:** PMN > 250; ⊖ culture. Treat as SBP.
- **Monomicrobial non-neutrocytic bacterascites:** PMN < 250; ⊕ culture. Treat if the patient becomes symptomatic for SBP.
- **Alcoholic hepatitis:** If PMN > 250, treat as SBP. If < 250, treat as SBP for 48 hours and discontinue treatment if all cultures are ⊖.
- **Perforated viscus:** PMN > 250; multiple organisms found on culture. The presence of 2 of the following suggests 2° bacterial peritonitis: total protein > 1 g, LDH higher than normal for serum, and glucose < 50.

Diagnosis

Diagnosis is established by a PMN count > 250, a ⊕ **culture** of ascitic fluid obtained via paracentesis, and exclusion of a surgical infection.

Treatment

- **Cefotaxime (or other third-generation cephalosporin):** Administer IV with an **albumin** infusion (to ↓ the incidence of hepatorenal syndrome).
- **Prophylaxis:**
  - **Prior SBP:** Norfloxacin QD, TMP-SMX QD, or ciprofloxacin 750 mg weekly.
  - **GI bleeding in the setting of cirrhosis:** Norfloxacin or TMP-SMX × 7 days (there is an ↑ risk of SBP in these patients).
  - **Ascites and ascitic protein < 1 g/dL OR bilirubin > 2.5 mg/dL:** Norfloxacin QD, TMP-SMX QD, or ciprofloxacin 750 mg weekly.

HEPATORENAL SYNDROME

- Characterized by **progressive renal failure** and < 500 mg/dL of **proteinuria** in the presence of **advanced liver failure** and **portal hypertension** with no other explainable cause.
- Believed to be caused by intense renal vasoconstriction, presumably resulting from failure of renal vasodilator synthesis. Also defined by lack of response to a fluid bolus or diuretic withdrawal. Can be rapidly progressive (type I, often as consequence of SBP) or insidious (type II).

- **Treatment:**
  - **Supportive care:** IV albumin, with octreotide and midodrine to ↑ mean arterial pressure by 15 mmHg.
  - **Liver transplantation:** Survival is essentially zero without liver transplantation.
  - Hemodialysis alone does not improve patient outcome and is used only for patients awaiting transplantation.

HEPATIC ENCEPHALOPATHY

Causes are multifactorial, but the **ammonia hypothesis** is still the predominant etiology. **Usually has a precipitating cause,** including GI bleeding (↑ urea levels and ammonia levels); hyponatremia; hypokalemia (↓ renal ammonia excretion); alkalosis (favors $NH_4 \rightarrow NH_3$, which crosses the blood–brain barrier); infection; TIPS placement; or constipation (↓ GI clearance of ammonia). Exacerbated by hypoxia and sedatives/tranquilizers.

SYMPTOMS/EXAM/DIAGNOSIS

Initially presents as sleep disturbances but progresses to disorientation and confusion, with asterixis and other neurologic signs. Usually diagnosed clinically; ↑ **ammonia** is common, but the level does not correlate with severity.

TREATMENT

- **Correct the precipitating event**—eg, NG lavage, potassium.
- **Pharmacotherapy: Lactulose;** a retention enema can be used if oral lactulose is not well tolerated. **Antibiotics** (eg, neomycin, rifaximin) can be used; flumazenil can be considered if symptoms are worsened by benzodiazepines.

HEPATOPULMONARY SYNDROME

Characterized by the triad of (1) chronic liver disease, (2) an ↑ alveolar-arterial (A-a) O_2 gradient on room air, and (3) intrapulmonary vascular dilatations leading to right-to-left intrapulmonary shunts. Thought to be caused by failure of the liver to clear pulmonary vasodilators.

SYMPTOMS/EXAM

Usually characterized by dyspnea; **platypnea** and **orthodeoxia** (shortness of breath and deoxygenation in the upright position) are suggestive. There is a correlation between hepatopulmonary syndrome and the presence of **spider angiomata.**

DIAGNOSIS

- **Contrast-enhanced echocardiography:** A useful screen for pulmonary vascular dilatations. **Macroaggregated albumin lung perfusion scanning** is more specific and is used to confirm the diagnosis.
- High-resolution CT scanning may also detect dilatations.

TREATMENT

Methylene blue may improve oxygenation (inhibits nitric oxide–induced vasodilation). **Liver transplantation** may reverse the syndrome.

TABLE 5.7.   **Child-Pugh Scoring System**

	1 POINT	**2 POINTS**	**3 POINTS**
Encephalopathy grade	None	Mild confusion/lethargy	Marked confusion/coma
Bilirubin (mg/dL)	< 2	2–3	> 3
Ascites	None	Mild-moderate	Severe or refractory
Albumin (mg/dL)	> 3.5	2.8–3.5	< 2.8
INR	< 1.7	1.7–2.3	> 2.3

Total Points	**Classification**	**1-Year Survival**	**2-Year Survival**
5–6	Class A	100%	85%
7–9	Class B	80%	60%
10–15	Class C	45%	35%

END-STAGE LIVER DISEASE (ESLD)

Etiology: Alcohol and chronic viral hepatitis. Other etiologies include autoimmune, metabolic (hemochromatosis, Wilson disease, α_1-antitrypsin), biliary (1° biliary cirrhosis, 1° sclerosing cholangitis), and vascular (Budd-Chiari, nonalcoholic fatty liver disease) disorders.

SYMPTOMS/EXAM

Jaundice, spider angiomata, icterus, palmar erythema, asterixis, ascites, splenomegaly, peripheral edema.

DIAGNOSIS

- Clinical history (alcohol abuse, IV drug use, known hepatitis, family history of liver disease).
- **Labs:** Hypoalbuminemia, ↑ INR, thrombocytopenia, macrocytic anemia, hyperbilirubinemia.
- **Radiology:** Evidence of fibrosis on ultrasound or CT scan.
- **Biopsy:** Shows cirrhosis.

PROGNOSIS

- MELD score: A scoring system reflecting total bilirubin, INR, and creatinine. Directly correlates with mortality. System used for assigning rank for patients listed for liver transplant. Calculators can be used to determine 90-day mortality risk.
- Child-Pugh classification system: A scoring system used to rank severity of cirrhosis and predict survival. Used by surgeons to determine pre-op risk stratification (see Table 5.7).

ESOPHAGEAL VARICES

A 52-year-old man with recently diagnosed HBV with cirrhosis establishes care with you. He does not have ascites but did have an EGD showing esophageal varices. What do you recommend?
Propranolol titrated to ↓ his heart rate by 25% or to 50–60 bpm.

Dilated submucosal veins due to portal hypertension that may bleed. Approximately one-half of all cirrhotic patients have varices, and one-third of all varices bleed. The mortality rate associated with variceal bleed is 20%; risk factors include size, the presence of "red color" markings, high Child-Pugh class, and active alcohol use. Gastric varices are also common.

SYMPTOMS/EXAM/DIAGNOSIS

Asymptomatic unless there is acute hemorrhage (see the discussion of upper GI bleeding below). Patients with cirrhosis should be screened with endoscopy.

TREATMENT

See the section on upper GI bleeding below.

- **Banding and sclerotherapy:** Acute therapy for bleeding varices. Both measures arrest and prevent rebleeding, although their effect on in-hospital mortality is unclear.
- **Prophylaxis against SBP** or other serious infection (see section on SBP above).
- **Somatostatin or octreotide drips:** ↓ splanchnic flow and portal pressures.
- **Balloon tube tamponade** (Minnesota, Sengstaken-Blakemore tubes): Have a high complication rate (esophageal ulceration, aspiration, perforation); used when bleeding cannot be controlled medically or endoscopically while awaiting TIPS/portosystemic shunt.
- **TIPS/portosystemic shunt:** Create a decompressive shunt between the portal and hepatic veins. Associated with high mortality rates.
- **1° prophylaxis for variceal hemorrhage:** Prophylaxis with nonselective β-blockers (propranolol, nadolol) is preferable to prophylactic banding therapy and offers a slightly better reduction in the risk of bleeding, but is more invasive. The goal for medical prophylaxis is generally to ↓ resting heart rate by 25% or to 50–60 bpm. Nitrates are **not** recommended.

KEY FACT

Approximately one-half of cirrhotic patients have varices, and one-third of varices bleed. The mortality rate associated with bleed is 20%.

Biliary Disease

GALLSTONES AND ACUTE CHOLECYSTITIS

Caused by **aberrations in the solubilization of cholesterol.** More common in women and Native Americans. Risk factors include obesity, insulin resistance, rapid weight loss, and pregnancy. Cholecystitis is usually caused by an impaction of a gallstone (90% of cases).

SYMPTOMS

- **Cholelithiasis:** May be asymptomatic or may cause variable amounts of **RUQ or epigastric pain,** often after eating.
- **Acute cholecystitis:** Presents with **fever** and **severe RUQ or epigastric pain** that may radiate to the infrascapular area. Symptoms are usually precipitated by a large or fatty meal and typically resolve after 12 hours. Vomiting is common.

EXAM

- Usually normal or may reveal mild RUQ tenderness in cholelithiasis.
- In acute cholecystitis, exam reveals RUQ tenderness, a ⊕ **Murphy sign,** guarding, and rebound pain. The gallbladder may be palpable, and jaundice may be present.

DIFFERENTIAL

- **Biliary dyskinesia:** Biliary colic in the setting of ⊖ initial radiographic studies. Usually caused by undetected stenosis, adhesions, or kinking in the cystic duct. Diagnosed by ↓ gallbladder emptying on scintigraphy following cholecystokinin injection. Cholecystectomy is curative.
- **Acalculous cholecystitis:** Patients at high risk include those who have undergone major surgery and critically ill patients without enteral feeding for prolonged periods.
- **Infectious cholecystitis:** Found in HIV-⊕ patients, those with CMV, and those with crypto- or microsporidiosis.
- **Cholangitis:** Highly suspicious if jaundice is present (a component of Charcot triad, along with fever and RUQ pain).
- See the acute abdomen discussion in the Surgery chapter for a comprehensive differential.

DIAGNOSIS

- **Labs:** Labs are usually normal in cholelithiasis. In acute cholecystitis, there may be leukocytosis along with ↑ serum bilirubin, aminotransferases, and alkaline phosphatase.
- **Imaging:**
  - **RUQ ultrasound:** Most frequent first-line test (see Figure 5.10). Demonstrates the presence of stones in cholelithiasis. Can demonstrate cholelithiasis, gallbladder wall thickening, pericholecystic fluid, and a sonographic Murphy sign. **Contrast-enhanced CT** also shows good performance in making this diagnosis and can be used when ultrasound is not available.
  - **HIDA scan:** Can demonstrate obstruction in the cystic duct, but reliable only if **bilirubin is < 5 mg/dL.**
- **Cholangiography:** Usually performed intraoperatively to rule out choledocholithiasis or preoperatively by ERCP or MRCP.

TREATMENT

- **Asymptomatic gallstones:** Cholecystectomy is indicated if the **gallbladder wall appears calcified, or in young patients with sickle-cell disease and in patients with rapid weight loss.**
- **Symptomatic gallstones:** Laparoscopic cholecystectomy is indicated.
- Cheno- and ursodeoxycholic acids can dissolve some cholesterol stones in patients who refuse cholecystectomy or are poor surgical candidates.

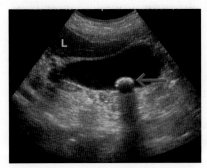 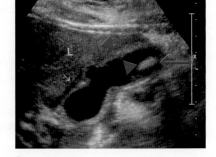

A   B

FIGURE 5.10. Gallstone disease. (A) Cholelithiasis. Ultrasound image of the gallbladder shows a gallstone *(arrow)* with posterior shadowing. (B) Acute cholecystitis. Ultrasound image shows a gallstone *(red arrow)*, a thickened gallbladder wall *(arrowheads)*, and pericholecystic fluid *(white arrow)*. L = liver. (Reproduced, with permission, from USMLERx.com.)

- **Acute cholecystitis: NPO, IV fluids, pain control, antibiotics.** Laparoscopic cholecystectomy is indicated after acute illness resolves. Percutaneous cholecystostomy/ultrasound-guided aspiration may be considered in patients with a high operative risk.

COMPLICATIONS

- **Gangrene:** Suggested by progression of symptoms, including severe abdominal pain, fever, vomiting, and hypotension. Cholecystectomy is mandatory.
- **Perforation:** Develops a picture of generalized peritonitis, although it usually remains anatomically localized. Cholecystectomy is mandatory.
- **Gallstone ileus:** Mechanical obstruction by a stone in the bowel (usually the ileocecal valve) caused by passage of a gallstone through a cholecystenteric fistula.
- **Repeated episodes** can cause chronic inflammation, leading to choledocholithiasis, fistulization to the bowel, pancreatitis, and, rarely, carcinoma of the gallbladder.

CHOLEDOCHOLITHIASIS AND CHOLANGITIS

- **Choledocholithiasis:** Presence of gallstone in the common bile duct (occurs in 15% of patients with gallstones).
- **Cholangitis:** An infection within the common bile duct, usually (85% of the time) resulting from a common bile duct stone.

SYMPTOMS/EXAM

- Symptoms develop if **obstruction occurs** and causes biliary colic and jaundice.
- **Pain, jaundice,** and **fever (Charcot triad)** are classic findings in cholangitis.
- In acute suppurative cholangitis, patients may also present with **confusion and hypotension (Reynolds pentad).**
- Exam reveals RUQ tenderness, icterus, and hepatomegaly.

DIFFERENTIAL

Carcinoma; Mirizzi syndrome (gallbladder neck stone compressing the common bile duct); benign biliary stricture; cholestatic liver disease (1° sclerosing cholangitis, 1° biliary sclerosis, drug-induced cholestasis); external obstruction; congenital disease (biliary atresia, choledochal cysts); parasites (*Ascaris lumbricoides*, *Echinococcus* spp).

DIAGNOSIS

- **Ultrasound:** The usual initial test to detect bile duct dilation.
- **ERCP:** Determines the cause, location, and extent of biliary obstruction; also preferred for interventions. **MRCP** for patients who cannot undergo ERCP.
- **Labs:** ↑ bilirubin, alkaline phosphatase, GGT, and PT/INR. Elevation of aminotransferases in the 1000s may be seen if acute necrosis of hepatocytes occurs.

TREATMENT

- **Choledocholithiasis:** Endoscopic papillotomy and stone extraction followed by cholecystectomy.

- **Choledocholithasis with cholangitis:** Broad-spectrum antibiotics with ERCP, sphincterotomy, and stone extraction on an urgent or emergent basis.
- Vitamin K to correct coagulopathy may be required.

Pancreatic Disease

ACUTE PANCREATITIS

Disease ranges from edematous to necrotizing pancreatitis. The most common etiologies are **biliary disease** and **alcohol.** Other etiologies include drugs (2%–5%), postoperative or post-ERCP, trauma, hypertriglyceridemia, viral infection (eg, mumps), vasculitis, pancreas divisum, sphincter of Oddi dysfunction, and hypercalcemia. May also be idiopathic.

SYMPTOMS

- Presents with a steady abdominal pain, with radiation to the back, chest, and lower abdomen.
- The pain worsens in a supine position and improves in a fetal position.
- Nausea, vomiting, distention due to GI hypomobility, and chemical peritonitis are common.

EXAM

- Patients appear distressed, with fever, tachycardia, hypotension, and shock as well as with variable degrees of abdominal tenderness and rigidity.
- Diminished bowel sounds are noted.
- **Cullen sign** (ecchymosis at the umbilicus) and **Grey Turner sign** (ecchymosis of the flanks) point to severe necrotizing pancreatitis.
- Occasionally, left pulmonary rales and/or pleural effusion may be present.

DIFFERENTIAL

Perforated viscus (peptic ulcer), acute cholecystitis, biliary colic, acute intestinal obstruction, mesenteric vascular occlusion, renal colic, MI, dissecting aortic aneurysm, vasculitis, pneumonia, DKA (causing false elevation of amylase).

DIAGNOSIS

- Labs:
  - **Serum lipase:** Specificity is 85%–100%.
  - CBC may show leukocytosis and anemia (due to hemorrhage); chemistry may show hyperglycemia and hypocalcemia. LFTs may reveal transient elevation of AST, alkaline phosphatase, and bilirubin. An **ALT > 150** is 96% sensitive for gallstone-related pancreatitis. An albumin level < 3.0 suggests greater severity and higher mortality.
  - **ABGs:** Reveal hypoxemia in cases of impending ARDS.
  - **Ranson criteria:** Used to assess severity of acute pancreatitis (see Table 5.8).
- Imaging:
  - **AXR:** Important for excluding other diagnoses. Can assess for bowel obstruction or free intraperitoneal air.
  - **Ultrasound:** Often used for initial investigation if pancreatitis is suspected. Efficacy is limited by obesity and intestinal gas.

KEY FACT

In patients < 35 years of age with a strong family history and recurrent episodes of pancreatitis, consider genetic causes.

MNEMONIC

Causes of acute pancreatitis:

I GET SMASHED

Idiopathic
Gallstones
Ethanol
Trauma
Steroids
Mumps
Autoimmune (PAN)
Scorpion stings
Hyperlipidemia/**H**ypercalcemia
ERCP
Drugs (including azathioprine and diuretics)

TABLE 5.8.   Ranson Criteria

Presence of ≥ 3 of the following factors on admission is 60%–80% sensitive for severe necrotizing pancreatitis:	Development of the following factors in the first 48 hours indicates a worse prognosis:
Age > 55 years	Hematocrit decrease > 10%
WBC > 16,000	BUN increase > 5
Glucose > 200	$Pao_2 < 60$
LDH > 350	Ca < 8
AST > 250	Base deficit > 4
	Estimated fluid sequestration > 6 L

One point for each criteria; with each point, the mortality rate increases:
0–2 = 1%
3–4 = 16%
5–6 = 40%
7–8 = 100%

- **CT scan** (IV contrast preferred): The best imaging study. Can confirm the diagnosis when amylase levels are normal; also indicates severity. Not as sensitive or specific as serum lipase level. CT scan is not indicated unless pancreatic necrosis or other developing complication is suspected or the diagnosis of pancreatitis is in doubt (see Figure 5.11).
- **Contrast-enhanced dynamic CT:** Indicated in the presence of > 2 Ranson criteria as well as for patients who are seriously ill or clinically deteriorating.
- **MRI/MRCP:** Increasingly used. Advantages include absence of ionizing radiation, excellent assessment for fluid collections, and detection of choledocholithiasis rivaling ERCP.

TREATMENT

- **NPO** and **IV fluids; NG tube** if needed.
- **Analgesics:** Typically morphine or fentanyl PCA.
- **Early refeeding** (with fat restriction): Increasingly supported by evidence.
- **Early enteral nutrition (jejunum).**
- **Antibiotics:** Broad-spectrum antibiotics for severe cases. **Fungicides** may also be needed with prolonged antibiotic use.
- For gallstone pancreatitis, urgent ERCP with papillotomy; planned cholecystectomy.

COMPLICATIONS

- **Infected pancreatic necrosis** 1–2 weeks after onset.
- **Pancreatic abscess** 4–6 weeks after onset (see Figure 5.11C.)
- **Pseudocysts** may develop over 1–4 weeks, diagnosed by sonography or CT; resolves in 25%–40% of patients; drainage considered if complicated (ie, infection) or if > 5 cm and persists for > 6 weeks (see Figure 5.11B).
- **Pancreatic ascites** is caused by an internal fistula between a duct or pseudocyst and the peritoneal cavity.
- **Pancreatic pleural effusions** are caused by a fistula between the duct and pleural space.

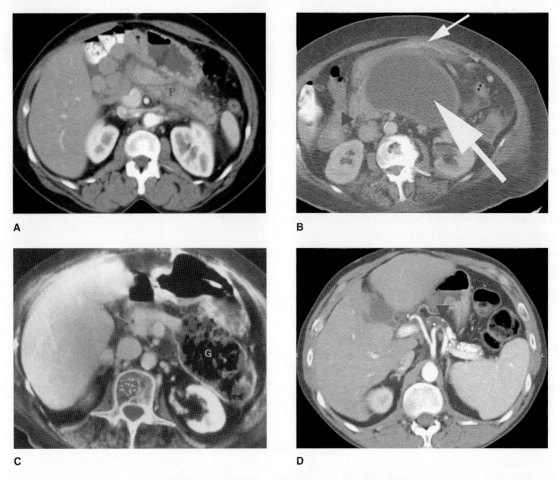

FIGURE 5.11. **Transaxial contrast-enhanced CT evaluation of acute and chronic pancreatitis.** (A) Uncomplicated acute pancreatitis. Peripancreatic fluid and fat stranding can be seen *(arrows)*. P = pancreas. **(B)** Pancreatic pseudocyst *(large arrow)*. The stomach is compressed anteriorly *(small arrow)*. The arrowhead indicates the pancreatic head. **(C)** Pancreatic abscess. A rim-enhancing collection of fluid and air (G) replaces the body and tail of the pancreas. The arrowhead indicates the pancreatic head. **(D)** Chronic pancreatitis. Note the dilated pancreatic duct *(arrowhead)* and pancreatic calcifications *(arrow)*. (Images A and D reproduced, with permission, from USMLERx.com. Image B reproduced, with permission, from Doherty GM. *Current Diagnosis & Treatment: Surgery,* 13th ed. New York: McGraw-Hill, 2010, Fig. 26-3B. Image C reproduced, with permission, from Chen MY, et al. *Basic Radiology.* New York: McGraw-Hill, 2004, Fig. 11-67.)

MNEMONIC

Causes of chronic pancreatitis:

TIGAR-O

Toxic/metabolic (alcohol, hypercalcemia, severe protein-calorie malnutrition)
Idiopathic
Genetic
Autoimmune
Recurrent severe/acute
Obstructive

CHRONIC PANCREATITIS

The causes of chronic pancreatitis are outlined in the mnemonic **TIGAR-O**. The majority of cases are associated with alcoholism.

Symptoms/Exam

May present with symptoms identical to those of acute pancreatitis; however, the pain pattern may be variable and located in the upper quadrants of the back or upper abdomen. Late symptoms and signs include weight loss, steatorrhea, and DM.

Differential

Same as acute pancreatitis (see above).

Diagnosis

- Labs:
  - **Amylase and lipase:** May be ↑ or **normal.**
  - ↑ alkaline phosphatase or bilirubin is seen if inflammation leading to ductal obstruction is present.

- ↑ fasting glucose, ↑ fecal fat, and cobalamin malabsorption are seen in later stages.
- **Classic triad: Pancreatic calcifications, steatorrhea,** and **DM** are pathognomonic.
- **Secretion stimulation test:** Perform if the classic triad is not present (⊕ when 60% of exocrine function is lost).
- Serum trypsinogen is low.
- **Imaging:** Sonography, CT, and ERCP (to delineate anatomy and to find a possible source amenable to intervention) are also used (see Figure 5.11).

> **KEY FACT**
>
> Approximately 70%–80% of chronic pancreatitis cases are associated with alcoholism.

TREATMENT

- **Treat pain:** Avoid alcohol and large fatty meals; narcotics may be needed for pain management.
- Pancreatic enzyme replacement; treat DM.
- Ductal decompression or pancreatic resection in selected cases.

COMPLICATIONS

Associated with ↑ risk of pancreatic carcinoma.

GI Malignancies

ESOPHAGEAL CANCER

Most often affects patients 50–70 years of age, with a male-to-female ratio of 3:1. **Squamous cell carcinoma** is strongly associated with chronic alcohol use and smoking and is also more common in blacks. In the majority of cases, **adenocarcinoma** develops from Barrett esophagus. A diet low in fruits and vegetables is a risk factor, as is obesity.

SYMPTOMS/EXAM

- Presents with solid food dysphagia that progresses over weeks to months. Weight loss is common.
- Cough on swallowing, chest or back pain, and voice hoarseness are seen with invasive disease.

DIAGNOSIS

- **Endoscopy with biopsy:** Disease is usually incurable at the time of diagnosis (see Figure 5.12).

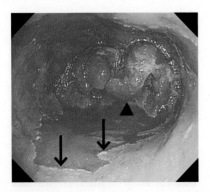

FIGURE 5.12. **Esophageal cancer.** An esophageal adenocarcinoma *(arrowhead)* is seen on endoscopy against a background of the pink tongues of Barrett esophagus *(arrowheads)*. (Reproduced, with permission, from Fauci AS, et al. *Harrison's Principles of Internal Medicine,* 17th ed. New York: McGraw-Hill, 2008, Fig. 285-3D.)

- **CT of the chest and liver:** For disease staging.
- If CT is ⊖, endoscopic ultrasound should be performed to evaluate wall involvement as well as local mediastinal and lymph node involvement (in conjunction with FNA). Bronchoscopy to evaluate airways for invasive disease.

TREATMENT

- **Early-stage disease:** May be cured by **surgery alone** (transhiatal esophagectomy with anastomosis of the stomach with cervical esophagus). Radiation plus chemotherapy with cisplatin or 5-FU is more effective than radiation alone.
- **Advanced local spread or distant metastases:** Surgery is not warranted. Palliative treatment should be directed toward dysphagia and pain relief. Radiation and chemotherapy have significant side effects and may be considered in otherwise healthy patients with good functional status and minimal medical problems.
- Prognosis is poor, with a 5-year survival rate of 15%.

GASTRIC CANCER

Adenocarcinoma is the most common form of gastric cancer. Mean age at diagnosis is 63 years; uncommon in patients < 40 years of age. The male-to-female ratio is 2:1. It is more common among patients of Hispanic, black, and Asian descent. Additional risk factors include chronic *H pylori* gastritis (responsible for 35%–90% of distal cases), chronic atrophic gastritis, pernicious anemia, and a history of partial gastric resection.

SYMPTOMS/EXAM

- Presents with dyspepsia, vague epigastric pain, anorexia, early satiety or vomiting, weight loss, occult fecal blood (and iron deficiency anemia), hematemesis, and melena. A gastric mass is palpable in 20% of cases.
- Metastatic spread may reveal palpable **left supraclavicular or umbilical nodes** (Virchow and Sister Mary Joseph nodes, respectively), a **rigid rectal shelf** (Blumer shelf), or **ovarian metastases** (Krukenberg tumor).

DIAGNOSIS

- **Endoscopy with brush cytology and biopsy:** Should be performed on any patient > 50 years of age with dyspepsia who does not respond to a short course of acid suppression (see Figure 5.13).
- **Staging:** Performed with abdominal CT and endoscopic ultrasound.

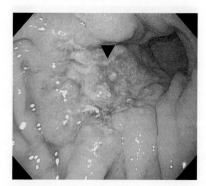

FIGURE 5.13.   Gastric cancer. A malignant gastric ulcer (*arrowhead*) involving the greater curvature of the stomach is seen on endoscopy. (Reproduced, with permission, from Fauci AS, et al. *Harrison's Principles of Internal Medicine,* 17th ed. New York: McGraw-Hill, 2008, Fig. 285-2B.)

TREATMENT

- **Localized disease: Surgical resection** (depending on the location and extent of disease) can be curative. Chemotherapy and radiation confer no additional benefit.
- **Advanced disease:** Patients may have palliative tumor resection or, for unresectable tumors, a gastrojejunostomy (to prevent bleeding and obstruction by tumor). Chemotherapy may be used for palliation (single or multiagent with fluorouracil, doxorubicin, cisplatin, or mitomycin).
- **Prognosis:** 15% 5-year survival rate. However, long-term survival is > 45% in patients who undergo curative resection.

COLORECTAL CANCER

A 44-year-old male construction worker comes to your office to establish care. He is generally healthy but tells you that he occasionally sees blood on the toilet paper following a bowel movement. When asked about a family history of colorectal cancer, he recalls that his father had in fact been diagnosed with "cancer in his rectum" when he was 52 years of age. Anoscopy reveals internal hemorrhoids. What is the next appropriate step?

The patient is at high risk for colorectal cancer, and screening should have begun at 42 years of age. You refer your patient for colonoscopy, which is normal, aside from revealing internal hemorrhoids. You advise the patient to use stool softeners and to avoid excessive straining at work, and his hemorrhoids subsequently improve. You remind him that he needs to be screened in another 5 years or, if he has any symptoms, sooner.

Colorectal cancer is the **second leading cause of death due to cancer** in the United States, with a 6% lifetime risk. Almost all cases are **adenocarcinomas,** and slightly < 50% are distal to the splenic flexure. Colorectal cancer is believed to arise from transformation of adenomatous polyps. Risk factors include age > 45 years (incidence ↑ sharply), IBD, a diet high in fats and red meat, black race, and a ⊕ family history (risk doubles if a first-degree relative has been diagnosed, quadruples if 2 family members have been diagnosed, and ↑ further if relatives were diagnosed at an early age). **Predisposing conditions** include the following:

- **Adenomatous polyps:** Present in 35% of patients > 50 years of age. The risk of progression to cancer ranges from < 4% to > 10%, depending on size and histologic features (larger size and villous features carry an ↑ risk). Commonly removed by colonoscopic polypectomy.
- **Familial adenomatous polyposis (FAP):** An autosomal-dominant syndrome characterized by **> 100 colonic adenomatous polyps.** Polyps appear by 15 years of age, adenomatous polyps by 35 years of age, and **colorectal cancer by 50 years of age.** Colectomy or proctocolectomy is indicated before 20 years of age.
- **Hereditary nonpolyposis colorectal cancer (HNPCC):** An autosomal-dominant syndrome; also ↑ risk for endometrial and other cancers. Associated with a **70%–80% lifetime risk of colorectal cancer.** Typically, only a **few adenomas** develop, but these tend to be villous, with high-grade dysplasia. If cancer is found, treatment is subtotal colectomy.

SYMPTOMS/EXAM

- Presents with occult bleeding, hematochezia from the right colon, colicky abdominal pain, and altered bowel habits from obstruction in the left colon.
- Rectal cancers may present with tenesmus, urgency, and hematochezia. Weight loss is uncommon.
- Rectal exam may reveal a mass or fixation. Abdominal masses may be palpable, and the liver edge may be enlarged in the presence of metastases.

DIAGNOSIS

- **Colonoscopy:** The procedure of choice, as it permits biopsy. If the cecum cannot be reached, CT colonography or barium enema may be considered (see Figure 5.14).
- **CEA:** ↑; a level of > 5 ng/mL is predictive of a poorer prognosis.
- **Labs: Iron deficiency anemia with blood loss; liver enzymes may be ↑** if metastases are present.
- **Staging:**
  - **Colon cancer:** CT of the abdomen and pelvis +/– CXR or chest CT.
  - **Rectal cancer:** Pelvic MRI or endorectal ultrasound and chest CT.

TREATMENT

- **Resection and regional lymph node dissection:** Even in advanced disease, a palliative resection can ↓ the likelihood of complications such as obstruction or bleeding. Transanal resections may be performed for some rectal cancers. Resection of isolated liver or lung metastases (1–3 sites) may improve survival.
- **Adjuvant chemotherapy and radiation:**
  - **Colon cancer:** Chemotherapy can be appropriate for node-⊕ disease. Radiation may be considered with locally advanced disease.
  - **Rectal cancer:** Treatment is more aggressive, involving **combination chemotherapy** and **radiation** with locally advanced disease.
- **Surveillance in survivors:**
  - **Colon cancer:** Evaluate every 3–6 months for 3–5 years with a history and exam, FOBT, LFTs, and CEA. Colonoscopy should be performed 6–12 months after surgery and every 3–5 years thereafter.
  - **Rectal cancer:** As with colon cancer, but sigmoidoscopy every 6–12 months for 3 years.
  - Any change in the clinical picture warrants a CXR and an abdominal CT to look for metastases.

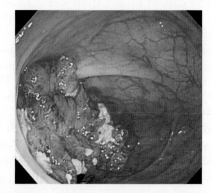

FIGURE 5.14. **Colon cancer.** Colonoscopy reveals an adenocarcinoma growing into the lumen of the colon. (Reproduced, with permission, from Fauci AS, et al. *Harrison's Principles of Internal Medicine,* 17th ed. New York: McGraw-Hill, 2008, Fig. 285-6.)

PREVENTION

Measures of **1° prevention** include the following:

- **Screening methods:** Annual FOBT; flexible sigmoidoscopy every 5 years; FOBT plus flexible sigmoidoscopy every 5 years; colonoscopy every 10 years or barium enema every 5–10 years. CT colonography may emerge in the coming years as an alternative screening method.
- Screen according to level of risk:
  - **Average risk:** No family history or 1 second- or third-degree relative with cancer. Begin screening at 50 years of age.
  - **Elevated risk:** Refers to patients with a first-degree relative diagnosed with cancer/adenoma at > 60 years of age or 2 or more second-degree relatives with cancer only. Begin screening at 40 years of age.
  - **High risk:** Describes patients with a first-degree relative diagnosed with cancer/adenoma at < 60 years of age or 2 first-degree relatives with cancer/adenoma. Begin screening at 40 years of age or when the patient is 10 years younger than the family member's age at diagnosis; repeat every 5 years.
- **Adenomatous polyp on screening colonoscopy:** Repeat colonoscopy in 5 years, unless polyp was > 9 mm in size or there were 3 or more adenomatous polyps found, in which case repeat in 3 years.
- **FAP:** Genetic testing offered to first-degree family members after 10 years of age; if inconclusive, sigmoidoscopy performed beginning at 12 years of age. Upper endoscopic evaluation of the duodenum/periampullary area every 1–3 years.
- **HNPCC:** Offer genetic counseling and testing if the family history is suggestive. If testing is ⊕, screen with colonoscopy every 1–2 years starting at 25 years of age or when the patient is 5 years younger than the age of the family member at diagnosis. Also screen annually for endometrial cancer among patients 25–35 years of age with endometrial aspirate or transvaginal ultrasound (or consider prophylactic TAH-BSO).
- **IBD:** No consensus; the general recommendation is colonoscopy every 1–2 years beginning 8 years after a diagnosis of IBD.
- **Prognosis:** The long-term prognosis is 90% with early-stage cancer but is < 5% with metastatic disease. The prognosis for rectal cancer worsens with each stage.

HEPATOCELLULAR CARCINOMA (HCC)

Associated with cirrhosis in general, especially HBV/HCV and alcoholic liver disease. Other associations include aflatoxin exposure, hemochromatosis, α_1-antitrypsin deficiency, and tyrosinemia.

SYMPTOMS/EXAM

- Patients typically present in a deteriorated state, with cirrhosis, cachexia, weakness, and weight loss.
- Bloody ascites may occur suddenly (suggesting portal or hepatic vein thrombosis or bleeding from a tumor).
- Exam may show hepatomegaly or a palpable mass. A bruit may be audible over the tumor.

DIAGNOSIS

- α-fetoprotein (AFP) is ↑ in 70% of cases but is **nonspecific.**
- **Triple- or quad-phase liver CT scan:** Preferred initial imaging studies (see Figure 5.15).

KEY FACT

HCC usually develops in the setting of cirrhosis, except in chronic HBV.

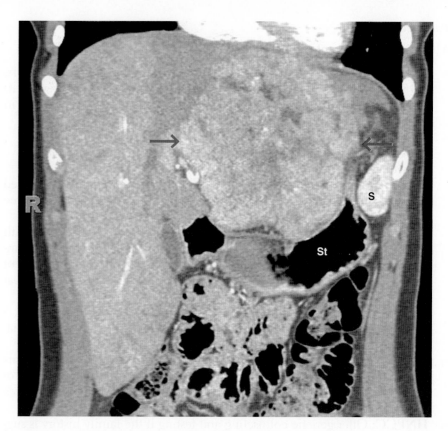

FIGURE 5.15. **Hepatocellular carcinoma.** Coronal reformation from a contrast-enhanced CT shows a large HCC in the left hepatic lobe *(arrows)*. St = stomach; S = spleen. (Reproduced, with permission, from USMLERx.com.)

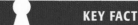

KEY FACT

A ⊕ imaging test with ↑ AFP > 200 µg/L is adequate for the diagnosis of HCC.

- **Liver biopsy:** Diagnostic, but imaging with ↑ AFP can be sufficient. Biopsy may be deferred if surgical resection is planned because of possible seeding of the needle tract.

TREATMENT

- **Surgical resection:** May result in cure, but not possible in advanced cirrhosis or when the tumor is multifocal. Chemotherapy with sorafenib (a tyrosine kinase inhibitor) may help to prolong survival by up to 3 months.
- **Liver transplantation:** Associated with 5-year survival in up to 75% of cases.
- **Palliative measures:** Include chemoembolization via the hepatic artery; small tumors may be amenable to ethanol injection, radiofrequency ablation, or cryotherapy.

PREVENTION

- Screening for liver cancer is controversial.
- **AFP:** Often ↑ in HCC, but levels do not correlate with size or stage. Also ↑ in pregnancy, gonadal tumors, and chronic liver disease (especially HCV). At low cutoff values, the test is nonspecific; at high cutoffs, the test loses sensitivity despite high specificity (> 500 µg/L in high-risk patients is virtually diagnostic).
- **Ultrasound:** Noninvasive and widely available, but sensitivity range is 40%–78%.
- Despite these limitations, many clinicians measure AFP and ultrasonography **every 6 months** in patients with Child-Pugh class A cirrhosis or

chronic HBV who would be suitable candidates for partial hepatectomy, liver transplantation, or other percutaneous therapies.

- Others recommend imaging alone every 6–12 months, either by ultrasound, CT, or MRI.
- **Prognosis:** For locally resectable disease, 5-year survival is 56%. For unresectable disease, 5-year survival is virtually zero.

PANCREATIC CANCER

Risk factors include age, obesity, tobacco use, prior abdominal radiation, and a ⊕ family history of pancreatic cancer.

SYMPTOMS/EXAM

- Presents with vague, diffuse pain in the epigastrium or LUQ (if the tail is involved) with occasional radiation to the back. Pain that is relieved by sitting or leaning forward suggests inoperable spread of disease. However, may also be painless.
- Diarrhea may be an early symptom; weight loss and depression are late signs.
- May also present with pancreatitis, and jaundice (sometimes painless) may be present with obstruction. A palpable gallbladder (**Courvoisier sign**) may be present. A hard, fixed epigastric mass may be palpable.

DIAGNOSIS

- **Multiphase thin-cut spiral CT or MRI:** Detects most tumors, demonstrates vessel invasion, delineates the extent of disease, and allows for FNA. **ERCP or MRCP** can aid in diagnosis if CT or MRI is ambiguous.
- **Endoscopic ultrasonography:** Also aids in diagnosis by demonstrating venous or gastric invasion.
- **Labs: CA 19-9** has not proved sensitive enough (70%) for early detection. Specificity is 87%; ↑ values are also found in acute and chronic pancreatitis and cholangitis.
- **Other:** Mild anemia, impaired glucose intolerance, and ↑ amylase/lipase may be seen. LFTs may suggest obstructive jaundice.

PREVENTION

In patients with a ⊕ family history, consider screening with **spiral CT or endoscopic ultrasound** beginning 10 years earlier than the age of the family member at diagnosis.

TREATMENT

- **Lesions limited to the head, periampullary zone, and duodenum:** Resection by a **Whipple procedure** (pancreaticoduodenectomy) is associated with a 20%–25% 5-year survival rate, increasing to 40% in the presence of ⊖ margins and lymph nodes. Adjuvant chemotherapy with fluorouracil or gemcitabine is beneficial.
- **Unresectable lesions:** Treatment is palliative. Treat jaundice with endoscopic stenting of the bile duct or cholecystojejunostomy; duodenal obstruction can be treated or prevented by gastrojejunostomy or endoscopic placement of a self-expandable duodenal stent. Combined irradiation and chemotherapy may be used for palliation of unresectable cancer confined to the pancreas.
- **Metastatic disease:** Chemotherapy has been disappointing in metastatic pancreatic cancer, although improved response rates have been reported with gemcitabine.

- Celiac plexus nerve block or thoracoscopic splanchnicectomy may improve pain control.
- **Prognosis** is poor, with a 2%–5% 5-year survival rate for masses in the body and tail and a 20%–40% rate for ampullary lesions.

GI Bleeding

ACUTE UPPER GI BLEEDING

More common in patients > 60 years of age. Associated with a mortality rate of 10%, but mortality is usually due to complications of underlying disease, not exsanguination. Etiologies include peptic ulcers, varices, Mallory-Weiss tears, erosive esophagitis, gastritis (eg, NSAIDs, alcohol) and duodenitis, malignancy, vascular anomalies (ectasias, Dieulafoy lesion), aortoenteric fistula, and hemobilia (see Figure 5.16).

SYMPTOMS/EXAM

- Commonly presents as **melena** or **hematemesis** (bright red or coffee-ground emesis). Melena develops with as little as 50–100 mL of bleeding.
- Ten percent of cases present with hematochezia, but this requires > 1000 mL of bleeding.
- Symptoms and signs of predisposing diseases may be present (eg, a history of retching; stigmata of liver disease).

DIAGNOSIS/TREATMENT

- **Initial resuscitation and stabilization:**
  - Patients should be **NPO; discontinue aspirin, NSAIDs,** and any **anticoagulants.**
  - Place two 18-gauge IVs and initiate **aggressive fluid resuscitation** if there is hemodynamic compromise.
  - Place an **NG tube** for lavage. Aspiration of red blood or coffee-ground emesis confirms an upper GI source, but clear aspirate does not exclude it (eg, duodenal bleed). An aspirate that clears with lavage suggests lower-risk bleeding, whereas failure to clear points to a high-risk bleed.
- **Type and cross red blood cells.**
- The decision to transfuse should be based on the following criteria:
  - **Hematocrit:** Consider transfusion if hematocrit is < 25%–30% or if the patient is bleeding briskly, regardless of hematocrit. Hematocrit takes

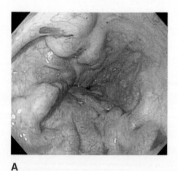
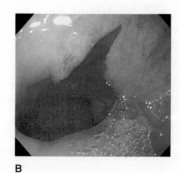
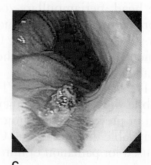
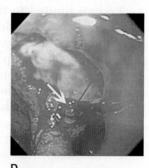

A   B   C   D

FIGURE 5.16. **Causes of upper GI bleed at endoscopy.** (A) Esophageal varices. (B) Mallory-Weiss tear. (C) Gastric ulcer with protuberant vessel. (D) Duodenal ulcer with active bleeding *(arrow)*. (Reproduced, with permission, from Fauci AS, et al. *Harrison's Principles of Internal Medicine,* 17th ed. New York: McGraw-Hill, 2008, Figs. 285-16, 285-18, and 285-15D and E.)

48–72 hours to equilibrate, so a normal value should not be considered reassuring in acute GI bleeding.

- **Platelets:** Transfuse if the platelet count is < 50,000 or if bleeding is due to platelet dysfunction.
- **INR:** Transfuse with FFP for values > 1.5. One unit of FFP is required for every 5 units of packed RBCs transfused.
- Send laboratory studies based on suspicion for disease etiology (eg, *H pylori*, LFTs, INR, BUN, creatinine).

- **Triage:**
    - **Discharge:** Healthy patients with normal hemodynamics, an aspirate that clears with NG lavage, and normal labs may be discharged. Endoscopy should be scheduled as an outpatient procedure. The risk of rebleeding is low if the patient presents < 48 hours after the event.
    - **Admit to the hospital:** All other patients must be admitted for observation and/or endoscopy.
    - **ICU admission:** Active bleeders, those with > 5 units of blood loss, and those with advanced liver disease or serious comorbidities must be admitted to the ICU.
- **Endoscopy:** All patients except those at low risk, as well as those with continued active bleeding, should have endoscopy within 12 hours of resuscitation and stabilization. Endoscopy is **diagnostic, prognostic,** and **therapeutic** (cautery, injection, or endoclips; injection of a sclerosant or application of a rubber band to the bleeding varix). Surgical intervention may be necessary if endoscopic interventions fail.
- **Other medical therapy:**
    - **IV PPIs:** ↓ the risk of rebleeding in peptic ulcers with high-risk features following endoscopic treatment. High doses of oral PPIs may also be effective.
    - **Octreotide infusion:** ↓ splanchnic blood flow and portal BP; effective in the initial control of variceal bleeding.
    - **Desmopressin (DDAVP):** Administer to uremic patients (those with dysfunctional platelets) with active bleeding.
    - **Refractory bleeding: Surgical intervention;** intra-arterial embolizations/vasopressin; **TIPS** for acute variceal hemorrhage.

ACUTE LOWER GI BLEEDING

Defined as bleeding occurring below the ligament of Treitz. Approximately 95% of cases arise from the colon. Lower GI bleeds tend to have a **more benign course** than upper GI bleeds, largely because there is less likelihood of hemodynamic compromise (see Table 5.9 for other factors that distinguish upper from lower GI bleeding). Etiologies correlate with age:

- **Patients < 50 years of age:** Associated with infectious colitis, hemorrhoids, fissures, and IBD.
- **Patients > 50 years of age:** Associated with diverticulosis, vascular ectasias, neoplasm/malignancy, ischemia, and recent polypectomy (generally 2 weeks postprocedure).

SYMPTOMS/EXAM

- Black stools (melena) indicate bleeding proximal to the ligament of Treitz; maroon stools point to the right colon or small intestine. Brown stools mixed or streaked with blood indicate a source in the rectosigmoid or anus.
- In 20% of acute bleeding episodes, no source of bleeding can be identified.

KEY FACT

Ten percent of cases of hematochezia are due to a brisk upper GI bleed and usually have concomitant hypotension and shock.

TABLE 5.9.   Upper vs. Lower GI Bleed

	CAUSES	SYMPTOMS/SIGNS
Upper GI bleed	Peptic ulcer disease (30%–50%). Mallory-Weiss tear (15%–20%). Varices (10%–20%). Gastritis (10%–15%). Esophagitis (5%–10%). Angiodysplasia (5%). Cancer (1%–2%).	Epigastric pain. Hematemesis (fresh blood or coffee-ground emesis). Melena.
Lower GI bleed	Diverticulosis (30%–40%). Bowel ischemia (6%–18%). Anorectal disease (6%–16%). Colon cancer (7%–11%). Angiodysplasia (1%–3%). IBD (2%–4%). Infectious diarrhea.	Hematochezia. Abdominal pain. Tenesmus. Maroon-colored stools. Physical exam may reveal hemorrhoids, fissures, mass.

DIAGNOSIS/TREATMENT

- **Initial resuscitation and stabilization:** Measures are the same as those for upper GI bleeding. An upper tract source should be excluded by NG lavage and possibly by EGD, especially if the patient is hemodynamically unstable.
- **Triage:**
  - For patients > 45 years of age or those with recurrent/persistent bleeding, colonoscopy is required.
  - For patients < 45 years of age with an isolated episode, anoscopy and sigmoidoscopy are sufficient if a cause is found; otherwise, colonoscopy.
- **Diagnostic and treatment options:**
  - **Colonoscopy:** Diagnostic, prognostic, and therapeutic (epinephrine injection, cautery, or application of metallic endoclips). Diagnostic accuracy is ↓ with inadequate prep (eg, with severe, active bleeding).
  - **Nuclear bleeding scan** (technetium-labeled RBC scan) or **angiography:** Can identify the bleeding site for arterial embolization or bowel resection, but has poor diagnostic accuracy unless bleeding is brisk.
  - **Small intestine push enteroscopy** (a small-diameter endoscope that can reach the distal jejunum)/**wireless capsule imaging:** May help identify a source of persistent recurrent bleeding.
  - **Surgery:** Indicated with ongoing bleeding that requires > 4–6 units of blood within 24 hours or > 10 units in total. May also be indicated in patients with 2 or more hospitalizations for diverticular hemorrhage.

DIVERTICULOSIS AND DIVERTICULITIS

- **Diverticulosis:** Outpocketings of the colonic mucosa in the wall of the colon; most commonly in the sigmoid colon. Risk factors include low-fiber/high-fat diet, increased age, constipation, and connective tissue disorders (eg, Marfan syndrome). Often asymptomatic. No specific treatment necessary, but a high-fiber diet may help.

- **Diverticulitis: Infection within the diverticula.** Colonoscopy and barium enema are contraindicated because of the ↑ risk of perforation. Clinical features include fever, LLQ pain, and leukocytosis with left shift. Treatment includes antibiotics against colonic flora (oral or IV, depending on severity) and keeping patient NPO. Surgery with resection or diverting colostomy is indicated if patient has not responded to medical therapies or has had repeat episodes, abscess or fistula formation, obstruction, or peritonitis.

DIAGNOSIS

Colonoscopy, barium enema, CT, and MRI (for a CT image of diverticulitis, see Figure 12.4 in the Surgery chapter).

MESENTERIC ISCHEMIA

An acute vascular insult that causes ischemia in the bowel. The 4 main causes are arterial embolism (often the SMA), arterial thrombosis (from preexisting vascular disease), nonocclusive etiology (low cardiac output with mesenteric vasoconstriction), and venous thrombosis.

DIAGNOSIS

- Clinical history (with postprandial abdominal pain and "food fear").
- Signs include abdominal pain out of proportion to physical exam.
- **Labs:** Leukocytosis, hemoconcentration, ↑ amylase, ↑ LDH.
- **Imaging:** KUB may show "thumbprinting" of the bowel wall (seen in < 40% of cases); CT may show thickened bowel wall, bowel wall hemorrhage, and/or nonenhancing bowel wall and may show arterial or venous occlusion.

TREATMENT

- Fluid resuscitation.
- General surgery and interventional radiology consultation.
- Treat underlying condition as indicated.
- Consider anticoagulation if there are no contraindications and if patient is not going to surgery (talk to a surgeon first!).
- Prognosis is 50% mortality if diagnosed within 24 hours of symptom onset; > 70% if diagnosis is delayed beyond 24 hours.

CHAPTER 6

Infectious Diseases

Jack Chase, MD

Central Nervous System Infections

A 45-year-old woman presents to the ER after 5 days of fever, cough, pleuritic chest pain, and purulent sputum. Her family brought her to the hospital today because she began complaining of a headache and neck pain. The family also notes that she has been acting strangely and seems confused. On physical exam, you note a temperature of 40.4°C (104.7°F) and nuchal rigidity. The patient is oriented only to self. What would you do first?

Perform a noncontrast head CT, order an LP, and then start empiric antibiotics (ceftriaxone and vancomycin)—all within the first 60 minutes of presentation. Also consider steroids before the first dose of antibiotics. Also give steroids before or with the first dose of antibiotics if at least moderate suspicion for pneumococcal meningitis. If the CT scan or LP is delayed, **do not delay antibiotics,** as CSF cultures usually remain positive for the first few hours after antibiotics are given. The CSF Gram stain and chemistries will still be useful, even if the cultures have been rendered negative.

ACUTE BACTERIAL MENINGITIS

A purulent leptomeningeal infection associated with a profound inflammatory response. Without treatment, mortality can be > 50%. Survivors usually have severe morbidity. Typical bacterial pathogens include *Streptococcus pneumoniae*, *Neisseria meningitidis*, group B streptococci, and *Listeria monocytogenes*. Demographic factors and comorbidities predispose patients to specific pathogens (see Table 6.1).

SYMPTOMS/EXAM

- Symptoms include headache, photophobia, and nausea/vomiting. Neonates may present with fever or hypothermia and subtle signs, including lethargy, poor feeding, and/or bulging fontanelles.
- Less common presentations are rash (petechiae and palpable purpura in disseminated intravascular coagulation from meningococcal meningitis); cranial nerve palsies; cerebral involvement in the form of seizures, aphasia, or focal neurologic deficits (eg, **syphilitic meningitis**); and coma.
- Traditional signs thought to correlate with meningeal irritation include **Kernig sign** (with the thigh and knee flexed, passive leg extension leading to pain) and **Brudzinski sign** (passive flexion of the neck leading to spontaneous flexion of the hip and knees). However, these signs are not sensitive for the diagnosis of bacterial meningitis.
- Atypical presentations are common in neonates, infants, the elderly, and immunocompromised patients.

DIFFERENTIAL

- Other forms of meningitis, such as viral, fungal (*Cryptococcus neoformans*), tuberculous, and aseptic (absence of bacteria on routine examination and culture, eg, medication-induced, autoimmune).
- Viral encephalitis or bacterial encephalitis (eg, Rocky Mountain spotted fever, Lyme disease).

KEY FACT

The classic triad of bacterial meningitis consists of fever, altered mental status, and nuchal rigidity. Virtually all patients have at least one of these symptoms.

KEY FACT

Meningeal signs:
K is for *K*ernig and *K*nee.
You "**K**need" to move the knee to test for **K**ernig.

TABLE 6.1.   Causes and Treatment of Bacterial Meningitis

AGE/TREATMENT GROUP	COMMON MICROORGANISMS	EMPIRIC ANTIBIOTICS—FIRST CHOICE	SEVERE PENICILLIN ALLERGY
< 1 month of age	Group B strep, *E coli, Listeria*.	Ampicillin and cefotaxime/ gentamicin.	N/A.
1 month to 50 years of age	*S pneumoniae, N meningitidis, H influenzae*.[a]	Ceftriaxone/cefotaxime + vancomycin.	Aztreonam or carbapenem[b] + vancomycin.
> 50 years of age	*S pneumoniae, Listeria*, gram-⊖ bacilli.	Ceftriaxone/cefotaxime + ampicillin + vancomycin.	FQ or aztreonam or carbapenem[b] (*N meningitidis*) + TMP-SMX (*Listeria*) + vancomycin.
Impaired cellular immunity (or alcohol abuse)	*S pneumoniae, L monocytogenes*, gram-⊖ bacilli.	Ceftazidime or cefepime + ampicillin + vancomycin.	TMP-SMX + vancomycin.
Postneurosurgery or post– head trauma	*S pneumoniae, S aureus*, gram-⊖ bacilli (incl. *Pseudomonas*).	Meropenem, cefepime, or ceftazidime + vancomycin (if MRSA risk).	Aztreonam or ciprofloxacin + vancomycin.

Adapted, with permission, from Tierney LM, et al. *Current Medical Diagnosis & Treatment*, 44th ed. New York: McGraw-Hill, 2005: 1251.

[a]*H influenzae* type B has much decreased in pediatrics as a result of vaccination.

[b]Agent choice depends on patient age and clinical situation.

- A parameningeal focus such as epidural, subdural, or intraparenchymal abscess. **Epidural abscess** may present as headache, back pain, and neurologic deficits 2° to cord compression. Consider in patients with a history of IV drug abuse.
- Noninfectious causes include SAH, vasculitis, and connective tissue disease.

DIAGNOSIS

- History and physical examination.
- **Labs:** Leukocytosis with PMN predominance or leukopenia (associated with severe infection). Thrombocytopenia and coagulopathy can be seen in DIC (think of meningococcemia; see Figure 6.1).
  - **CSF:**
    - Opening pressure is typically ↑. Send CSF for cell count and differential, total glucose, protein, Gram stain, and bacterial culture (see Table 6.2).
    - In the appropriate setting, test CSF for viral PCR (HSV), viral culture, cryptococcal antigen, AFB culture, fungal culture, or VDRL (syphilis).
  - **Blood cultures:** Bacteremia is common and is seen in 40%–90% of patients with community-acquired bacterial meningitis.

TREATMENT

- Untreated, bacterial meningitis causes severe morbidity and mortality exceeds 50%. Begin antimicrobial therapy ASAP: within 60 minutes of presentation. Choose empiric therapy based on patient factors (see Table 6.1) and tailor to results of CSF culture.

KEY FACT

Consider neuroimaging before performing an LP if there is concern about ↑ ICP (ie, mass effect with shift) in patients with focal neurologic findings, papilledema, or immunocompromise.

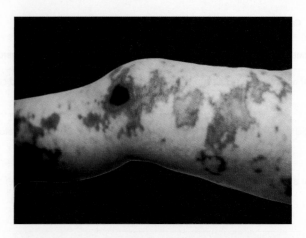

FIGURE 6.1. **Palpable purpura due to disseminated intravascular coagulation (DIC) in a patient with fulminant meningococcal meningitis and septicemia.** (Reproduced, with permission, from Wolff K, et al. *Fitzpatrick's Dermatology in General Medicine,* 7th ed. New York: McGraw-Hill, 2008, Fig. 180-1.)

- Unless allergic, all patients should receive a third-generation cephalosporin. For patients > 1 month of age, add vancomycin to cover penicillin-resistant *S pneumoniae* infection. Ampicillin should be added in very young, elderly, or immunocompromised patients to cover *L monocytogenes.*
- Consider giving corticosteroids (dexamethasone) *in the 30 minutes before antibiotics.* Steroids ↓ mortality and morbidity in adults with pneumococcal meningitis and ↓ hearing loss in children with *H influenzae* meningitis. Steroids may also ↓ other adverse outcomes in children with bacterial meningitis.

TABLE 6.2. **CSF Profiles in Common CNS Diseases**

DIAGNOSIS	RBC (per L)	WBC (per L)	GLUCOSE (mg/dL)	PROTEIN (mg/dL)	OPENING PRESSURE (cm H₂O)	APPEARANCE
Normal[a]	< 10	< 5	About 2/3 of serum level	15–45	10–20	Clear
Bacterial meningitis	Normal	↑ (PMNs)	↓	↑	↑	Cloudy
Aseptic/viral meningitis, encephalitis	Normal (may be ↑ in encephalitis)	↑ (lymphs)[b]	Normal	Normal or ↑	Normal or ↑	Usually clear
Chronic meningitis (TB, fungal)	Normal	↑ (lymphs)[b]	↓	↑	↑	Clear or cloudy
Spirochetal meningitis (syphilis, Lyme disease)	Normal	↑ (lymphs)[b]	Normal	↑	Normal or ↑	Clear or cloudy
Neighborhood reaction[c]	Normal	Variable	Normal	Normal or ↑	Normal or ↑	Usually clear
SAH, cerebral contusion	↑↑	↑	Normal	↑↑	Normal or ↑	Yellow or red

[a] With traumatic tap, usually have 1 WBC/800 RBCs and 1 mg protein/1000 RBCs.

[b] May have PMN predominance in early stages.

[c] May be seen with brain abscess, epidural abscess, vertebral osteomyelitis, sinusitis/mastoiditis, septic thrombus, and brain tumor.

- Patients with features of rickettsial meningitis (Lyme disease, Rocky Mountain spotted fever) may benefit from early antibiotics (ceftriaxone for Lyme disease and doxycycline for Rocky Mountain spotted fever). Patients suspected of TB meningitis should be isolated, and early antimycobacterial therapy and steroids initiated in consultation with an infectious disease specialist and a neurologist.
- **Do not delay antibiotics** while waiting for imaging or LP. Cultures usually remain positive for the first few hours after antibiotics are given. The CSF Gram stain and chemistries will still be useful, even if the cultures have been rendered negative.

COMPLICATIONS

- Systemic complications result primarily from bacteremia and include septic shock, DIC, ARDS, and septic or reactive arthritis.
- Neurologic complications include cerebral edema and ↑ ICP, hydrocephalus, seizures, cognitive impairment, hearing loss and other cranial neuropathies, subdural effusion, empyema, epidural abscess, and SIADH. Permanent neurologic morbidity may occur.

VIRAL MENINGITIS AND ENCEPHALITIS

Viruses infiltrate the CNS in various ways, including hematogenous and axonal spread, causing a range of disease processes, including meningitis (Table 6.3) and encephalitis as well as postinfectious autoimmune demyelination.

TABLE 6.3. Etiologic Agents in Viral Meningitis

VIRUS	INCIDENCE	SOURCE	SUSCEPTIBLE POPULATION	SEASONALITY, ASSOCIATED SYMPTOMS, LABORATORY FINDINGS
Echoviridae	30%.	Fecal-oral.	Children, family contacts.	Summer/fall. Rash, gastroenteritis common.
Coxsackievirus A/B	A: 10%; B: 50%.	Fecal-oral.	Children, family contacts.	Summer/fall. Rash, gastroenteritis, herpanagina (in A) serositis, myocarditis, orchitis (in B).
Mumps virus	15%.	Inhalation.	Children, male more than female.	Winter/spring. Parotitis, orchitis, oophoritis, pancreatitis. CSF glucose may be ↑ or ↓.
Herpes simplex virus (type 2)	Uncommon.	Genital infection.	Neonates with affected mothers.	Vesicular genital lesions.
Adenovirus	Uncommon.	Inhalation.	Infants, children.	Pharyngitis, pneumonia.
Lymphocytic choriomeningitis virus	Uncommon.	Mouse.	Laboratory workers.	Late fall/winter. Pharyngitis and pneumonia. Marked CSF pleocytosis.
Hepatitis viruses	Uncommon.	Fecal-oral, venereal, transfusion.	IV drug users, high-risk sexual activity, transfusion recipients.	Jaundice, arthritis, LFT abnormalities.

(continues)

TABLE 6.3. Etiologic Agents in Viral Meningitis *(continued)*

VIRUS	INCIDENCE	SOURCE	SUSCEPTIBLE POPULATION	SEASONALITY, ASSOCIATED SYMPTOMS, LABORATORY FINDINGS
Epstein-Barr virus (infectious mononucleosis)	Uncommon.	Oral contact.	Teenagers, young adults.	Atypical lymphocytes, ⊕ heterophil, LFT abnormalities, lymphadenopathy, pharyngitis, splenomegaly, skin/palatal rash.
Flaviviruses (West Nile, Japanese B, St. Louis, yellow fever)	Uncommon.	Mosquitoes.	Rural, near standing water.	Variable geographic distribution. Rash, myocarditis, hepatitis, pancreatitis.
Alphaviruses (Eastern/ Western/Venezuelan equine)	Uncommon.	Mosquitoes.	Rural, near standing water.	Neurologic sequelae common in EEE, uncommon in WEE and VEE.
Orbivirus (Colorado tick fever)	Uncommon.	Ticks.	Western and Rocky Mountain states.	Rash.
Rabies	Rare.	Rodent, bat, canine, feline vectors.	Worldwide; individuals bitten/ scratched by animal vectors (dogs in most of world; bats in the United States).	Invariably fatal unless treated promptly with vaccine and antiserum before symptoms.

Adapted, with permission, from Aminoff MJ, et al. *Clinical Neurology*, 6th ed. New York: McGraw-Hill, 2005: 27.

SYMPTOMS/EXAM

- Presents with altered mental status, motor/sensory deficits, and speech/ movement abnormalities.
- Overlap between symptoms of meningitis and encephalitis can occur. Both can have rash (meningococcus, Rocky Mountain spotted fever, Lyme disease, VZV), fever, headache, nausea/vomiting, seizures, or focal neurologic deficits (flaccid paralysis in West Nile virus). However, photophobia and stiff neck are less common findings in pure encephalitis.
- HSV encephalitis can cause bizarre behavior such as olfactory hallucinations and aphasia. This is due to the predilection for involvement of the **medial temporal lobes** (see Figure 6.2).

DIFFERENTIAL

See the differential for bacterial meningitis above as well as other common causes of altered mental status.

DIAGNOSIS

- The 1° goal is to **distinguish HSV from other causes.**
- A thorough history is essential and should include season, sexual activity, travel, and insect or animal bites.
- **MRI is the optimal imaging study** to visualize brain parenchyma. CT scan is an acceptable alternative, if MRI is unavailable or contraindicated.

KEY FACT

HSV encephalitis may cause high RBCs in CSF.

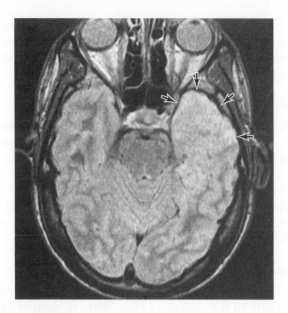

FIGURE 6.2.   MRI in HSV encephalitis. (Reproduced, with permission, from Aminoff MJ, et al. *Clinical Neurology*, 6th ed. New York: McGraw-Hill, 2005: 30.)

TREATMENT

- Untreated HSV encephalitis is associated with high morbidity and mortality. Therefore, in suspected cases of encephalitis without an obvious source, **empiric IV acyclovir** should be used until this is ruled out. Young children and the immunocompromised are at greatest risk for HSV disease.
- Supportive measures are the mainstay of treatment for all other types of viral encephalitis.
- If rabies exposure is possible by history, consult infectious disease clinicians and consider administration of antiserum and rabies vaccine.
- Failure to improve within **48 hours** should prompt reevaluation of the diagnosis.

COMPLICATIONS

Rates of morbidity and mortality vary by type of viral encephalitis.

KEY FACT

With rare exceptions, HSV is currently the only treatable type of viral encephalitis. IV acyclovir is the drug of choice.

Head and Neck Infections

A 15-year-old boy is being seen in urgent care for a 1-day history of right eye pain and swelling. On exam, you note significant erythema and periorbital swelling, and the patient reports pain when asked to look to his left. What is your next step in this patient's management?

Perform a CT scan of the orbits, obtain blood cultures, and admit to the hospital for IV antibiotics.

ORBITAL AND PERIORBITAL CELLULITIS

Bacterial infection of the soft tissues surrounding the eye following a URI, sinusitis, dental infection, or trauma. Common causative agents include *Staph-*

ylococcus spp, *Streptococcus* spp, and, until recently, *H influenzae* (now a less common cause, with routine vaccination). An important clinical distinction is made between periorbital (ie, preseptal) and orbital cellulitis (around and posterior to the globe).

SYMPTOMS/EXAM

- **Periorbital (preseptal) cellulitis:** Presents with swelling and erythema of the eyelids, minimal pain, and fever. Conjunctivitis, proptosis, restricted eye movements, and visual deficits are **not** generally present (see Figure 6.3).
- **Orbital cellulitis:** Presents with very painful erythematous swelling of the eyelid, **conjunctivitis,** proptosis with **ophthalmoplegia,** and fever. Patients may also have ↓ visual acuity, pain with eye movement, and an afferent pupillary defect.

DIAGNOSIS/TREATMENT

- Consider CT scan of the orbit to evaluate for postseptal extension or **abscess** (imperative in the presence of symptoms or signs of orbital cellulitis; see Figure 6.4). Patients with low clinical suspicion of orbital extension do not require a CT scan.
- If concern for associated cavernous sinus thrombosis, an MRI with venous phase is indicated.
- Consider blood cultures, although these are generally ⊖.
- Usually requires hospital admission and IV antibiotics (broad-spectrum antistaphylococcal and antistreptococcal coverage). Typically, vancomycin and ceftriaxone or ampicillin plus sulbactam (if low suspicion for MRSA).
- Prompt drainage of an abscess or the paranasal sinuses is indicated if vision deteriorates despite antibiotic therapy.

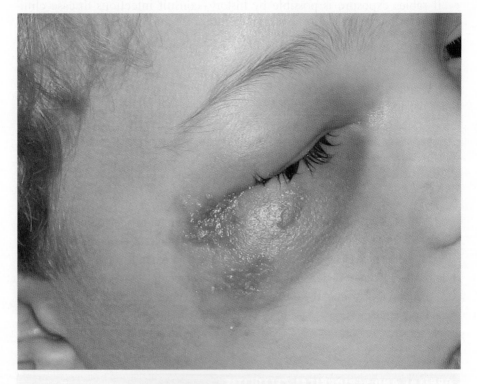

FIGURE 6.3. **Periorbital cellulitis in a 7-year-old boy with recent upper respiratory infection and 3-day history of progressive eye swelling and pain.** (Reproduced, with permission, from USMLERx.com.)

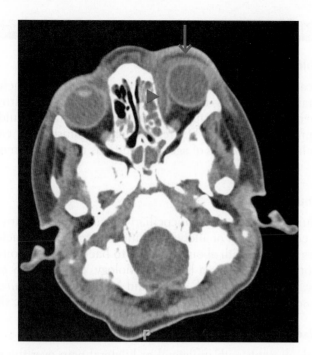

FIGURE 6.4. **Orbital cellulitis.** Left periorbital inflammation (*arrow*) with preseptal extension into the medial orbit (*arrowhead*). (Reproduced, with permission, from USMLERx.com.)

COMPLICATIONS

Abscess, blindness, or extension into the CNS, causing meningitis or septic cavernous sinus thrombosis.

CONJUNCTIVITIS

The most common cause of a red eye, infectious etiologies of conjunctivitis include both viruses and bacteria. Although usually a self-limited infection, it occasionally requires treatment (see Table 6.4).

TABLE 6.4.   Manifestations and Treatment of Infectious Conjunctivitis

	VIRAL	**BACTERIAL**
Etiologies	Adenovirus, HSV.	*Staphylococcus* spp., *Streptococcus* spp., *H influenzae*, *Neisseria gonorrhoeae* (GC), *Chlamydia trachomatis* (CT).
Symptoms/exam	Erythema, watery discharge, photophobia. Frequently bilateral. Concomitant URI. "Pink eye."	Erythema, mucopurulent discharge, "morning crustiness." Usually unilateral.
Treatment	Symptomatic; cold compresses.	Topical erythromycin, bacitracin-polymyxin, trimethoprim, fluoroquinolone. For GC, ceftriaxone IM/IV × 1. For CT, erythromycin syrup PO.
Prevention	Frequent hand washing (highly contagious).	Frequent hand washing.
Complications	Corneal abrasion 2° to rubbing.	Untreated *C trachomatis* conjunctivitis is a common cause of **blindness** worldwide.

NOSE AND SINUS INFECTIONS

Common Cold

- Usually caused by **rhinoviruses.** Other viruses implicated include coronavirus, parainfluenza virus, RSV, influenza virus, and adenoviruses.
- **Tx:** Generally treat with supportive measures, including fluids, rest, and contact precautions. The FDA recommends against OTC cold preparations in children < 2 years of age and cautious use in children 2–11 years of age.

Bacterial Sinusitis

Sinusitis results from impaired mucociliary clearance and obstruction of the osteomeatal complex; viral or allergic rhinitis is a predisposing factor. The majority of cases are viral, with about **20% due to bacteria.** Infections lasting > 1 week are more likely to have a bacterial etiology, commonly *S pneumoniae,* *H influenzae,* and occasionally *S aureus* and *Moraxella catarrhalis. Pseudomonas aeruginosa* and anaerobes are implicated in cases of **chronic sinusitis.**

SYMPTOMS/EXAM

- Frequently presents with unilateral or bilateral pain over the maxillary sinuses or teeth as well as with fever and nasal discharge (at times purulent).
- Acute sinusitis can last 1–4 weeks; sinusitis > 4 weeks is considered chronic.
- Transillumination of the sinuses may be attempted but is an insensitive test.

DIFFERENTIAL

- **Zygomycosis:** A rare but dangerous fungal infection that occurs in immunocompromised patients—eg, those with diabetes, end-stage renal disease, bone marrow transplants, lymphoma, or AIDS.
- Presents as **facial pain** with a necrotic eschar of the nasal mucosa and subsequently with cranial nerve palsies.
- Early diagnosis is paramount because the infection can spread rapidly. Treat emergently with antifungal therapy (traditionally amphotericin B; possibly posaconazole) and surgical debridement.
- **Other:** In chronic or resistant sinusitis, consider anatomic obstruction, common variable immunodeficiency, a CF variant, Wegener granulomatosis, or periodontal or dental infection.

DIAGNOSIS

- Usually made by the history and physical exam.
- **Routine imaging is not indicated** in uncomplicated acute sinusitis. However, in chronic, resistant, or complicated sinusitis, CT scan is much more sensitive than x-rays. Imaging may identify air-fluid levels, bony abnormalities, and extension outside of the paranasal sinuses.

TREATMENT

- **General:** Oral and/or nasal decongestants (eg, oral pseudoephedrine, intranasal oxymetazoline).
- **Acute bacterial sinusitis:** 5–10 days of amoxicillin or a macrolide are standard therapy. However, antibiotics offer limited clinical benefit in this disease. Consider amoxicillin/clavulanate if risk factors for anaerobes or β-lactamase-producing organisms (eg, *H influenzae* [30% produce

β-lactamase] and *M catarrhalis*) are present. Risk factors include diabetes, other immunocompromised states, and recent antibiotic use.

- **Chronic sinusitis:** Amoxicillin/clavulanate for at least 3–4 weeks along with intranasal glucocorticoids.

COMPLICATIONS

Complications are rare but include extension into the CNS and orbital or periorbital cellulitis.

OROPHARYNGEAL INFECTIONS

Pharyngitis

> An otherwise healthy 25-year-old woman presents to the urgent care clinic with a very sore throat, subjective fever, and swollen glands in her neck. The patient has a temperature of 38.5°C (101.3°F). On exam, you note palatal petechiae, purulent tonisllar exudates, and tender cervical lymphade-nopathy. What is your treatment plan?
>
> You employ the Centor criteria and treat the patient empirically for group A streptococcus (*S pyogenes*) pharyngitis with a 10-day course of oral penicillin.

An infection or irritation of the pharynx and/or tonsils. Etiologies include the following:

- **Bacterial:** The most important bacterial etiology is group A streptococcus (GAS, or *Streptococcus pyogenes*), causing "strep throat" (see below). Other bacterial agents include groups C and G streptococcus, *N gonorrhoeae*, *Mycoplasma pneumoniae*, *Chlamydia pneumoniae*, and, rarely, *Corynebacterium diphtheriae*.
- **Viral:** Viruses are the most common etiology of pharyngitis (see below). These include rhinovirus, coronavirus, adenovirus, and many others. Pharyngitis may also occur 2° to systemic viral infections such as mononucleosis (EBV), herpangina (coxsackievirus), and acute retroviral syndrome (HIV).
- **Other:** Allergy, gastroesophageal reflux, trauma, toxins, malignancy.

Bacterial Pharyngitis, Including *S pyogenes*/GAS (Strep Throat)

SYMPTOMS/EXAM

- Prominent sore throat and odynophagia. Patients with acute bacterial pharyngitis typically have purulent **tonsillar exudates.**
- In cases of **gonococcal** or **chlamydial** pharyngitis, patients may have associated **GU symptoms** (dysuria, discharge, etc) or **joint complaints.**
- Testing and treatment for GAS, the major cause of bacterial pharyngitis, are based on the **Centor criteria:**
  - Temperature > 38.0°C (100.4°F).
  - Tender anterior cervical lymphadenopathy.
  - Absence of cough.
  - Presence of pharyngotonsillar exudates.

DIAGNOSIS

- If needed, the **test of choice** for GAS is the **rapid antigen test,** which has > 90% sensitivity. Use in patients with 2–3 positive features of the Centor criteria. If rapid test is $\ominus$ but continued suspicion, send a GAS culture. Pharyngitis due to GAS is more common in children than adults.

- A routine bacterial culture is not indicated unless there is high suspicion of a bacterial infection other than GAS (eg, gonococcal pharyngitis.)

TREATMENT

- Treatment for GAS is based on results of rapid testing and the Centor criteria:
  - **4 of 4:** PPV 60%. Treat empirically without a rapid test.
  - **2–3 of 4:** Test and treat only if the rapid test is $\oplus$; if $\ominus$, send a confirmatory culture.
  - **0–1 of 4:** NPV 70+%. No test, no antibiotics. Supportive care for viral pharyngitis unless alternative diagnosis.
- For GAS, give 1 dose IM benzathine penicillin or a 10-day course of oral penicillin VK or erythromycin (for penicillin-allergic patients). Other antistreptococcal antibiotics (eg, cefuroxime or amoxicillin) may be used, but the efficacy of these drugs in the prevention of rheumatic fever has not been adequately studied.
- Patients may return to work or school 24 hours after initiation of therapy.
- For uncomplicated **gonococcal** pharyngitis, treat with ceftriaxone or azithromycin. If complicated by pelvic or joint infection, treatment may require IV antibiotics and hospitalization. For **chlamydia**, doxycycline or azithromycin can be used as first-line therapy.

COMPLICATIONS

- Complications include peritonsillar abscess, and, rarely, pharyngeal abscesses.
- In GAS, postinfectious phenomena can occur, including **acute rheumatic fever** (see Special Topics: Acute Rheumatic Fever, at the end of this chapter) and glomerulonephritis.

Viral Pharyngitis

As above, suggested by upper respiratory symptoms and the absence of tonsillar exudates. Usually due to common viral causes of upper respiratory infection including adeno-, corona- and rhinoviruses. Pharyngitis 2° to other systemic viral infections presents as follows:

- **Mononucleosis:** Characterized by the triad of **lymphadenopathy, fever,** and **tonsillitis.** Symptoms also include severe fatigue, headache, and malaise. More common in young adults. Transmitted in saliva and may persist for up to 18 months after 1° infection (see Figure 6.5).
- **Herpangina:** Presents with fever, sore throat, myalgias, and a vesicular exanthem on the soft palate. Commonly caused by coxsackievirus A16 (see Figure 6.6) and may be associated with vesicular rash on the palms and soles in hand-foot-mouth disease.
- **Acute retroviral syndrome:** Nonexudative pharyngitis and fever are common symptoms of this syndrome, which develops several weeks after infection with HIV.

DIAGNOSIS

- **Mononucleosis:** Diagnosed with a $\oplus$ heterophil antibody (Monospot) test or a high anti-EBV antibody titer.
- Consider HIV or other viral testing.

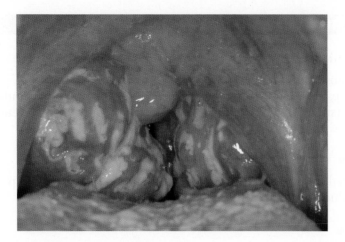

FIGURE 6.5. **Mononucleosis pharyngitis.** (Reproduced, with permission, from Knoop KJ, et al. *The Atlas of Emergency Medicine,* 3rd ed. New York: McGraw-Hill, 2010, Fig. 5.36. Photo contributor: Lawrence B. Stack, MD.)

TREATMENT

- **Supportive care, including** acetaminophen or NSAIDs and saltwater gargling for symptomatic relief. Oral steroids may occasionally be needed for severe pharyngitis.
- Patients may return to work or school when fever resolves and they are well enough to participate in normal activities.

COMPLICATIONS

- **Mononucleosis:** Complications include hepatitis, a morbilliform rash following antibiotic administration (especially ampicillin/amoxicillin), and splenomegaly occurring within the first 3 weeks. To ↓ the risk of **splenic rupture,** noncontact sports must be avoided for 3–4 weeks and contact sports for 4–6 weeks after the onset of symptoms.
- For **HIV** disease, see section on HIV.

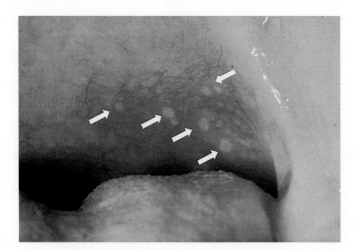

FIGURE 6.6. **Herpangina.** Acute, multiple papulovesicular lesions progress to form shallow ulcerations, with brisk marginal erythema. (Reproduced, with permission, from Wolff K, et al. *Fitzpatrick's Dermatology in General Medicine,* 7th ed. New York: McGraw-Hill, 2008, Fig. 192-18.)

DENTAL AND PERIODONTAL INFECTIONS

Dental Caries

- The most common chronic childhood disease.
- For a patient to develop caries, 3 factors must be present: a **host**, a **substrate (sucrose)**, and **bacteria**. The most common bacterial agent is *Streptococcus mutans*.

PREVENTION

Fluoridated water, good oral hygiene, and regular dental follow-up are effective in reducing dental caries.

DIFFERENTIAL

Isolated gingival infections, sinus disease, trigeminal neuralgia.

COMPLICATIONS

- Acute pulpitis, periapical abscess, granuloma, or cyst. Abscesses may track and lead to serious infections.
- **Ludwig angina:** A life-threatening infection of the sublingual and submandibular spaces that causes brawny sublingual edema, potentially leading to airway obstruction. Requires hospitalization and IV antibiotics, ampicillin/ sulbactam, clindamycin, or high-dose penicillin plus metronidazole.
- **Lemierre syndrome:** A suppurative thrombophlebitis of the internal jugular vein located in the posterior compartment of the lateral pharyngeal

TABLE 6.5. Differential of Common Mouth Ulcers

	APHTHOUS ULCER (CANKER SORE)	**HERPES STOMATITIS**
Cause	Common; unknown cause (possible association with HHV-6).	Common; HSV.
Symptoms	Pain up to 1 week; heals within a few weeks.	Initial burning, followed by small vesicles and then scabs.
Exam	Small ulcerations, with yellow centers surrounded by red halos on **nonkeratinized** mucosa (buccal and lip mucosa).	Vesicles, scabs.
Treatment	Anti-inflammatory: topical steroids.	No need for treatment, but oral **acyclovir** × 7–14 days may shorten the course and postherpetic pain.
Prognosis	Recurrent.	Resolves quickly; frequent reactivation in immunocompromised patients.
Differential diagnosis	If large or persistent, consider erythema multiforme, HSV, pemphigus, Behçet disease, IBD, or SCC.	Aphthous ulcer, erythema multiforme, syphilis, cancer.

space caused by *Fusobacterium necrophorum*. Can lead to bacteremia, septic pulmonary emboli, and other septic embolic complications.

TREATMENT

- Antibiotics that cover oral flora include penicillins (Pen VK, amoxicillin), clindamycin, and erythromycin for penicillin-allergic patients.
- Referral to a dentist or oral surgeon for dental extraction or incision and drainages as appropriate.

Oral Lesions

Table 6.5 outlines the differential diagnosis of common mouth ulcers.

Cardiovascular Infections

A 33-year-old man is brought to the ER complaining of fever and shortness of breath of 3 days' duration. On exam, the only pertinent findings are warm skin and some track marks in the left antecubital fossa. The nurse tells you that his current temperature is 39.5°C (103.1°F). You order a CXR, a UA, and blood cultures. Six hours later, the patient's blood cultures are ⊕ for gram-⊕ cocci. You ask the lab about the bacterial morphology (eg, clusters vs. pairs and chains). On reexamination, you note a II/VI systolic ejection murmur. Which antibiotics would be the most appropriate empiric choice?
Start vancomycin. Order an echocardiogram.

ENDOCARDITIS

An infection of the endothelium of the heart that most frequently involves the valves. A vegetation consists of bacteria, platelets, fibrin, and inflammatory cells. Endocarditis is classified as acute vs. subacute and **native-valve endocarditis (NVE)** (see Figure 6.7) vs. **prosthetic-valve endocarditis (PVE)**. IV drug users are a special population at risk, particularly for tricuspid valve endocarditis (see Table 6.6).

SYMPTOMS

- **Acute bacterial endocarditis:** Presents with high fever (80%) and chills and can cause symptoms related to embolic phenomena (< 50%) and CHF.
- **Subacute endocarditis:** Presents with fever, weight loss, and poor appetite; has an indolent course. May also have signs or symptoms of CHF.

EXAM

- Fever and a heart murmur are most commonly seen (85% have heart murmurs, but only 5%–10% have a new murmur).
- Other symptoms and signs are as follows:
  - **Osler nodes:** Tender nodules on the finger and toe pads.
  - **Janeway lesions:** Nontender hemorrhagic macules on the palms and soles.
  - **Splinter hemorrhages:** Reddish-brown streaks in the proximal nail beds (see Figure 6.8).

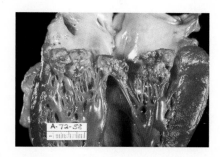

FIGURE 6.7. Purulent valvular vegetations in acute bacterial endocarditis.
(Reproduced, with permission, from USMLERx.com.)

TABLE 6.6.   **Etiologies of Endocarditis**

Type	Etiology (Incidence)
NVE	*S aureus* (32%), viridans group streptococci (18%), *Enterococcus* (11%), coagulase-⊖ staphylococci (10%), *S bovis* (6.5%), HACEK group (1.7%), culture ⊖ (8.1%).
PVE	*S aureus* and coagulase-⊖ staphylococci, gram ⊖s, and fungi (in valves < 2 months old), agents similar to NVE in valves > 2 months old, except more coagulase-⊖ staphylococci.
IV drug use	*S aureus* (60%), unusual gram ⊖s, and fungi.
Notes	**HACEK** organisms (*Haemophilus, Actinobacillus, Cardiobacterium, Eikenella, Kingella*) previously required special media or longer incubation time. Consider *Candida* and *Aspergillus* in IV drug users and patients with long-term indwelling catheters or immunosuppression. Causes of culture-⊖ infective endocarditis: *Chlamydia psittaci*, the "ellas" (*Bartonella, Legionella, Brucella, Coxiella*), Whipple disease, and recent antibiotic use.

Adapted, with permission, from Le T, et al. *First Aid for the Internal Medicine Boards*, 2nd ed. New York: McGraw-Hill, 2008: 431.

KEY FACT

Osler nodes are *painful* nodules. Think **OUCH**ler nodes.

- **Roth spots:** Retinal hemorrhages seen with an ophthalmoscope.
- Petechiae, especially conjunctival and mucosal.
- Signs of right or left heart failure or CVA may also be seen.

DIFFERENTIAL

Atrial myxoma, marantic endocarditis (nonbacterial thrombotic endocarditis, seen in cancer and chronic wasting diseases), Libman-Sacks Endocarditis (autoantibodies to heart valve, seen in **SLE**), acute rheumatic fever, suppurative thrombophlebitis, catheter-related sepsis, renal cell carcinoma, carcinoid syndrome.

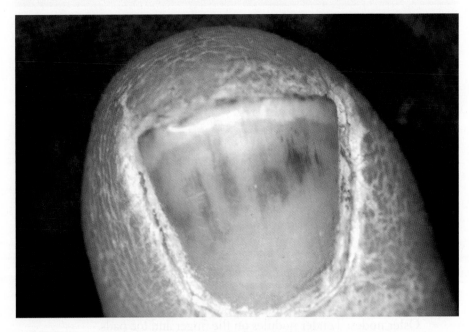

FIGURE 6.8.   Splinter hemorrhage of infective endocarditis. 60-year-old man, three months status-post aortic valve replacement. (Reproduced, with permission, from USMLERx.com.)

DIAGNOSIS

- **Duke criteria:** Clinical diagnosis of endocarditis must meet 2 major, 1 major plus 3 minor, or 5 minor criteria (see Table 6.7). Duke criteria sensitivity is 95%.
- **Labs:** Leukocytosis with left shift, mild anemia, and ↑ ESR.
- **Blood cultures:** Critical in establishing the diagnosis; ⊕ in 85%–95% of cases. It is recommended that **3 sets** of blood cultures be taken at least **1 hour apart** before antibiotics if subacute endocarditis is suspected.
- **Echocardiogram:** In NVE, transthoracic echo (TTE) is 60%–75% sensitive, whereas transesophageal echo (TEE) is 95% sensitive. Both are 95% specific. TTE is insensitive (15%–30%) with prosthetic valves—use TEE.
- **ECG:** May show varying degrees of **heart block** if the conduction system is involved. Consider perivalvular abscess if PR prolongation is present.
- **CXR:** May show multiple peripheral infiltrates with cavitation or effusions from septic emboli in patients with right-sided heart valve involvement.

TREATMENT

- In general, therapy must be bactericidal, IV, and administered for prolonged periods. The choice of antibiotic should be guided by clinical and

TABLE 6.7.   Duke Criteria for the Clinical Diagnosis of Infective Endocarditis

MAJOR CRITERIA

1. A ⊕ blood culture:
   - A typical microorganism consistent with infective endocarditis from 2 separate blood cultures, as follows:
     - Viridans streptococci, *S bovis,* HACEK group, *S aureus* **OR**
     - Community-acquired enterococci in the absence of a 1° focus **OR**
   - A persistently ⊕ blood culture, defined as recovery of a microorganism consistent with infective endocarditis from:
     - 2 or more blood cultures drawn > 12 hours apart **OR**
     - All of 3 or a majority of 4 or more separate blood cultures, with the first and last drawn at least 1 hour apart **OR**
   - A single ⊕ blood culture for *Coxiella burnetii* or anti–phase 1 IgG antibody titer of > 1:800.
2. Evidence of endocardial involvement:
   - A ⊕ echocardiogram, defined as follows:
     - An oscillating intracardiac mass on the valve or supporting structures, in the path of regurgitant jets, or in implanted material in the absence of an alternative anatomic explanation **OR**
     - Abscess **OR**
     - New partial dehiscence of a prosthetic valve **OR**
   - New valvular regurgitation (an ↑ or change in a preexisting murmur is not sufficient).

MINOR CRITERIA

1. **Predisposition:** A predisposing heart condition or IV drug use.
2. **Fever:** ≥ 38.0°C (≥ 100.4°F).
3. **Vascular phenomena:** Major arterial emboli, septic pulmonary infarcts, mycotic aneurysm, intracranial hemorrhage, conjunctival hemorrhages, Janeway lesions.
4. **Immunologic phenomena:** Glomerulonephritis, Osler nodes, Roth spots, RF.
5. **Microbiologic evidence:** A ⊕ blood culture but not meeting major criteria as noted previously[a], or serologic evidence of active infection with an organism consistent with infective endocarditis.

[a]Excluding single ⊕ cultures for coagulase-⊖ staphylococci and diphtheroids, which are common culture contaminants, and organisms that do not cause endocarditis frequently, such as gram-⊖ bacilli.

epidemiologic clues in the absence of culture data or before culture data are available.

- **NVE (empirical therapy):** Starting with vancomycin plus ceftriaxone is reasonable before blood culture results are available. Adjust antibiotics on the basis of culture results and treat for 4–6 weeks. Uncomplicated right-sided, methicillin-sensitive staphylococcal endocarditis (with no systemic embolic disease and with intact pulmonary function) can be treated with nafcillin and gentamicin for 2 weeks.
- **PVE (empirical therapy):** Vancomycin plus rifampin plus gentamicin initially for *S aureus* and coagulase-$\ominus$ staphylococci. Adjust antibiotics in accordance with culture results and treat for 6 weeks.
- **Persistent fever** after 1 week suggests a septic embolic focus or inadequate antibiotic coverage.
- Reappearance of fever **after initial defervescence** suggests septic emboli, drug fever, or, less commonly, the emergence of antimicrobial resistance.
- **Indications for surgery** are individualized. Common indications include refractory CHF, valvular obstruction, myocardial abscess, perivalvular extension (new conduction abnormalities), persistent bacteremia, fungal endocarditis, and most cases of PVE.

PREVENTION

- **Antibiotic prophylaxis:** Recommended only for patients at the highest risk with prosthetic valve, patch, devices; surgical systemic pulmonary shunts; unrepaired cyanotic congenital heart defects, including palliative shunts; or prior endocarditis; and also for patients < 6 months of age post cardiac surgery with prosthetic material, or cardiac transplantation with valvulopathy.
- **Procedures requiring prophylaxis:** Dental procedures involving manipulation of gingiva, oral mucosa, or periapical regions of teeth; respiratory tract procedures; procedures on infected skin or soft tissues. No longer required for GI or GU procedures.
    - **Dental or respiratory tract procedures:** PO amoxicillin or clindamycin 1 hour before procedure. If giving parenterally, IV ampicillin or IV clindamycin 30 minutes before procedure.

COMPLICATIONS

- **CHF:** Caused by valvular destruction or myocarditis. The **most common cause of death** due to endocarditis.
- **Embolic phenomena:** Mycotic aneurysms, infarction, or abscesses in the CNS, kidney, coronary arteries, or spleen. Right-sided disease can lead to pulmonary emboli, but if a patent foramen ovale is present, it can also lead to systemic emboli ("paradoxical embolus").
- **Conduction abnormalities:** Include arrhythmia and heart block.
- **Myocardial or perivalvular abscess:** May extend to cause pericarditis and tamponade. Most common with *S aureus*.

MYOCARDITIS

Defined as inflammation of the myocardium; postulated to be a common cause of "idiopathic" dilated cardiomyopathy. The typical patient is young and healthy and may have had a recent viral URI. Can be a cause of sudden cardiac death. Etiologies include the following:

- **Infectious:** Usually **viral** (eg, coxsackievirus, HIV, influenza) but may also be caused by other pathogens, including bacteria such as *Borrelia burgdorferi* in Lyme disease (most commonly on the East Coast and in the Rocky

Mountain regions of the United States) and parasites such as *Trypanosoma cruzi* in Chagas disease (almost exclusively found in Central and South America) (see Figure 6.9).

- **Immune mediated:** Medication allergy, sarcoidosis, scleroderma, SLE, and others.
- **Toxin related:** Medications (anthracyclines), EtOH, heavy metals, and others.
- **Postpartum.**

SYMPTOMS/EXAM

- Nonspecific. Flulike symptoms, fever, arthralgias, and malaise may be seen. In severe cases, patients may present with chest pain, dyspnea, and symptoms of heart failure.
- Physical exam may be normal or may exhibit findings consistent with heart failure.

DIFFERENTIAL

CAD/MI, aortic dissection, pericarditis, pulmonary embolism, other pulmonary and GI processes.

DIAGNOSIS

- **Endomyocardial biopsy:** The **gold standard.** However, the test is insensitive because of the patchy involvement of the myocardium. Also, by the time most patients seek care, fibrosis is the only notable finding.
- **ECG:** Can be abnormal, but is neither sensitive nor specific.
- **Cardiac enzymes:** May be ↑ in the acute phase.
- **Echocardiogram:** May reveal focal wall motion abnormalities and ↓ ejection fraction, but findings are nonspecific.
- Cardiac catheterization: To exclude CAD.

TREATMENT

- No specific therapy. Treatment can be focused if there is a known cause (eg, a parasite). Steroids have not been shown to be of use, except in small studies of autoimmune disease–mediated myocarditis (eg, sarcoidosis).

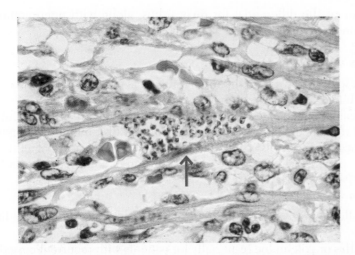

FIGURE 6.9. *Trypanosoma cruzi* **in the heart muscle of a child who died of acute Chagas myocarditis.** An infected monocyte containing several dozen *T cruzi* amastigotes *(arrow)*.
(Reproduced, with permission, from Fauci AS, et al. *Harrison's Principles of Internal Medicine,* 17th ed. New York: McGraw-Hill, 2008, Fig. 206-1.)

- Treat heart failure.
- Consider cardiac transplantation in severe cases.

COMPLICATIONS

Dilated cardiomyopathy, CHF, arrhythmias, death.

PERICARDITIS

Defined as inflammation of the pericardium that leads to chest pain, pericardial friction rub, and typical ECG changes. It is often accompanied by a pericardial effusion, which can lead to tamponade.

Infectious etiologies include:

- **Viral:** Coxsackievirus A and B, echovirus, mumps, adenovirus, hepatitis, HIV, EBV, VZV, HSV.
- **Bacterial:** *S pneumoniae* and other streptococci, *S aureus*, *Neisseria* spp, *Legionella* spp, *Mycobacterium tuberculosis*, *Treponema pallidum*.
- **Fungal:** Histoplasmosis, coccidioidomycosis, *Candida* spp, blastomycosis.

Noninfectious etiologies of pericarditis include:

- **Autoimmune:** Most commonly rheumatoid arthritis and lupus (SLE).
- **Malignant:** Most commonly lung, breast, or metastatic disease.
- **Posttraumatic** (aka Dressler syndrome): After surgery, an MI, or radiation therapy.
- **Metabolic:** Dialysis-related or from uremia.

SYMPTOMS/EXAM

- Classically described as sharp, **pleuritic** chest discomfort that worsens when patients are supine and **eases when they lean forward.**
- On exam, a pericardial **friction rub** is the hallmark. The rub is classically described as having 3 components: atrial contraction, ventricular contraction, and ventricular filling.

DIFFERENTIAL

The same as the differential for myocarditis, along with pneumothorax and costochondritis.

DIAGNOSIS

- Look for a history of chest pain that is typical of acute pericarditis.
- Listen for the presence of friction rub.
- Typical ECG changes (diffuse ST-segment elevation, PR-segment depression) are **not** compatible with a single coronary distribution (see Figure 6.10).
- Echocardiography is useful to exclude a large pericardial effusion, but many patients will have only a small effusion or a normal echocardiogram.

TREATMENT

- Usually supportive, although treatment should be directed to the likely etiology.
- NSAIDs or colchicine (especially for patients with recurrent episodes).
- Steroids are often used as a last resort when patients do not respond to other therapies.
- Monitor for signs of enlarging pericardial effusion and/or tamponade (hypotension and elevated JVP)—a medical emergency requiring pericardiocentesis and/or a surgical pericardial window.

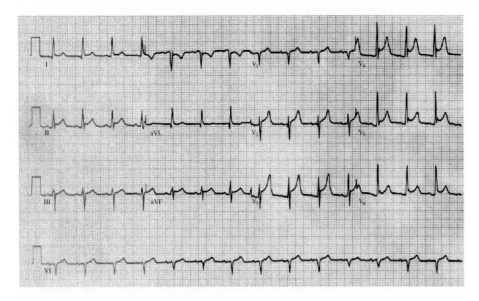

FIGURE 6.10. **ECG in acute pericarditis.** (Reproduced, with permission, from Crawford MH, et al. *Current Diagnosis & Treatment in Cardiology*, 3rd ed. New York: McGraw-Hill, 2009, Fig. 17-2.)

Pulmonary Infections

ACUTE BRONCHITIS

A nonspecific term used to describe an acute productive cough without evidence of pneumonia in patients with or without underlying lung disease. By definition, the inflammation is limited to the trachea and to large and medium-sized bronchi. The most common causative organisms are respiratory viruses (RSV; rhino-, corona-, and adenoviruses; influenza and parainfluenza viruses) and, to a lesser extent, atypical bacteria (*M pneumoniae*, *C pneumoniae*, *Bordetella pertussis*).

SYMPTOMS/EXAM

- Cough (productive or not) may persist for 1–3 weeks, often with initial URI symptoms (rhinorrhea or sore throat).
- Lung exam findings range from clear to wheezes (from bronchospasm) or rhonchi.

DIFFERENTIAL

- Rule out community-acquired pneumonia.
- Consider *B pertussis* in children with a "whooping" cough and in adults with a severe paroxysmal cough. Recent studies show that adolescents and young adults with waning immunity are a reservoir to infect unvaccinated or inadequately vaccinated children with pertussis. The Td vaccine has been expanded to Tdap (one booster for patients 19–64 years of age).
- Other conditions that may lead to chronic cough include GERD, asthma, postnasal drip, foreign body, malignancy, CHF, and TB. Chronic cough may also be a side effect of ACEI use.

DIAGNOSIS

Diagnosis is made clinically. CXR is not routinely indicated except possibly to rule out pneumonia.

TREATMENT

- Because the most common etiologies are viral, antibiotics are **not generally indicated** except in the setting of a COPD exacerbation.
- Expectorants can be used for symptomatic treatment.
- Bronchodilators may be used if there is a reactive airway component.

INFLUENZA

A 23-year-old woman, otherwise healthy, develops a fever of 39.5°C (103.1°F) and diffuse myalgias the day after returning from a business trip. On the second day of her illness, she develops cough, rhinorrhea, and shortness of breath. Her O$_2$ saturation in your office is 95% on room air. What should you do next?

The differential diagnoses include CAP and influenza, among other etiologies. Obtain a CXR and a rapid test for influenza, discuss the treatment options and precautions with the patient, and consider early initiation of the antiviral medication oseltamivir.

An acute viral respiratory infection caused by influenza A and B, members of the Orthomyxoviridae family. Infection and mortality are most common in winter. Transmission via aerosolized droplets is highly contagious. Influenza is responsible for many **local epidemics as well as historical pandemics.**

Influenza infectivity and virulence vary yearly, related to the surface proteins hemagglutinin (H) and neuraminidase (N). Different combinations of H + N create a given influenza A serotype (eg, H1N1, or "swine flu").

Influenza A strains are harbored by animal reservoirs—pigs and birds—which can be asymptomatic carriers. New combinations of H + N are due to **antigenic shift:** the reassortment of H + N when virus serotypes exchange genetic material in a host animal or person.

SYMPTOMS/EXAM

- Presentation usually includes **abrupt onset** of fever (up to 5 days), chills, headache, myalgias, fatigue, anorexia, dry cough, sore throat, and/or clear rhinorrhea. Abdominal pain and diarrhea may be seen as well.
- Physical findings are nonspecific and may include hyperemic pharyngeal mucosa without exudates, lymphadenopathy, and scattered rhonchi or rales on lung exam.

DIFFERENTIAL

Other respiratory viruses, atypical bacteria (*M pneumoniae, Chlamydia pneumoniae*), bacterial pneumonia or pharyngitis, exacerbation of underlying comorbidities such as COPD.

DIAGNOSIS

- **Viral testing:** Rapid tests can be collected from the nasopharynx to detect viral particles within 30 minutes. In general, these tests are more specific than sensitive. Viral cultures and PCR for identification are usually available, but can take up to 3–5 days for results.
- **Blood tests:** WBC counts can vary from mild leukopenia to mild leukocytosis. Significant leukocytosis should prompt consideration of a bacterial etiology.

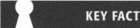

KEY FACT

Birds are the primary reservoir for influenza A; swine are the putative "mixing vessel" where antigenic shift can occur. This shift can lead to a pandemic if a strain becomes easily transmissible in humans and there is little existing immunity.

TREATMENT

- **Symptomatic treatment:** Treat fever, headache, and myalgias with acetaminophen. Avoid salicylates in patients < 18 years of age because of the risk of **Reye syndrome.** Antitussives can be used sparingly. Encourage rest and hydration.
- **Antiviral therapy:** Most effective when administered within the first 6 hours of symptom onset. When used within the first 48 hours of illness, antivirals may ↓ the duration of illness by 1–2 days and in some studies ↓ the subjective symptom severity.
- Since 2005, widespread resistance to the antivirals amantadine and rimantidine has developed, but influenza A and B remain mostly sensitive to oseltamivir and zanamivir (neuraminidase inhibitors).
- Consider hospitalization if there is concern about hydration and oxygenation or if the patient has significant comorbidities. Whereas zanamivir is used for postexposure prophylaxis, oseltamivir is generally used for hospitalized patients.

KEY FACT

Reye syndrome is a rare complication of influenza with concurrent aspirin use in children. Fatty liver and encephalopathy lead to a mortality rate of 30%.

PREVENTION

- **Universal yearly vaccination** is now recommended for all patients > 6 months of age (see Table 6.8). The vaccine is produced in eggs and thus is **contraindicated in serious egg allergy.**
- Chemoprophylaxis with antiviral medication may be considered in very-high-risk individuals during an influenza epidemic but is not an evidence-based approach except in certain settings, such as skilled nursing facilities.

COMPLICATIONS

With the majority of influenza strains, complications are common in very young patients, in patients > 65 years of age with comorbid conditions, and

TABLE 6.8.   Recommendations for Influenza Vaccination

The CDC recommends **universal vaccination** for all patients > 6 months of age.

Type of vaccine for administration:

- Two types of influenza vaccine are currently available: live attenuated influenza vaccine (**LAIV**) and trivalent influenza vaccine (**TIV**).
- LAIV contains weakened live virus, which can cause mild symptoms such as malaise, rhinorrhea, and cough. It is administered by nasal spray.
- TIV contains killed virus and cannot cause infection. It is administered by injection.

Vaccination of specific populations:

- LAIV should only be administered to healthy, nonpregnant patients 2–49 years of age.
- TIV should be administered to all other patients, including pregnant women, any person with chronic illness > 6 months of age, and adults > 50 years of age.
- Because of the theoretical risk of transmission of live influenza virus, LAIV should not be administered to the contacts or caregivers of the severely immunocompromised, such as recipients of hematopoietic stem cell transplant while they require care in a protective environment (eg, positive pressure room).
- LAIV may be administered to contacts of pregnant women and moderate-risk patients (eg, those with chronic illness, including cancer and AIDS). There have not been any documented cases of severe influenza via transmission from an LAIV recipient.

Notes on children: Children 6 months to 8 years of age who have not been previously vaccinated should receive two sequential vaccine doses in their first year of vaccination.

Notes on H1N1: H1N1 has been incorporated into the seasonal influenza vaccine since the 2010–2011 season.

during the second or third trimester of pregnancy. H1N1 influenza A, the most recent epidemic strain, was unusual in that it caused severe illness in relatively healthy, young people.

- **Pulmonary:** ARDS, leading to hypoxemic respiratory failure, secondary bacterial pneumonia (including a higher relative risk of *Streptococcus pneumoniae* and *S aureus* pneumonia).
- **Musculoskeletal:** Myositis, rhabdomyolysis, and myoglobinuria are rare.
- **Cardiopulmonary:** Myocarditis (especially in younger patients), pericarditis, and exacerbations of COPD, asthma, or CHF.
- **Neurologic:** Encephalitis, transverse myelitis, Guillain-Barré syndrome.
- In rare cases, influenza can cause ARDS and multiorgan failure. The majority of cases are not nearly as severe, and many cases are self-limited and likely go without specific diagnosis.
- **Reye syndrome:** Children present with nausea and vomiting, followed by CNS changes several days after a viral illness. Currently, Reye syndrome is uncommon due to ↓ aspirin use in children.

ACUTE BACTERIAL PNEUMONIA

A purulent infection of the lung parenchyma and airspaces. Caused by a diverse array of pathogens. The most common infectious cause of disease and death in the United States, responsible for 50,000–60,000 deaths yearly. Treatment is based on severity of symptoms, presumed pathogen, and the risk of multidrug resistance (MDR) in a given patient.

SYMPTOMS/EXAM

- Symptoms include shortness of breath, productive cough, pleuritic chest pain, fever and chills, or rigors.
- Hyperthermia or hypothermia, tachypnea, tachycardia, and hypoxia are common clinical findings. Severe cases may present with cyanosis and altered mental status and can advance to sepsis and multiorgan failure.
- In addition to altered air movement and rhonchi or rales on lung exam, special findings due to lung consolidation may include egophony, whispered pectoriloquy, and tactile fremitus.

DIFFERENTIAL

- **Infectious causes:** Viral or fungal pneumonia (including *Pneumocystis jiroveci*, formerly known as *Pneumocystis carinii*); TB, postobstructive pneumonia, septic emboli from right-sided endocarditis.
- **Noninfectious causes:** Malignancy, foreign body, pulmonary infarct from emboli, collagen vascular disease with vasculitis leading to hemorrhage and hypersensitivity, radiation, chemical pneumonitis, aspiration pneumonitis.

DIAGNOSIS

- **Chest imaging:** CXR is recommended for diagnosis and helps to avoid overtreatment; may characterize pneumonia severity, extent, and whether the pneumonia is complicated (see Figure 6.11). CT scan of the chest can provide more detailed information, but it is recommended only in complicated cases or if the diagnosis is unclear.
- **Sputum Gram stain and culture: Recommended for inpatients** with productive cough; usually not necessary in outpatients. Must have > 10 squamous cells to be considered an adequate sample.

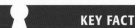

KEY FACT

Egophony is E to A change. Whispered pectoriloquy means the patient whispers and the doctor hears the chest (pectus) speaking ("loquy" from the Latin root to speak).

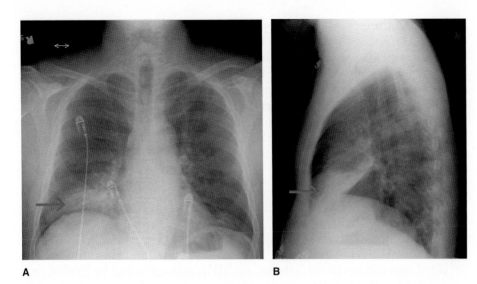

A   B

FIGURE 6.11.   **Community-acquired pneumonia.** Frontal (**A**) and lateral (**B**) radiographs show airspace consolidation in the right middle lobe *(red arrows)* in a patient with community-acquired pneumonia. (Reproduced, with permission, from USMLERx.com)

TABLE 6.9.   **Causative Organisms and Historical Features of Community-Acquired Pneumonia**

ORGANISM	CAUSE (%)	SUGGESTIVE HISTORICAL FEATURES
Streptococcus pneumoniae	20–60	Acute onset; often follows URI or influenza; underlying COPD.
Haemophilus influenzae	3–10	Often follows URI; COPD.
S aureus	3–5	May follow influenza infection; cavitary disease. May be methicillin resistant (MRSA), especially in HAP/HCAP or VAP.
Legionella spp.	2–8	Exposure to humidifier, hot tub, or air-conditioning cooling towers; pleuritic chest pain and pleural effusion are common; diarrhea; hyponatremia.
Klebsiella, other gram-⊖ rods	3–10	Ethanol abuse, diabetes, patients in long-term care, aspiration, VAP. Some may display broad MDR (eg, ESBL).
Mycoplasma pneumoniae	1–6	Young adults in summer and fall; associated rash and bullous myringitis.
Chlamydia pneumoniae	4–10	Young adults; often follows prolonged sore throat.
Pseudomonas aeruginosa	Rare	Important cause of VAP, high rate of morbidity from chronic lung disease and mortality.
Stenotrophomonas and *Acinetobacter*	Rare	Additional causes of VAP; can display broad resistance patterns; usually require 14+ days of antibiotics.
Q fever (*Coxiella burnetii*)	Rare	Exposure to livestock (cattle, goats, sheep); elevated LFTs.
Chlamydia psittaci	Rare	Exposure to birds, including parrots, pigeons, and chickens; headache; temperature-pulse dissociation.

■ **Blood cultures:** Collect in hospitalized patients before antibiotic therapy. Provide reliable data and allow for the tailoring of antimicrobial therapy if cultures are ⊕. However, cultures are ⊕ in only 10% of cases.

■ **Tests for specific etiologies:** If there is a high clinical suspicion for a specific etiologic organism, seek appropriate available testing (see Table 6.9).

■ In ventilated patients, obtain **endotracheal sample** (via bronchoalveolar lavage or tracheal aspirate) before antibiotic administration. Quantitative culture can provide more specific information if a pathogenic organism is present.

TREATMENT

■ The type of pathogen in a given patient depends on comorbidities and setting (see Table 6.9).

■ Per Infectious Diseases Society of America (IDSA) and American Thoracic Society (ATS) guidelines, acute bacterial pneumonia treatment is divided into settings by risk category for MDR pathogens and by level of care needed (see Table 6.10).

■ Local antibiograms and infectious disease specialist recommendations can be helpful in choice of initial antibiotic therapy. For initial therapy, use the IDSA/ATS consensus guidelines (Table 6.10).

■ **β-lactams** include: high-dose amoxicillin +/– clavulanate, ampicillin +/– sulbactam, and piperacillin + tazobactam (antipseudomonal); and cephalosporins such as ceftriaxone, cefotaxime, cefuroxime, and cefepime (antipseudomonal).

TABLE 6.10. **Definition of Pneumonia and Initial Antibiotic Therapy**

TYPE OF PNEUMONIA	DEFINITION	INITIAL ANTIBIOTIC THERAPY
Community-acquired (CAP)	Dx within 48 hours of admission; does not fit HCAP/HAP or VAP criteria.	Outpatient: macrolide (ML) or doxycycline. If chronic disease, immunocompromised, or antibiotics in past 3 months: respiratory fluoroquinolone (RF) or β-lactam + ML or doxycycline. Inpatient: RF or β-lactam + ML or doxycycline.
Health care–associated (HCAP) or hospital-acquired (HAP)	> 2 days acute hospitalization within past 90 days. Exposed to antibiotics, chemotherapy, or wound care within 30 days of current illness. Reside in LTC facility. Hemodialysis at hospital or clinic. Home nursing care. Contact of patient with MDR infection.	If no MDR risk factors: monotherapy with β-lactam, ertapenem, or RF. If MDR risk factors: antipseudomonal (AP) β-lactam or carbapenem + RF. If MRSA risk factors: add vancomycin, consider consolidation to 2 agents, depending on presumed pathogen (eg, vancomycin + AP β-lactam).
Ventilator-associated (VAP)	Develops > 48 hours after endotracheal intubation or < 48 hours of extubation.	Same as above regimen for MDR risk factors.
Aspiration	Largely the same therapy for CAP and HAP/HCAP, but potentially greater risk for anaerobes if severe periodontal disease or macroscopic aspiration event (alcoholism, neuromuscular impairment). Differentiate between pneumonitis (a transient inflammatory infiltrate *not requiring* antibiotics) and pneumonia.	No consensus guideline, some expert opinions recommend: AP β-lactam, carbapenem, or AP cephalosporin. RF or β-lactam + clindamycin or metronidazole.

- **RFs** include levofloxacin (antipseudomonal), gemifloxacin, and moxifloxacin.
- **MLs** include azithromycin and clarithromycin (an erythromycin used less commonly and usually not as monotherapy for pneumonia).
- **Carbapenems** include ertapenem, meropenem (antipseudomonal), imipenem +/– cilastatin (antipseudomonal), and doripenem (anti-pseudomonal).
- **Treatment setting:** Outpatient therapy is appropriate in low-risk patients. By assigning risk categories, indices such as the pneumonia PORT severity index (PSI) and CURB-65 can help determine which patients are appropriate for outpatient care and which should be hospitalized (see Tables 6.11 and 6.12).
- **Response to treatment:** Antimicrobial therapy initiated within **4–8 hours** of presentation is associated with improved outcomes.
- **Early conversion** from parenteral to oral therapy is appropriate once a patient has improved clinically, is hemodynamically stable, and is able to take oral medication.
- Tailor antibiotic therapy to the narrowest coverage possible per available bacteriologic results (culture, specific serologies) to limit future resistance. For some organisms, minimum inhibitory concentration (MIC) data, found via bacterial culture, may be important for dosing of antibiotics.
- **Duration of treatment** varies by organism and setting, but 5–7 days is adequate for most cases of pneumonia, with at least 48–72 hours afebrile before discontinuing antibiotics.
- Longer courses (**at least** 2 weeks) may be required for infections due to MRSA, *Legionella*, *Mycoplasma*, *Chlamydia*, *Pseudomonas*, *Acinetobacter*, or *Stenotrophomonas* spp.
- If inadequate response after 48–72 hours, consider resistance, an alternative pathogen (atypical or rare bacteria, virus, fungi), a complicated pneumonia (abscess or empyema), or an alternative diagnosis.
- **Repeat chest imaging is not required** during hospitalization, except when complications are suspected (eg, ongoing fever, hypoxia, clinical deterioration).
- Consider CXR in 4–8 weeks in patients with risk factors for persistent infection or underling malignancy (eg, smokers and patients > 65 years of age).
- Patients may be discharged without delay at the time of conversion to oral therapy if they meet criteria (see Table 6.13).

PREVENTION

- Smoking cessation is key to improving mucociliary clearance and to ↓ risk of COPD and lung malignancy.
- Administer the pneumococcal vaccine to patients > 65 years of age, to patients with chronic disease such as diabetes or cardiopulmonary disease, and to asplenic patients.
- Basic infection control (eg, frequent hand hygiene and sterilization of ventilation equipment) is paramount, as the mortality rate for HCAP/HAP and VAP may reach 40%.

COMPLICATIONS

- Severe pneumonia can progress to **sepsis, ARDS,** shock, and multiorgan failure. If shock (eg, hypotension, organ failure), respiratory failure, or CXR consistent with ARDS is present on presentation, the patient should be directly admitted to ICU, with critical care consultation as appropriate.
- **Pleural effusion/empyema/lung abscess:** Approximately 40% of patients with CAP have an effusion on CXR/CT. Thoracentesis should be per-

TABLE 6.11. **Scoring System for Risk Class Assignment of Community-Acquired Pneumonia (PSI)**[a]

PATIENT CHARACTERISTIC	POINTS ASSIGNED
Demographic factor:	
Age: men	Number of years
Age: women	Number of years minus 10
Nursing home resident	10
Comorbid illnesses:	
Neoplastic disease[b]	30
Liver disease[c]	20
CHF[d]	10
Cerebrovascular disease[e]	10
Renal disease[f]	10
Physical examination finding:	
Altered mental status[g]	20
Respiratory rate ≥ 30 breaths/min	20
Systolic BP < 90 mmHg	
Temperature ≤ 35°C (95°F) or ≥ 40°C (104°F)	15
Pulse ≥ 125 bpm	10
Laboratory or radiographic finding:	
Arterial pH < 7.35	30
BUN ≥ 30 mg/dL	20
Sodium < 130 meq/L	20
Glucose > 250 mg/dL	10
Hematocrit < 30%	10
Arterial Po$_2$ < 60 mmHg	10
Pleural effusion	10

[a]A total point score for a given patient is obtained by summing the patient's age in years (age minus 10 for women) and the points for each applicable characteristic.

[b]Any cancer except basal or squamous cell carcinoma of the skin that was active at the time of presentation or diagnosed within 1 year before presentation.

[c]Clinical or histologic diagnosis of cirrhosis or another form of chronic liver disease.

[d]Systolic or diastolic dysfunction documented by history, physical examination and CXR, echocardiogram, multigated angiogram (MUGA) scan, or left ventriculogram.

[e]Clinical diagnosis of stroke or TIA or stroke documented by MRI or CT scan.

[f]History of chronic renal disease or abnormal BUN and creatinine concentration documented in the medical record.

[g]Disorientation (to person, place, or time, not known to be chronic), stupor, or coma.

TABLE 6.12. **Recommendations for Site of Care for Community-Acquired Pneumonia by Point Score**

POINT SCORE	RECOMMENDED TREATMENT SETTING
≤ 70	Outpatient
71–90	Outpatient or brief inpatient
> 90	Inpatient

TABLE 6.13. **Criteria for Discharge in Community-Acquired Pneumonia**

Clinical stability:

- Improvement in cough/dyspnea.
- Adequate O₂ saturation (> 90%).
- Afebrile (temperature < 37.8°C [100°F]).
- Resolution of tachycardia (< 100 bpm).
- Resolution of tachypnea (RR < 24).
- Resolution of hypotension (SBP > 90 mmHg).
- No evidence of complicated infection (eg, extrapulmonary or pleural involvement).
- Ability to tolerate oral medications.

formed if the effusion is impairing oxygenation or ventilation or if the patient is septic or is not responding to antimicrobial therapy. For empyema, complicated parapneumonic effusions, or a lung abscess, consultation with pulmonology, interventional radiology, or thoracic surgery should be obtained for percutaneous or surgical drainage.

- **Necrotizing pneumonia:** Destruction of the lung parenchyma and airspaces due to infection and inflammation; can lead to fibrosis and chronic lung disease. Consult with a pulmonologist.
- **Recurrent pneumonia:** Recurrent CAP in the same anatomic location within 2 years may be due to an obstruction (ie, mass or foreign body). If recurrence is in a new location, consider an immunodeficiency workup and a chest CT to rule out bronchiectasis or obstructive lesion.

TUBERCULOSIS (TB)

A 36-year-old man from Burma presents to his primary care doctor with increasing cough over the past 6 weeks, associated with a 15-pound weight loss and night sweats. He moved to the United States 9 months ago and had a 20-mm PPD skin test during his first primary care visit. On exam, he is febrile to 38.4°C (101.2°F) and has decreased breath sounds and scattered supraclavicular and axillary lymphadenopathy. What is your next step?

Place a mask on the patient and have him wait in an isolation room, ideally with a negative pressure system. All staff in the area should wear appropriately sized N95 respirator masks. Order a CXR and contact your area TB controller for diagnostic and treatment recommendations.

The largest single cause of infectious disease morbidity and mortality worldwide. A slow-growing, acid-fast bacillary infection caused by *Mycobacterium tuberculosis* (mTB). TB can affect nearly any system in the body, most commonly the lungs, and is transmitted by airborne respiratory droplets from patients with active pulmonary disease. TB can cause **primary, latent, and reactivation infection.** Symptoms and capacity for transmission depend on location and activity of disease.

SYMPTOMS/EXAM

- Symptoms vary, depending on location and type of infection. **Latent disease: asymptomatic.**
- In **active pulmonary TB**, patients may experience cough, hemoptysis, shortness of breath, weight loss, and pleuritic chest pain.

- In **skeletal TB,** symptoms include bone pain, arthritis of affected joints, pathologic fracture in advanced disease, and paralysis in 50% of patients with undiagnosed vertebral tuberculosis (Pott disease).
- Other sites can include the GI and GU tracts, lymph nodes (called scrofula in the cervical nodes; see Figure 6.12), skin, eyes, and CNS (causing various manifestations, most commonly a basilar meningitis resulting in headache, altered mental status, possible cranial nerve abnormalities, and potential for cerebrovascular accident).

DIFFERENTIAL

Depends on location: In pulmonary disease, TB can mimic pneumonia, fungal infection, malignancy, postinfectious scar, autoimmune disease (sarcoidosis, Wegener granulomatosis, etc), and pulmonary fibrosis.

DIAGNOSIS

- Imaging studies to evaluate patients with suspected mTB disease should be guided by symptoms and may include **CXR or CT scan** (see Figure 6.13).
- Findings on imaging, especially in pulmonary tuberculosis, are highly variable and nonspecific:
  - Primary pulmonary infection can display segmental or lobar consolidation, hilar or mediastinal LAD, effusion, atelectasis. **CXR is normal in approximately 15%** of patients with 1° pulmonary TB.
  - Individuals with latent TB often have the classic Ghon complex (a peripheral calcified nodule and hilar lymphadenopathy).
  - Reactivation disease in immunocompetent individuals, including HIV-⊕ patients with CD4+ cell count > 400 cells/mm^3, usually causes upper lung zone disease with apical cavitation.

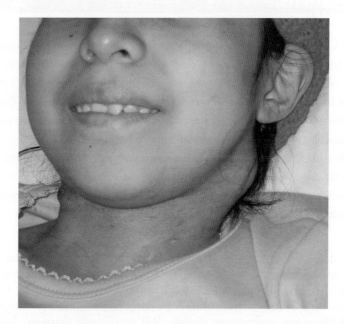

FIGURE 6.12. Tuberculosis adenopathy. Bilateral cervical adenopathy (scrofula) in a Peruvian child with documented TB. Cervical adenopathy in a child in highly endemic areas is strongly suggestive, and is the most common form, of extrapulmonary TB. (Reproduced, with permission, from Knoop KJ, et al. *The Atlas of Emergency Medicine,* 3rd ed. New York: McGraw-Hill, 2010, Fig. 21.56. Photo contributors: Seth W. Wright, MD and Universidad Peruana Cayetano Heredia, Lina, Peru.)

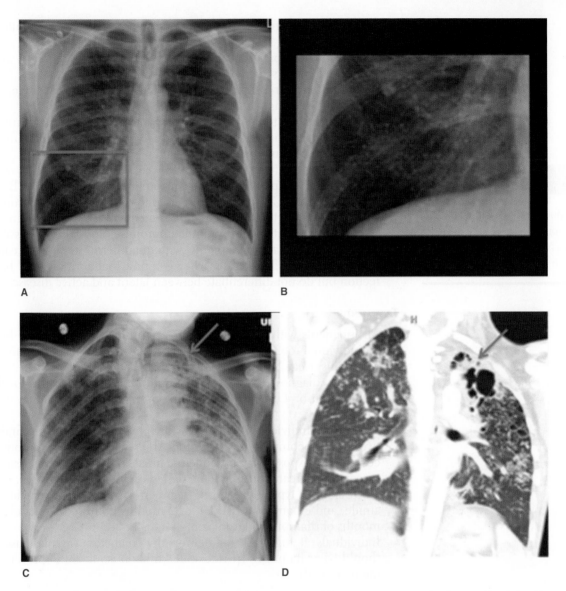

FIGURE 6.13. **Pulmonary tuberculosis.** (A) Frontal CXR demonstrating diffuse 1- to 2-mm nodules due to miliary TB. (B) A zoomed-in view corresponding to the area delineated by the red box in Image A. (C) Frontal CXR demonstrating left apical cavitary consolidation *(red arrow)* and patchy infiltrates in the right and left lungs in a patient with reactivation TB. (D) Coronal reformation from a noncontrast chest CT in the same patient as Image C, better demonstrating left apical cavitary consolidation *(red arrows)* and other areas of parenchymal abnormality corresponding to the endobronchial spread of TB. (Reproduced, with permission, from USMLERx.com.)

- Immunocompromised patients, including those with AIDS with CD4+ cell count < 200 cells/mm³, have variable manifestations such as diffuse disease with miliary, lower lung zone, or hilar/mediastinal foci.
- For potential foci of extrapulmonary TB (more common in immunocompromised patients), imaging and sample/biopsy must be guided by the location and probability of disease.

DIAGNOSIS

- Can be challenging. In suspected pulmonary TB, **sputum samples should be collected on 3 consecutive mornings,** with the patient NPO after midnight before each sample if it is being induced. Patients without cough may have sputum induced by inhalation of hypertonic saline.

- In young children, early-morning gastric aspirates can substitute for sputum samples.
- In an intubated patient, samples can be obtained by tracheal aspirations performed 8 hours apart.
- If sputum or gastric samples are unobtainable, bronchoscopy can be performed for washings +/– biopsies.
- All samples need to be sent specifically for mycobacterial culture (see Figure 6.14). mTB may take up to 8 weeks to grow in a traditional mycobacterial culture, although it often grows in 2–3 weeks.
- Sputum cultures must be $\ominus \times 3$ for 8 weeks to definitively rule out growth of TB in the sample. Because of the variable appearance of TB on imaging, a $\ominus$ x-ray or CT should not be used to rule out active pulmonary TB.
- Evidence of infection can be demonstrated with PPD skin testing (false $\ominus$ possible in patients with immunocompromise, and false $\oplus$ possible in recent BCG vaccination recipients) with quantiferon serology (greater specificity than PPD.) These tests, when $\oplus$, show that an individual has TB infection but do not differentiate between latent and active disease.

TREATMENT

- All inpatients with concern for active pulmonary TB must be isolated in an individual room with a negative pressure system. Persons who enter the room must wear N95 masks to minimize chance of infection.
- All newly diagnosed cases of TB should be **reported to the local health department** or TB controller. The reporting requirements may vary by location.
- In high-risk individuals (positive history/physical/radiographic findings, active immunocompromise including AIDS with CD4+ cell count < 200 cells/ mm^3, exposure in TB-endemic areas, history of homelessness or incarceration), treatment should be started on the first day of care.
- TB therapy is typically a 4-drug regimen of rifampin, isoniazid, pyrazinamide, and ethambutol (RIPE) for 2 months, followed by an additional 4 months of rifampin and isoniazid.
- Individuals at high risk for neuropathy (diabetes, vascular disease, etc) should take vitamin B$_6$ (pyridoxine) while on isoniazid to prevent worsening neuropathy.

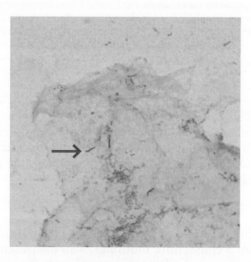

FIGURE 6.14. *Mycobacterium tuberculosis* on AFB smear. (Courtesy of the Centers for Disease Control and Prevention, Atlanta, GA.)

- Therapy depends on the risk of MDR or XDR TB, and consultation with the local TB controller should be obtained before beginning anti-TB therapy for all patients.
- For patients with extrapulmonary TB, therapy is determined by the site and complications of disease, and appropriate specialty consultation should be employed.

PREVENTION

- Health care providers and exposed individuals (family members or caregivers of individuals with active disease) should have yearly PPD testing to check for infection.
- Individuals with latent disease can usually be treated with isoniazid alone, but consultation with local health department/TB controller is recommended before starting therapy.

Gastrointestinal Infections

GASTROENTERITIS AND COLITIS

> A 39-year-old woman calls you at home complaining of 18 hours of intense abdominal pain, nausea, vomiting, and profuse, nonbloody, watery diarrhea. On further questioning, she states that she just returned from a trip to the Bahamas and adds that her sister has been experiencing similar symptoms. She is unable to take any liquids by mouth because of vomiting, and she has had 10 bowel movements in the past 12 hours. You instruct the patient to take her pulse, and she states that it is 120 bpm. After recommending that the patient go to the ER for IV fluids, you call the ER attending. What do you tell her is your leading diagnosis?
>
> Traveler's diarrhea caused by enterotoxigenic *E coli*.

An acute infection of the gastrointestinal tract with multiple pathogenic etiologies, primarily characterized by diarrhea and vomiting. Globally, diarrheal illnesses are the second leading cause of death behind cardiovascular disease and are the leading cause of death in children. However, most cases are mild and self-limited. Enteric pathogens are transmitted via the fecal-oral route, and risk factors for acquisition include travel, AIDS/immunocompromise, institutional care, and recent antibiotic use. Historical clues and diarrhea descriptions can be helpful in determining the etiologic agent.

The most common bacterial causes of inflammatory enteritis in the United States are *Campylobacter jejuni*, *Salmonella* spp, and *Shigella* spp. *Clostridium difficile* is a health care–associated pathogen acquired by 20% of hospitalized patients, and the most common cause of antibiotic-associated diarrhea in the United States. See Table 6.14 for additional etiologies.

SYMPTOMS

- **Noninflammatory diarrhea:** Pathogens act primarily in the **small intestine** to induce fluid secretion. Patients have **large-volume, watery diarrhea** and nausea, vomiting, cramping, and minimal fever.
- **Inflammatory diarrhea:** Pathogens induce inflammation in the **colon** via invasion or cytotoxins. Patients present with fever, **small-volume stools containing blood or mucus,** tenesmus, and lower abdominal cramping.

KEY FACT

The most common cause of infectious diarrhea in U.S. children is rotavirus. Noroviruses are the most common cause overall.

TABLE 6.14.   Microbiology of Infectious Diarrhea

Inflammatory Diarrhea	Noninflammatory Diarrhea	Grossly Bloody Diarrhea	Diarrhea in HIV/AIDS Patients	Traveler's Diarrhea
Bacteria:	**Bacteria:**	**Bacteria:**	**Bacteria:**	**Major causes:**
■ *Campylobacter jejuni*	■ *S aureus*	■ Enterohemorrhagic *E coli*	■ *Campylobacter jejuni*	■ Enterotoxigenic *E coli*
■ *Shigella* spp	■ *Bacillus cereus*	■ *Shigella* spp	■ *Shigella* spp	
■ Enterohemorrhagic *E coli*[a]	■ *Clostridium perfringens*	■ *Campylobacter jejuni*	■ *Salmonella* spp	**Less common causes:**
■ *C difficile*	■ Enterotoxigenic *E coli*		■ *C difficile*	■ *Campylobacter jejuni*
■ *Vibrio parahaemolyticus*[b]	■ *Vibrio cholerae*	**Protozoa:**	■ Enteroaggregative *E coli*	■ *Shigella* spp
■ *Listeria monocytogenes*	■ *Mycobacterium avium* complex	■ *Entamoeba histolytica*	■ *Mycobacterium avium* complex	■ *Salmonella* spp
■ *Yersinia enterocolitica*	■ *Aeromonas hydrophila*			■ Rotavirus
■ Enteroinvasive *E coli*	■ *Plesiomonas shigelloides*		**Viruses:**	■ Norwalk virus
■ Enteroaggregative *E coli*			■ CMV	■ *Vibrio parahaemolyticus*
	Viruses:		■ Enteric adenovirus	■ *Entamoeba histolytica*
Viruses:	■ Rotavirus		■ Caliciviruses	■ *Giardia lamblia*
■ CMV	■ Enteric adenovirus		■ HIV enteropathy	■ *Cryptosporidium parvum*
	■ Caliciviruses			■ *Cyclospora cayetanensis*
Protozoa:	■ Norwalk virus		**Protozoa:**	
■ *Entamoeba histolytica*	■ CMV		■ *Cryptosporidium parvum*	
			■ *Isospora belli*	
	Protozoa:		■ *Cyclospora cayetanensis*	
	■ *Cryptosporidium parvum*		■ *Microsporidia* spp	
	■ *Giardia lamblia*			
	■ *Cyclospora cayetanensis*			
	■ *Isospora belli*			
	■ *Microsporidia* spp			

[a]Cases can have no fever or focal leukocytes.

[b]May also cause a noninflammatory syndrome.

Reproduced, with permission, from Wilson WR. *Current Diagnosis & Treatment in Infectious Diseases*, 1st ed. New York: McGraw-Hill, 2001: 261.

Exam

- Signs of dehydration, abdominal tenderness, and distention are commonly seen. In neonates and infants, sunken fontanelles and lethargy are important signs of severe illness.
- Fever > 38.5°C (101.3°F), abdominal guarding or rigidity (acute abdomen), and systemic signs (hypotension, tachycardia, altered mental status) are seen in severe illness.

Differential

Noninfectious causes include drugs, food allergies, IBD, malabsorption, and motility disorders.

DIAGNOSIS

- The history and physical are paramount.
- Further evaluation is indicated in the setting of severe symptoms and signs as above, bloody diarrhea, immunocompromised hosts, age > 70 years, or severe dehydration.
- Specific testing is not needed in patients without the above warning signs.
- **Blood tests:** CBC, electrolytes, amoeba serologies.
- **Stool tests:** Leukocytes (when present, suggest colonic inflammation and inflammatory diarrhea), lactoferrin (another marker of colonic inflammation), O&P (in recent travelers or immunocompromised hosts), *Giardia* antigen, *C difficile* toxin, bacterial culture. Let the lab know of suspected causative bacteria, as different media are required for the various possibilities.
- **Endoscopy:** Flexible sigmoidoscopy or colonoscopy with biopsy for chronic diarrhea or in select cases of unclear acute infection. Notable findings in *C difficile* colitis include pseudomembrane formation (see Figure 6.15).

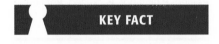

> **KEY FACT**
>
> Incidence of **community-acquired** *C difficile* diarrhea is increasing.

TREATMENT

- **Mild diarrhea:**
  - Oral rehydration therapy with oral glucose-electrolyte solutions.
  - A BRAT diet (bananas, rice, applesauce, toast) is recommended but is not evidence based.
  - **Antidiarrheals:** Loperamide. Use with caution in infectious diarrhea, as it may prolong the duration of symptoms, lead to toxic megacolon, and ↑ the risk of hemolytic-uremic syndrome (HUS). Not recommended in children.
- **Severe diarrhea:** Oral or IV rehydration. Consider hospital admission.

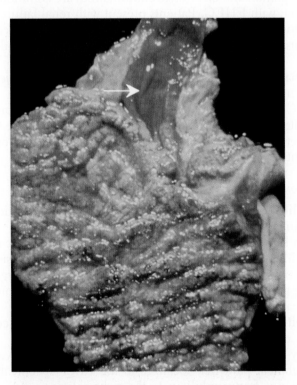

FIGURE 6.15. *Clostridium difficile* **colitis.** Autopsy specimen showing confluent pseudomembranes covering the cecum of a patient with pseudomembranous colitis. Note the sparing of the terminal ileum *(arrow)*. (Reproduced, with permission, from Fauci AS, et al. *Harrison's Principles of Internal Medicine,* 17th ed. New York: McGraw-Hill, 2008, Fig. 123-1.)

- **Antibiotics:**
  - Use only in the presence of fever, tenesmus, bloody stool (unless enterohemorrhagic *E coli* [EHEC] is suspected), fecal leukocytes, or cultures/antigen tests ⊕ for bacteria or protozoa.
  - Empiric treatment for bacterial enteritis/colitis consists of ciprofloxacin 500 mg PO or 400 mg IV BID × 3–5 days.
  - Antibiotics are **not** recommended for nontyphoidal *Salmonella* (may prolong shedding), *Aeromonas*, *Yersinia*, or *E coli* O157:H7 infections. Antibiotics **are** recommended for *Campylobacter* infection, shigellosis, cholera, extraintestinal salmonellosis, severe traveler's diarrhea, *C difficile* colitis (stop other antibiotics if possible and start metronidazole or vancomycin), giardiasis (metronidazole), amebiasis (metronidazole), and AIDS-related infectious diarrhea.

PREVENTION

- For infectious gastroenteritis or colitis, frequent hand washing with soap and water is critical, especially for care providers, and before eating or preparing meals. (Note: *C difficile* spores are not killed by alcohol-based hand sanitizers. However, in other circumstances, hand gels are more effective than soap and water in decreasing bacterial colony counts on the hands.)
- Avoid excessive or unnecessary antibiotic use: *C difficile* is largely an iatrogenic infection.
- Vaccinate appropriate neonates against rotavirus, a 2–3-dose series given in the first 6 months of life. Notable rare complication of intussusception with vaccination. See ACIP guidelines from 2009 for full details.

COMPLICATIONS

- Volume depletion and electrolyte abnormalities are common.
- **HUS** is seen with **EHEC**. Patients present with renal failure, microangiopathic hemolytic anemia, and thrombocytopenia. Antibiotics and antimotility agents may ↑ the risk. Risk of HUS is greatest in children and the elderly.
- Guillain-Barré syndrome is a potential complication of *C jejuni* and presents with ascending paralysis.
- In severe *C difficile* colitis, the bowel mucosa can be compromised, leading to peritonitis requiring surgical management (see Figure 6.15).
- Some enteroviruses can cause encephalitis (see discussion of encephalitis in the Central Nervous System Infections section above).

SPECIAL SITUATIONS

- **Diverticulitis** is a bacterial infection of preexisting diverticulosis (small outpouchings) of the colon, most commonly the sigmoid.
- Treat with IV antibiotic coverage for gram-⊖ and anaerobic organisms. In patients with a severe or complicated case (perforation, sepsis) or multiple (usually more than three) uncomplicated cases, interval surgical resection (when the patient is not infected) is indicated for prevention of recurrent severe disease.
- **Appendicitis** is a bacterial infection of the appendix coli (see Figure 12.2 in Surgery chapter).
  - **History and exam:** Hallmarks are anorexia, nausea, fever, and initial periumbilical pain that localizes to the RLQ (specifically, two-thirds the distance from umbilicus to the right anterior superior iliac spine, called the McBurney point). The patient may have peritoneal signs.
  - **Imaging:** CT or ultrasound.
  - **Tx:** Surgery, with interval antibiotics if surgery is delayed.

HEPATIC DISEASE

Hepatitis A (HAV)

Most common in developing countries. The infection occurs sporadically or in epidemics associated with **seafood, especially shellfish.** HAV is **transmitted via the fecal-oral route** and causes acute hepatitis. Although rare, it can cause severe disease, including fulminant hepatic failure, especially in immunocompromised individuals and pregnant women. Severe disease is more common in individuals with hepatitis C coinfection. Symptoms and mortality vary with patient age.

KEY FACT

Hepatitis A and E are transmitted by the fecal-oral route.

SYMPTOMS/EXAM

- Adults present with flulike illness, RUQ pain, jaundice, and pruritus. Children may be asymptomatic.
- Physical exam reveals jaundice and RUQ tenderness.

DIFFERENTIAL

- **Viral infections:** HAV, HCV, mononucleosis (EBV), CMV, HSV.
- **Nonviral infections:** Spirochetal disease (leptospirosis, syphilis), rickettsial disease (Q fever), acute bacterial gastroenteritis.
- **Noninfectious causes:** Autoimmune hepatitis, alcoholic hepatitis, fatty liver disease, hemochromatosis, Wilson disease, gallbladder disease.

DIAGNOSIS

Anti-HAV IgM will be ⊕ in acute infection, whereas IgG will be ⊕ in prior infection or immunization.

TREATMENT/PREVENTION

- Treatment is supportive. Patients with severe symptoms such as dehydration from GI losses or signs of liver failure should be hospitalized and appropriate diagnostic and treatment measures given.
- Vaccination (a series of 2) should be given to travelers going to endemic regions, men who have sex with men (MSM), IV drug users, patients with chronic liver disease, food handlers, and day care center workers. HAV vaccine is a formalin-killed vaccine. This is now a routine vaccine for children.
- Anti-HAV immune globulin may be given to household contacts of infected patients and to those who have eaten uncooked food prepared by an infected individual. However, in many circumstances, HAV vaccine can be used for postexposure prophylaxis in place of immune globulin.

Hepatitis B (HBV)

Chronic infection with HBV is present in > 400 million people worldwide. **Transmission occurs via exposure to infected body fluids**—ie, blood and semen. Although most individuals clear the infection, 5%–10% of infected individuals will become chronic HBV carriers. Of all patients with chronic HBV, 15%–20% will develop cirrhosis and 10%–15% will develop hepatocellular carcinoma (HCC). In mothers with acute HBV or those who carry HBsAg and HBeAg, the rate of virus acquisition by the infant is about 90%. Almost all of these infants will become chronic carriers unless passive immunization is given. Coinfection with hepatitis D virus is associated with a worse prognosis.

SYMPTOMS

- **Acute HBV:** Flulike symptoms—eg, malaise, anorexia, weakness, low-grade fever, nausea, and vomiting. RUQ pain and jaundice will also be present.
- **Chronic HBV:** Usually asymptomatic.
- **Extrahepatic manifestations:** Serum sickness–like rash, polyarteritis nodosa, glomerulonephritis.

EXAM

- **Acute HBV:** Scleral icterus, jaundice, RUQ tenderness, arthralgias.
- **Chronic HBV:** Stigmata of cirrhosis—eg, spider angiomata, palmar erythema, gynecomastia, caput medusae, and ascites.

DIFFERENTIAL

See the differential for HAV above.

DIAGNOSIS

- ↑ transaminases, bilirubin, and PT/PTT.
- Serologic markers are the gold standard (see Table 6.15):
    - **HBsAg:** Surface antigen. Indicates **acute** or chronic HBV infection.
    - **Anti-HBs:** Antibody to surface antigen. Serves as the **protective** antibody and indicates past viral infection or immunization.
    - **Anti-HBc:** Antibody to core antigen. IgG indicates **prior or current HBV infection.** IgM indicates acute infection.
    - **HBeAg:** Envelope antigen. Proportional to the quantity of intact virus—a sign of infectivity.
    - HBV DNA can be used to measure active replication.
- Liver biopsy is not routinely needed but should be considered if the diagnosis is in question or to rule out other processes.

TREATMENT

- **Acute exposure/postexposure prophylaxis:** The CDC recommends that hepatitis B immune globulin (HBIG) be given in the first 24 hours, along

TABLE 6.15. Commonly Encountered Serologic Patterns of HBV

HBsAg	Anti-HBs	Anti-HBc	HBeAg	Anti-HBe	Interpretation
+	−	IgM	+	−	Acute hepatitis B.
+	−	IgG[a]	+	−	Chronic hepatitis B with active viral replication.
+	−	IgG	−	+	Chronic hepatitis B with low viral replication.
+	+	IgG	+ or −	+ or −	Chronic hepatitis B with heterotypic anti-HBs (about 10% of cases).
−	−	IgM	+ or −		Acute hepatitis B.
−	+	−	−	−	Vaccination (immunity).
−	−	IgG	−	−	False ⊕; infection in remote past and anti-HBs has waned; window period; low-level chronic infection.

[a]Low levels of IgM anti-HBc may also be detected.

with the first dose of vaccine, if the patient was not previously immunized. Babies born to infected women should receive HBIG and HBV vaccine in the first 24 hours of life, followed by 3 doses of the vaccine in the first 6 months of life (prevents infection in 85%–95% of infants exposed).

- **Chronic active HBV:** The AASLD/IDSA published a consensus guideline in *Hepatology* (2009) for consideration of HBV treatment. The risk-to-benefit ratio of treatment depends on the presence of HBeAg, viral load, and transaminitis, with recommendations to treat patients who show persistent VL elevation or transaminitis or parenchymal damage without alternative cause on liver biopsy. The following agents are used for treatment:
  - **Interferon-α:** Given SQ for 4–6 months. Confers long-term benefit in 33% of cases but has many side effects and is contraindicated in some cases (eg, advanced cirrhosis and decompensated psychiatric disease).
  - **Antiviral agents:** Lamivudine given PO is well tolerated but resistance develops when used as a single drug. Adefovir, entecavir, telbivudine, and tenofovir are alternatives for 1° therapy and may have activity against lamivudine-resistant virus.
  - **Corticosteroids:** Not indicated for viral hepatitis.
  - **Liver transplant:** In eligible patients with decompensated cirrhosis.
  - Chronic carriers should be encouraged to avoid hepatotoxic agents, including EtOH and high-dose acetaminophen.

PREVENTION

- 1° prevention is accomplished by the HBV vaccine, a recombinant vaccine. A series of three vaccines provides detectable HBsAb levels in > 95% of individuals.
- Patients with known HBV should be vaccinated against HAV.

COMPLICATIONS

- HCC can develop **before** cirrhosis in HBV patients (this is not the case in HCV).
- Approximately 0.1% of patients develop fulminant hepatic failure.

Hepatitis C (HCV)

A 46-year-old man presents to the ER with cellulitis of his leg from IV heroin use. He has a 25-year history of IV drug use. On physical examination, he has multiple tattoos, his liver edge is firm and nodular under the right costal margin, and caput medusa is noted on the anterior abdominal wall. He is treated for cellulitis with standard therapy. Given his history, what tests would you recommend to his PCP to evaluate the findings of his abdominal physical exam?

Hepatitis serologies, including a hepatitis C antibody, HIV antibody, LFTs, CBC, and coagulation profile. Consider abdominal imaging and ensure PCP follow-up for further evaluation and treatment.

Generally transmitted via blood. Before screening, HCV was the most common cause of posttransfusion hepatitis, accounting for 90% of all such cases. Today, most infections occur 2° to IV drug use, but occupational exposure as well as sexual and vertical transmission may also be seen. Chronic HCV infection occurs in about 75% of those exposed; the remaining patients clear the virus without sequelae. Approximately 20% of carriers will develop cirrhosis within 20 years. HCC risk is 1%–4% per year of cirrhosis. Rates of coinfection with HIV in high-risk populations can exceed 50%, and HIV coinfection accelerates the risk of cirrhosis and HCC.

SYMPTOMS

- **Acute HCV:** Generally asymptomatic or symptoms are very mild.
- **Chronic HCV:** Mostly asymptomatic as well, but may include renal failure, vasculitic skin rash, and arthralgias, all 2° to cryoglobulinemia and sicca syndrome.
- Symptoms of cirrhosis may also be seen.

EXAM

See the HBV exam findings above.

DIFFERENTIAL

See the HAV differential above.

DIAGNOSIS

- Diagnosis is usually made after ↑ liver enzymes are noted on routine blood testing.
- **HCV antibody** will be present 4–6 weeks after infection. If qualitative PCR is used, antibody may appear as soon as 2 weeks postinfection. Recombinant immunoblot assay (RBA) can be used to rule out false ⊕s, but viral load is now used more commonly.
- Liver biopsy can be used to determine extent of cirrhosis, giving prognostic information. Biopsy is not required before initiating therapy.

TREATMENT

- **Acute exposure/postexposure prophylaxis:** Not recommended. Early treatment may be indicated if acute infection develops, as it appears to ↓ the risk of chronic carriage.
- Treatment is indicated for patients > 18 years of age and those with compensated liver disease, ⊕ HCV RNA test, biopsy showing bridging fibrosis or more severe pathology, and willingness to adhere to treatment requirements. Consensus guidelines on HCV management were updated in 2009 by the AASLD.
- **First-line treatment:**
  - Pegylated interferon-α SQ + ribavirin PO × 6–12 months. Treatment response is 40%–80%, depending on viral genotype (types 2 and 3 are considered favorable).
  - Up to 90% of virologic response occurs within the first 12 weeks of therapy. Side effects can be limiting and include flulike symptoms and depression.
- **Contraindications:** Major uncontrolled psychiatric disease, solid organ transplantation, severe concurrent medical disease (CAD/CVD, COPD, uncontrolled diabetes), decompensated cirrhosis, seizure disorders, autoimmune diseases, pregnancy or inability to use birth control, age < 2 years. Patients with active alcohol or drug dependence are generally required to establish sobriety before treatment.

Hepatic Abscess

The liver is the most common organ for abscess development, aside from the skin. Pyogenic liver abscesses can develop through bacterial invasion from the biliary tree (most common), portal vein, or hepatic artery as well as through direct trauma or adjacent bacterial infection. Approximately 15%–40% of abscesses have no known cause and are termed cryptogenic. Predisposing factors include advanced age, male gender, diabetes, malignancy, IBD, and a history of diverticulitis or cirrhosis. Bacterial abscesses are polymicrobial in > 50% of cases. Common organisms include *E coli*, *Klebsiella pneumoniae*, *Proteus vulgaris*, *Enterobacter aerogenes*, and other gram-⊖ and anaerobic organisms. Streptococci may also be present. It is important to consider other etiologies as well—eg, *Entamoeba histolytica* in immigrants and travelers and *Candida* spp in neutropenic hosts.

SYMPTOMS

- Onset is generally insidious. **Fever** is the most common presenting symptom.
- RUQ/epigastric pain, chills, nausea/vomiting, and weight loss are additional symptoms. Referred right shoulder pain occurs as well.

EXAM

Fever, jaundice, RUQ tenderness.

DIFFERENTIAL

Cholelithiasis, cholecystitis, cholangitis, hepatitis, gastritis, pancreatitis.

DIAGNOSIS

- **Labs:** CBC, LFTs (nonspecific elevations, but alkaline phosphatase will be ↑ in 70% of patients), and blood cultures (⊕ in 33%–100% of cases).
- **Imaging:** Abdominal CT with contrast is the imaging modality of choice, but ultrasound, MRI, and/or tagged WBC scan can detect hepatic abscesses as well (see Figure 6.16).

TREATMENT

- **Antibiotics:**
  - Aim to cover gram-⊖ organisms and anaerobes—ie, use a third-generation cephalosporin and metronidazole or a carbapenem. Treat-

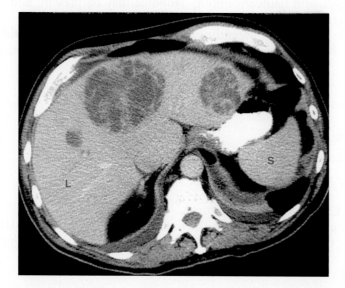

FIGURE 6.16. **Multiple pyogenic liver abscesses.** L = liver; S = spleen. (Reproduced, with permission, from Brunicardi FC, et al. *Schwartz's Principles of Surgery*, 9th ed. New York: McGraw-Hill, 2010, Fig. 31-19.)

ment should be initiated by IV, and total course duration should be 6–12 weeks. Treatment is often continued until radiographic resolution for bacterial liver abscesses.

- Additional empiric choices are available, and therapy should be tailored to culture results.

- **Interventions:** Drain if the abscess is ≥ 5 cm or is slow to respond to antibiotics. Drainage is usually percutaneous but may require surgery.

- Serology is very likely to be positive in amoebic liver abscess. Treatment is with metronidazole followed by by paromomycin (or iodoquinol). Clinical response is usually prompt, but imaging improvement/resolution lags and should not lead to prolonged or repeated treatment.

BILIARY INFECTIONS: CHOLECYSTITIS, CHOLANGITIS

A 43-year-old woman presents to the ER with acute onset of fever, chills, and right shoulder pain. She reports vomiting an hour ago after eating lunch. In the ER, her exam is remarkable for fever of 39°C (102.2°F), blood pressure 105/60, ⊕ Murphy sign, and rigors. What is your next step?

Obtain a CBC, blood cultures, and an ultrasound or abdominal CT scan with contrast. Begin empirical antibiotics with ceftriaxone and metronidazole and admit for further treatment.

Infections of the biliary tree are most commonly caused by gram-⊖ enteric pathogens in the setting of biliary obstruction (gallstones, biliary or pancreatic mass). **Cholecystitis** is an acute or chronic purulent infection of the gallbladder, causing surrounding pericholecystic inflammation. **Cholangitis** is a purulent infection of the biliary tree, specifically the common bile duct, and is associated with a higher degree of morbidity and mortality.

SYMPTOMS

- In cholecystitis, classic symptoms include RUQ/epigastric pain worst immediately postprandial (due to contraction of an inflamed gallbladder), fever/rigors, and nausea/vomiting. Jaundice may be present, and pain may be referred to the right shoulder due to the phrenic nerve.

- **Classic findings in ascending cholangitis** are termed **Reynolds pentad** (fever, RUQ pain, jaundice, altered mental status, and hypotension).

EXAM

Fever, jaundice, RUQ tenderness.

DIFFERENTIAL

Cholelithiasis, hepatitis, gastritis, pancreatitis, hepatic abscess.

DIAGNOSIS

- **Labs:** CBC, LFTs, blood cultures.
- **Imaging:** Ultrasound, CT with contrast, or nuclear medicine HIDA scan can be used to visualize the gallbladder and biliary tree (see Figure 6.17).

TREATMENT

- **Antibiotics:** Initial coverage should include activity against gram-⊖ and anaerobic pathogens (β-lactam or cephalosporin or fluoroquinolone plus metronidazole; or monotherapy with carbapenem).

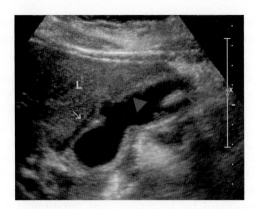

FIGURE 6.17. **Acute cholecystitis.** Ultrasound image shows gallstone *(red arrow)*, gallbladder wall thickening *(arrowheads)*, and pericholecystic fluid *(white arrow)*. L = liver. (Reproduced, with permission, from USMLERx.com.)

- ERCP with sphincterotomy may be employed to allow passage of obstructing gallstones and infected bile. If abscess is present and not relieved by endoscopic intervention, it may be drained by percutaneous cholecystostomy and, less commonly, open surgical approaches. If duct stenosis is present, biopsies and brushings via ERCP are often taken to rule out malignancy as the cause of stenosis.
- Admission to ICU for patients with hypotension or evidence of shock or concomitant organ failure.
- Patients with acute infection should have a surgical consult for cholecystectomy. Timing is often delayed until after resolution of acute infection (termed interval cholecystectomy).

COMPLICATIONS

- Abscess or necrosis of the biliary tree, including biliary extravasation into the peritoneum requiring surgical exploration and wash-out.
- Severe sepsis and ARDS, more commonly in the setting of ascending cholangitis +/– concomitant pancreatitis.

Genitourinary Disorders

URINARY TRACT INFECTION (UTI)

A 24-year-old woman comes into your clinic with fever, nausea, and mild dysuria. She says that she has had 2 bladder infections in the past, but she adds that this feels "a little different." On exam, her temperature is 38.0°C (100.4°F), and she has mild epigastric pain and moderate CVA tenderness on the right side. UA shows ⊕ leukocyte esterase, 20–50 WBCs, and more than 3 bacteria. What would be the most appropriate choice of antibiotic for this patient?

Ciprofloxacin/levofloxacin or TMP-SMX, depending on local resistance patterns. Be sure to give the patient instructions to return if she does not improve.

Infection along the urinary tract, from the renal parenchyma to urethra. Commonly divided into cystitis (when isolated to the bladder and distal structures) and pyelonephritis (when affecting the kidneys +/– other structures). Generally more common in women. A UTI in a man should prompt consideration for a urologic workup. UTIs can be classified as complicated or uncomplicated:

- **Uncomplicated:** Cystitis in a young, healthy, nonpregnant woman. The most common organisms are *E coli* and *Staphylococcus saprophyticus*. Less common are *Proteus mirabilis*, *Klebsiella* spp, and *Enterococcus* spp.
- **Complicated:** Defined as cystitis in anyone else—eg, male, elderly, hospitalized, and pregnant patients; or pyelonephritis in any patient. Complicating factors may include an indwelling catheter, recent catheterization, anatomic abnormalities, recent antibiotics, symptoms > 1 week, immunosuppression, diabetes, recurrent UTI, or a history of resistant UTI. Culture data will be important for treatment, and duration of therapy should be longer.

SYMPTOMS

- **Cystitis** commonly presents with a triad of dysuria, frequency, and urgency. Gross hematuria, fever, or suprapubic pain may also be present.
- **Pyelonephritis** presents with flank or back pain and fever. These are usually accompanied by one or more of the symptoms of cystitis, beginning 1–2 days prior. Patients may also have nausea, vomiting, abdominal pain, and/or diarrhea.

EXAM

- In cystitis, suprapubic tenderness may be present; **fever is uncommon.**
- Pyelonephritis findings include fever, CVA tenderness, mild to severe abdominal tenderness, and, in severe cases, hypotension and organ failure.
- Consider a pelvic exam in sexually active women if STIs are being considered in the differential.
- A rectal exam should be done in men to rule out prostatitis; however, vigorous prostate massage can lead to bacteremia and should be avoided.

DIFFERENTIAL

- **Prostatitis:** In acute prostatitis, men present with fever, chills, dysuria, frequency, and perineal and low back pain. Exam will reveal an exquisitely tender prostate. Although it is most often caused by *E coli*, other *Enterobacteriaceae* are common as well. Treatment should continue for 4 weeks.
- **Other:** Pyelonephritis, epididymitis, STIs, vaginitis (including atrophic), nephrolithiasis, interstitial cystitis, "bubble-bath" urethritis, and bladder tumors.

DIAGNOSIS

- UA typically shows leukocyte esterase, protein, blood, WBCs, and RBCs. With infection due to ammonia splitting bacteria, such as *E coli*, nitrites may be positive.
- Additional tests may include focused STI testing, wet mount, and KOH if there is a concern for vaginitis.
- Need for other laboratory evaluation in UTI depends on severity of illness.
- **CBC:** In ill-appearing patients, CBC may reveal leukocytosis with left shift.
- **Culture:** Urine culture is usually ⊕ and may help to guide therapy. At least 10,000 colony-forming units of a pathogenic single organism should be present, although less than this may be significant in men, or in complicated UTI in women. Blood cultures are ⊕ in 10%–20% of cases.

TREATMENT

- **Outpatient:** For **uncomplicated cystitis,** 3 days of treatment with TMP-SMX or a fluoroquinolone is adequate. Nitrofurantoin or cephalexin may also be used and should be given for 7 days. **Phenazopyridine** can be used for symptomatic treatment of severe dysuria for up to 2 days. (Note that fluoroquinolones are contraindicated in pregnancy and TMP-SMX is not recommended in the first and third trimesters.)
- In **complicated UTI** in outpatients, fluoroquinolone × 7–14 days can be used. Second-line therapy consists of either amoxicillin/clavulanate or TMP-SMX for the same duration. Susceptibility results should be confirmed.
- **Inpatient:** Patients may require hospitalization if they are unable to tolerate PO treatment, if signs of urosepsis are present, or if pregnant. Antibiotic therapy should be initiated early and guided by local antibiotic sensitivities.
- IV ceftriaxone is a reasonable empiric choice for most patients; however, resistance is developing, especially among *E coli* (ESBL strains; see Emerging Antibiotic Resistance section).
- Add ampicillin to regimen if **enterococcus** is suspected.
- Radiologic evaluation for complications may be necessary in patients who are severely ill, are immunocompromised, or are not responding to treatment, as well as for patients in whom complications are likely (eg, pregnant patients, patients with diabetes, and those with nephrolithiasis, reflux, transplant surgery, or other GU surgery).
- Plain films can detect radiopaque stones (uric acid and indinavir stones are radiolucent), some masses, and abnormal gas collections.
- Ultrasound can examine the ureters and kidneys for fluid collections and stones. Ultrasound and voiding cystoureterography can evaluate patients suspected of having reflux disease.
- CT with and without contrast is most sensitive but may be contraindicated in those with impaired renal function.

COMPLICATIONS

- Perinephric abscess should be considered in patients who remain febrile 2–3 days after appropriate antibiotics (see Figure 6.18). Patients with large abscesses or those who have failed antibiotics alone are treated by percutaneous or surgical drainage.
- Intrarenal abscess (eg, infection of a renal cyst) < 5 cm usually responds to antibiotics alone.
- Patients with diabetes may develop emphysematous pyelonephritis. This condition once required urgent nephrectomy because of its high mortality rate, but now it is often treated medically with percutaneous drainage. In pregnant patients, pyelonephritis is associated with ↑ risk of preterm delivery and maternal complications.
- **Recurrence:**
  - Any patient with new symptoms of a UTI > 2 weeks after resolution of a prior UTI has a recurrence. Patients with two or more recurrences in a 6-month period may need suppression. There are several antibiotics of choice for recurrent UTI, including daily nitrofurantoin, trimethoprim, or TMP-SMX. Postcoital antibiotics are an option for sexually active women.
  - In patients with recurrent complicated UTIs, consider discussion with a urologist and imaging with IVP, renal ultrasound, or CT to rule out anatomic abnormalities or nephrolithiasis, which may act as a nidus for infection. Struvite stones (staghorn calculi) are associated with recurrent UTIs due to urease-producing bacteria (*Proteus, Pseudomonas,* and *Klebsiella*).

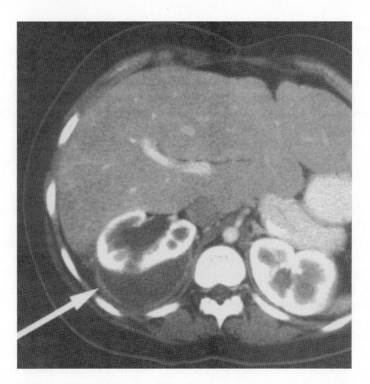

FIGURE 6.18. Perinephric abscess. Acute right pyelonephritis complicated by right perinephric abscess *(arrow)*. (Reproduced, with permission, from Tanagho EA, McAninch JW. *Smith's General Urology*, 17th ed. New York: McGraw-Hill, 2008, Fig. 13-4.)

PREVENTION

Data are limited, but patients with recurrent UTIs are commonly instructed to clean themselves away from the urethra and to void immediately after intercourse. Data suggest that these maneuvers are not helpful. Drinking cranberry juice, which ↓ bacterial adherence to the uroepithelium, has been shown to be helpful in some studies. Diaphragm and spermicide use and douching in women should be avoided. Topical estrogen can be considered in postmenopausal women. There is ↑ frequency of UTIs in uncircumcised infant males.

Skin, Soft Tissue, and Orthopedic Infections

CELLULITIS AND SKIN ABSCESS

Common skin and soft tissue infections (SSTIs) of the dermis, either diffusely infiltrative in cellulitis or creating a loculated purulent focus in abscess. The two can coexist and are usually 2° to bacterial entry into a laceration, abrasion, or irritated skin without a macroscopic defect. SSTIs are most commonly due to S *aureus* and group A streptococci (S *pyogenes*). Other causes of SSTIs are erysipelas and impetigo, most common in children, and human and animal bite wounds.

SYMPTOMS

Pain, warmth, and redness of the skin. Swelling or pus drainage from the skin. Fever constitutes a complicated case with systemic illness.

EXAM

- Erythema (reticular pattern in mild cases, circumferential in more severe cases, sometimes tracking via lymphangitic spread), induration, warmth; in abscess, fluctuance may be found. Regional lymphadenopathy is common.
- **Erysipelas,** due to group A streptococci, typically displays a well-demarcated, tender, intensely erythematous plaque, with possible lymphangitic spread. It is most commonly found on the face and in one-third of cases follows streptococcal pharyngitis.
- Impetigo typically causes one or more demarcated plaques or ulcers, with a "honey-colored" crust. It can cause bullae, which rupture and form plaques. Often found around the external nares and mouth of children. Impetigo may be caused by S *aureus* or group A streptococcus.
- Pain out of proportion to exam, systemic toxicity, or rapidly progressive exam findings should prompt consideration of necrotizing fasciitis, requiring hospital admission with emergent surgical consult.

DIFFERENTIAL

Burns, dermatitis (atopic, contact, photosensitivity), chronic stasis dermatitis (in lower extremities), erythema multiforme, and varicella. Streptococcal and staphylococcal toxic shock syndromes create diffuse erythema (erythroderma). Although gangrene and necrotizing fasciitis are much less common, they have much greater morbidity and mortality and need to be considered in appropriate settings.

DIAGNOSIS

- Cellulitis, abscess, and associated skin infections are clinical diagnoses.
- Skin biopsy can be obtained in cases with unclear diagnosis.
- In abscess, deep wound culture can help tailor antibiotic therapy. Culture of cellulitis is not helpful; however, with an abscess, deep wound culture in the setting of incision and drainage, carefully obtained without skin flora contamination, can help tailor antibiotic therapy.
- Common etiologies are group A streptococcus and S *aureus* (including, most commonly, erysipelas implicating GAS and impetigo, implicating S *aureus* or GAS). In immunocompromised hosts, gram-$\ominus$ flora are a possible cause (see section on Diabetic Foot Infections). In neonates, group B streptococci are a possible cause and can present with sepsis. β-hemolytic streptococci other than GAS (most commonly, group B streptococci and group G streptococci) may cause SSTI in older persons or those with underlying illness. Rarely, fungus or other atypical bacteria can cause skin and soft tissue infection. Risk factors for SSTI include immunocompromise, homelessness, and frequent skin trauma, as in IVDU.

TREATMENT

- Uncomplicated cellulitis can be treated with oral antibiotic therapy to cover streptococci and staphylococci, such as cephalexin or nafcillin. Because of the rising prevalence of MRSA, antibiotics with MRSA coverage such as TMP-SMX, doxycycline, or clindamycin should be considered, based on local antibiogram. TMP-SMX and doxycycline do not have adequate coverage for group A streptococci.
- Uncomplicated abscess is treated definitively by incision and drainage and does not require antibiotics, unless complicated by surrounding cellulitis or systemic symptoms.

- Erysipelas and impetigo are effectively treated with similar medications, which have activity against streptococcal and staphylococcal bacteria (again, consider agents with activity against MRSA). Mild cases of impetigo can be treated with topical antibiotics, such as mupirocin, and polymyxin B plus neomycin.
- Infected animal or human bite wounds are typically polymicrobial and include aerobic and anaerobic flora. While the specific biting organism's oral flora may differ (humans include *Eikenella corrodens*; dogs and cats include *Pasteurella multocida*, among others), the initial antibiotic coverage is largely similar: oral amoxicillin/clavulanate or intravenous ampicillin/sulbactam or carbapenems. For patients with severe PCN allergy, a fluoroquinolone plus clindamycin is generally recommended.
- Treatment of immunocompromised hosts may requires broader-spectrum coverage (eg, coverage of both gram-⊕ and gram-⊖ flora).
- Current guidelines for necrotizing fasciitis recommend potent agents against streptococci, staphylococci, and anaerobes empirically; coverage for MRSA where appropriate (although this is a less common etiology); and clindamycin (because of its inhibition of bacterial protein synthesis). Surgical debridement and sometimes amputation are frequently employed in severe necrotizing fasciitis to prevent widespread, life-threatening infection.

COMPLICATIONS

If not properly treated, superficial SSTIs can progress by lymphatic or hematogenous spread to cause gangrene, necrotizing fasciitis, or sepsis.

PREVENTION

In both active infection and for prevention, general good hygiene should be practiced. Agents such as topical chlorhexidine are frequently prescribed in the setting of recurrent SSTI, but their efficacy is unclear.

SEPTIC ARTHRITIS

A 54-year-old man presents to the urgent care center with a very painful right knee. The day before, he was cleaning his house and cut his knee with a nail while kneeling on the floor. The knee became painful, warm, and swollen over the past 24 hours. On exam, you find decreased and exquisitely painful range of motion, tenderness, warmth, and erythema of the skin. No other joints are affected, and he has no prior history of these symptoms. What should you do?

Obtain a joint aspirate, call for an orthopedic consult, and begin empiric antibiotics for septic arthritis.

KEY FACT

If a young, sexually active adult presents with acute monoarticular joint pain, think about disseminated gonococcal disease.

An infection of the joint space that is usually spread by hematogenous seeding from another site. Risk factors for infection include trauma, diabetes, rheumatoid arthritis (RA), malignancy, frequent glucocorticoid injections, prior joint surgery, and IV drug use. The most common organism is *S aureus*, but other etiologic agents include *H influenzae*, gram-⊖ bacilli, *S pneumoniae*, β-hemolytic streptococci, and *N gonorrhoeae*.

SYMPTOMS

Presents with acute onset of a painful, warm, swollen joint. Fever, chills, ↓ ROM, and skin rash may be seen.

EXAM

- Although monoarticular more common, may be polyarticular. Most commonly involves the knee and hip; less commonly involves the shoulder, elbow, and small joints. If the sacroiliac or sternoclavicular joints are involved, screen the patient for IV drug use (the most common risk factor for these sites).
- Findings include fever, warmth, intra-articular effusion, ↓ ROM, tenderness to palpation, and rash.

DIFFERENTIAL

- **Infectious:** Osteomyelitis, cellulitis, Lyme disease, fungal infection.
- **Rheumatologic:** Gout, pseudogout, SLE, RA, psoriatic arthritis.
- **Other:** Degenerative joint disease, internal derangement, arthritis 2° to serum sickness, reactive arthritis (formerly Reiter syndrome), or poststreptococcal infection (may be a manifestation of rheumatic fever).

DIAGNOSIS

- **Labs:** CBC; consider ESR and CRP (serial monitoring of CRP provides evidence of response to treatment); obtain blood cultures (⊕ in < 30% of cases).
- **Arthrocentesis:** Send synovial fluid for cell count, Gram stain (typically ⊖ in N gonorrhoeae septic arthritis), culture, uric acid crystals, and calcium pyrophosphate dehydrate crystals (see Table 6.16).
- **Imaging:** Plain films may show soft tissue swelling but are otherwise unhelpful, except in excluding other diagnoses. Consider bone scan or MRI if there is concern for osteomyelitis.
- **Other:** Urethral/cervical testing for N gonorrhoeae.

TABLE 6.16.   Examination of Synovial Fluid

	NORMAL	NONINFLAMMATORY	INFLAMMATORY	SEPTIC
Clarity	Transparent.	Transparent.	Cloudy.	Cloudy.
Color	Clear.	Yellow.	Yellow.	Yellow.
WBC/μL	< 200.	< 200–2000.	200–50,000.	> 50,000.
PMNs (%)[a]	< 25.	< 25.	> 50.	> 50.
Culture	Negative.	Negative.	Negative.	> 50% positive.
Crystals	None.	None.	Multiple or none.	None.
Associated conditions		Osteoarthritis, trauma, rheumatic fever.	Gout, pseudogout, spondyloarthropathies, RA, Lyme disease, SLE.	Nongonococcal or gonococcal septic arthritis.

[a]WBC count and percent PMNs are affected by a number of factors, including disease progression, affecting organism, and host immune status. The joint aspirate WBC and PMNs should be considered part of a continuum for each disease, particularly septic arthritis, and should be correlated with other clinical information.

Reproduced, with permission, from Tintinalli JE, et al. *Emergency Medicine: A Comprehensive Study Guide*, 6th ed. New York: McGraw-Hill, 2004: 1795.

TREATMENT

- Joint infection:
  - Drainage can be accomplished by open surgical wash-out (preferred by many orthopedists), arthroscopic wash-out, or percutaneous needle drainage. Surgical wash-out is usually necessary only once, but repeated procedures may be needed. Preferred method of drainage is not clearly established.
  - Start empirical antibiotics after cultures have been sent. Ideally, treat parenterally for 2–4 weeks.
  - Empirical antimicrobial choice is dependent on the age of the patient, regardless of sexual activity and Gram stain results.
  - Vancomycin +/– a third-generation IV cephalosporin is appropriate first-line therapy.
  - Because of the rising prevalence of fluoroquinolone-resistant gonococcal disease, agents such as cipro- and levofloxacin are no longer recommended unless susceptibility is confirmed. For N *gonorrhoeae* arthritis, ceftriaxone can be used as initial therapy, and can be transitioned after 48–72 hours of improvement to oral cephalosporins, such as cefpodoxime or cefixime. All individuals with N *gonorrhoeae* arthritis should be tested and treated for *Chlamydia* infection because of the high rate of coinfection.
- **Special situations:** Patients with **prosthetic joints** usually require orthopedic intervention.

ACUTE OSTEOMYELITIS

An infection of the bone or bone marrow. In adults, 80% of osteomyelitis cases result from contiguous spread. These cases often become chronic. This is seen in patients with diabetes, prosthetic joints, decubitus ulcers, trauma, and recent surgery. In 20% of cases, the infection is hematogenous in origin. Risk factors include IV drug use, sickle cell disease, and advanced age. Etiologies are as follows:

- **Common organisms:** S *aureus* (most common), coagulase-⊖ staphylococci (prosthetic joints or postoperative infections), streptococci and anaerobes (bites, diabetic foot infections, decubitus ulcers), *Pasteurella* spp (animal bites), *Eikenella corrodens* (human bites), P *aeruginosa* (IV drug use and nail punctures).
- **Other causes:** *Salmonella* spp (sickle cell patients), *Mycobacterium tuberculosis* (foreign immigrants, HIV), *Bartonella* spp (HIV), *Brucella* spp (unpasteurized dairy products).
- **By location:** P *aeruginosa* affects the sternoclavicular joint and symphysis pubis (in IV drug use); *Brucella* spp affect the sacroiliac joint, knee, and hip; and TB affects the lower thoracic vertebrae (Pott disease).

SYMPTOMS

Fever is more common in hematogenous osteomyelitis; localized pain and swelling of the affected extremity or area.

EXAM

Fever, tenderness, erythema, and swelling over the affected bone. May present as a chronic draining wound that tracks to bone.

DIFFERENTIAL

Cellulitis, RA, osteoarthritis, diskitis, bone cyst/tumor, septic arthritis, simple skin ulcer.

DIAGNOSIS

- **Labs:** CBC, ESR, CRP (serial monitoring of CRP may provide evidence of response to treatment), and blood cultures (⊕ in 10%–50% of cases where hematogenous spread in suspected). Serology for atypical causes can be ordered on an individual basis.
- **Imaging: Plain films** are frequently normal but may reveal periosteal elevation or bony erosions (see Figure 6.19). Three- or 4-phase **bone scans** are helpful to distinguish bone from soft tissue inflammation. **MRI** is quickly becoming the preferred modality, especially for vertebral osteomyelitis (see Figure 6.20).
- **Surgery:** Bone biopsy and culture is the gold standard and will in some cases reveal an etiologic agent. Very helpful if ⊕, but frequently ⊖. Swabs of exposed bone are generally not helpful, as the organisms isolated do not correlate well with organisms in the bone. May be used to determine if *S aureus* is present.

TREATMENT

- Empiric antibiotics such as vancomycin plus a third-generation cephalosporin should be started **after** all cultures have been obtained. The regimen should be directed toward the most likely organism(s). After culture results are received, therapy may be narrowed.
- IV antibiotics should be given for 4–6 weeks, although some patients may be treated with PO regimens, as guided by culture results.
- Surgery is indicted for spinal cord decompression, bony stabilization, removal of necrotic bone, and reestablishment of vascular supply.
- Complications include epidural abscess and diskitis (with vertebral osteomyelitis). Most osteomyelitis that has invaded contiguous foci is chronic by the time it is diagnosed.

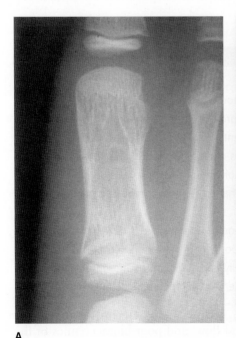
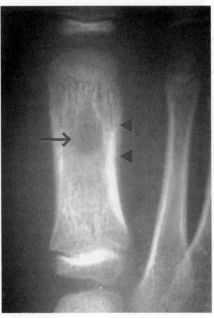
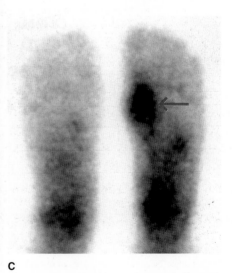

A   B   C

FIGURE 6.19. **Acute osteomyelitis after puncture wound.** (A) Radiograph of first metatarsal of right foot after puncture injury, showing no foreign body and no evidence of osteomyelitis. (B) Follow-up radiograph after 2 weeks of treatment with oral antibiotics, showing interval development of focal lucency *(red arrow)* and periosteal reaction *(red arrowheads)*, consistent with acute osteomyelitis. (C) Plantar image of both feet from bone scan performed at the same time as radiography in (B) shows increased radiotracer uptake in the region of the first metatarsal of the right foot *(red arrow)* in comparison with the normal left foot, confirming osteomyelitis. (Reproduced, with permission, from Skinner HB. *Current Diagnosis & Treatment in Orthopedics,* 4th ed. New York: McGraw-Hill, 2006, Fig. 8-8.)

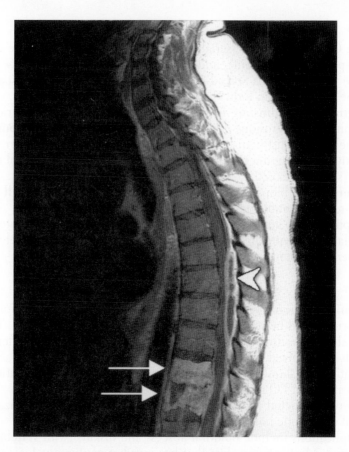

FIGURE 6.20. **Diskitis-osteomyelitis.** Sagittal postcontrast MR image show diskitis-osteomyelitis *(arrows)* and a rim-enhancing epidural abscess *(arrowhead)*, compressing the spinal cord. (Reproduced, with permission, from Tintinalli JE, et al. *Tintinalli's Emergency Medicine: A Comprehensive Study Guide,* 6th ed. New York: McGraw-Hill, 2004, Fig. 305-5.)

DIABETIC FOOT INFECTIONS

While you are finishing nursing home rounds, a nurse asks you to inspect a male patient's foot. As you approach the man, you note that he is one of your colleague's elderly patients with diabetes. Exam reveals an erythematous 1.5-cm foot ulcer. The ulcer is draining yellow, foul-smelling material. Pulses in the foot are palpable, but monofilament testing reveals peripheral neuropathy. The patient has been afebrile. What is the most appropriate management of this patient's infection?

Obtain a radiographic study to rule out osteomyelitis. If no osteomyelitis is found, start a first-generation cephalosporin and metronidazole or amoxicillin/clavulanate. The patient should be serially examined, and, if no improvement is seen, admitted to the hospital for debridement and IV antibiotic therapy.

Because of neuropathy, abnormal blood flow, and poor biomechanics of the feet, patients with diabetes are prone to foot ulcers and infections, including osteomyelitis. With these infections come significant morbidity and mortality. Although most infections are polymicrobial, common organisms include S *aureus*, streptococci (often group B), gram-$\ominus$ aerobes, and anaerobic bacteria.

Symptoms

May be asymptomatic because of neuropathy or may present with significant pain. Ulcer with eschar is frequently present.

Exam

Exam reveals an ulcer on the foot that may have indurated edges, erythema, swelling, and/or drainage. The plantar surface of the foot is the most common site of infection. Fever is possible.

Differential

Cellulitis, noninfected ulcer, peripheral artery disease, venous stasis ulcer.

Diagnosis

- **Labs:** CBC, ESR, CRP, HbA_{1c}.
- **Specimen:** Culture taken from a debrided ulcer or bone is most helpful.
- **Imaging:** Plain films are of some use, but a 3-phase bone scan, a tagged WBC scan, and MRI are more helpful. Arterial flow to the foot should also be assessed.

Treatment

- **Wound care:** Can range from daily dressing changes to bedside or intraoperative debridement.
- **Antibiotics:** Mild infections can be treated on an outpatient basis with PO agents to cover, at a minimum, streptococcal and staphylococcal infections (MRSA must be considered) and close follow-up. More extensive infections should be treated with hospitalization and IV antibiotics such as cefepime, piperacillin/tazobactam, or carbapenems. Given the risk of MDR organisms in patients with chronic illness or in long-term care facilities, strongly consider coverage for MRSA, resistant gram-⊖ rods, and vancomycin-resistant *Enterococcus* (VRE). Typically, 1–2 weeks of therapy is sufficient for mild to moderate infection (with IV switched to PO after 48–72 hours) and 2–4 weeks in patients with severe or complicated infection.

Prevention

In addition to reasonable glycemic control: frequent foot exams, proper footwear, and routine monofilament neuropathy screening.

Complications

Osteomyelitis, sepsis, need for amputation.

Human Immunodeficiency Virus (HIV)

 A 35-year-old man with a 6-year history of known HIV comes into your clinic for a routine follow-up. He states that in the past 2 months he has had worsening dysphagia with both solids and liquids. On exam, you notice a moderate amount of thrush on his tongue and oropharynx. In addition to treating his candidal infection, you check a CD4+ cell count, which has ↓ to 150 cells/mm³. Which chemoprophylactic agents should be started today?

TMP-SMX for PCP prophylaxis. Given that your patient is taking antiretroviral medication, you consider the possibility of resistance or nonadherence. First, discuss adherence with the patient and test for viral load and genotyping/resistance pattern. Then consider the current HAART regimen.

Since the initial cases in 1981, more than 50 million people have been infected with HIV, and more than 25 million people have died of AIDS and related complications. The virus targets and destroys CD4+ T lymphocytes, which leads to AIDS (acquired immune deficiency syndrome, a state of immunocompromise causing increased vulnerability to infection and malignancy). HIV research continues to discover new complications of immune dysregulation in seropositive patients that result in noninfectious complications such as metabolic disorders, increased rates of coronary heart disease, and endocrinopathies.

HIV transmission is via exposure to contaminated body fluids. Risk factors include unprotected sexual intercourse, IV drug use, maternal infection, and accidental needlesticks. In contrast to the demographics in the early years of the AIDS epidemic, women account for 50% of all adults with HIV worldwide. Markers used to measure progression are CD4+ count and HIV RNA viral load. The CD4+ count measures the degree of immune compromise and predicts the risk of opportunistic infections. Viral load measures HIV replication rate, and genotypic and phenotypic resistance testing can predict the efficacy of specific antiretrovirals.

With the advent of highly active antiretroviral medication (HAART or ARV), HIV can be a chronic disease, with infected individuals living for decades. However, individual patient outcomes in HIV/AIDS remain largely determined by economics; only 42% of the > 10 million people in resource-limited nations who are in immediate need of lifesaving treatment receive HAART (according to UNAIDS, 2009). HIV/AIDS is one of the most polarizing geopolitical and medical issues in our time.

SYMPTOMS/EXAM

- 1° HIV infection:
    - Often asymptomatic or may present with **acute retroviral syndrome**, which consists of fever, sore throat, lymphadenopathy, and a truncal maculopapular rash or mucocutaneous ulceration occurring 2–6 weeks after initial infection.
    - Other signs and symptoms include myalgias, arthralgias, diarrhea, headache, nausea, vomiting, weight loss, and thrush.
- **Chronic HIV infection:**
    - Suspect and test for in patients with thrush (see Figure 6.21), oral hairy leukoplakia, herpes zoster, seborrheic dermatitis, oral aphthous ulcers, or recurrent vaginal candidiasis. Signs and symptoms of opportunistic infections and HIV/AIDS-related malignancy are variable; see the section on AIDS and Opportunistic Infections.
    - Other symptoms may be vague and may include fatigue, fevers, night sweats, diarrhea, dysphagia, dyspnea, persistent lymphadenopathy, weight loss, and altered mental status.

DIFFERENTIAL

- Acute retroviral syndrome resembles viral URI, influenza, infectious mononucleosis, acute CMV infection, aseptic meningitis, and syphilis.

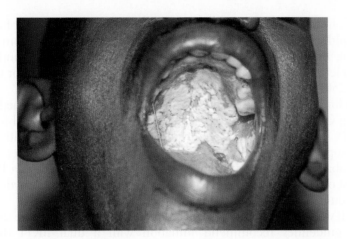

FIGURE 6.21. **Oral candidiasis.** Removable whitish plaques on the palate are seen in this HIV patient with pseudomembranous candidiasis. (Reproduced, with permission, from Knoop KJ, et al. *The Atlas of Emergency Medicine*, 3rd ed. New York: McGraw-Hill, 2010, Fig. 20.4. Photo contributor: Thea James, MD.)

■ Depending on the manifestation, chronic HIV infection may resemble malignancy, subacute bacterial endocarditis, connective tissue disease, depression, eating disorders, IBD, or malabsorption syndromes.

DIAGNOSIS

■ The CDC now recommends HIV testing of all persons 13–64 years of age in all health care settings, unless HIV prevalence is known to be < 0.1%. Patients may opt out of testing. Separate written consent should not be required.
■ **ELISA/enzyme immunoassay (EIA):** Used to diagnose HIV by detecting antibodies to the virus in serum. In most cases, ELISA will be ⊕ 3 months after infection. Approximately 95% of infected patients will be ⊕ by 6 months. ⊕ tests must be confirmed by **Western blot** (a protein electrophoresis to determine presence of HIV proteins in a patient's cells). **The combination of ELISA and confirmatory Western blot is the gold standard for diagnosis of HIV.**
■ CD4+ cell count should **not** be used for screening, as it can be ↓ in many conditions other than HIV, including acute illness.
■ **HIV-1 RNA viral load** (PCR, or nucleic acid amplification testing [NAAT]) determination may be used when Western blot is indeterminate. False ⊕s do occur. It is not a first-line test for HIV diagnosis.
■ Additional testing for **p24 core antigen** is approved by the FDA for diagnosis in the first few weeks after infection, but it is less sensitive than either ELISA with confirmatory Western blot or PCR. It is not a first-line diagnostic test for HIV.

TREATMENT

■ Decisions regarding treatment of HIV are complex, and a comprehensive discussion is outside the scope of this review. Treatment guidelines differ by locale, including resource-rich vs. resource-poor settings. The main goals of treatment are to suppress viremia and prevent immunosuppression and other HIV-related systemic complications, such as malignancy and noninfectious dysregulatory sequelae.
■ IAS-USA guidelines (2010) recommend treatment for **all adult patients with a CD4+ count < 500 and consideration of treatment for all HIV-⊕ patients, regardless of CD4+ count.**
　■ Treatment of HIV-⊕ children is determined by age, with treatment recommended for all HIV-⊕ children < 12 months of age, regardless

of clinical status, CD4+ cell count, or viral load. Treatment for HIV-⊕ children > 12 months of age is based on presence of symptoms (if present, then HAART is indicated), HIV-related conditions, and/or serologic markers such as CD4+ cell count < 350 cells/ mm^3 or CD4+ % < 25% and HIV-1 RNA > 100,000 copies/mL.

■ Before treatment initiation, additional tests should be obtained, including CBC and complete metabolic panel (hepatic and renal function), HIV viral load, HIV genotype/resistance testing, hepatitis/syphilis/toxoplasmosis, and HLA-B5701 serotype (for abacavir hypersensitivity if abacavir use is planned). If not already obtained, check a PPD skin test or quantiferon serology for TB. Gonococcal and chlamydial testing should be used as appropriate.

■ For HIV-⊕ adult and adolescent treatment-naive patients, the 2010 IAS-USA guidelines recommend initiation with a dual nRTI (tenofovir/emtricitabine or abacavir/lamivudine) component and a third agent NNRTI (efavirenz), PI (atazanavir, darunavir, fosamprenavir, lopinavir), INSTI (raltegravir), or CCR5 inhibitor (maraviroc).

■ Table 6.17 is a brief summary of HAART mechanisms, side effects, and considerations.

TABLE 6.17. HAART Medications in HIV Treatment

Antiretroviral Class	Method of Action	Examples	Common Side Effects	Specific Considerations
Nucleoside reverse transcriptase inhibitors (NRTIs)	Malfunctioning substrate for HIV reverse transcriptase (RT), preventing viral DNA formation.	Zidovudine (AZT), lamivudine, didanosine, stavudine, abacavir, and emtricitabine (tenofovir = nucleotide RTI).	Peripheral neuropathy, GI (anorexia, diarrhea), pancreatitis; these are drug specific.	Abacavir can cause a fatal hypersensitivity syndrome; check for risk with HLA-B5701 test.
Nonnucleoside reverse transcriptase inhibitors (NNRTIs)	Bind directly to RT, preventing viral DNA formation.	Delavirdine, efavirenz, and nevirapine.	Rash, vertigo, myalgia.	Efavirenz causes vivid dreams and may exacerbate underlying psychiatric illness.
Protease inhibitors (PIs)	Interfere with viral maturation by preventing cleavage of viral protein precursors.	Indinavir, darunavir, nelfinavir, ritonavir (used for boosting other PIs), saquinavir, fosamprenavir, atazanavir, tipranavir, and lopinavir + ritonavir.	Metabolic abnormalities and GI side effects, including diarrhea.	
Integrase inhibitors	Prevent insertion of HIV genome into host DNA by integrase.	Raltegravir.	Diarrhea, nausea, HA, fever.	
CCR5 inhibitors	Prevent HIV virus binding to CD4 cell surface by coreceptor CCR5.	Maraviroc.	Diarrhea, nausea, HA.	HIV strains divide into R5 (susceptible) and X4 classes (resistant); must do tropism assay before using.
Fusion inhibitors	Prevent fusion of the virus to CD4 cell membrane.	Enfurtivide (SQ injection).	Injection-site reactions, GI upset.	

- During **pregnancy**, HIV-⊕ women should be offered standard therapy as above for infected adults/adolescents. In women who do not need immediate HAART initiation for their own health, consider starting after 10–14 weeks of gestation to minimize the risk of teratogenicity.
- **Intrapartum, all HIV-⊕ women should receive IV zidovudine infusion to prevent transmission.** In the United States, for women who have had prenatal HIV-1 RNA > 1000 copies/mL (suboptimal suppression), C-section is indicated to prevent perinatal transmission.
- **Strict adherence** to antiretroviral treatment is necessary for the success and longevity of certain regimens, although modern options have alleviated this problem somewhat. Patients should be counseled regarding the importance of adherence.
- **HAART failure** (demonstrated by rising viral load or decreasing CD4+ cell count, despite medication adherence) or **reinitiation of HAART** after discontinuation requires **HIV specialty consultation** because of the risk of ↑ medication resistance and the complexity of medication choice.

PREVENTION

- **Prevention counseling:** Needle exchange programs for IV drug users; safe sex practices; universal HIV testing; universal precautions for health care workers.
- **Postexposure prophylaxis (PEP):** Rapid initiation of PEP and nonoccupational postexposure prophylaxis (nPEP) are paramount to ↓ the risk of infection. A common regimen for PEP and nPEP is Combivir (zidovudine plus lamivudine). Individualized treatment should be formulated for high-risk exposures to highly resistant viruses.

AIDS AND OPPORTUNISTIC INFECTIONS (OIS)

Patients with HIV, especially those with AIDS, are vulnerable to complications of immunosuppression, including infections atypical in the immunocompetent host, metabolic complications, and a higher rate of certain types of malignancy. This section provides a short description of such complications of advanced HIV and AIDS.

AIDS is defined as HIV infection and a CD4+ cell count < 200 cells/mm³. Additionally, a seropositive person is diagnosed with AIDS in the presence of any AIDS-defining condition (ADC)—a set of 20 infectious, degenerative, or malignant diseases associated with advanced HIV disease. Some of the most common ADCs are discussed below.

SYMPTOMS/EXAM/TREATMENT

- Notable OIs include:
  - **Candidiasis:** Although common in infants and in localized candidal dermatitis in immunocompetent hosts, AIDS can predispose patients to esophageal and diffuse oropharyngeal candidiasis. Treat with antifungal medication, such as fluconazole.
  - *Pneumocystis jiroveci* **pneumonia** (previously *Pneumocystis carinii* pneumonia; still called PCP for *Pneumocystis* pneumonia): A rapidly progressive fungal pneumonia, typified by severe hypoxemia out of proportion to exam and radiologic findings (see Figure 6.22). Treat with TMP-SMX and steroids, such as prednisone.
  - **Toxoplasmosis:** An infection, usually reactivation in the CNS, by *Toxoplasma gondii*, a protozoan parasite. Exam findings include fever, altered mental status, and focal neurologic deficits. Diagnosis is made

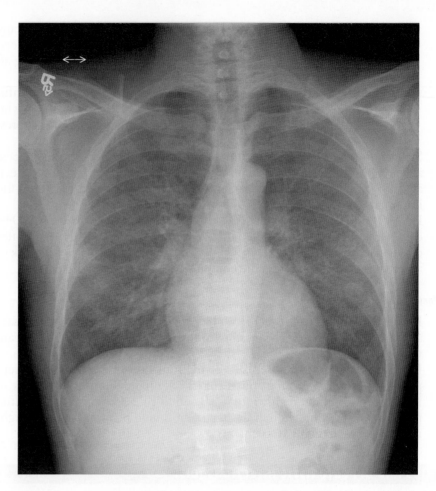

FIGURE 6.22. ***Pneumocystis jiroveci (carinii)* pneumonia.** Portable AP radiograph showing diffuse, bilateral interstitial infiltrates in a 50-year-old HIV-⊕ woman with a CD4+ cell count of 55 cells/mm³, who presented with significant arterial hypoxemia. Broncheoalveolar lavage was positive for *Pneumocystis jiroveci*. (Reproduced, with permission, from USMLERx.com.)

by anti-toxoplasmosis IgG serology and CT, showing ring-enhancing lesions in the brain parenchyma. Treat with pyrimethamine + sulfadiazine or clindamycin. Treatment nonresponders after 7–14 days (diagnosed by reimaging of CNS) require a brain biopsy for further evaluation (rule out lymphoma, TB, bacterial abscess, atypical cryptococcosis, other parasites).

- **Cryptococcal meningitis:** An infection of the CNS by the fungus *Cryptococcus neoformans*. Presents with fever and progressively worsening headache. Diagnose with lumbar puncture sent for CSF cryptococcal antigen and culture. Serum cryptococcal antigen also aids in diagnosis. ↑ ICP is associated with worse outcomes. Treat with ICP management (serial LP, or, rarely, a drainage device) and antifungal therapy with amphotericin or amphotericin B and flucytosine, followed by fluconazole suppression until adequate immune reconstitution, or if this does not occur, indefinitely.

- **Cytomegalovirus:** Infection, usually reactivation, of a human herpesvirus (HHV-5), leading to colitis and chorioretinitis (see Figure 6.23), with other manifestations somewhat less common. Treat with ganciclovir, valganciclovir, or foscarnet (cidofovir is a second-line agent). Occurs at low CD4+ counts (< 50).

- **TB:** See section on TB.

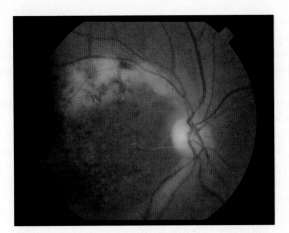

FIGURE 6.23.   Retinal changes in HIV infection. White retinal plaques with local hemor-rhage in cytomegalovirus retinitis. (Reproduced, with permission, from Riordan-Eva P, Whitcher JP. *Vaughan & Ash-bury's General Ophthalmology*, 17th ed. New York: McGraw-Hill, 2008, Fig. 15-33.)

- **Viral hepatitis:** Coinfection of HIV and hepatitis is common and is as-sociated with worse outcomes from HBV- and HCV-related complica-tions. Vaccination for HAV and HBV are indicated, and prevention/risk reduction is imperative.
- **Notable AIDS-related malignancies include:**
  - **Kaposi sarcoma:** A vascular lymphatic tumor, rare except in Mediter-ranean and African populations before HIV disease; due to unchecked infection with HHV-8. KS lesions are red, purple, vascular-appearing nodules, typically found on the skin and mouth, but can affect the re-spiratory and GI tracts (see Figure 6.24). Treat with HAART, local ther-apy (radiation, cryotherapy, retinoids), and systemic therapy, including interferon and chemotherapy.
  - **Lymphoma:** Related to immune dysregulation and susceptibility to on-cogenic viruses; patients with HIV disease have increased susceptibility to lymphoma, especially diffuse large B cell lymphoma.

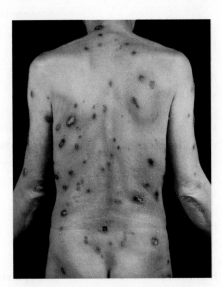

FIGURE 6.24.   Kaposi sarcoma in a patient with AIDS. Multiple lesions at all stages of development (macules, papules, nodules) are present on the trunk. Note that the lesions follow the skin's relaxed tension lines. (Reproduced, with permission, from Wolff K, et al. *Fitzpatrick's Dermatology in General Medicine*, 7th ed. New York: McGraw-Hill, 2008, Fig. 128-3.)

- **Invasive anogenital cancer** (including cervical cancer): ↑ prevalence and progression of squamous cell carcinoma caused by human papillomavirus (HPV) due to ↓ immune surveillance and ↓ endogenous antineoplastic capability. Treat with surgical excision, chemotherapy, and radiation therapy, depending on staging and location.
- **Notable metabolic disorders promoted by immune dysregulation in HIV include:**
  - **HIV wasting syndrome:** A hypermetabolic state, characterized by anorexia, leading to muscle atrophy and weight loss, often worsened by GI complications of advanced HIV. Treatment options include nutritional counseling, appetite stimulants, and recombinant human growth hormone.
  - Metabolic syndrome/dyslipidemia.
  - Advanced coronary atherosclerosis.

TABLE 6.18.   Prophylaxis Against AIDS-Related Opportunistic Infections

Pathogen	Indication for Prophylaxis	Medication	Comments
Pneumocystis jiroveci cystic pneumonia (PCP)	CD4+ cells < 200/mm³ or a history of oral thrush. Prophylaxis may be stopped if CD4+ cells > 200/mm³ for ≥ 3 months on HAART.	TMP-SMX or dapsone +/– pyrimethamine or pentamidine nebulizers or atovaquone.	Single-strength tablets of TMP-SMX are effective and may be less toxic than double-strength tablets.
Mycobacterium avium complex (MAC)	CD4+ cells < 50/mm³. Prophylaxis may be stopped if CD4+ cells > 100/mm³ for ≥ 3 months on HAART.	Azithromycin or clarithromycin or rifabutin.	Azithromycin can be given once weekly; rifabutin can ↑ hepatic metabolism of other drugs.
Toxoplasma	CD4+ cells < 100/mm³ and *Toxoplasma* IgG ⊕. Prophylaxis may be stopped if CD4+ cells > 100–200/mm³ for ≥ 3 months on HAART.	TMP-SMX or dapsone +/– pyrimethamine or atovaquone.	Covered by all PCP regimens except pentamidine.
Mycobacterium tuberculosis	PPD > 5 mm; history of ⊕ PPD that was inadequately treated; close contact to a person with active TB.	INH sensitive: INH × 9 months (include pyridoxine).	For INH-resistant strains, use rifampin or rifabutin +/– pyrazinamide.
Candida	Frequent or severe recurrences.	Fluconazole or itraconazole.	
Herpes simplex virus (HSV)	Frequent or severe recurrences.	Acyclovir or famciclovir or valacyclovir.	
Pneumococcus	All patients.	Pneumococcal vaccine. Repeat when CD4+ cells > 200/mm³.	Some disease may be prevented with TMP-SMX, clarithromycin, and azithromycin.
Influenza	All patients.	Influenza vaccine.	
HBV	Generally, all susceptible patients; depends on immune status.	Hepatitis B vaccine (3 doses).	
HAV	All susceptible patients at ↑ risk for HAV infection or with chronic liver disease (eg, chronic HBV or HCV).	Hepatitis A vaccine (2 doses).	IV drug users, MSM, and hemophiliacs are at ↑ risk.

DIAGNOSIS/TREATMENT

Depends on disease process and exam findings. A guiding principle is that HAART and maintenance of an undetectable viral load and high CD4+ cell count largely prevent the above complications, even when a patient has previously been diagnosed with AIDS.

PREVENTION

See Table 6.18 for OI prophylaxis and testing/treatment guidelines.

Vector-Borne Infections

MOSQUITO-BORNE INFECTIONS

Table 6.19 lists common types of mosquito-borne infections.

TABLE 6.19. **Mosquito-Borne Zoonotic Infections**

DISEASE	CLINICAL FEATURES	GEOGRAPHIC DISTRIBUTION	COMMENTS
Malaria (*Plasmodia* spp)	Fever, hemolysis, meningoencephalitis.	Worldwide, largely in para-equitorial distribution. Highest mortality in sub-Saharan Africa and Southeast Asia.	Causes 1–3 million deaths yearly, predominantly in under-resourced nations. Artemisinin derivatives now standard of care for antimalarial therapy in most settings. Widespread resistance to older agents, such as choloroquine. Prophylaxis recommended for travel in endemic areas.
Dengue fever (flaviviruses)	Two common presentations: "Breakbone fever" = myalgia, fever, HA, petechial rash; and less commonly, hemorrhagic fever, with thrombocytopenia, spontaneous hemorrhage, and shock.	Central and South America, sub-Saharan Africa, Southeast Asia.	Endemic in > 100 countries. No cure; treatment is supportive.
Yellow fever (flavivirus)	Most cases 3–4-day self-limited febrile illness. Second phase with jaundice due to hepatitis. Can cause acute hemorrhage illness, accounting for majority of mortality.	Tropical and subtropical areas of Africa and South America.	Vaccine is available. WHO estimates 200,000 cases and 30,000 deaths yearly in unvaccinated populations. Treatment is supportive.
Encephalitides Alphaviruses			
Eastern equine	Encephalitis, peripheral neuropathy.	United States (Atlantic and Gulf coasts), Caribbean, South America.	Children are usually affected; mortality is 50%–75%; neurologic sequelae are common.

(continues)

TABLE 6.19. **Mosquito-Borne Zoonotic Infections** *(continued)*

DISEASE	CLINICAL FEATURES	GEOGRAPHIC DISTRIBUTION	COMMENTS
Western equine	Encephalitis.	Western and central United States, South America.	Infants and adults > 50 years of age are usually affected; mortality is 5%–15%; neurologic sequelae are uncommon, except in infants.
Venezuelan equine	Encephalitis.	Florida, southwestern United States, Central and South America.	Adults are usually affected; mortality is 1%; neurologic sequelae are rare.
Flaviviruses			
Japanese B	Encephalitis.	China, Southeast Asia, India, Japan.	A vaccine is available.
St. Louis	Encephalitis.	United States (rural west and midwest states, New Jersey, Florida, Texas), Caribbean, Central and South America.	Adults > 50 years of age are most often affected; mortality is 2%–20%; neurologic sequelae occur in about 20% of cases.
West Nile	Encephalitis, polymyelitis-like, peripheral neuropathy.	Middle East, Africa, Europe, Central Asia, United States.	

Adapted, with permission, from Aminoff MJ, et al. *Clinical Neurology*, 6th ed. New York: McGraw-Hill, 2005: 28.

TICK-BORNE INFECTIONS

A 45-year-old woman returns from visiting her relatives in Cape Cod, Massachusetts. On her trip, she went camping and mountain biking in a state park. She comes to your primary care office today for left knee pain and swelling. She recently had a target-shaped rash on her leg (Figure 6.25), which has disappeared. On ROS, you elicit a history of fatigue and subjective fevers. On exam, her temperature is 37.7°C (99.8°F), and her left knee is erythematous, with a moderate effusion and mild tenderness to palpation. You discover an erythematous targetoid lesion on her lateral left thigh 15 cm in diameter. What do you do?

Send anti-Lyme IgM and IgG tests, and if ⊕, order a confirmatory Western blot. (If negative, it may be too early for a serologic result.) Consider an ECG and begin early doxycycline for a presumptive diagnosis of Lyme disease.

Table 6.20 outlines the presentation of tick-borne zoonoses.

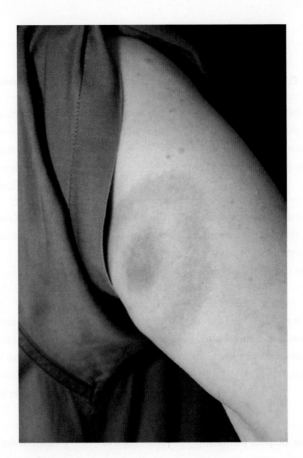

FIGURE 6.25. **Lyme disease.** The classic "target" or "bull's-eye" lesion of erythema migrans is seen. (Courtesy of James Gathany, Public Health Image Library Centers for Disease Control and Prevention.)

TABLE 6.20. **Tick-Borne Zoonotic Infections**

DISEASE	VECTOR	ANIMAL RESERVOIR	CLINICAL FEATURES	ANTIBIOTIC TREATMENT	GEOGRAPHIC DISTRIBUTION
Babesiosis	*I scapularis, I pacificus.*	Cattle, horses, dogs, cats, rodents, deer.	Fatigue, malaise, anorexia, nausea, HA, sweats, rigors, abdominal pain, emotional lability, depression, dark urine, hepatomegaly, fever, petechiae, ecchymosis, occasionally rash and pulmonary edema.	For the seriously ill, atovaquone and azithromycin, or quinine plus clindamycin.	Coastal areas of Massachusetts, Rhode Island, and New York; also in Maryland, Virginia, Minnesota, Wisconsin, Georgia, Washington, and Mexico.
Colorado tick fever	*Dermacentor andersoni.*	Deer, marmots, porcupines.	Fever, chills, HA, myalgias, nausea, vomiting, photophobia, abdominal pain, and occasional sore throat; also may have conjunctivitis, lymphadenopathy, hepatosplenomegaly, stiff neck, retro-orbital pain, weakness, and lethargy.	Supportive care.	Western and northwestern United States and southwestern Canada.

(continues)

TABLE 6.20. **Tick-Borne Zoonotic Infections** *(continued)*

Disease	Vector	Animal Reservoir	Clinical Features	Antibiotic Treatment	Geographic Distribution
Human granulocytic anaplasmosis	*Ixodes scapularis.*	Dogs, deer, other mammals.	Fevers, chills, malaise, HA, nausea, muscle aches, cough, sore throat, and pulmonary infiltrates (especially in children).	Doxycycline or tetracycline.	Japan, Malaysia, and the eastern, northeastern, and north central United States; some cases in western United States.
Human monocytic ehrlichiosis	*Amblyomma americanum* (Lone Star tick) and *D variabilis.*	Dogs, deer, other mammals.	Fevers, chills, malaise, HA, nausea, muscle aches, cough, sore throat, and pulmonary infiltrates (especially in children).	Doxycycline or tetracycline.	Japan, Malaysia, and southern United States.
Lyme disease (*Borrelia burgdorferi*)	*Ixodes dammini.*	Deer, sheep, deer mice.	Erythema migrans (see Figure 6.25), meningitis, encephalitis, neuropathy, and joint and heart symptoms.	Doxycycline, amoxicillin, cefuroxime, erythromycin, ceftriaxone, or cefotaxime.	Atlantic central and north central United States, occasional in western United States; separate species in Europe.
Rocky Mountain spotted fever (*Rickettsia rickettsii*)	*Dermacentor andersoni* (wood tick) and *D variabilis* (dog tick).	North American mammals.	Petechiae, purpura, pulmonary infiltrates, jaundice, myocarditis, hepatosplenomegaly, meningitis, encephalitis, and lymphadenopathy.	Doxycycline or chloramphenicol.	Most of the continental United States; more prevalent in the southeast and south central United States.
Relapsing fever (*Borrelia* spp)	*Ornithodoros* spp (actually human body lice, not ticks)	Wild rodents.	Fever, chills, HA, myalgias, and arthralgias; pain, nausea, vomiting, and hypotension.	Erythromycin or doxycycline.	Worldwide.
Tularemia (*Francisella tularensis*)	*Dermacentor* spp and *Amblyomma* spp.	Rabbits, deer, dogs.	Pneumonia, regional lymphadenopathy and HA, cough, myalgias, arthralgias, nausea, vomiting, ulceration at inoculation site, and ocular findings.	Tobramycin or gentamicin; chloramphenicol for meningitis.	United States (except Hawaii) and Canada.

Reproduced, with permission, from Tintinalli JE, et al. *Emergency Medicine: A Comprehensive Study Guide*, 6th ed. New York: McGraw-Hill, 2004: 372.

Special Topics

SEPSIS AND INFECTIONS IN THE CRITICAL CARE SETTING

A 64-year-old man with diabetes is brought to the ER by ambulance. His wife found him in bed this morning, delirious and sweating, and called 911. EMS arrived to find an obtunded, obese male, GCS 10 in bed, diaphoretic, and with mottled skin. BP en route was 85/palpation, and his pulse was 125 bpm. Peripheral IV access was established prehospital. The patient's wife notes that he was complaining of fever and malaise yesterday but had no other specific complaints. After a focused physical exam, including assessment of airway, breathing, and circulation, you feel that infection is the most likely cause. What do you do?

Begin aggressive intravenous rehydration with isotonic fluids, obtain labs (including CBC, chemistry panel, and a lactate), blood and urine cultures, and CXR, and begin empirical broad-spectrum antibiotics for septic shock.

Significant research about sepsis has occurred in the past 2 decades. Choice of resuscitation fluids, amount of fluid, type of vasopressor, and choice of empirical antibiotics have all been investigated, among other topics. The current algorithm for early goal-directed therapy emphasizes the importance of aggressive fluid resuscitation prior to beginning vasopressor agents and consideration of other therapies, such as colloid repletion (transfusion), steroids, and drotrecogin alfa (activated protein C). Some of these measures remain controversial.

- For early goal-directed therapy, patients must meet **at least 2 of 4** systemic inflammatory response syndrome (SIRS) criteria:
  - Core temperature $> 38.0°C$ ($100.4°F$) or $< 36°C$ ($96.8°F$).
  - Heart rate > 90 bpm.
  - Respiratory rate > 20, $PCO_2 < 32$ mmHg, or need for mechanical ventilation.
  - WBC $> 12,000/mm^3$ or $< 4000/mm^3$, or $> 10\%$ bands.
- And **1** of the following criteria:
  - Lactate > 4 mmol/L.
  - Systolic BP < 90 mmHg after 20–30 mL/kg fluid resuscitation.

Additionally, the organisms causing infections in critically ill patients may differ, depending on length of hospitalization, antecedent hospitalizations, risk factors for multidrug resistant organisms (MDRO), indwelling devices, and immunocompromise, among other variables. Consideration of MDRO should occur (see next section) and may influence choice of empirical antibiotic coverage. The same types of infections occur, and the same principles of selecting and tailoring antimicrobial coverage apply, whether in the ICU setting or in the outpatient or medical/surgical ward setting.

EMERGING ANTIBIOTIC RESISTANCE

Because of antibiotic use as well as endogenous genetic mutation and transmission of resistance genes between organisms, antibiotic resistance has become a topic of intense focus. Development of antibiotic resistance is not a new phenomenon, but because of the increasing availability of many types of antimicrobial agents, you must **carefully consider the choice and spectrum of agent and length of therapy** to both ensure coverage and limit resistance.

Methicillin-resistant *Staphylococcus aureus* (MRSA) is both a nosocomial and community-acquired pathogen. Much research is ongoing to characterize resistance factors and develop treatment algorithms for MRSA, as well as other emerging MDR organisms, such as vancomycin-resistant enterococci (VRE), *Pseudomonas aeruginosa, Stenotrophomonas maltophilia, Acinetobacter,* and others. Brief descriptions of 3 common MDR organisms are presented here.

- **MRSA:**
  - MRSA is present in both nosocomial and community settings (CA-MRSA, usually with the strain USA-300). Primarily responsible for SSTIs, MRSA can also cause pneumonia (especially in patients post-influenza, with a history of smoking methamphetamine, and in the critical care setting, especially mechanically ventilated patients). The following antibiotics may be used, depending on local resistance profiles and degree of illness: clindamycin, TMP-SMX, ciprofloxacin (if susceptibility confirmed) + rifampin, tetracycline derivatives, linezolid, vancomycin, and daptomycin.
  - Carriage of MRSA occurs in the nares and other skin sites; however, studies examining the efficacy of decolonization have been disappointing. In patients with a history of severe or recurrent MRSA infection, decolonization may be attempted with intranasal mupirocin and chlorhexidine-containing body washes.
- **VRE:**
  - VRE infections are primarily found in nosocomial settings among patients who have previously received antibiotics. Enterococci are part of the gastrointestinal flora and have both endogenous and acquired antibiotic resistance.
  - VRE strains, most commonly *E faecium*, are responsible for infections of the urinary tract, catheter-related infections, endocarditis, intra-abdominal and wound infections, among others.
  - Risk factors for VRE infection include recent antibiotics, critical illness, immunocompromise (organ transplant, hematologic malignancy, corticosteroid use, neutropenia, chemotherapy), prior VRE colonization, and parenteral nutrition. Before treatment, all indwelling devices (CVC, urinary catheters, etc) should be removed and any abscesses drained.
  - Antibiotics should be tailored by antibiogram and culture results, as the susceptibility of VRE strains is variable. Common agents such as doxycycline, nitrofurantoin, and chloramphenicol were used in the past, but the newer agents linezolid, daptomycin, and tigecycline are more commonly used now. Infectious disease consultation is advised.
- ***Pseudomonas aeruginosa:***
  - A gram-$\ominus$ rod, *Psuedomonas* is an opportunistic microbe common in nosocomial infections of the urinary tract, lungs (especially in mechanically ventilated patients), and CNS and in bacteremia among patients with or without indwelling devices. It is typically found after > 7 days of hospitalization and in patients who are immunocompromised.

- Other than its presence as a nosocomial pathogen, *Pseudomonas* has been a long-treated microbe in patients with cystic fibrosis and in otitis externa among swimmers (swimmer's ear).
- Often produces a blue-green pigment, leading to the description of the blue purulent exudate sometimes found in infected tissue (not a sensitive finding).
- Treatment for *Pseudomonas* coverage varies by severity and site of infection. Outpatient treatment is appropriate in non-life-threatening infections. For hospitalized patients, single coverage with an antipseudomonal agent (β-lactams such as ticarcillin and piperacillin; cephalosporins such as cefepime; or fluoroquinolones such as ciprofloxacin) is usually adequate. Double coverage is probably not indicated in most circumstances. When given, it is recommended to use a β-lactam with an aminoglycoside or with a fluoroquinolone (either ciprofloxacin or levofloxacin).

THE SPLENECTOMIZED PATIENT

Patients who have undergone a splenectomy are at ↑ risk for serious bacterial infections, especially with encapsulated organisms such as *S pneumoniae*, *N meningitidis*, and *H influenzae*. The highest risk is in the first 3 years after splenectomy. The most feared complication is overwhelming **postsplenectomy sepsis**. Patients present after a short viral-like prodrome that is followed by abrupt decompensation and shock. Vaccination against pneumococcus, *H influenzae*, and *N meningitidis* should be given 2 weeks prior to elective splenectomy or at hospital discharge for emergent cases.

All splenectomized patients should be counseled that new fever is a medical emergency and that they should seek attention immediately. Penicillin prophylaxis is controversial, given that the only data are based on sickle-cell anemia patients with functional asplenia. Recommendations are strongest for children < 5 years old in the first year postsplenectomy, and those with additional underlying immunodeficiency. PCN prophylaxis is not routinely recommended in adults. These patients are also at ↑ risk for parasitic infections, specifically, babesiosis and malaria.

COMMON FUNGAL INFECTIONS

Table 6.21 lists the presentation and treatment of common fungal infections.

CATHETER-RELATED INFECTIONS

A category of infections that includes catheter-related bloodstream infections as well as exit-site, tunnel, and pocket infections. The most commonly isolated etiologic agents are coagulase-⊖ staphylococci, *S aureus*, *Enterococcus* spp, and *Candida* spp. In the United States, 5 million central venous catheters (CVCs) are placed per year, and more than 200,000 nosocomial bloodstream infections occur per year. Risk of infection varies by type and site of catheter, with CVC first (1.6–6.8 infections/1000 catheter days), then PICC (peripherally inserted central catheter), then peripheral IV (0.2/1000 catheter days). Among CVCs, risk of infection is lowest with subclavian lines, and risk of infection in femoral = internal jugular CVCs.

MNEMONIC

To remember the appearance of **B**lastomyces under the microscope, think of **B**road-based, **B**udding yeast.

KEY FACT

In hemodialysis patients, *S aureus* is the most common etiology for catheter-related infections.

TABLE 6.21. **Clinical Presentation and Treatment of Selected Fungal Infections**

FUNGUS	GEOGRAPHY	MANIFESTATION	TREATMENT	NOTES
Candida spp	Common yeast on the skin worldwide.	Thrush, esophagitis, intertrigo, vaginitis, candiduria, hepatosplenic candidiasis (in postneutropenic chemo patients), disseminated candidiasis.	Topical antifungals for mucosal disease. Oral fluconazole for esophagitis; IV or PO fluconazole, amphotericin formulation, or echinocandin for disseminated disease. Remove vascular catheters.	*Candida glabrata* is frequently resistant to azole therapy.
Aspergillus spp	Widespread in soil, water, compost, potted plants, and ventilation ducts.	Allergic bronchopulmonary aspergillosis; aspergilloma of the lung or sinuses; invasive aspergillosis.	Voriconazole, echinocandin, or amphotericin for invasive disease (combination therapy is sometimes used); surgical excision of aspergilloma in the setting of hemoptysis.	A common infection in neutropenic patients or post-transplant.
Cryptococcus	Worldwide in bird droppings (especially pigeons).	Meningitis, especially in HIV patients with CD4+ cells < 100 mm³ and in atypical pneumonia.	For meningitis, amphotericin and 5-flucytosine, followed by fluconazole; fluconazole for mild lung disease.	Cryptococcal antigen on CSF and serum.
Coccidioides	Soil of the southwestern United States and San Joaquin Valley.	"Valley fever," flulike syndrome, pneumonia. Disseminated disease in 1%–5%.	Supportive therapy for valley fever; fluconazole or amphotericin for disseminated disease.	Check for *Coccidioides* antibody titer.
Histoplasma	Bird and bat droppings in the Mississippi and Ohio River valleys and in Central America.	Pulmonary infection, disseminated disease.	Supportive therapy for lung disease; itraconazole or amphotericin for disseminated disease.	Risk factors include spelunking and contact with chicken coops.
Blastomyces	Upper Midwest and Great Lakes region.	Most commonly pneumonia; occasionally skin infections, osteomyelitis, and epididymitis/prostatitis.	Itraconazole or amphotericin.	Risk factor is exposure to forests and streams.
Sporothrix	Found in soil, especially rose bushes.	Most commonly SSTI. Can also cause disseminated disease.	Itraconazole for mild disease; amphotericin for severe disease.	

SYMPTOMS/EXAM

- Clinical findings are **unreliable.**
- Fever and chills are sensitive but not specific.
- Inflammation and purulence around the catheter are specific but not sensitive.

DIAGNOSIS

- **Blood cultures:** Obtain 2 sets of cultures, at least 1 set drawn percutaneously.

- **Catheter tip culture:** Should be performed if line sepsis is suspected. The semiquantitative (roll plate) method is most commonly used. After the catheter has been removed from the patient, the tip is rolled across an agar plate. A colony count of > 15 after overnight incubation suggests catheter-related infection when blood cultures are also ⊕. Alternative methods for diagnosis include time to positivity and quantitative cultures.

TREATMENT

- **Catheter removal:** Used in most cases of nontunneled catheters. For tunneled catheters and implantable devices, removal should be considered in the presence of severe illness or documented infection (especially *S aureus*, gram-⊖ rods, or *Candida* spp) or if complications occur.
- **Initial antibiotic choice:** Empirical treatment should include vancomycin to cover *S aureus* (including MRSA) and coagulase-negative staphylococci until culture data are available.
- **Duration of therapy:** Patients with uncomplicated bacteremia should be treated for 10–14 days. Patients with complicated infections (eg, those with persistent ⊕ blood cultures after catheter removal, endocarditis, septic thrombophlebitis, or osteomyelitis) should be treated for 4–6 weeks.

PREVENTION

Recent trials have shown that good practices at the time of insertion decrease CVC-associated bloodstream infection: Use gloves, gown, mask, full drape, and cap, with hand hygiene at the time of insertion. Inpatients with CVC should be assessed daily to see if a central line is still necessary.

COMPLICATIONS

Septic thrombophlebitis, infective endocarditis, septic pulmonary emboli, osteomyelitis, or other complications due to septic emboli.

FEVER OF UNKNOWN ORIGIN (FUO)

Defined as a temperature > 38.3°C (100.9°F) for ≥ 3 weeks that remains undiagnosed despite evaluation over 3 outpatient visits or 3 hospital days. Common etiologies include infection (25%–40%), cancer (25%–40%), and autoimmune disease (10%–15%). Infection is more likely if the patient is older or from a developing country, as well as in cases of nosocomial, neutropenic, or HIV-associated FUO. In approximately 10%–15% of cases, no diagnosis will be discovered, and the fever will resolve spontaneously.

SYMPTOMS

Fever; otherwise variable, but a careful history should be taken on serial visits to elucidate any clues to a diagnosis.

EXAM

Repeated physical exams may yield subtle findings in the fundi, conjunctivae, sinuses, temporal arteries, and lymph nodes. Heart murmurs, splenomegaly, and perirectal or prostatic fluctuance/tenderness should be assessed.

DIFFERENTIAL

- **Infectious:** TB, endocarditis, and **occult abscesses** are the most common infectious causes of FUO in immunocompetent patients. Consider 1° HIV infection or OIs due to unrecognized HIV. In rare cases, the cause is babesiosis or other tick-borne diseases.

- **Neoplastic: Lymphoma** and **leukemia** are the most common cancers causing FUO. Other causes include hepatoma, renal cell carcinoma, and atrial myxoma.
- **Autoimmune:** Adult Still disease, SLE, cryoglobulinemia, polyarteritis nodosa, and temporal arteritis (especially in the elderly).
- **Other:** Drug fever, thyroiditis, granulomatous hepatitis, sarcoidosis, Crohn disease, Whipple disease, familial Mediterranean fever, recurrent pulmonary embolism, retroperitoneal hematoma, factitious fever.

DIAGNOSIS

- Ask about HIV risk factors, cardiac valve disorders, drug use, travel, exposure to animals/insects, occupational history, recent medications, sick contacts, and a family history of fever.
- Obtain routine labs and CXR. Blood cultures should be drawn off antibiotics and held for 2 weeks. Place a PPD (or check a gamma interferon release assay). If indicated, obtain cultures of other body fluids (sputum, urine, stool, CSF). If travel history is present, obtain a blood smear (malaria, babesiosis). Do an HIV test.
- Perform echocardiography to look for vegetations. If neoplasm or abscesses are suspected, order a CT/MRI.
- Use other tests selectively (ANA, RF, viral cultures, antibody/antigen tests for viral and fungal infections).
- Invasive procedures are generally low yield except for temporal artery biopsy in the elderly, liver biopsy in patients with LFT abnormalities, and bone marrow biopsy in HIV with pancytopenia.

TREATMENT

- If there are no other symptoms, treatment may be deferred until a definitive diagnosis is made.
- Give broad-spectrum antibiotics if the patient is severely ill or neutropenic.
- Again, 10%–15% of cases will spontaneously resolve.

ACUTE RHEUMATIC FEVER

A postinfectious autoimmune complication of GAS pharyngitis. Acute rheumatic fever was once a common cause of acquired valvular disease. Rare in

TABLE 6.22.   The Jones Criteria for Rheumatic Fever

MAJOR CRITERIA	MINOR CRITERIA
Carditis	Clinical:
Migratory polyarthritis	Fever
Sydenham chorea	Arthralgia
Subcutaneous nodules	Laboratory:
Erythema marginatum	Elevated acute-phase reactants
	Prolonged PR interval
Plus:	
Supporting evidence of a recent group A streptococcal infection (eg, a ⊕ throat culture or rapid antigen detection test and/or an elevated or increasing streptococcal antibody test).	

the era of antistreptococcal antibiotics, the incidence of rheumatic fever is 0.5%–1%.

DIAGNOSIS

The Jones criteria are used for diagnosis of acute rheumatic fever (see Table 6.22). **Two major criteria** or **1 major criterium plus 2 minor criteria** must be present.

TREATMENT

A course of penicillin (minimal evidence base); NSAIDs for inflammation, preferably salicylates; bed rest for cardiac complications; IV immunoglobulin for severe inflammatory states; and antiepileptics, specifically, valproic acid for severe chorea.

NOTES

CHAPTER 7

Hematology/Oncology

Sachiko Kaizuka, MD

Anemia

APPROACH TO ANEMIA

Definition: Low oxygen-carrying capacity of blood, shown by low level of hemoglobin or low number of circulating RBCs in blood.

SYMPTOMS

Symptoms depend on acuity, severity, and the age of patient:

- Acute anemia: Symptoms of hypovolemia (**postural hypotension** and **tachycardia** or shock).
- Chronic anemia: Often asymptomatic if mild and chronic; but **fatigue, DOE, postural lightheadedness, pallor, and headache** if moderate to severe.
- The elderly: May exhibit worsening angina, claudication, and possibly heart failure.

DIAGNOSIS

Workup: Begin by categorizing the possible causes by typical MCV and reticulocyte count (hyper- or hypoproliferative). The etiology is often multifactorial, but the basic algorithm and possible causes are shown in Figure 7.1 and Table 7.1.

MICROCYTIC ANEMIA

Iron Deficiency Anemia (IDA)

Etiologies generally include blood loss (eg, GI, hemolysis, surgical blood loss, hookworm infestation), malabsorption (eg, gastrectomy, sprue, IBD), iron-deficient erythropoiesis (hemodialysis, pregnancy, malabsorption), iron-store depletion (rapid growth, menstrual blood loss, inadequate diet).

- Assume GI bleed for males and postmenopausal females until proven otherwise!
- Menstrual blood loss is the most common cause in premenopausal women.

SYMPTOMS/EXAM

- Mostly asymptomatic if mild.
- If severe: Fatigue, pallor, ↓ exercise capacity.

<table>
<tr><td>**MNEMONIC**</td></tr>
</table>

Causes of microcytic anemia:

TICS

Thalassemia
Iron deficiency
Chronic disease
Sideroblastic anemia

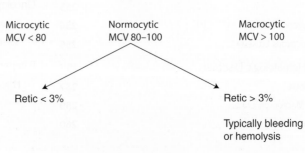

Anemia

| Microcytic | Normocytic | Macrocytic |
| MCV < 80 | MCV 80–100 | MCV > 100 |

Retic < 3%   Retic > 3%

Typically bleeding
or hemolysis

FIGURE 7.1.   Algorithm for categorizing anemia.

TABLE 7.1. Classification of Anemia by MCV

MICROCYTIC (MCV < 80)	NORMOCYTIC (MCV 80–100)	MACROCYTIC (MCV > 100)
Iron deficiency anemia.	**Hypoproliferative:**	**Megaloblastic:**
Anemia of chronic disease.	Anemia of chronic disease.	B_{12} or folate deficiency.
Sideroblastic anemia.	Bone marrow disease.	Drug-induced bone marrow suppression (methotrexate,
Thalassemia.	Renal failure.	phenytoin, phenobarbital, zidovudine).
Lead poisoning.	Hypersplenism.	**Nonmegaloblastic:**
	Infection: HIV, *Mycoplasma,* EBV.	Liver disease.
	Any early or mixed process of anemia.	Alcoholism.
	Hyperproliferative:	Hypothyroidism.
	Hemolysis.	Reticulocytosis.
	Acute blood loss.	Some bone marrow diseases (aplastic anemia, myelodysplastic syndrome, myeloma).

- If severe and prolonged (seen in IDA):
  - **Angular cheilosis:** Fissures at the corners of the mouth.
  - **Atrophic glossitis.**
  - **Pica:** Craving for nonnutritive substances.
  - **Koilonychia:** Spooning of the fingernails.
  - **Plummer-Vinson syndrome:** Esophageal webs and atrophic glossitis, leading to dysphagia.

These symptoms are not sensitive or specific; lab studies should be done to diagnose IDA.

DIAGNOSIS

- CBC with smear: ↓/normal MCV, ↑ RDW, microcytic, hypochromic RBCs, and variation in RBC size (anisocytosis) or shape (poikilocytosis). No target cells!
- Iron studies: ↓ serum iron, ↑ transferrin iron-binding capacity (TIBC), ↓ transferrin sat, and ↓ serum ferritin.
- DDx (See Table 7.2):
  - Thalassemia: ⊕ target cells, normal RDW, microcytosis/hypochromia before anemia is moderate to severe, leads to ↑ Fe, TIBC, and ferritin, ↑ HbA_2 on electrophoresis.
  - Anemia of chronic disease (ACD): ↓ Fe and TIBC, ↓ transferrin sat, and ↑ serum ferritin.
  - Sideroblastic anemia: Mitochondrial functional defect, ringed sideroblast, normal to high Fe, normal TIBC, ↑ transferrin sat and ferritin.

TABLE 7.2. ACD vs. IDA vs. Thalassemia

	MCV	RDW	FE	TIBC	FERRITIN	TRANSFERRIN SATURATION	TRANSFERRIN
IDA	↓/normal	↑	↓	↑	↓	Low	↑
ACD	↓/normal	Normal	↓	Normal/↓	Normal/↑	Normal	Normal
Thalassemia	↓	Normal	Normal/↑	Normal	Normal	Normal	Normal

TREATMENT

If possible, correct the underlying cause (eg, GI bleed, malabsorption).

- **Oral Fe replacement:** Adequate for ↑ physiologic needs, inadequate dietary Fe intake, or pregnancy. Ineffective in GI malabsorption. Poor response in continuing blood loss, ESRD, inflammatory illness, or damaged marrow. Generally takes 6 months to rebuild iron stores. Reticulocyte count should ↑ 3–4 days after the initiation of treatment and peaks at about 10 days.
- **Parenteral Fe therapy:** Use to adequately deliver Fe for patients unable to tolerate PO iron or unable to correct iron deficiency with PO iron.

Sideroblastic Anemia

Defective heme biosynthesis in RBC precursors, leading to impaired erythropoiesis, which in turn leads to accumulation of iron in mitochondria and then "ringed sideroblasts."

- **Hereditary:** X-linked or autosomally inherited. Manifests in infancy.
- **Acquired:** Lead poisoning, INH, alcoholism, copper deficiency, and chloramphenicol.

DIAGNOSIS

- Variable RBC morphology and MCV.
- Check peripheral smear with siderocytes: Hypochromic RBCs with basophilic stippling that stains ⊕ for iron (ie, Pappenheimer bodies).
- Bone marrow with ringed sideroblasts (pathognomonic).
- ↑ Fe, transferrin sat, and ferritin; ↓ transferrin (= Fe overload).

TREATMENT

- Treat any reversible causes.
- Transfuse periodically for severe anemia.
- Supplement pyridoxine for some hereditary forms.
- Iron chelation Tx or therapeutic phlebotomy for Fe overload.

NORMOCYTIC ANEMIA

Anemia of Chronic Disease (ACD)

Caused by multiple factors (cytokine release in inflammation), including ↓ EPO production/release, ↓ EPO response, inhibition of Fe delivery from reticuloendothelial cells, and erythroid precursor growth, leading to the failure of bone marrow to respond to anemia. Hepcidin is the negative regulator of iron absorption. In anemia of inflammation, hepcidin production is increased, and this may account for the defining feature of this condition, sequestration of iron in macrophages.

DIAGNOSIS

↓/normal MCV, normal RDW, ↓ reticulocyte, ↓ Fe and TIBC, transferrin sat normal (in renal disease) or ↑ in inflammation ferritin. Table 7.2 outlines factors that distinguish ACD from IDA and thalassemia.

TREATMENT

- Treat the underlying cause if possible.
- Give EPO for ACD (including renal disease), with adequate Fe stores if ↓ serum EPO levels.

Hemolytic Anemia

Premature destruction of RBCs before their normal life span of 90–120 days. Various causes:

- RBC interior abnormalities (become trapped in spleen) and RBC membrane abnormalities (lysis in vessels).
- Extrinsic factors: Antibodies mainly trapped in spleen and some lysis in vessels, mechanical destruction, toxins leading to lysis in vessels.

SYMPTOMS/EXAM

- General symptoms of anemia (such as fatigue) plus jaundice, red-brown urine (hemoglobinuria) +/– splenomegaly.
- **Labs:** ↑ reticulocytes, ↑ I-Bil (up to 5 mg/dL), ↓ haptoglobin, ↑ LDH. (*Note:* No urine Bil.)
- Hemolytic anemia can be classified as extravascular or intravascular, based on the site of RBC destruction (see Table 7.3).
- **Major causes of hemolytic anemia:**
    - **Autoimmune hemolytic anemia (warm AIHA):** An acquired disorder in which an IgG autoantibody binds to the RBC membranes, causing RBC destruction by macrophages or spleen. Direct lysis by complements is rare. Spherocytosis and reticulocytosis are seen on the peripheral smear. ⊕ direct Coombs test. Indirect Coombs test may be ⊕ or ⊖. 50% idiopathic. Other causes: SLE, chronic lymphocytic leukemia, lymphoma. 10% with immune thrombocytopenia (Evans syndrome). Treated with steroids, immunosuppressants, rituxan, splenectomy.
    - **Cold agglutinin disease (cold AIHA):** Acquired hemolytic anemia 2° to an IgM autoantibody, which occurs only in cooler parts of the body such as fingers, nose, and ears. IgM binds to RBC and fixes complement. Lysis is rare. RBCs with complement are sequestered by Kupffer cells in the liver. Mostly idiopathic. Other cases associated with lymphoproliferative disorders, nonlymphoid malignancies, and acute infections (mycoplasmal pneumonia, infectious mononucleosis). ⊕ direct Coombs test for complement only.
    - **Microangiopathic hemolytic anemia:** Intravascular destruction of RBCs, with RBC fragmentation. ⊕ hemoglobinemia, hemoglobinuria, and methemalbuminemia if severe. ⊖ Coombs test. ⊕ fragmented

TABLE 7.3. Extravascular vs. Intravascular Hemolytic Anemia

	EXTRAVASCULAR	INTRAVASCULAR
Site of RBC destruction	Macrophage (spleen, liver).	Blood vessels.
Serum haptoglobin	↓	↓↓
Serum LDH	↑	↑↑
Urine hemosiderin	⊖	⊕
Urine hemoglobin	⊖	⊕ if severe.
Peripheral smear	Spherocytes.	Schistocytes.
Etiologies	Warm AIHA, hypersplenism, delayed hemolytic transfusion reaction, hemoglobinopathies.	Cold AIHA, acute hemolytic transfusion reaction, microangiopathic hemolysis, G6PD deficiency, PNH, hemoglobinopathies.

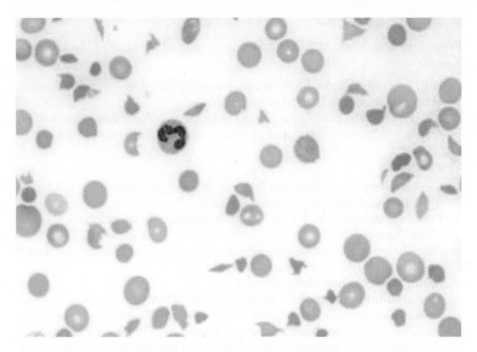

FIGURE 7.2.   Schistocytes and helmet cells in a patient with DIC. (Reproduced, with permission, from USMLERx.com.)

RBCs (schistocytes, helmet cells) on the peripheral smear (see Figure 7.2). Etiologies include TTP, DIC, malignant hypertension, HELLP syndrome, and prosthetic cardiac valves.

- **Glucose-6-phosphate dehydrogenase (G6PD) deficiency:** X-linked, recessive. ↑ susceptibility of RBCs to oxidative stress, causing episodic hemolytic anemia in response to oxidant drugs (dapsone, sulfonamides, antimalarias, nitrofurantoin), acute infections, or foods (fava beans). ⊕ Heinz body (precipitants formed by denatured oxidized hemoglobin) and "bite cells" on the peripheral smear. Seen in 10%–15% of American black males. Remember that testing G6PD levels during acute hemolysis episode may yield false ⊖ results since G6PD deficient cells are often destroyed, leaving only healthy RBCs to test.
- **Paroxysmal nocturnal hemoglobinuria (PNH):** Acquired disorder in stem cell, leading to ↑ RBC sensitivity to complement and episodes of intravascular hemolysis and hemoglobinuria. Patients are prone to thrombosis (especially mesenteric, hepatic, CNS, and skin veins). May lead to aplastic anemia, myelodysplasia, or acute myelogenous leukemia. ⊕ urine hemosiderin. WBC and PLT may be ↓.
- **Sickle cell anemia:** See the discussion of hemoglobinopathies below.

MACROCYTIC, MEGALOBLASTIC ANEMIA

Results from impaired DNA synthesis 2° to vitamin B$_{12}$ or folate deficiency or drug-induced bone marrow suppression (see Table 7.1).

DIAGNOSIS

- Anemia and ↑ MCV are usually found but are not required for diagnosis. Pancytopenia may sometimes be seen with severe disease.
- ↑ LDH and I-Bil 2° to ineffective erythropoiesis.

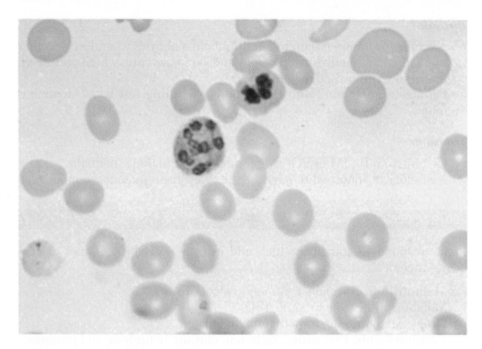

FIGURE 7.3. **Megaloblastic anemia.** Note macro-ovalocytes and prominent hypersegmented neutrophil. (Reproduced, with permission, from Fauci AS, et al. *Harrison's Principles of Internal Medicine,* 17th ed. New York: McGraw-Hill, 2008, Fig. 100-2A.)

- ↑ homocysteine (in both vitamin B_{12} and folate deficiency) and methylmalonic acid (vitamin B_{12} deficiency only) occur 2° to ↓ rate of metabolism.
- Hypersegmented neutrophils, macro-ovalocytes, and megaloblasts in the peripheral smear (see Figure 7.3).

VITAMIN B_{12} DEFICIENCY

Vitamin B_{12} is found in animal products and binds to intrinsic factor (IF) secreted by gastric parietal cells. The complex is absorbed in the terminal ileum.

- **Pernicious anemia:** Most common cause. ⊕ autoantibody against IF and gastric parietal cells, leading to chronic atrophic gastritis and ↓ production and function of IF. This can lead to ↑ **risk of gastric cancer and carcinoid tumors.**
- Other causes may include:
  - Malnutrition in individuals following a strict vegan diet.
  - ↓ **absorption:** Abnormal GI tract (including after bariatric surgery), metformin use, and PPI use.
  - ↑ competition for vitamin B_{12}, as seen in **fish tapeworm infestation** or bacterial overgrowth of the terminal ileum.

SYMPTOMS/EXAM

- **Symmetric peripheral neuropathy** with paresthesias and **ataxia**, leading to severe weakness, spasticity, and clonus.
- Memory loss, **personality changes**, and **dementia.**
- **Glossitis**, vaginal atrophy, and malabsorption.

DIAGNOSIS

- ↓ serum cobalamin (vitamin B_{12}). In subclinical cases when levels are low normal, check methylmalonic acid and homocysteine, which will be elevated in vitamin B_{12} deficient states.
- Pernicious anemia: ⊕ **anti-IF antibody** (**Schilling test** is not done anymore).

TREATMENT

- Give vitamin B_{12} IM or PO (IM required for pernicious anemia).
- Neurological abnormalities may not be reversible if present > 6 months.

KEY FACT

Neurologic symptoms of vitamin B_{12} deficiency may precede the anemia.

FOLATE DEFICIENCY

Folate is found in animal products and in leafy vegetables. Causes of deficiency include:

- **Malnutrition,** especially common in **alcoholism.**
- **Malabsorption:** Due to sprue, IBD.
- **Drugs:** Methotrexate, trimethoprim, phenytoin.
- ↑ **requirements: Pregnancy, lactation, chronic hemolysis,** and **psoriasis.**

DIAGNOSIS

↓ serum or RBC folate.

TREATMENT

- Give PO folate for 1–4 months or until the underlying condition resolves.
- Evaluate vitamin B_{12} deficiency before starting folate, as folate replacement may mask the hematologic manifestation of vitamin B_{12} deficiency while allowing neurologic damage to progress.

Hemoglobinopathies

THALASSEMIAS

Hereditary disorders caused by ↓ **production of globin chains** (α or β) of hemoglobin (normal adult hemoglobin [HbA] consists of 1 pair of α and β chains each [$\alpha_2\beta_2$]), leading to ↓ hemoglobin synthesis, which in turn leads to hypochromic microcytic anemia. (Remember abnormal RBCs are also hemolyzed.)

- **α-chain disorders:** Most commonly found in patients from **Southeast Asia** and **China,** and less commonly in those of African descent (see Table 7.4).
- **β-chain disorders:** Most commonly found in patients of **Mediterranean** origin and sometimes in Asians and those of African descent (see Table 7.5).

SICKLE CELL DISEASE

An autosomal-recessive disease due to a defect in the β-chain, leading to an unstable form of hemoglobin (called hemoglobin S: HbS). Deoxygenation of HbS leads to ↓ solubility, causing aggregation into long strands, which are the "sickled"-appearing RBCs. The sickled RBCs are less deformable and therefore less able to pass through microvasculature.

TABLE 7.4. α-Chain Disorders

ALLELES	DISEASE	CLINICAL RESULT
(−/−)	Hydrops fetalis.	Incompatible with life outside the uterus.
(a-/−)	Hemoglobin H disease.	Moderate to severe hemolytic anemia; splenomegaly. May require occasional transfusions.
(a-/a-)(aa/−)	Thalassemia minor or α-thalassemia-1 trait.	Mild microcytic anemia with a normal life expectancy.
(aa/a-)	Carrier/α-thalassemia-2 trait.	Patients are clinically normal.

SYMPTOMS/EXAM

Common manifestations are as follows (see also Figure 7.4 and Table 7.6):

- **Sickle cell crisis:**
  - The most common symptoms among patients > 2 years of age.
  - Most commonly affects the back and long bones of the extremities; lasts for days.
  - Often presents with fever, swelling, tenderness, hypertension, tachypnea, and nausea/vomiting. **Note: This cannot be diagnosed with labs.**
- **Acute chest syndrome:**
  - **New pulmonary infiltrate** in at least 1 whole lung segment; **chest pain, fever, and tachypnea, wheezing, or cough.**
  - Usually 2° to vaso-occlusion; may also be caused by infarction, embolism, or bacterial pneumonia.
  - Pulmonary complications: Most common cause of death in sickle cell disease.
- **Splenic sequestration crisis:**
  - Vaso-occlusion within the spleen leads to pooling of RBCs and ↓ peripheral hemoglobin concentration.
  - Massive splenomegaly.
  - Risk of hypovolemic shock.
  - Usually occurs in younger patients, as their spleens have not yet fibrosed.
  - **10%–15% mortality rate** and a **high rate of recurrence:** Recommended treatment is a splenectomy after the first episode.

KEY FACT

Patients with sickle cell disease have functional asplenia and are at ↑ risk for infection, especially from encapsulated organisms, such as *Streptococcus pneumoniae, Haemophilus influenzae* type b, and *Neisseria meningitidis.*

TABLE 7.5. β-Chain Disorders

β-CHAIN SYNTHESIS	DISEASE	CLINICAL RESULT
Near absence	β-thalassemia major.	Severe anemia dependent on **lifelong transfusions.** **Bony changes** 2° to bone marrow expansion. Hepatosplenomegaly. Manifests during the first year of life as hemoglobin F (HbF) declines. Patients typically die in the third or fourth decade because of sequelae of **iron overload.**
Moderate	β-thalassemia intermedia.	Mild bony changes and hepatosplenomegaly. May require transfusions.
Near normal	β-thalassemia minor.	Mild anemia but overall asymptomatic.

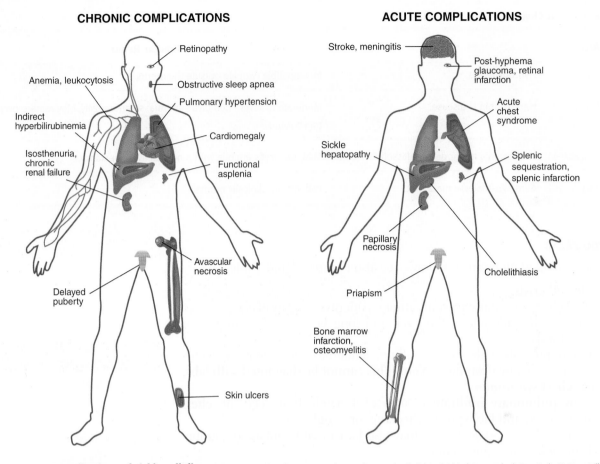

FIGURE 7.4. **Complications of sickle cell disease.** (Reproduced, with permission, from Hall JB, et al. *Principles of Critical Care,* 3rd ed. New York: McGraw-Hill, 2005, Fig. 108-1.)

KEY FACT

Factors that promote sickling:
- Cold
- Dehydration
- Hypoxia
- Infection
- Stress
- Menses
- Alcohol consumption

DIAGNOSIS

- Diagnosis made by hemoglobin electrophoresis.
- CBC shows normocytic anemia and reticulocytosis.
- Remember to check peripheral smear: Sickle cells, Howell-Jolly bodies, and target cells (see Figure 7.5).
- **Fish-mouth vertebrae** may be seen on L-spine films.

TREATMENT

- **Chronic treatment:**
  - Give pneumococcal vaccine (↑ risk of infection from encapsulated organisms due to functional asplenism).

TABLE 7.6. **Complications of Sickle Cell Disease by Etiology**

ACUTE VASO-OCCLUSIVE COMPLICATIONS	CHRONIC VASO-OCCLUSIVE COMPLICATIONS	CHRONIC HEMOLYTIC ANEMIA COMPLICATIONS
Acute pain crisis.	Retinopathy.	Cholelithiasis.
Acute chest syndrome.	Splenic infarction.	**Aplastic crisis** (precipitated by **parvovirus**
Splenic sequestration.	Avascular necrosis of the femoral or	**B19** infection).
Priapism.	humeral head.	
Stroke.	Chronic renal failure.	
Dactylitis (the most common initial symptom).		
Acute hepatic crisis.		

- Screen for retinopathy annually.
- Supplement folic acid 1 mg PO daily.
- Consider chronic hydroxyurea treatment to ↓ frequency of crises in patients with > 3 crises/year requiring hospitalization; this will ↑ production of hemoglobin F.
- **Acute treatment:**
- Start with hydration, O_2, and analgesia.
- Transfusion for aplastic or hemolytic crises. Consider exchange transfusion for acute vaso-occlusive crises (ie, intractable pain crises, acute chest syndrome, stroke, or recurrent priapism).

COMPLICATIONS

Patients have ↓ life expectancy, with the median age of death in the fifth decade. The most common causes of death include infection and splenic sequestration.

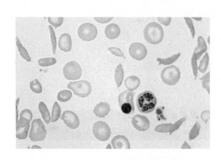

FIGURE 7.5. Sickled red blood cells. The elongated and crescent-shaped RBCs seen on this smear represent circulating irreversibly sickled cells. Target cells and a nucleated red blood cell are also seen. (Reproduced, with permission, from Fauci AS, et al. *Harrison's Principles of Internal Medicine*, 17th ed. New York: McGraw-Hill, 2008, Fig. 99-4.)

Platelet Disorders

THROMBOTIC THROMBOCYTOPENIC PURPURA (TTP)/HEMOLYTIC-UREMIC SYNDROME (HUS)

Platelet aggravation and microthrombi formation in the microvasculature, leading to thrombocytopenia and microangiopathic hemolytic anemia. TTP and HUS are likely 2 variants of the same disease (see Table 7.7), with TTP more strongly associated with CNS involvement and HUS more strongly associated with renal involvement. Both are associated with the following conditions:

- **Pregnancy** and postpartum state.
- **HIV.**
- **Medications: Estrogens,** quinine, ticlopidine, clopidogrel, bleomycin, cisplatin, cyclosporine, tacrolimus.
- **Autoimmune disorders:** SLE, antiphospholipid antibody syndrome (APS), scleroderma.
- **Enterohemorrhagic** *E coli* **(O157:H7).**

KEY FACT

Drugs associated with thrombocytopenia:
- Heparin
- Acetaminophen
- H_2 blockers
- Sulfa drugs
- Furosemide
- Captopril
- Digoxin
- β-lactams
- Gold
- Quinine

TABLE 7.7. TTP vs. HUS

	TTP	HUS
Fever	⊕ in 75% of patients.	Usually ⊖.
Renal insufficiency	Mild/absent in some patients.	⊕ in all patients.
Neurological defects	⊕ in most patients.	⊕ in 50% of patients.
Epidemiology	Mostly in adults.	Mostly in children.
Precipitating factor	Idiopathic (viral illness or familial in some).	Antecedent hemorrhagic enteritis in most patients.

Adapted, with permission, from McPhee SJ, Papadakis MA. *Current Medical Diagnosis and Treatment*, 49th ed. New York: McGraw-Hill, 2010: 485.

SYMPTOMS/EXAM

All of the **5 classic features** are present in only 25% of patients:

- **Microangiopathic hemolytic anemia,** leading to schistocytes, ↑ LDH and T-Bil (see Figure 7.2).
- **Thrombocytopenia,** leading to purpura (see Figure 7.6), petechiae, and/ or bleeding.
- **Fever.**
- **Acute renal insufficiency.**
- **Neurologic abnormalities:** Usually confusion or headache; occasionally seizures, aphasia, or hemiparesis.

DIFFERENTIAL

Other causes of ↓ platelets include DIC, idiopathic thrombocytopenic purpura (ITP), HIV, SLE, heparin-induced thrombocytopenia (HIT), microangiopathies, mechanical destruction, hypersplenism, bone marrow suppression, drug-induced thrombocytopenia, and platelet clumping.

DIAGNOSIS

Made clinically. If the diagnosis is unclear, a renal biopsy may be helpful to rule out other causes of renal failure.

TREATMENT

- Initiate urgent **plasma exchange** to reverse platelet consumption (mortality > 95% if untreated).
- Do not transfuse platelets unless there is life-threatening bleeding and only after plasmapheresis is underway.
- Consider **corticosteroids** for inadequate response to plasmapheresis.
- Consider **splenectomy** for recurrent cases.

COMPLICATIONS

- Survival with plasma exchange: 80% at 6 months.
- High rate of relapse after remission (especially in the first year).

MNEMONIC

Features of TTP:

FAT RN

Fever
Anemia
Thrombocytopenia
Renal insufficiency
Neurologic abnormality

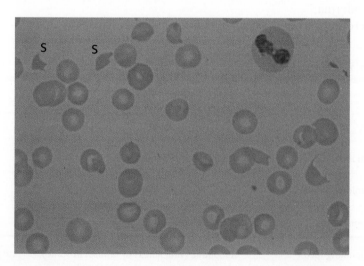

FIGURE 7.6. Thrombotic thrombocytopenic purpura. Note the schistocytes (S) and paucity of platelets. TTP is characterized by microangiopathic hemolytic anemia, thrombocytopenia, fever, neurologic abnormalities, and renal failure. (Courtesy of Dr. Peter McPhedran, Yale Department of Hematology.)

- About 25% of patients develop chronic renal failure.
- Complications of treatment: Local infection, bacteremia, hypotension, and urticaria.

IDIOPATHIC THROMBOCYTOPENIC PURPURA (ITP)

A 27-year-old woman presents complaining of frequent nosebleeds over the past week. She denies any gingival or GI bleeding. Her last period may have been slightly heavier than normal. She has no history of easy bleeding or bruising and denies any family history. On physical exam, you note petechiae over her lower legs bilaterally. There is no splenomegaly. Her platelet count is 9000, but the rest of her CBC is within normal limits. Her peripheral smear shows an isolated thrombocytopenia and occasional megathrombocytes. What is the most likely diagnosis?

In the absence of a history and exam suggesting another alternative, the probable diagnosis is idiopathic thrombocytopenic purpura.

An autoimmune platelet disorder in which antibodies against platelets lead to platelet clearance and decreased platelet production in the bone marrow, resulting in thrombocytopenia. Most commonly affects women < 40 years of age (female-to-male ratio = 3:1). There is an acute form that children can get after a viral infection.

SYMPTOMS/EXAM

Related to bleeding 2° to thrombocytopenia:

- **Petechiae, purpura,** and ecchymoses.
- **Mucosal bleeding** (epistaxis, gingival bleeding, menorrhagia).
- Rarely, GI bleeding and gross hematuria may be seen.

DIAGNOSIS

- Exclude other DDx by history, physical, and tests. This is a diagnosis of exclusion.
- Check CBC with smear: **Isolated thrombocytopenia** and **large platelets.**
- Order ANA to rule out SLE.
- Also consider abdominal ultrasound to rule out sequestration in liver or spleen as cause of low platelets.
- Order tests for hepatitis, CMV, EBV, toxoplasma, and HIV if hepatic or splenic enlargement, lymphadenopathy, or atypical lymphocytes.
- An HIV test should be done in patients with risk factors.
- A bone marrow examination should be done in patients > 60 years of age to rule out myelodysplasia.

TREATMENT

- Acute treatment (for platelets < 20,000–30,000 or if significant bleeding) involves **corticosteroids.**
- **IVIG** if refractory to steroids or for life-threatening bleeding. Platelet transfusions may also be tried for life-threatening bleeding. Also consider Rho (D) immune globulin for Rh+ patients.
  - A **splenectomy** may be necessary for patients with more serious manifestations refractory to treatment.
  - Rituximab can also be considered. Optimal sequence of therapy to try has not been determined.

- Chronic treatment: Danazol, cyclophosphamide, azathioprine, or vincristine/vinblastine for cases that last > 3 months and are refractory to splenectomy.

COMPLICATIONS

Fatalities are rare. Most patients achieve remission with corticosteroids. Cerebral hemorrhage is a rare but the most serious complication.

HEPARIN-INDUCED THROMBOCYTOPENIA (HIT)

Acquired disorder caused by formation of IgG antibodies to heparin-platelet factor 4 (PF4) complexes: IgG antibodies bind to platelets, leading to activation of platelets, which results in thrombocytopenia and a prothrombotic state. Affects 3% of patients on unfractionated heparin and 0.6% of patients on low-molecular-weight heparin (LMWH). Older terminology distinguished between 2 forms of HIT: type 1 (mild, non–immune-mediated, and self-limiting ↓ in platelets) and type 2 (later-onset immune disorder). Currently, the term HIT is used without a modifier to describe the immune-mediated severe form.

SYMPTOMS/EXAM

- New-onset thrombocytopenia within **5–10 days** of exposure to heparin: A ↓ of ≥ 50% from baseline platelet count is regarded as compatible with HIT.
- Lower incidence with the use of LMWH than unfractionated heparin.
- **Venous and arterial thrombosis,** especially DVT, is common.

DIAGNOSIS

Clinically:

- **New-onset** thrombocytopenia of ≥ 50% from the baseline platelet count within 5–10 days of exposure to heparin.
- **Rapid-onset HIT** can occur in patients previously (past 100 days) exposed to heparin who formed heparin-PF4 antibodies within 1–4 days of reexposure.
- **Confirmation:** Clinical diagnosis, supported by ⊕ heparin-PF4 antibody by ELISA, functional assay (serotonin release assay).

TREATMENT

- Immediately **stop all heparin** products, including flushes and LMWH.
- Begin treatment with direct thrombin inhibitor (**lepirudin** or **argatroban**) to prevent possible thrombosis.
- Perform Doppler ultrasound of lower extremities to rule out subclinical thrombosis if indicated.
- Do not start warfarin until the patient is on direct thrombin inhibitor and platelet count > 100,000, as it may transiently worsen hypercoagulability. Continue warfarin for at least 30 days, even after platelet recovery, and for 3 months if documented thrombosis.

Bleeding Disorders

HEMOPHILIA A AND B

X-linked recessive disorder that causes excessive bleeding due to clotting factor deficiencies. Severity depends on the extent of the deficiency.

- Hemophilia A: Factor VIII deficiency.
- Hemophilia B (also called **Christmas disease**): Factor IX deficiency.

MNEMONIC

Hemophilia clotting factor deficiencies:

A8 (factor **VIII**)
B9 (factor **IX**)

SYMPTOMS/EXAM

- Patients typically become symptomatic by 2 years of age.
- Many patients are diagnosed by excessive bleeding following a circumcision.
- Common sites of spontaneous bleeding: Joints (80% of hemorrhage), muscles, and GI tract.
- **Spontaneous hemarthrosis: Stiffness,** warmth, pain, and swelling, often in knees or ankles.
- Excessive bleeding following invasive procedures or injuries may be the initial manifestation in patients with mild or moderate disease.

DIAGNOSIS

- Isolated, reproducibly low factor VIII or factor IX activity level (without other conditions). Severe: < 1%; moderate: 1%–5%; mild: > 5% activity.
- Normal platelet count, normal PT, typically ↑ **APTT** (especially in severe hemophilia), which is **corrected when mixed with normal plasma,** unless an inhibitor is present.
- Many cases are diagnosed on the basis of family history but **one-third of patients have no family history.**

TREATMENT

- Administer purified or recombinant **factor VIII or IX concentrate** during acute bleeding or prophylactically before invasive procedures (or FFP if specific factor concentrate is unavailable). Children with severe disease receive regular, long-term infusions to prevent recurrent joint bleeding.
- Patients with mild hemophilia A may respond to **DDAVP (desmopressin),** which ↑ release of factor VIII from endothelial storage, leading to ↑ circulating factor VIII level.
- **Antifibrinolytic therapy (such as aminocaproic acid)** can be used to stabilize mucosal bleeding and is usually used adjunctively.
- **Chronic treatment:** Avoid high-impact activities or surgical risks for trauma. Screen for hepatitis and HIV. Advise vigilant preventive dental care. The COX-2 selective NSAID celecoxib can be used for joint pain but other NSAIDs and aspirin should be avoided because of the ↑ risk of bleeding.

COMPLICATIONS

- **Hemophiliac arthropathy:** Synovitis and joint destruction, leading to chronic pain and ↓ ROM. Usually avoided in patients who have received long-term prophylaxis with factor concentrate in childhood.
- Blood-borne infections from factor concentrates (hepatitis C and HIV in the 1980s).
- Development of antibodies inhibiting the deficient factor (**inhibitors**), leading to ↓ response to factor concentrates.

VON WILLEBRAND DISEASE (VWD)

A 24-year-old woman comes to your office with a complaint of easy bruising. She had a history of frequent epistaxis as a child that resolved in adolescence. She describes her periods as moderately heavy, and her dentist has told her that she bleeds somewhat more than the typical patient. Her father and aunt have both told her that they have a similar problem with easy bleeding. Initial laboratory work is significant for a slightly ↑ PTT. Her platelet count and INR are normal. What is the most likely diagnosis?

The most common inherited bleeding disorder is von Willebrand disease. The diagnosis can be confirmed by checking plasma von Willebrand factor antigen and factor VIII activity.

The **most common inherited bleeding disorder.** Characterized by ↓ production or activity of von Willebrand factor (vWF), produced by megakaryocytes and endothelial cells. vWF forms a platelet plug and acts as a carrier protein for factor VIII, prolonging the half-life of factor VIII. vWF is the only clotting factor not synthesized by the liver. vWD is usually inherited but may be acquired. There are 3 major types of inherited vWD; the most common type is a quantitative deficiency of vWF that is inherited in an autosomal-dominant pattern, causing mild to moderate disease.

SYMPTOMS/EXAM

- Bleeding patterns similar to those seen in platelet disorders: **Easy bruising, mucosal bleeding,** heavy menses, and excessive bleeding after trauma or dental or surgical procedures.
- **Bleeding following aspirin or NSAID use** is common.

DIAGNOSIS

- **Screening tests:** Variable plasma vWF antigen levels, depending on the type, ↓ plasma vWF activity (ristocetin cofactor activity), ↓ factor VIII activity, ↑ or normal PTT. Bleeding time is rarely performed any more.
- Send vWF multimer analysis and ristocetin-induced platelet aggregation (RIPA) for subtyping of vWD.

TREATMENT

- **Desmopressin (DDAVP)** indirectly ↑ the release of vWF from endothelial storage and can be used prophylactically before invasive procedures or during acute bleeding episodes. The effect is variable, depending on disease type and subtype.
- **vWF replacement therapy** via **recombinant vWF** or **factor VIII concentrates** rich in vWF can be used in patients with more severe disease.

PROGNOSIS

Good. Severe disease is rare and can be managed with replacement therapy.

DISSEMINATED INTRAVASCULAR COAGULATION (DIC)

Consumptive coagulopathy that occurs as a complication of an underlying illness, leading to **bleeding and thrombosis.** Common underlying illnesses include sepsis, transfusion reaction, neoplasia, trauma, and obstetric complications.

SYMPTOMS/EXAM

- **Bleeding:** Petechiae, ecchymoses, oozing from wounds and IV sites, and mucosal bleeding.
- **Thrombosis:** DVT, migratory thrombophlebitis, digital ischemia, renal cortical necrosis.
- **End-organ damage:** Acute renal failure (ARF), hepatic dysfunction, and CNS dysfunction can occur 2° to microthrombi, hypotension, and sepsis.

DIAGNOSIS

- ↑ fibrin split products (FDP), D-dimer, and PT/PTT.
- ↓ fibrinogen, platelets, and hematocrit.
- Don't forget to check the peripheral smear for schistocytes.

TREATMENT

- Correct the underlying disease.
- If no serious bleeding or thrombosis is present or anticipated, then no specific coagulopathy treatment is required.
- **Transfuse platelets** for platelet counts < 20,000 or < 50,000 with serious bleeding.
- Consider **cryoprecipitate** to maintain a fibrinogen concentration > 100 mg/dL.
- Give **activated protein C (APC)** for patients with severe sepsis.
- In patients with thrombotic manifestations, **heparin** can be used to achieve a goal PTT of about 45 seconds.

PROGNOSIS

Prognosis varies widely, depending on the ability to correct the underlying disease.

Clotting Disorders

APPROACH TO THROMBOPHILIA

The differential diagnoses of clotting disorders are outlined in Table 7.8. Consider inherited hypercoagulability in patients with the following:

- Idiopathic venous thrombosis at < 50 years of age.
- Recurrent thrombosis.
- A first-degree relative with idiopathic thromboembolism at < 50 years of age.
- Thrombosis associated with pregnancy or OCPs.
- Thrombosis in an unusual location.

DIAGNOSIS

- Perform **CBC with peripheral smear** to evaluate for myeloproliferative disorders and thrombotic microangiopathies.
- Check **PTT** to screen for antiphospholipid antibody syndrome.
- Order age-appropriate malignancy screening.
- **Screen for inherited hypercoagulability:**
  - **Factor V Leiden** mutation.
  - **Homocysteine level** for hyperhomocysteinemia.
  - **Antiphospholipid antibody tests,** including anticardiolipin antibody test and lupus anticoagulant antibody assays.

TABLE 7.8.   Differential Diagnoses of Clotting Disorders

ARTERIAL AND VENOUS	VENOUS ONLY	ARTERIAL ONLY
Malignancy.	Factor V Leiden.	Atherosclerosis.
HIT syndrome.	Prothrombin 20210 mutation.	Vasculitis.
Hyperhomocysteinemia.	Protein C or S deficiency.	
Paroxysmal nocturnal hemoglobinuria.	Antithrombin III deficiency.	
Myeloproliferative disease.	Hormonal.	
APS.	Postsurgical, pregnancy, immobilization.	

- Prothrombin 20210 mutation for deficiency.
- If an inherited thrombophilia is strongly suspected, include **functional assays for protein C, protein S, and antithrombin III activity** as well. These tests should be done **2 weeks after completion of anticoagulation therapy.**

FACTOR V LEIDEN DEFICIENCY

A mutation in the gene for clotting factor V leads to a gene product called factor V Leiden, which is resistant to cleavage by APC, leading to slower inactivation. It is the most common cause of inherited hypercoagulability in the white population: about 5% among whites. Heterozygotes have a 7-fold ↑ risk of thrombosis, and homozygotes have a 50–80-fold ↑ risk.

SYMPTOMS/EXAM

DVT, PE, cerebral vein thrombosis, and unexplained pregnancy loss.

DIAGNOSIS

Order genotyping for **factor V Leiden mutation.**

TREATMENT

- Avoid smoking and OCPs.
- Anticoagulation after the first thrombotic event:
  - Heterozygotes should be treated like any other patient.
  - Homozygotes should be considered for anticoagulation.

PROGNOSIS

Despite the ↑ risk of thromboembolic events, there is no evidence of ↑ mortality.

ANTIPHOSPHOLIPID ANTIBODY SYNDROME (APS)

Characterized by thrombosis and/or pregnancy morbidity associated with antibodies to plasma proteins that are bound to phospholipids. May be associated with SLE or other rheumatic diseases.

SYMPTOMS/EXAM

- May present with arterial and venous thrombosis, thrombocytopenia, recurrent spontaneous abortions, livedo reticularis, and hemolytic anemia.
- Catastrophic APS presents with widespread thrombotic disease, with multiorgan failure.

DIAGNOSIS

Diagnostic criteria are as follows:

- **Thrombosis OR pregnancy morbidity AND**
- **Anticardiolipin antibody OR lupus anticoagulant** present in serum on 2 or more occasions at least 6 weeks apart.
- Other lab findings include: ↑ PTT (not corrected by mixing the patient's plasma with normal plasma), biological false-⊕ syphilis test.

TREATMENT

- Start anticoagulation with **LMWH,** since **PTT** cannot be used to titrate unfractionated heparin.
- Continue warfarin anticoagulation for a minimum of 6 months after the first thrombotic event. Consider lifelong therapy. Use aspirin if warfarin is discontinued (eg, in pregnancy).
- Continue lifelong anticoagulation with warfarin in patients with recurrent thrombotic events.
- **Goal INR: 2–3.**
- For asymptomatic, nonpregnant, non–aspirin-allergic patients, start **prophylactic aspirin therapy** (81 mg/day), particularly if concomitant SLE or history of miscarriage.

PROGNOSIS

APS is associated with premature death from thromboembolic disease as well as from associated comorbidities.

Transfusion Medicine

A 46-year-old male patient becomes febrile 14 hours after a transfusion of 2 units of packed RBCs. He then develops chills, flank pain, and hypotension. His urine appears brown but is negative for nitrites and leukocyte esterase, and no bacteria are seen. What is the appropriate treatment? This clinical history is consistent with an acute hemolytic transfusion reaction. Aggressive hydration should be initiated to prevent acute tubular necrosis.

BLOOD PRODUCTS

Table 7.9 compares the categories of blood products used in transfusion medicine.

PRETRANSFUSION TESTING

- **Type and cross:** The recipient's blood and the donor's blood are crossmatched (via indirect Coombs test) for reactivity from recipient plasma.
- **Type and screen:** Obtained when transfusion is possible. An indirect Coombs test on a **standardized reference RBC** panel to test for reactivity from recipient plasma.
- Weigh the need for transfusion against the risks:
  - Transfusion reactions (see Table 7.9).
  - **Risk of infection** in decreasing order of risk: **CMV, HBV, HCV,** and **HIV.**

TABLE 7.9. Types of Blood Products

Product and Description	Comments
Whole blood	Provides volume expansion. Used in patients with **acute massive blood loss.**
Packed RBCs	Concentrated. Each unit should ↑ hematocrit by 3%–4%.
Washed RBCs	Removes the small amount of residual plasma from packed RBCs. Used for the following: ■ Patients with a history of severe or recurrent allergic **transfusion reactions.** ■ Patients with IgA deficiency if RBCs from IgA-deficient donors are unavailable. ■ Patients with complement-dependent AIHA.
Irradiated RBCs	Prevents donor T lymphocytes from dividing in the recipient. Used in **immunodeficient or immunosuppressed patients at risk for graft-versus-host disease (GVHD).**
Leukocyte-depleted RBCs	Used because WBCs lead to **HLA** alloimmunization and cytokine release and carry **CMV.** Used for the following: ■ Patients who are **chronically transfused.** ■ Potential **transplant recipients.** ■ Patients with a history of febrile nonhemolytic transfusion reactions. ■ Patients in whom CMV-seronegative components are desirable but not available.
Pooled random donor platelets	Used for the following: ■ Prophylactic transfusion for platelet counts < 20,000. ■ Transfusions for platelet counts < 50,000 in bleeding patients or those undergoing major surgery.
Single-donor platelets	Used in patients refractory to random donor platelets 2° to alloimmunization.
FFP	Contains all coagulation factors. Used for the following: ■ Patients with documented **coagulation factor deficiencies** who are actively bleeding or are scheduled for an invasive procedure. ■ **Reversal of warfarin** anticoagulation if significant bleeding or risk of bleeding is present. ■ Treatment of **TTP.**
Cryoprecipitate	Prepared from plasma and containing fibrinogen, vWF, factor VIII, factor XIII, and fibronectin. Used for the following: ■ Patients with significant **hypofibrinogenemia** (< 100 mg/dL) who are actively bleeding or are scheduled for an invasive procedure. ■ Replacement of factor VIII or vWF when specific factor concentrates are unavailable.

TRANSFUSION REACTIONS

Manage transfusion reactions as follows (see also Table 7.10):

■ Immediately discontinue the transfusion.
■ Alert the blood bank and check for clerical errors.
■ From the **other arm, draw blood** for CBC, direct antiglobulin test, plasma free hemoglobin, LDL, haptoglobin, I-Bil, and PT/PTT. Repeat type and crossmatch and blood culture.
■ Save a **urine sample** for UA and urine hemoglobin.
■ Send all untransfused blood with attached tubing back to the blood bank.

TABLE 7.10. Types of Transfusion Reactions

TYPE	RISK	CLINICAL FEATURES	TREATMENT	CAUSE	COMMENTS
Febrile nonhemolytic reactions	1/100	Fever, chills, mild dyspnea within 6 hours of transfusion.	Antipyretics +/− meperidine.	Antibodies against donor WBCs and cytokine buildup.	The **most common reaction.**

Allergic reactions
  Urticaria
 	
  Anaphylaxis
	1/100	Hives.
		
		Bronchospasm, angioedema, hypotension. Occurs within seconds to minutes.
			Diphenhydramine.
			
			Epinephrine.
				Allergic reaction to plasma proteins.
				Anti-IgA antibodies in **IgA-deficient patients.**	

Delayed hemolytic transfusion reaction	1/1000	Fever, ↓ hematocrit, hyperbilirubinemia, spherocytosis within 2–10 days of transfusion.	Supportive care. Evaluate for new alloantibody and avoid in the future.	An anamnestic response to undetected alloantibodies against minor antigens.	Occurs with re-exposure to an antigen encountered during prior transfusion, transplantation, or pregnancy.
Transfusion-related acute lung injury (TRALI)	1/5000	Noncardiogenic pulmonary edema, ARDS, hypotension, and fever, usually within 6 hours of transfusion.	Supportive care as in ARDS.	Donor antibodies to recipient WBCs in pulmonary capillaries.	Recovery is usually complete within 96 hours.
Acute hemolytic transfusion reaction	1/250,000	Fever, chills, flank pain, red or brown urine, hypotension, and tachycardia within 24 hours of transfusion. DIC if severe.	Vigorous hydration to prevent ATN. Maintain urine output with diuretics, mannitol, or dopamine.	Preformed antibodies against donor RBCs. Usually 2/2 ABO incompatibility.	Usually due to an error.

Myeloproliferative Disorders

POLYCYTHEMIA VERA (PV)

A clonal proliferation of myeloid cells distinguished by ↑ RBC mass.

SYMPTOMS/EXAM

- Symptoms related to ↑ blood volume and ↑ blood viscosity: Headache, dizziness, tinnitus, blurred vision, fatigue.
- Other symptoms include: **Pruritus** (2° to histamine from basophilia), epistaxis (mucosal engorgement and platelet dysfunction), **erythromelalgia** (burning pain in feet or hands, with erythema, pallor, and cyanosis), PUD, **acute gouty arthritis.** Can be associated with venous or arterial thrombosis, including unusual locations such as splenic or mesenteric vein thrombosis, or Budd-Chiari syndrome.
- Exam: **Plethora, engorged retinal vein, splenomegaly, HTN.**

DIFFERENTIAL

- Distinguish PV from reactive erythrocytosis, which can be caused by hypoxia, smoking, COPD, high altitude, sleep apnea, and renal and liver lesions.
- Other myeloproliferative diseases (eg, chronic myelogenous leukemia [↑↑ WBC]), myelofibrosis (abnormal RBC morphology), essential thrombocytosis (↑ platelets only).

DIAGNOSIS

- Must meet both major criteria and 1 minor criterion OR the first major criterion and 2 minor criteria (2008 WHO criteria):
  - **Major criteria:**
    - Hemoglobin > 18.5 g/dL (males) or >16.5 g/dL (females) or other evidence of ↑ RBC volume.
    - **JAK2 mutation** (JAK2V617F or similar mutation): ⊕ in nearly all patients.
  - **Minor criteria:**
    - **Bone marrow biopsy:** Hypercellularity for age with trilineage growth (panmyelosis), with ↑ erythroid, granulocytic, and megakaryocytic proliferation.
    - **↓ serum EPO.**
    - Endogenous erythroid colony formation in vitro.
- Other lab findings include ↑ WBC, ↑ platelets, eosinophilia, iron deficiency, ↑ vitamin B_{12}, ↑ uric acid.

TREATMENT

- Perform **serial phlebotomy** to maintain hematocrit < 45% in males and < 42% in females (avoid Fe supplementation, even if iron deficiency develops).
- Recommend low-Fe diet.
- Give **hydroxyurea** in patients at ↑ risk for thrombosis: > 60 years of age, prior thrombosis, CV risk factors, or platelet count > 1,500,000. (Avoid alkylating agents, as they may ↑ conversion to acute leukemia.)
- Consider **anagrelide** in patients with platelet count > 1,500,000 and refractory to hydroxyurea.
- Give **low-dose daily ASA** in all patients to prevent thrombosis.
- Use **allopurinol** in patients with symptomatic ↑ uric acid or ↑ risk of uric acid calculi (↑ uric acid excretion).

COMPLICATIONS

- Venous or arterial **thrombosis** (due to ↑ viscosity and abnormal platelet function).
- Hemorrhage (due to abnormal platelet function).
- Transformation to **acute myelogenous leukemia/myelodysplastic syndrome** in 5% of cases.
- Transformation to **myelofibrosis/myeloid dysplasia** in 15% of cases. Risk ↑ with disease duration and most commonly occurs after 10 years.

PROGNOSIS

Indolent disease course. The median survival is 10–15 years. The major cause of morbidity and mortality is arterial thrombosis.

MYELOFIBROSIS

A clonal proliferative disorder of myeloid cells that leads to reactive bone marrow fibrosis, causing extramedullary hematopoiesis. Seen in adults > 50 years of age.

SYMPTOMS/EXAM

- **Ineffective erythropoiesis,** leading to cytopenias, causing **fatigue and bleeding.**
- **Extramedullary hematopoiesis** (may occur in any organ):
    - **Massive splenomegaly** leads to abdominal fullness and abdominal pain (splenic infarction) and early satiety.
    - Hepatomegaly leads to abdominal fullness and portal HTN, ascites, esophageal varices.
- Bone pain (especially in the upper legs).
- Transverse myelitis (2° to myelopoiesis in the epidural space).
- Tumor bulk and ↑ cell turnover lead to **constitutional "B" symptoms** (fever, night sweats, and weight loss).

DIAGNOSIS

There are no uniformly accepted criteria, but the 2008 WHO criteria state that patients must meet all 3 major criteria and 2 minor criteria:

- **Major criteria:**
    - Megakaryocyte proliferation and atypia (small to large megakaryocytes with an aberrant nuclear-to-cytoplasmic ratio and hyperchromatic, bulbous, or irregularly folded nuclei and dense clustering), usually with reticulin and/or collagen fibrosis, or if ⊖, significant reticulin fibrosis; the megakaryocyte changes must have ↑ bone marrow cellularity, characterized by granulocytic proliferation and often ↓ erythropoiesis (ie, prefibrotic cellular-phase disease).
    - Not meeting WHO criteria for PV, BCR-ABL1+ chronic myelogenous leukemia, myelodysplastic syndrome, or other myeloid neoplasms.
    - Demonstration of JAK2V617F or other clonal marker (eg, MPLW515L/K), or if ⊖ clonal marker, no evidence that the bone marrow fibrosis or other changes are 2° to infection, autoimmune disorder, or other chronic inflammatory condition; hairy cell leukemia or other lymphoid neoplasm; metastatic malignancy; or toxic (chronic) myelopathies.
- **Minor criteria:**
    - Leukoerythroblastosis (nucleated RBCs and immature WBCs).
    - ↑ serum LDH.
    - Anemia.
    - Splenomegaly.
- Other findings include:
    - Peripheral smears: Poikilocytosis, **teardrop cells,** and giant granulated platelets.
    - Bone marrow aspirate: A **"dry tap."**

TREATMENT

- Treat anemia with androgens, periodic transfusions, and EPO.
- Use thalidomide or lenalidomide +/− steroids.
- Consider splenectomy for symptomatic splenomegaly and anemia requiring frequent transfusions.
- Allogenic hematopoietic stem cell transplantation (HSCT) provides the only potential cure and may be considered for young patients with an appropriate donor available.

PROGNOSIS

- Median survival: 5 years. Three-year survival rate: 50%.
- Transformation into acute myelogenous leukemia < 5%, with a much worse prognosis.
- Common causes of death: Bleeding (2° to thrombocytopenia) and liver failure (2° to liver hematopoiesis and subsequent portal HTN).

ESSENTIAL THROMBOCYTOSIS

Marked proliferation of megakaryocytes in the bone marrow, leading to non-reactive ↑ platelets. Median age 50–60 years.

SYMPTOMS/EXAM

- Often asymptomatic at presentation and diagnosed incidentally.
- May present with thrombosis and hemorrhage.
- Vasomotor symptoms: Headache, lightheadedness, atypical chest pain, acral paresthesia, and erythromelalgia (erythema, warmth, and burning of the hands and feet).
- Palpable splenomegaly may be present on exam.

DIAGNOSIS

Must meet all 4 criteria (2008 WHO criteria):

- Sustained platelet count ≥ 450,000.
- Bone marrow biopsy specimen showing ↑, mainly of the megakaryocytic lineage, with ↑ enlarged, mature megakaryocytes. No significant ↑ or left shift of neutrophil granulopoiesis or erythropoiesis.
- Not meeting WHO criteria for PV, primary myelofibrosis, BCR-ABL1-⊕ chronic myelogenous leukemia, myelodysplastic syndrome, or other myeloid neoplasms.
- ⊕ JAK2V617F or other clonal marker, or if JAK2V617F-⊖, no evidence of reactive thrombocytosis (2° to iron deficiency, splenectomy, surgery, infection, inflammation, connective tissue disease, metastatic cancer, or lymphoproliferative disorders).

TREATMENT

- Patients < 60 years of age with no history of thrombosis or hemorrhage and platelet count < 1,500,000: Follow-up only or treat with low-dose ASA.
- Patients > 60 years of age or those with history of thrombosis: Treat with **hydroxyurea** (preferred) or **anagrelide.**

KEY FACT

Patients with essential thrombocytosis have a normal survival rate.

PROGNOSIS

Survival does not greatly differ from that of the control population. Low rate of transformation.

CHRONIC MYELOGENOUS LEUKEMIA (CML)

A myeloproliferative disorder characterized by proliferation of myeloid cells that are capable of differentiation. Associated with the **Philadelphia chromosome t(9;22)**, producing the **fusion gene** *bcr/abl.* Median age at presentation is 55 years.

The clinical course may be divided into 3 phases, defined by the number of blasts:

- **Chronic phase:** Blasts < 10%.
- **Accelerated phase:** Blasts 10%–20%.
- **Blast phase:** Blasts > 20%.

SYMPTOMS/EXAM

- Approximately **85% of patients present in the chronic phase and are typically asymptomatic.**
- Patients become ↑ symptomatic as they progress through the accelerated and blast phases.
- Common symptoms include fatigue, weight loss, night sweats, LUQ pain, early satiety, and bone pain.
- Hepatosplenomegaly is common.
- Symptoms of leukostasis (blurred vision, respiratory distress, priapism) may be seen in the blast phase.

DIAGNOSIS

- Peripheral smear shows ↑↑ WBC (left shifted) and may show anemia, thrombocytopenia (but could be ↑ before blast phase), basophilia, and eosinophilia.
- As noted above, **the number of blasts seen determines the phase.**
- **Leukocyte alkaline phosphatase is low** (in contrast to other myeloproliferative disorders).
- The **Philadelphia chromosome** is present in **95% of patients** and may be diagnosed via cytogenetics or PCR for the *bcr-abl* gene product.

TREATMENT

- **Allogenic HSCT** is the only curative treatment and should be considered in the **chronic phase** for younger patients who have a suitable donor available.
- **Imatinib mesylate (Gleevec)** is an oral tyrosine kinase inhibitor targeted to the fusion gene product. It may be used for patients in the accelerated or blast phase or for chronic phase patients who are not candidates for HSCT. It is associated with a 95% rate of complete hematologic remission.
- Dasatinib and nilotinib are second-generation inhibitors that compare favorably to Gleevec.
- Interferon-α (IFN-α) plus cytarabine may be tried in patients who do not respond to imatinib, but is associated with greater toxicity and fewer treatment responses.

PROGNOSIS

CML used to have a poor prognosis, with a median survival of 4–6 years. However, with imatinib and other molecular targeted agents, > 80% of patients remain alive and without disease progression at 7 years.

Miscellaneous Hematologic Disorders

MULTIPLE MYELOMA (MM)

A neoplastic clonal proliferation of plasma cells, producing a monoclonal IgG and IgA. Median age is 65 years.

SYMPTOMS/EXAM

- The most common complaints are **bone pain** (especially back or ribs), weakness, fatigue, and weight loss.
- Symptoms of **anemia, hypercalcemia, renal insufficiency, and lytic bone lesions.**
- Symptoms of hyperviscosity: Mucosal bleeding, vertigo, nausea, visual disturbances, altered mental status.
- Neurologic disease may lead to radiculopathy, peripheral neuropathy, cord compression, and CNS involvement (vertebral fracture).
- Amyloidosis, leading to enlarged tongue, neuropathy, CHF, or hepatomegaly.
- ↑ infection.

DIAGNOSIS

- Must meet the following 3 criteria:
  - A **bone marrow aspirate or biopsy with clonal plasma cells ≥ 10%** or the presence of a plasmacytoma (see Figure 7.7).
  - A **monoclonal (M) protein** in serum or urine on electropheresis (need ≥ 3 g/dL in serum or ≥ 300 mg/24 hr in urine of monoclonal protein to define it as MM).
  - Evidence of 2° organ or tissue impairment such as lytic bone lesions, renal insufficiency, anemia, or hypercalcemia.
- **Skeletal survey will identify lytic lesions in the majority of patients** (will not be seen on bone scan, as they are not osteoblastic; see Figure 7.8).

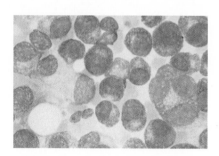

FIGURE 7.7. Multiple myeloma bone marrow aspirate. (Reproduced, with permission, from Fauci AS, et al. *Harrison's Principles of Internal Medicine,* 17th ed. New York: McGraw-Hill, 2008, Fig. 106-2.)

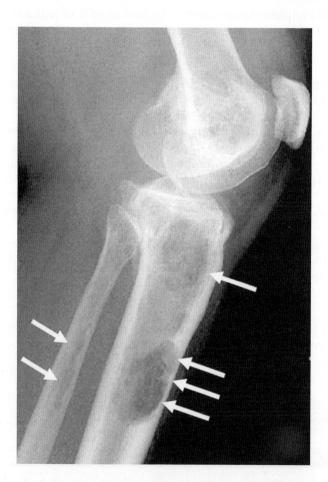

FIGURE 7.8. Typical x-ray appearance of focal lytic lesions resulting from multiple myeloma *(arrows)* **seen in a lateral view of the tibia and fibula.** (Reproduced, with permission, from Lichtman MA, et al. *Williams Hematology,* 8th ed. New York: McGraw-Hill, 2010, Fig. 109-13A.)

- β$_2$-microglobulin usually ↑. Higher values—more advanced staging (poorer prognosis).
- Check β$_2$-microglobulin and albumin levels for staging.
- The presence of M-protein < 3 g/dL, with < 10% clonal plasma cells in the bone marrow, and without organ or tissue impairment seen in MM, is called monoclonal gammopathy of undetermined significance (MGUS). Periodic follow-up is recommended, as MGUS can progress at 1%/year to MM or a related B-cell disorder, such as macroglobulinemia, amyloidosis, or lymphoma.

TREATMENT

No treatment for smoldering multiple myeloma (ie, no end-organ damage). The main options for therapy include:

- Chemotherapy: **Melphalan, Doxil.**
- Immune modulators: **Thalidomide, lenalidomide,** and bortezomib. These agents may be used in combination with standard chemotherapy agents and steroids.
- **Corticosteroids** such as prednisone or dexamethasone.
- **Stem cell (bone marrow) transplantation.**
- Regimens and combinations are chosen based on the risk of the disease and whether bone marrow transplantation is a possibility.
- Prevention and treatment of complications, including:
  - **Hypercalcemia:** Hydration, prednisone, or a bisphosphonate.
  - **Skeletal lesions: Bisphosphonates,** chemotherapy, local radiation, or surgical fixation.
  - **Infection:** Immunization with pneumococcal and influenza vaccines and aggressive treatment of bacterial infections. Consider prophylactic antibiotics and IVIG for recurrent infections.
  - **Renal failure:** Hydration, prednisone, allopurinol, avoidance of NSAIDs and IV contrast, and plasmapheresis for acute failure.
  - **Hyperviscosity syndrome:** Plasmapheresis.
  - **Anemia:** EPO.

PROGNOSIS

Median survival is 4–6 years, depending on the level of tumor burden and the availability of stem cell transplantation. Newer combinations of agents can often show 90+% response rates, so median survival will likely increase dramatically in the near future.

WALDENSTRÖM MACROGLOBULINEMIA

Lymphoplasmacytic lymphoma in the bone marrow and an IgM monoclonal gammopathy in the blood. The median age at diagnosis is 60s. Majority of cases are sporadic, and some (20%) are familial. Etiology is unknown. Symptoms are mainly related to lymphoplasmacytic infiltration and IgM monoclonal gammopathy.

SYMPTOMS/EXAM

- Anemia, leading to fatigue, weakness, pallor.
- Constitutional symptoms such as weakness, fatigue, weight loss, fever, night sweats.
- Lymphadenopathy and/or organomegaly.
- Oronasal and GI bleeding from engorged blood vessels and platelet dysfunction.

- Hyperviscosity in serum, leading to vision change, headache, ataxia, dementia, stroke, or coma.
- Peripheral neuropathy.
- Fundoscopic abnormalities: "Sausage link appearance" of retinal veins seen in 34% of patients.

DIAGNOSIS

- Must meet the following 3 criteria:
  - A bone marrow biopsy sample with > **10% plasmacytic lymphocytes.**
  - An IgM monoclonal gammopathy in the serum (any size).
  - The bone marrow infiltrate shows the typical immunophenotype.
- Other labs include anemia, neutropenia, thrombocytopenia, $\uparrow$ LDH, $\uparrow$ β_2-microglobulin, $\uparrow$ ESR, $\uparrow$ serum viscosity.
- Smear typically shows rouleaux formation.

TREATMENT

- Asymptomatic patients: No treatment is indicated.
- Symptomatic patients: Standard treatment is not established. Treat hyperviscosity with plasmapheresis emergently. For tumors, many experts have incorporated rituximab into the initial treatment, alone or in combination with other chemotherapeutic agents. Hematopoietic cell transplantation is also considered.

PROGNOSIS

Medial survival is approximately 5 years from the time of diagnosis. Poor prognostic factors are older age, cytopenias, and an elevated β_2 microglobulin level.

APLASTIC ANEMIA

Hypoplastic or aplastic bone marrow (with no dysplasia), leading to pancytopenia. Biphasic distribution, with a peak in adolescent and elderly years. May be congenital (rare) or acquired. Etiologies of acquired diseases are as follows:

- **Idiopathic** (**most common** and probably autoimmune).
- Cytotoxic drugs and radiation.
- Idiosyncratic drug reactions to chloramphenicol, NSAIDs, and sulfa drugs.
- **Viral infections:** Parvovirus B19, EBV, HIV.
- **Immune disorders:** SLE, GVHD, thymoma.
- Paroxysmal nocturnal hemoglobinuria.
- Pregnancy.

SYMPTOMS/EXAM

- Anemia, leading to fatigue, weakness, pallor.
- Neutropenia, leading to recurrent infections.
- Thrombocytopenia, leading to mucosal and skin bleeding, purpura, petechiae.
- What should **not** be present: hepatosplenomegaly, lymphadenopathy, or bone tenderness.

DIAGNOSIS

- Labs: **Pancytopenia** and **absolute reticulocytopenia.**
- Bone marrow: **Hypocellular,** with morphologically normal residual hematopoietic precursor cells.

- For severe disease, at least 3 of the following 4 values must be present: Neutrophils < 500; platelets < 20,000, reticulocytes < 1%, and bone marrow cellularity < 20%.

TREATMENT

- Mild: Supportive care (RBC and platelet transfusions as needed).
- Hematopoietic cell (bone marrow) transplantation is the only definitive therapy (for children and young patients).
- Immunosuppression with antithymocyte globulin (ATG), cyclosporine, or prednisone for patients > 50 years of age or those without HLA-matched donors.

PROGNOSIS

Prognosis depends on the severity of the pancytopenia and the patient's age. In severe forms, the median survival without treatment is 3 months, and 1-year survival is 20%. If treated, the 5-year survival rate is 20%–80%.

Acute Leukemia

Neoplastic disorders characterized by proliferation of immature hematopoietic precursor cells in the bone marrow and later in the peripheral blood and other organs and tissues. If untreated, death usually occurs within 6 months of diagnosis. ↑ **risk** is associated with the following:

- **Congenital disorders:** Down syndrome, Bloom syndrome, Fanconi anemia, ataxia-telangiectasia.
- **Acquired disorders:** Myeloproliferative disorders, myelodysplastic syndromes, aplastic anemia.
- **Environmental exposure:** Alkylating agents, radiation, cigarette smoke, benzene, organic solvents.

SYMPTOMS/EXAM

Common presenting symptoms are 2° to anemia, thrombocytopenia, and neutropenia: Fatigue, fever, easy bruising and purpura/petechiae, and infection.

DIAGNOSIS

- **Peripheral smear:** ↑ circulating blasts (90% of patients), anemia, and thrombocytopenia.
- **Bone marrow:** ↑ blasts (> 20%).
- Immunohistochemistry, cytogenetics, and flow cytometry should also be done to aid in diagnosis, classification, and risk stratification.
- An **LP** on all patients with acute lymphocyte leukemia and any acute myelogenous leukemia patients with **CNS symptoms.**

ACUTE LYMPHOCYTIC LEUKEMIA (ALL)

Seen predominantly in children (the most common cancer in children). Bimodal distribution, with peaks at 3–7 years and 65 years of age. Classified as follows:

- Clonal cells may be B cells (75%) or T cells.
- Test patients with T-cell ALL for **HTLV-1.**
- **Burkitt leukemia:** Subtype of ALL with ↑ B cells. **t(8;14) translocation** is universally seen, leading to aberrant expression of the **c-myc oncogene.**

SYMPTOMS/EXAM

Findings that are more common in ALL than in acute myelogenous leukemia (AML) include the following:

- **Bone pain.**
- **Lymphadenopathy:** Occurs in > 50% of patients with ALL.
- **Hepatosplenomegaly:** Occurs in 66% of patients with ALL.
- CNS involvement.

TREATMENT

- Remission induction with combination chemotherapy to prevent resistance.
- **CNS prophylaxis** with **intrathecal chemotherapy** for all patients to prevent CNS relapse.
- Prolonged **postremission therapy** (1–3 years) to eliminate residual disease.

COMPLICATIONS

- Long-term disease-free survival rate: **30% for adults, 66%–85% for children.**
- Common sites of **solitary relapse (sanctuary sites): CNS and testes** (2° to poor penetration of chemotherapy).

ACUTE MYELOGENOUS LEUKEMIA (AML)

Represents 80% of all acute leukemia cases in adults. Most patients are > 65 years of age, and the incidence ↑ with age.

SYMPTOMS/EXAM

Findings that are more common in AML than in ALL include the following:

- **Leukostasis:** Sludging of blasts in the microvasculature, which occurs when the blast count in the peripheral blood > 100,000/mm³. Commonly leads to CNS symptoms (**somnolence, seizure, stroke**) and pulmonary symptoms (**dyspnea**).
- **DIC:** Commonly associated with the promyelocytic subtype.
- **Leukemia cutis:** Violaceous raised lesions of the skin 2° to infiltration of leukemic cells; associated with monocytic subtypes.

DIAGNOSIS

Auer rods are pathognomonic for AML (see Figure 7.9).

TREATMENT

- **Induction chemotherapy** with anthracycline (daunorubicin or idarubicin) + **cytarabine.**
- **Postremission therapy** options include the following:
  - **Consolidation chemotherapy.**
  - **Allogenic or autologous HSCT** may be considered, especially for patients with poor-risk cytogenetics or those who fail to achieve a complete remission or who relapse.

PROGNOSIS

Although approximately 60%–80% of patients (< 60 years of age) achieve complete remission, the overall 5-year survival rate is 10%–35%. The cure rate for older patients is very low (10%–15%).

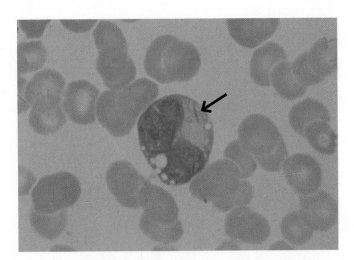

FIGURE 7.9. **Auer rod in acute myelocytic leukemia.** The red rod-shaped structure (*arrow*) in the cytoplasm of the myeloblast is pathognomonic. (Courtesy of Dr. Peter McPhedran, Yale Department of Hematology.)

ACUTE PROMYELOCYTIC LEUKEMIA (AML-M3 OR APL)

- Associated with t(15;17) translocation and fusion gene PML-RARα (retinoic acid receptor-α).
- Commonly associated with DIC.
- Anthracycline + *all*-trans retinoic acid induces complete remission in 90% of patients with APL.
- For high-risk patients, the addition of arsenic trioxide may be beneficial.

Chronic Leukemia

CHRONIC LYMPHOCYTIC LEUKEMIA (CLL)

A monoclonal proliferation of immunologically **incompetent mature B cells.** CLL is the **most common adult leukemia** in the Western world, representing 30% of all cases of leukemia. The median age of onset is 65 years.

SYMPTOMS/EXAM

- CLL is an **indolent** disease.
- Many patients are **asymptomatic at diagnosis.**
- Presenting symptoms include fever, night sweats, weight loss, fatigue, and weakness.
- **Generalized lymphadenopathy** and **hepatosplenomegaly** are common.
- Note ↑ incidence of autoimmune diseases, including AIHA, autoimmune thrombocytopenia, and pure red cell aplasia.

DIAGNOSIS

- **Peripheral smear shows isolated lymphocytosis.** Lymphocytes appear small and mature and are **monoclonal on flow cytometry.**
- **Smudge cells** are common on peripheral smear and occur when fragile malignant lymphocytes are disrupted during preparation of the smear (see Figure 7.10).

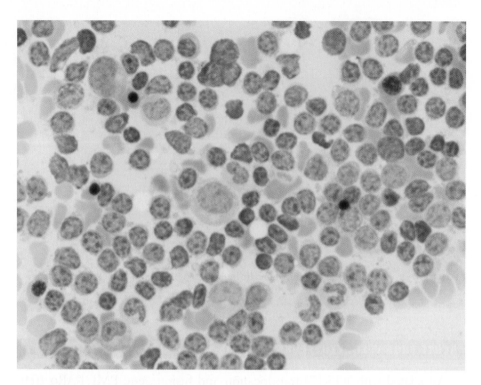

FIGURE 7.10. **Chronic lymphocytic leukemia.** The numerous small, mature lymphocytes and smudge cells are characteristic.

- Rai classification separates CLL into low-, intermediate-, and high-risk categories, which correspond with stages 0, I and II, and III and IV, respectively, depending on the presence of lymphadenopathy, organomegaly, anemia, or thrombocytopenia, in addition to lymphocytosis.

TREATMENT

- **Treatment is palliative.**
- Asymptomatic patients may be followed without treatment.
- **Alkylating agents** (chlorambucil or fludarabine) are the mainstay of therapy for symptomatic patients and those with rapidly progressive disease or complications.
- **Monoclonal antibodies** such as rituximab and alemtuzumab are options.
- Use **corticosteroids** for treatment of AIHA or autoimmune thrombocytopenia.
- **Radiation therapy** for large, bulky lymphoid masses.
- Nonmyeloablative **allogeneic bone marrow transplant** is being studied as an option.

PROGNOSIS

New therapies are changing the prognosis of CLL. The early-stage disease has a median survival of 10–15 years. For more advanced diseases, the 2-year survival has improved to > 90%.

CHRONIC MYELOGENOUS LEUKEMIA (CML)

CML is discussed as one of the myeloproliferative disorders.

MYELODYSPLASTIC SYNDROMES (MDS)

A group of malignant stem cell disorders characterized by cytopenia, dysplastic changes in the marrow, morphologic and cytogenetic abnormalities, and a variable risk of transformation to acute leukemia. The risk of developing MDS increases with age, with the median age > 65 years. MDS should be considered in any patient, particularly the elderly patient, with unexplained cytopenia(s) or monocytosis.

SYMPTOMS/EXAM

Signs and symptoms of MDS are nonspecific, and many patients are asymptomatic. Common presentations when patients are symptomatic include the following:

- Symptoms of anemia, including fatigue, weakness, dizziness, angina.
- Infection, easy bruising, or bleeding is less commonly seen.
- Fever, night sweats, and weight loss are uncommon.
- Pallor from anemia, petechia, and/or purpura are relatively common.

DIAGNOSIS

- Perform peripheral blood smear and bone marrow aspiration to define the subtypes. Many subtypes exist, including refractory anemia, refractory anemia with ringed sideroblasts, refractory anemia with excess blasts, chronic myelomonocytic anemia, and refractory anemia with excess blasts in transformation.
- Common findings include macrocytic red cells, reduced reticulocyte percentage, reduced neutrophil lobulation, and pancytopenia.
- Check vitamin B_{12} and folate levels to rule out megaloblastic anemia, which can show similar morphologic abnormalities of blood cells.

TREATMENT

- Due to the advanced age and comorbidities of most patients, supportive care is the mainstay of treatment, including antibiotics for infections, transfusion, and hematopoietic growth factors.
- Depending on the subtypes of MDS, patient age, functional status and prognostic scores, hematopoietic growth factors (EPO, G-CSF), immunosuppressive agents (antithymocyte globuline, cyclosporine), or other chemotherapeutic agents such as lenalidomide, cytarabine, or azacitidine may be used. Hematopoietic stem cell transplantation may also be considered. The 5q– subtype of MDS is particularly responsive to lenalidomide (Revlimid).

PROGNOSIS

The risk of transformation to AML depends on the percentage of blasts in the bone marrow. Survival could range from < 1 year to many years. Infection, transfusion refractoriness, and transformation to acute leukemia are common reasons for death.

Lymphoma

HODGKIN LYMPHOMA

A clonal **B-cell** malignancy in which **Reed-Sternberg cells** are the malignant cells. Bimodal age distribution, with peaks among patients in their 20s and in those > 50 years of age.

SYMPTOMS/EXAM

Common presentations include the following:

- A painless, enlarged, rubbery lymph node (70% of patients).
- A mediastinal mass on CXR, with possible retrosternal chest pain, cough, or shortness of breath.
- **B symptoms:** Fever, night sweats, and weight loss.
- Hepatosplenomegaly and pruritus are common.
- Pain in the affected lymph node after EtOH consumption is uncommon but suggestive.

DIAGNOSIS

- Perform **excisional lymph node biopsy** for definitive diagnosis (see Figure 7.11).
- Staging studies include CXR and CT of the chest, abdomen, and pelvis.
- Labs that may affect choice of therapy or staging include CBC with differential, ESR, LFTs, albumin, LDH, and calcium.
- Bone marrow biopsy.

TREATMENT

- Treat with irradiation and/or ABVD (Adriamycin, bleomycin, vincristine, dacarbazine), depending on the stage and on whether bulky mediastinal disease is present.
- Treat relapsed disease with conventional chemotherapy or high-dose chemotherapy plus autologous HSCT.

PROGNOSIS

The 10-year survival rate of patients with stage IA or IIA disease treated by radiotherapy is > 80%. Patients with disseminated disease (stage IIB, IV) have 5-year survival rates of 50%–60%.

NON-HODGKIN LYMPHOMA

Heterogeneous cancers of B and T cells. A number of different classification systems exist for lymphoma. The **WHO classification,** published in 2001 and updated in 2008, is the latest classification of lymphoma (see Table 7.11). This system attempts to group lymphomas by cell type (ie, the normal cell type that most resembles the tumor), defining phenotype, and molecular or cytogenetic characteristics.

Some major examples with the typical disease course are:

- **Indolent:** Typically not curable, but even if left untreated, survival is measured in years. Patients may have prolonged survival, even with partial treatment response.

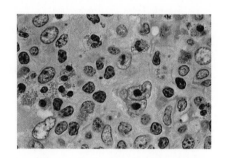

FIGURE 7.11.   Hodgkin lymphoma.
A Reed-Sternberg cell—a large cell with a bilobed nucleus and prominent nucleoli, giving an "owl's eye" appearance—can be seen near the center of the image. (Reproduced, with permission, from Fauci AS, et al. *Harrison's Principles of Internal Medicine,* 17th ed. New York: McGraw-Hill, 2008, Fig. 105-11.)

- **Follicular lymphoma:** Patients are typically middle-aged or older and present with painless peripheral lymphadenopathy.
- **Mucosa-associated lymphoid tissue (MALT) lymphoma:** A form of marginal zone lymphoma. Gastric tumors have been linked to *H pylori* infection, and the majority of patients regress with antimicrobial therapy. Patients with gastric tumors may present with PUD or abdominal pain.
- **Aggressive:** Typically curable, but survival is measured in months if untreated.
  - **Diffuse large B-cell lymphoma:** Patients are typically middle-aged or older and often present with a rapidly enlarging neck or abdominal mass.
- **Highly aggressive:** Typically curable, but survival is measured in weeks if untreated. There is a high risk of tumor lysis syndrome.
  - **Burkitt lymphoma:** Exists in endemic, sporadic, and immunodeficiency-related forms. It is endemic in Africa, with up to 90% of cases related to EBV infection; presents as a tumor of the jaw or facial bone. Of sporadic cases, only about 20% are related to EBV infection. Typically presents as bulky abdominal disease.

SYMPTOMS/EXAM

- B symptoms, including fever, weight loss, and sweats.
- Systemic lymphadenopathy is seen +/– hepatosplenomegaly.

DIAGNOSIS

- **Excisional lymph node biopsy** is preferable for definitive diagnosis and staging.
- Staging studies include CXR, CT of the chest/abdomen/pelvis, and bone marrow biopsy.
- Labs that may affect choice of therapy or staging include **LDH**, CBC with differential, peripheral smear, LFTs, chem 10, and serum protein electrophoresis.

TREATMENT

- **Indolent:** Treatment is aimed at alleviation of symptoms.
  - Early, asymptomatic disease may be observed or treated with locoregional or extended-field radiation therapy.
  - Options for more advanced disease include single-agent chemotherapy with chlorambucil, cyclophosphamide, or fludarabine; combination chemotherapy with CVP (cyclophosphamide, vincristine, and prednisone).
  - Monoclonal antibody therapy with rituximab used for B-cell lymphomas.
  - Radioimmunotherapy with yttrium-90 ibritumomab tiuxetan (Zevalin) or iodine 131 tositumomab (Bexxar) may also have a role in treatment.
- **Aggressive:** Treatment is aimed at cure.
  - Treat early disease with CHOP (cyclophosphamide, doxorubicin, vincristine, and prednisone), possibly followed by involved-field radiation.
  - Treat advanced disease with CHOP or a CHOP-like regimen.
  - Rituximab is used for aggressive B-cell lymphomas.
- **Highly aggressive:** May benefit from autologous HSCT early in the course.
- **Special forms of lymphoma:**
  - Burkitt lymphoma, lymphoblastic lymphoma: Require specific regimen tailored to each type.

TABLE 7.11. WHO-Proposed Classification of Non-Hodgkin Lymphoma

Precursor B
  B-cell lymphoblastic lymphoma
Mature B
  Diffuse large B-cell lymphoma
  Mediastinal large B-cell lymphoma
  Follicular lymphoma
  Small lymphocytic lymphoma
  Lymphoplasmacytic lymphoma
  Mantle cell lymphoma
  Burkitt lymphoma
  Marginal zone lymphoma
    MALT type
    Nodal
    Splenic
  Mucosal tissue associated
Precursor T
  T-cell lymphoblastic lymphoma
Mature T (and NK cell)
  Anaplastic T-cell lymphoma
  Peripheral T-cell lymphoma

KEY FACT

Burkitt lymphoma and Burkitt leukemia are considered manifestations of the same disease.

- Mantle cell lymphoma: Intensive initial chemotherapy, including autologous HSCT or reduced-intensity allogeneic HSCT.
- MALT lymphoma: Eradicate *H pylori* with antibiotics.

PROGNOSIS

The median survival with indolent lymphomas has been 6–8 years. Factors for poor prognosis are age > 60 years, ↑ serum LDH, stage III or IV disease, and poor performance status.

Brain Tumors

1° BRAIN TUMORS

Classified by predominant cell type:

- **Meningiomas:** Arise from cells in the arachnoid membrane. The vast majority are benign, but morbidity is caused by their mass effect (see Figure 7.12A).
- **Gliomas:** Tumors derived from glial cells—the most common 1° brain tumor (50%). Classified according to grade (glioblastomas are the highest/worst; see Figure 7.12B). Various genetic syndromes may lead to a predisposition to these tumors, including tuberous sclerosis, neurofibromatosis 1, and Li-Fraumeni syndrome.
- **Medulloblastomas:** Embryonal tumors, most often seen in children.

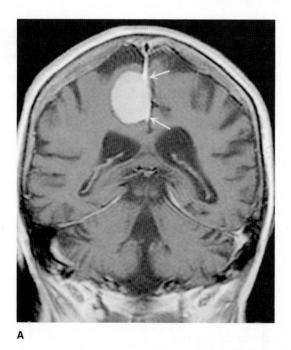
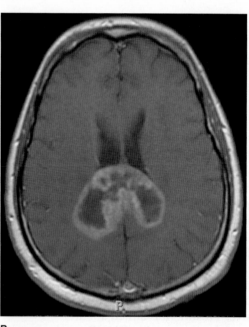

A B

FIGURE 7.12. **Meningioma (A) and glioblastoma multiforme (B).** (A) Coronal postcontrast T1-weighted MRI demonstrates an enhancing extra-axial mass arising from the falx cerebri *(arrows)*. (B) Transaxial contrast-enhanced image shows an enhancing intra-axial mass with central necrosis crossing the corpus callosum ("butterfly glioma"). (Image A reproduced, with permission, from Fauci AS, et al. *Harrison's Principles of Internal Medicine,* 17th ed. New York: McGraw-Hill, 2008, Fig. 374-5. Image B reproduced, with permission, from USMLERx.com.)

SYMPTOMS/EXAM

- Present with headaches, seizures, nausea and vomiting, syncope, disturbance in memory or mood, personality changes, muscle weakness, sensory deficits, and aphasia.
- Headache suggestive of a possible brain tumor: A change in a prior headache pattern, an abnormal neurologic exam, positional changes, and associated nausea and vomiting.

DIAGNOSIS

- **MRI** (preferred) or CT (diagnostic for meningioma), both +/– contrast.
- Tissue biopsy for histologic confirmation is often obtained at the time of resection or may be done via stereotactic biopsy in cases where resection will not improve survival.

TREATMENT

- Choose treatment depending on the type and location of the tumor and the condition of the patient.
- Treat malignant gliomas with maximal surgical resection and adjuvant radiation therapy and chemotherapy. Chemotherapeutic agents include temozolomide and the PCV regimen (procarbazine, CCNU, and vincristine). There is also an emerging role for targeted agents such as bevacizumab.
- Monitor asymptomatic meningiomas with serial neuroimaging every 3–6 months. If symptomatic, expanding, infiltrative, or associated with significant surrounding edema, resect the lesion. Adjuvant radiation therapy may be offered for patients with high-grade lesions or incomplete resection.
- Stereotactic radiosurgery may be used instead of surgical excision for small tumors in sites where complete excision is difficult.
- Give corticosteroids for cerebral edema before surgery. Treat hernia with dexamethasone and IV mannitol. Give anticonvulsants for seizures. Place shunting for obstructive hydrocephalus.

BRAIN METASTASES

Represent > **50% of intracranial tumors** in adults. Approximately 10%–15% of patients with solid tumors develop brain metastases.

SYMPTOMS/EXAM

Same as 1° brain tumors.

DIAGNOSIS

- Check **MRI and CT** (+/– **contrast**) with characteristic findings suggesting metastasis, including multiple lesions, circumscribed margins, vasogenic edema out of proportion to the size of the lesion, and location at the gray-white matter junction.
- Perform brain biopsy if the diagnosis is in doubt.
- Perform LP for patients with suspected carcinomatous meningitis.
- Order **CXR** to look for pulmonary metastasis or to establish a 1° site if it is unknown. About 60% of patients with brain metastases have either a lung 1° or pulmonary metastases from their 1° tumor.
- Don't forget mammography in women if 1° unknown.

MNEMONIC

Tumors that commonly metastasize to the brain:

"Pounds (LBS) Kilos (K)"

Lung
Breast
Skin (melanoma)
Kidney

TREATMENT/PROGNOSIS

- Patients with a **favorable prognosis** include those < 65 years of age with a high performance status, a controlled 1° tumor, and no extracranial metastases. Median survival is about 7 months. Aggressive treatment with **surgical resection or stereotactic radiosurgery** followed by **whole-brain radiation therapy** may be recommended.
- Patients with a **poor prognosis** have a poor performance status and a median survival of about 2 months. The following treatments are recommended:
    - Whole brain radiation therapy to improve neurologic deficits and prevent further neurologic deterioration.
    - Corticosteroids to control symptoms related to edema.

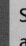

Squamous Cell Carcinoma (SCC) of the Head and Neck

Most commonly associated with tobacco and alcohol use. Other risk factors include radiation, occupational exposures, and chronic viral infection with EBV, HPV, HSV, or HIV.

SYMPTOMS/EXAM

- Neck mass.
- Ulcers or exophytic lesions in the nose, lips, mouth, or throat.
- Nasal obstruction, hoarseness, dysphagia, odynophagia, cervical lymphadenopathy, globus sensation, otalgia.

DIAGNOSIS

- Physical exam: Make sure to include bimanual examination of the tongue and the floor of the mouth and palpation of the neck.
- Panendoscopy: Perform laryngoscopy, bronchoscopy, and esophagoscopy to visualize the extent of tumor involvement.
- Check CT or MRI to determine the size/extent and location of lesions and nodes.
- Perform fine-needle biopsy of suspicious neck nodes (or of the visible tumors when scoped).

TREATMENT

Determine treatment by the resectability of the lesion and the extent of advancement. Treat early lesions with radiotherapy or surgery alone and more advanced lesions with concomitant chemotherapy.

NASOPHARYNGEAL CARCINOMA

- Cancer of the nasopharynx—SCC is the most common.
- Rare in the West and associated with tobacco and alcohol, as with other SCCs of the head and neck. Endemic in southern China and associated with EBV, genetic predisposition, and dietary factors such as nitrates, salted fish, and Chinese herbs. There are endemic areas in Southeast Asia and the Mediterranean as well.
- **Sx/Exam:** Neck mass, nasal obstruction, epistaxis, and otitis media.
- **Dx:** Same as for other SCCs of the head and neck; possible role for PET scan in staging. ↑ IgA to EBV.

- **Tx:** Concomitant chemoradiation with cisplatin and fluorouracil is commonly used. Selected cases of locally recurrent nasopharyngeal may be treated with repeat irradiation or surgery. Other SCCs are treated with a combination of surgery (when resectable) and irradiation.

Genitourinary Cancers

BLADDER CANCER

Second most common GU cancer. Affects men more than women. Mean age at diagnosis: 65 years. Risk factors for bladder cancer include cigarette smoking (60%), exposure to industrial dyes or solvents (15%), arsenic exposure, chronic cystitis, schistosomiasis, radiation, and cyclophosphamide use. In order of prevalence: urothelial cell carcinoma (90%), SCC (7%), and adenocarcinoma (2%).

SYMPTOMS/EXAM

- **Hematuria** is the most common presenting symptom (85%–90%).
- Irritative or obstructive voiding symptoms may be seen.
- Flank pain, suprapubic pain, hypogastric pain, and perineal pain may all result from invasive or metastatic disease.

DIAGNOSIS

- Assume hematuria in a patient > 40 years of age is urothelial cancer until proven otherwise and investigate with **cystourethroscopy, urine cytology,** and **CT with urography** or **IVP with renal ultrasound!**
- A CXR and bone scan may be used for screening patients with documented bladder cancer who are at high risk for metastasis.

TREATMENT

- **Superficial bladder cancer** (superficial to the muscularis propria):
  - Cystoscopic resection of visible tumor (**transurethral resection of the bladder tumor [TURBT]**).
  - If the superficial cancer is high risk based on histology, number of lesions or recurrences, or failure to completely resect, then intravesical therapy with BCG (live attenuated *Mycobacterium bovis*) or other chemotherapeutic agents is recommended.
  - Aggressive posttreatment surveillance with urine cytology and cystoscopy is recommended.
- **Invasive bladder cancer:**
  - **Radical cystectomy** with bilateral pelvic lymph node dissection.
  - **Neoadjuvant or adjuvant chemotherapy** is superior to radical cystectomy alone:
    - Gemcitabine plus cisplatin.
    - MVAC (methotrexate, vinblastine, doxorubicin, and cisplatin).

RENAL CELL CARCINOMA (RCC)

Risk factors include smoking, obesity, hypertension, and end-stage renal disease. Hereditary clear cell renal carcinoma is associated with von Hippel–Lindau syndrome and the von Hippel–Lindau gene mutation on chromosome 3.

SYMPTOMS/EXAM

- Remember: The classic triad—**flank pain, hematuria,** and a **palpable abdominal mass**—is found in only 10%–15% of patients.
- Increasingly diagnosed in asymptomatic patients during incidental abdominal imaging.

DIAGNOSIS

- Abdominal ultrasound is useful for distinguishing a benign cyst from a complex cyst or tumor.
- CT of the abdomen will show a multilocular mass, with thickened, irregular walls and septae, enhanced with contrast (see Figure 7.13).
- Percutaneous biopsy is occasionally used.

TREATMENT

- Patients with disease limited to the kidney (stages I and II) should undergo partial or radical (preferred if the condition allows) nephrectomy.
- Patients with limited invasion (stage III) should undergo radical nephrectomy; those with extensive invasion or metastasis (stage IV) may have palliative nephrectomy.

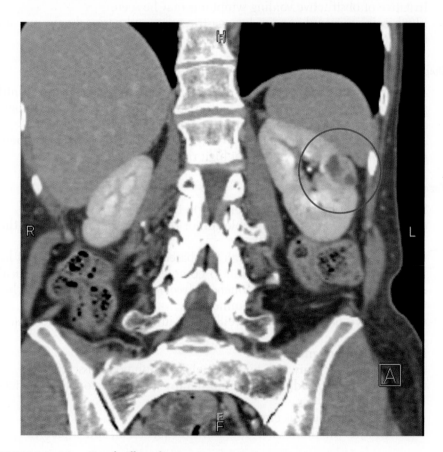

FIGURE 7.13. Renal cell carcinoma. (Reproduced, with permission, from USMLERx.com.)

- No chemotherapeutic regimen has been consistently shown to be effective in metastatic RCC.
- **Immunotherapy with IFN-α or interleukin-2** has been shown to induce an immune response against tumor cells and can be considered for metastatic RCC.
- Multikinase inhibitors such as **sorafenib** (Nexavar), a small-molecule Raf kinase and vascular endothelial growth factor (VEGF) multireceptor kinase inhibitor, and **sunitinib** (Sutent), have recently been approved by the FDA for the treatment of patients with advanced RCC and the treatment of metastatic kidney cancer that has progressed after a trial of immunotherapy, respectively.
- Many other targeted agents may benefit, including bevacizumab and others in clinical trials.

COMPLICATIONS

Fever, erythrocytosis, hypercalcemia, anemia, hepatopathy, and amyloidosis are all paraneoplastic syndromes associated with RCC.

KEY FACT

Risk factors for bladder cancer: chemicals, cigarette smoking, arsenic, chronic cystitis, schistosomiasis, radiation, cyclophosphamide.

KEY FACT

Workers in these industries are at ↑ risk: aluminum, dye, paint, petroleum, rubber, textiles.

Carcinoma of Unknown Primary

A term used when patients present with a metastatic site and initial evaluation fails to identify a 1° tumor. Represents 2%–5% of all cancer diagnoses. Classified in 1 of 5 histologic categories, based on light microscopy of biopsied tissue:

- Adenocarcinoma.
- SCC.
- Neuroendocrine carcinoma.
- Poorly differentiated carcinoma.
- Poorly differentiated neoplasm (the pathologist cannot differentiate between carcinoma and other cancers).

EXAM/DIAGNOSIS

- Begin with a complete history and physical (including genital and rectal exams).
- Include a CBC and UA in the initial lab.
- Include a CXR and CT of the chest, abdomen, and pelvis in the initial imaging.
- Biopsy with pathologic evaluation guides further studies. Examples:
  - Poorly differentiated carcinoma: HCG, AFP.
  - Adenocarcinoma: PSA, mammography, endoscopy.
  - SCC of cervical nodes: CT of the head and neck, laryngoscopy, nasopharyngoscopy, PET scan.

TREATMENT

Table 7.12 outlines the treatment options for carcinoma of unknown primary.

TABLE 7.12. **Empiric Treatment for Carcinoma of Unknown Primary**

PATIENTS WITH:	TREAT AS:
SCC in cervical lymph nodes.	Advanced head and neck cancer.
SCC in inguinal nodes.	Do a careful exam of the anal canal and genitalia and consider lymphadenectomy and postoperative radiation +/− chemotherapy.
Women with peritoneal carcinomatosis.	Advanced ovarian cancer.
Women with adenocarcinoma in axillary lymph nodes.	Stage II breast cancer.
Men with bone metastases or an ↑ PSA.	Advanced prostate cancer.
Young men with poorly differentiated carcinoma and a midline tumor.	Extragonadal germ cell tumor.
Poorly differentiated carcinoma.	Treat with empiric platinum/paclitaxel.
Poorly differentiated neuroendocrine carcinoma.	Treat with empiric platinum/etoposide +/− paclitaxel.

Chemotherapeutic Agents

Chemotherapeutic agents interfere with the cell cycle. They are divided into 2 categories based on kinetics:

- Cell-cycle-specific (CCS) drugs: Act specifically on cells that are cycling and are usually most active in one specific phase of the cycle.
- Cell-cycle-nonspecific (CCNS) drugs: Act on cells whether they are cycling or resting.

CLASSES OF CHEMOTHERAPEUTIC AGENTS

Drug classes are as follows:

- **Alkylating agents:** CCNS agents that alkylate nucleic acid bases, thus causing cross-linking, abnormal pairing, and breakage of DNA/RNA strands. Busulfan, chlorambucil, cyclophosphamide, ifosfamide, cisplatin, carboplatin.
- **Antimetabolites:** CCS agents that act primarily in the S phase of the cell cycle. They antagonize folate or nucleic acid bases, thus interfering with DNA/RNA synthesis. Methotrexate, mercaptopurine, thioguanine, cytarabine, fluorouracil, fludarabine, cytarabine, cladribine, gemcitabine, hydroxyurea.
- **Plant alkaloids:** CCS agents that are naturally occurring nitrogenous bases. Many act by inhibiting the mitotic spindle. Vinblastine, vincristine, etoposide, paclitaxel.
- **Antibiotics:** CCNS agents that intercalate adjacent nucleotides, thus causing DNA strand breaks. Doxorubicin, daunorubicin, bleomycin, mitomycin.
- **Hormonal agents:** Not directly cytotoxic, but they downregulate hormonally stimulated growth. Tamoxifen, Arimidex, letrozole, exemustane, leuprolide, goserelin, fulvestrant.
- **Immunotherapeutic agents:** Rituximab and other similar agents, IFN-α.

TOXICITIES

Selected toxicities of chemotherapeutic agents include the following:

- **Cardiomyopathy:** Doxorubicin, daunorubicin.
- **Pulmonary fibrosis:** Bleomycin.
- **Hemorrhagic cystitis:** Alkylating agents, especially cyclophosphamide and ifosfamide.
- **Peripheral neuropathy:** Paclitaxel, vincristine, vinblastine.

Acute Complications of Cancer Therapy

TUMOR LYSIS SYNDROME (TLS)

A syndrome of metabolic disarray that results from rapid lysis of cancer cells. Typically induced by chemotherapy or radiation, but may rarely be caused by spontaneous necrosis. Most commonly associated with poorly differentiated lymphomas (eg, Burkitt lymphoma) and with leukemias, especially ALL. Rare in solid tumors.

DIAGNOSIS

- Suspect the diagnosis in at-risk patients who develop ARF, ↑ uric acid, ↑ phosphate, and/or ↑ potassium.
- Laboratory diagnosis may be based on 2 of the following: 25% ↑ from baseline in uric acid, potassium, or phosphate; or 25% ↓ from baseline in calcium.

TREATMENT

- Pretreat patients at high risk for TLS before (as well as during and after) chemotherapy or radiation with allopurinol and fluids to maintain urine output > 2–3 L/day.
- Treatment includes management of electrolyte abnormalities, aggressive hydration, and diuretics to ↑ urine output.
- Hemodialysis may be needed for hyperkalemia, hyperphosphatemia, ARF, or fluid overload.

NEUTROPENIC FEVER

Defined as a single temperature > 38.3°C (101°F) or sustained temperature > 38°C (100.4°F) for 1 hour in a patient with an ANC < 500. Etiologies are as follows:

- **GNR** (especially *Pseudomonas*): The most common pathogens; however, **GPC** infections have recently become more common.
- Fungal infections, especially *Candida* and *Aspergillus*, are commonly found with prolonged and severe neutropenia and prolonged antibiotic use.
- Viral infections also occur, especially with **human herpesviruses.**

SYMPTOMS/EXAM

Perform a thorough review of systems and exam to localize the source of fever. Remember to examine the skin, mucous membranes, oropharynx, sinuses, and perirectal area.

KEY FACT

Risk factors for tumor lysis syndrome:
- Hyperuricemia
- Renal insufficiency
- Hypovolemia
- Chemosensitivity
- High tumor cell turnover
- Elevated LDH

DIAGNOSIS

- **Labs:** Include CBC with differential, chem 7, a hepatic panel, and UA.
- **Microbiology workup:** Obtain blood cultures through each line and 1 peripheral culture; urine Gram stain and culture. LP if indicated (although will need platelets > 100 to safely perform LP).
- **Imaging:** CXR; further imaging as indicated.

TREATMENT

- Start empiric antibiotic therapy:
  - **Monotherapy:** Ceftazidime, cefepime, or carbapenems.
  - **Combination therapy:** An antipseudomonal β-lactam (ceftazidime, cefepime, pip/taz, or carbapenem) plus an aminoglycoside (or a fluoroquinolone).
  - Vancomycin should be added in certain situations—eg, patients with a history of MRSA colonization or with hypotension, mucositis, possible skin or catheter site infection, or recent quinolone prophylaxis. Discontinue if cultures are ⊖ at 72 hours.
  - In patients with neutropenia and unexplained fever persisting for 5–7 days, an antifungal agent should be started.
  - Low-risk adult patients can use ciprofloxacin + amoxicillin/clavulanate, provided they are observed carefully and have access to medical care 24/7; ANC > 100; monocyte count > 100; normal CXR; normal LFTs and creatinine; no clinical IV site tunnel/exit site infection; temperature < 39.0°C (102.2°F); no abdominal pain; evidence of impending bone marrow recovery; no comorbidities; and neutropenia expected to last < 10 days.
- **Duration:**
- If the source is known, complete a standard course of treatment, even after ANC recovery.
- For an unknown source:
  - Continue empiric antibiotics until afebrile with ANC > 500 for at least 1 day and the patient is afebrile for 2 days, or complete a minimum of a 7-day course.
  - If the patient becomes afebrile but remains neutropenic, consider completing a 14-day course.
  - Persistent fever: If ANC > 500, discontinue antibiotics 4–5 days after ANC > 500 and reassess. If ANC < 500, continue for 14 days and reassess.

GRAFT-VERSUS-HOST DISEASE (GVHD)

A syndrome that is caused by immunocompetent cells from a graft targeting the receiving patient's cell antigens. Occurs most often after an allogeneic bone marrow transplantation. Rates of GVHD are 30%–40% among related donors and recipients and 60%–80% between unrelated donors and recipients. The greater the mismatch between donor and recipient, the greater the risk of GVHD.

There are 2 categories of disease:

- **Acute GVHD:** Presents within the first 100 days after transplantation and usually manifests in the skin, GI system, liver, and hematopoietic system.
- **Chronic GVHD:** Onset is > 100 days from the transplantation and usually manifests in the skin, GI system, liver, and lungs.

SYMPTOMS/EXAM

- Acute:
  - The most common presenting symptom is a **maculopapular rash** that may become confluent or form bullous lesions with diffuse desquamation.
  - Profuse watery or bloody **diarrhea, crampy abdominal pain,** nausea, vomiting, anorexia, and dyspepsia are also seen.
- Chronic:
  - Skin changes resemble those in scleroderma or SLE.
  - Also presents with dry oral mucosa with ulceration and pain, dysphagia, diarrhea, and weight loss.
  - Dyspnea and nonproductive cough are also seen.

DIAGNOSIS

- Labs show **hyperbilirubinemia** and ↑ ALK if the liver is involved.
- You can make a clinical diagnosis in patients with a characteristic presentation.
- Biopsies of affected organ systems can confirm.

TREATMENT

- Give **prophylaxis with methotrexate and cyclosporine** +/– T-cell depletion of the graft.
- Use **corticosteroids for treatment.** For chronic disease, cyclosporine or tacrolimus may be used as well.

Oncologic Emergencies

SPINAL CORD COMPRESSION

 A 63-year-old male patient presents with thoracic back pain 6 months after completion of treatment for RCC. He believes the pain started about 4 weeks ago, but he cannot recall precisely. He notices the pain more when he lies down in bed at night. He is afebrile, and his UA is unremarkable. Thoracic spine films show mild disk degeneration but are otherwise unremarkable. What is the next step?

An MRI of the spine should be immediately obtained. Plain films cannot rule out spinal cord compression.

Usually caused by metastasis to the vertebral bodies. The prostate, breast, and lung are the most common 1° sites.

SYMPTOMS/EXAM

- Consider the diagnosis in any patient with cancer who complains of **back pain.** It is usually the earliest symptom and may ↑ with recumbency, movement of the spine, or Valsalva maneuver.
- Note that functional deficits typically occur later and are progressive. They include weakness, sensory loss, and bowel and bladder dysfunction.
- There may be tenderness to palpation over the spine at the level of the lesion.
- Patients may be hyper- or hypotonic and hyper- or hyporeflexic, depending on the acuity of the lesion.

DIAGNOSIS

- Order **MRI** of the entire spine. Plain films cannot rule out compression.
- Bone scan may be useful for screening if the back pain symptoms are non-specific.
- Neurologic status at the time treatment is initiated is the most important prognostic factor, so evaluation in symptomatic patients should be prompt.

TREATMENT

- Give urgent **dexamethasone** 10–100 mg IV, followed by 4–6 mg IV or PO every 6 hours. (Patients with paraparesis or paraplegia may be given 100 mg, followed by 24 mg every 6 hours.) Treatment should be started before the MRI if neurologic deficits are present.
- Perform emergent neurosurgical evaluation for possible surgical decompression and biopsy if the primary cancer is unknown, followed by radiation therapy or radiation therapy alone if the patient is not a surgical candidate.
- Chemotherapy is occasionally used for sensitive tumors.

MNEMONIC

Tumors that commonly metastasize to bone:

BLT with Mayo, Mustard, and Kosher Pickle

Breast
Lung
Thyroid
Multiple **M**yeloma
Kidney (renal cell)
Prostate

SUPERIOR VENA CAVA (SVC) SYNDROME

A 32-year-old male smoker presents to your office with a complaint of a red face. On exam, you note distended neck veins in addition to his facial plethora. He denies dyspnea, and his O$_2$ saturation is 98% on room air. His CXR shows a widened mediastinum, and a contrast chest CT shows a mediastinal mass compressing the superior vena cava as well as suspicious mediastinal nodes. What is the next step?

If there is no evidence of airway obstruction, treatment can be delayed until a definitive tissue diagnosis is established.

Defined as compression of the SVC that is mainly caused by malignancy (non–small cell lung cancer: 50%; small cell lung cancer: 25%: lymphoma: 10%; and metastatic lesions: 10%) and thrombosis or nonmalignant conditions (35% of cases). Commonly associated with intravascular devices such as catheters or pacemakers. Mediastinitis from infections (syphilis, TB) or aneurysm can also be a rare cause.

SYMPTOMS/EXAM

- Typical presentation includes facial/neck/arm swelling, plethora (leading to edema that can cause cyanosis), headache, dizziness, visual disturbances, syncope (congestion and cerebral edema), dyspnea, and cough (edema of the larynx/pharynx). Symptoms are usually worse when patient is supine or bends over.
- Venous distention of the neck and chest wall is also seen.

DIAGNOSIS

- CXR may show mediastinal widening and a pleural effusion (⊕ in two-thirds of cases).
- **Contrast chest CT** is the study of choice.
- Perform biopsy of a peripheral lesion (such as lymph nodes), sputum cytology, thoracentesis, and pleural effusion cytology (50% diagnostic yield).

- Bronchoscopy (50%–70% diagnostic yield), transthoracic needle aspiration biopsy (75% diagnostic yield), mediastinoscopy/mediastinostomy (> 90% diagnostic yield).

TREATMENT

- SVC syndrome is a true **emergency only if central airway obstruction** is present. Otherwise, treatment may be delayed while an oncologic diagnosis is established, as chemoradiation may make subsequent diagnosis more difficult.
- Chemotherapy +/– radiation therapy is used for treatment-responsive tumors.
- An endovascular stent may be used for palliation in patients who are not good candidates for chemoradiation.
- Corticosteroids and loop diuretics are frequently used for symptomatic relief but have not been shown to be effective.

Paraneoplastic Syndromes

Table 7.13 outlines common paraneoplastic syndromes and their causes.

HYPERCALCEMIA

Affects 20%–30% of cancer patients—the most common paraneoplastic syndrome (see Table 7.13). The most common causes are myeloma, breast cancer, and non–small cell lung cancer +/– bone metastasis. Also related to PTH-related protein (PTH-rP).

SYMPTOMS/EXAM

Depends on the rate and degree of hypercalcemia.

- **Early:** Anorexia, nausea, fatigue, constipation, polyuria.
- **Late:** Muscular weakness, hyporeflexia, confusion, psychosis, tremor, lethargy.

TABLE 7.13.   Paraneoplastic Syndromes

SYNDROME	ASSOCIATED NEOPLASM	CAUSES
Lambert-Eaton syndrome	Small cell lung cancer, thymoma.	Autoantibodies against presynaptic calcium channels at the neuromuscular junction.
Erythrocytosis	RCC, hepatocellular carcinoma.	EPO.
Cushing syndrome	Small cell lung cancer, adrenal cancer, thymoma.	ACTH precursors.
SIADH	Small cell lung cancer, intracranial neoplasms, pancreatic cancer.	ADH or atrial natriuretic factor.
Hypercalcemia	Breast cancer, non–small cell lung cancer, and other solid tumors metastatic to bone. Multiple myeloma, lymphoma. Lymphoma, squamous cell lung cancer.	Local osteolysis by tumor cells. Osteoclast activating factors. PTH-related protein.

DIAGNOSIS

- ↑ calcium (correct with the serum albumin level or check the ionized/free calcium).
- When calcium > 12 mg/dL, ↑ risk of arrhythmia or sudden cardiac death. Check ECG (shortening of QT).

TREATMENT

- Hydrate immediately with NS at 100–200 mL/hr.
- Use bisphosphonate if normal kidney function: Pamidronate 60–90 mg IV over 2–4 hours, or zoledronic acid 4 mg IV over several minutes.
- Treat underlying cancer if possible.
- For refractory hypercalcemia: calcitonin, corticosteroids (with myeloma and lymphoma).

CHAPTER 8

Pulmonary

Bethany C. Calkins, MD

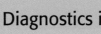

Diagnostics in Pulmonary Medicine

LUNG VOLUMES

Used to assess for restrictive lung disease, to show evidence of hyperinflation in obstructive lung disease, and to interpret the diffusing capacity for carbon monoxide (DL_{CO}).

Common definitions pertinent to the measurement of lung volume are as follows (see also Figure 8.1):

- **Residual volume (RV):** Air in the lung at maximal expiration.
- **Expiratory reserve volume (ERV):** Air that can be exhaled after normal expiration.
- **Tidal volume (TV):** Air entering and exiting the lungs during normal respirations.
- **Inspiratory reserve volume (IRV):** Air in excess of TV that enters the lungs at full inspiration.
- **Functional reserve capacity (FRC):** RV + ERV.
- **Inspiratory capacity (IC):** TV + IRV.
- **Total lung capacity (TLC):** RV + ERV + TV + IRV.

PULMONARY FUNCTION TESTS (PFTS)

Assessing lung function is important in pulmonary disease, and PFTs may aid significantly in diagnosis. The components of PFTs include spirometry, measurement of lung volume (as discussed above), and quantitation of diffusing capacity. Indications for testing include the following (see also Tables 8.1 and 8.2):

- Evaluation of various forms of pulmonary disease or for the presence of disease in patients with 1 or more risk factors (eg, smoking).
- Evaluation of chronic persistent cough, wheezing, dyspnea, or exertional cough/chest pain.
- Objective assessment of bronchodilator therapy.

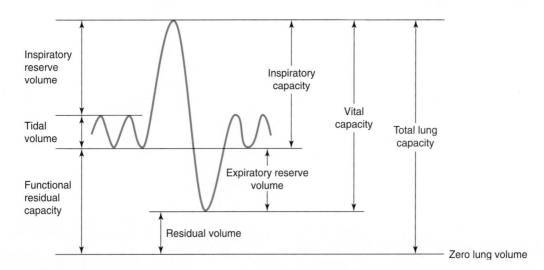

FIGURE 8.1.   **Lung volumes.** Lung volumes shown above as represented by spirogram tracing. (Reproduced, with permission, from Morgan GE Jr, et al. *Clinical Anesthesiology,* 4th ed. New York: McGraw-Hill, 2006, Fig. 22-5.)

TABLE 8.1. Diagnostic Applications of PFTs

MODALITY	MEASURES	PATIENT SELECTION
Spirometry	FEV$_1$, FVC, SVC.	All smokers > 45 years of age to screen for COPD.
Forced inspiratory maneuvers	FIVC.	Stridor heard over the neck or unexplained dyspnea.
Postbronchodilator spirometry	FEV$_1$, FVC.	Obstruction on spirometry or suspicion of asthma.
Lung volumes	TLC.	Interstitial lung disease.
Diffusing capacity	DL$_{CO}$.	Restrictive/obstructive disease.

- Evaluation of work exposures.
- Assessment of risk before major surgery.
- Objective assessment of impairment/disability.

Spirometry

Spirometry is the most useful and readily available of the PFTs. It includes measurement of forced expiratory volume in 1 second (FEV$_1$) and forced vital capacity (FVC). It may also include slow vital capacity (SVC), a measure that is useful when FVC is ↓, as slow exhalation causes less airway narrowing, and lung volumes are normal (which can screen for possible restrictive disease).

- **Forced inspiratory maneuvers** (ie, forced inspiratory vital capacity [FIVC]) can help detect variable airway obstruction, as is seen with vocal cord paralysis or dysfunction (see Figure 8.2).
- **Postbronchodilator spirometry** refers to the use of albuterol by metered dose inhaler (MDI) during initial workup if baseline spirometry indicates obstruction or if asthma is suspected. Repeat spirometry 10 minutes after treatment and advise patients that proper MDI use is essential. An ↑ in FVC$_1$ > 12% and at least > 0.2 L indicates acute bronchodilator responsiveness.

Diffusing Capacity

Measurement of single-breath DL$_{CO}$. Can be used in restrictive disease to distinguish intrinsic lung disease (DL$_{CO}$ is ↓) from other causes of restriction

TABLE 8.2. PFTs in Common Settings

SETTING	FEV$_1$/FVC	TLC	DL$_{CO}$
Asthma	Normal/low	Normal	Normal/high
COPD	Low	High/normal	Normal/high
Fibrotic disease	Normal/low	Low	Low
Extrathoracic restriction	Normal	Low	Normal

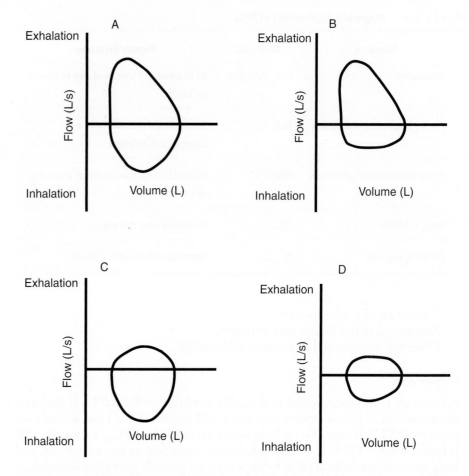

FIGURE 8.2. Flow volume loops. (A) Normal pattern. **(B)** Variable extrathoracic obstruction. **(C)** Variable intrathoracic obstruction. **(D)** Fixed obstruction. (Reproduced, with permission, from Le T, et al. *First Aid for the Internal Medicine Boards,* 2nd ed. New York: McGraw-Hill, 2008: 607.)

in which DL_{CO} is typically normal. In obstructive disease, diffusing capacity helps differentiate emphysema (characterized by a low DL_{CO}) from other causes of chronic airway obstruction. Obstruction from bronchitis typically has a normal DL_{CO}, whereas obstruction associated with asthma has a normal to high DL_{CO}.

Pulmonary Physiology

HYPOXEMIA

- **Hypoxia** is defined as **insufficient delivery of O_2** to the tissues.
- **Hypoxemia** is defined as an **abnormally low arterial O_2 tension.**
  - Generally, a PaO_2 of < 80 is considered hypoxemic (normal range: 80–100).
  - With age, this number ↓ according to the formula: $80 - [(age - 20)/4]$.
- Under most conditions, cardiac output is within a normal range, and **hypoxemia** is the most common cause of hypoxia.

- Hypoxemia is the result of any combinations of 5 separate mechanisms:
  1. **Hypoventilation:**
     - Many causes, but commonly due to oversedation from medications and responds well to O_2 therapy.
     - ↓ in **minute ventilation** (TV × breaths/minute) cause an ↑ in $Paco_2$ and a **normal** alveolar-arterial (A-a) O_2 gradient.
  2. **Right-to-left shunt:**
     - Blood bypasses the ventilated lung (eg, vascular malformations or intracardiac shunts) or perfuses a nonventilated lung (eg, pulmonary consolidation or pulmonary atelectasis) before returning to systemic circulation. This can be seen in the case of massive pulmonary embolus, PFO, or PDA.
     - Always involves an ↑ in the A-a O_2 gradient. $Paco_2$ may be low because of hyperventilation.
     - Characteristically, levels will not improve with supplemental O_2, as blood is flowing past the nonventilated lung. Use positive pressure ventilation.
     - Definitive treatment of a right-to-left shunt requires removal of the underlying cause.
  3. **Ventilation-perfusion (V/Q) mismatch:**
     - Failure to perfuse a ventilated lung (eg, in pulmonary embolism, asthma, COPD, pneumonia).
     - Associated with an ↑ A-a O_2 gradient. Hypoxemia usually **improves** with supplemental O_2 (↑ Fio_2 [the fraction of inspired O_2] in the ventilated lung will ↑ O_2 diffusion in the blood).
  4. **Diffusion impairment:**
     - Occurs when there is a ↓ in the diffusion of gas across the alveolar-capillary membrane and is associated with a very low DL_{CO}.
     - Occurs in interstitial lung disease or parenchymal disease.
     - Associated with an ↑ A-a O_2 gradient; hypoxemia improves with supplemental O_2.
  5. **Low inspired O_2:**
     - ↓ ambient O_2 pressure leads to hypoxemia.
     - Seen at high altitudes—ie, with lowered atmospheric pressure but preserved Fio_2 (21%). May also be seen in closed-space rescues or structural fires.
     - Characteristically has a normal A-a gradient and responds to O_2 supplementation.

SYMPTOMS/EXAM

- Neurologic findings include agitation, headache, somnolence, coma, and seizures. Motor dysfunction may also be seen.
- Tachypnea and hyperventilation are frequent signs, but don't rely on cyanosis. Patients may complain of pleuritic chest pain.
- With chronic hypoxemia, polycythemia, and pulmonary cachexia (weight loss as a result of ↑ energy requirements unbalanced by dietary intake) may be present. At very low values of Pao_2 (< 20 mmHg), depression of the central respiratory drive is seen, and death usually results from respiratory failure.

DIAGNOSIS

- Get an ABG and CXR. Pulse oximetry, although noninvasive, is limited in that it does not assess ventilation and may delay identifying clinically significant hypoxemia.
- Narrow the differential by calculating the A-a O_2 gradient, given by the formula $Pio_2 - (Pao_2 - Paco_2 / 8)$.

TABLE 8.3.   Physical Findings Associated with Common Lung Conditions

	COPD	PNEUMONIA	ATELECTASIS	PNEUMOTHORAX	PLEURAL EFFUSION	TUMOR
Barrel chest (AP diameter > transverse)	+	–	–	–	–	If associated COPD
Retractions	+	+/–	–			–
Tracheal deviations	–	Ipsilateral	Ipsilateral	Contralateral	Contralateral (if large)	–
Fremitus	↓	↓↑	↓	↓	↓	↑
Percussion	Hyperresonant	Dull	Dull	Resonant to hyperresonant	Dull	Dull
Breath sounds	Distant	Bronchial	↓	↓ or absent	↓ or absent (based on size)	↓
Egophony	–	Ipsilateral	–	–	+ or –	–

KEY FACT

Fremitus: Palpable vibration on chest while talking.

KEY FACT

When you hear a high-pitched "bleating" sound on auscultation, think **egophony.** This is compression of the lung tissue by consolidation or effusion.

TREATMENT

- If possible, treat the underlying condition.
- Patients are eligible for (and should be treated with) long-term O_2 therapy when their arterial Pao_2 is ≤ **55 mmHg** or their arterial O_2 saturation (Sao_2) is ≤ **88%.**
- If there is evidence of cor pulmonale, right heart failure, or erythrocytosis (hematocrit > 55%), patients who have a Pao_2 of 56–59 mmHg or an Sao_2 of 89% should also receive long-term O_2.
- If sleep or exercise causes O_2 desaturation as above, O_2 therapy is warranted.

LUNG PHYSICAL FINDINGS

Table 8.3 outlines physical findings commonly associated with various lung conditions.

Pulmonary Imaging Modalities

CHEST X-RAY (CXR)

- High clinical utility for identifying infectious diseases as well as for identifying masses in those patients at high risk for lung cancer.
- Can show infiltrates, nodules, masses, effusion, and, to a lesser extent, mediastinal and hilar abnormalities (see Tables 8.4 and 8.5).
- Generally includes both PA and lateral views.

TABLE 8.4. **Masses Found on CXR**

Anterior Mediastinal	Posterior Mediastinal
Teratoma	Bronchial cysts
Thymoma	Enterogenic cysts
Thymolipoma	Abscess
Thymic carcinoma/carcinoid	Non-Hodgkin lymphoma
Thymic cyst	Neurogenic tumors
Thoracic thyroid	Pericardial cysts/plasmacytoma
Terrible lymphoma	Hodgkin lymphoma

Reproduced, with permission, from Le T, et al. *First Aid for the Internal Medicine Boards,* 2nd ed. New York: McGraw-Hill, 2008: 604.

- Lateral decubitus views are used to look for free-flowing pleural fluid, and apical lordotic views visualize the lung apices more effectively than the standard PA view.
- Portable views for acutely ill or otherwise bed-bound patients yield an AP view.

COMPUTED TOMOGRAPHY (CT)

- **Advantages of CT** over standard CXRs include the following:
    - Cross-sectional images show fluid collections, distinguish soft tissue structures, eliminate overlap, and define mediastinal structures.
    - CT scan can show detailed imaging of airways, vasculature, and parenchyma.
    - Helical scans with IV contrast can detect pulmonary emboli or aortic dissection, and, with reconstruction, detailed bronchial views.
    - High-resolution scans with thin slicing (1–2 mm) demonstrate bronchiectasis, emphysema, and interstitial lung disease.
- **Disadvantages** include cost, radiation exposure, and adverse reactions to IV contrast media.

TABLE 8.5. **Infiltrates Found on CXR**

Upper Lobe	Lower Lobe
Ankylosing spondylitis	Bronchiectasis
Sarcoidosis	Aspiration
TB	Dermatomyositis/polymyositis
Eosinophilic granulomatosis	Asbestosis
Cystic fibrosis	Idiopathic pulmonary fibrosis
Silicosis	Pneumonia
Pneumonia	

Reproduced, with permission, from Le T, et al. *First Aid for the Internal Medicine Boards,* 2nd ed. New York: McGraw-Hill, 2008: 603.

VENTILATION/PERFUSION (V/Q) SCAN

- An imaging modality that aids in the diagnosis of pulmonary embolism using radioactive isotopes and a gamma camera.
- Albumin labeled with technetium-99m is injected and lodges in the pulmonary capillaries, showing the distribution of blood flow in the lung.
- Radiolabeled xenon gas can be inhaled to demonstrate the distribution of ventilation.
- In pulmonary embolism, defects in perfusion are not accompanied by a corresponding defect in ventilation and are thus called **mismatched defects.**

PULMONARY ANGIOGRAPHY

- Considered the **gold standard** for diagnosis of pulmonary embolism, although rarely used in clinical practice anymore.
- Radiopaque contrast medium is injected into the pulmonary artery, allowing visualization of **filling defects** (defects in the lumen of a vessel) or an abrupt termination ("**cutoff**") of the vessel.
- Use this if you suspect an occult pulmonary arteriovenous malformation (AVM) or to embolize a known AVM.
- The **disadvantage** is that it is invasive. Rarely used since CT angiography delivers rapid imaging in a safer way.

BRONCHOSCOPY

- Allows for evaluation of the airway/bronchial tree through direct visualization.
- **Flexible bronchoscopy:** Performed on awake but sedated patients; can identify endobronchial pathology (eg, tumors, granulomas, bronchitis, foreign bodies, bleeding sites) up to the level of subsegmental bronchi.
- Samples can be obtained via washing, brushing, needle aspiration endobronchial biopsy, and transbronchial biopsy.
- **Bronchial alveolar lavage** can reach the more distal pulmonary parenchyma and can recover organisms or cancer cells from the alveolar spaces.
- **Rigid bronchoscopy:** Requires general anesthesia and is performed for massive bleeding and for the removal of large foreign bodies, blood clots, and tumors that may be obstructing airways.
- Complications stemming from bronchoscopy include hemorrhage, fever, transient hypoxemia, and pneumothorax.

Common Respiratory Complaints

COUGH

Cough is one of the most common reasons patients visit their physicians. Healthy individuals rarely cough because mucociliary mechanisms are sufficient to clear normal bronchial secretions. Cough is useful for clearing foreign bodies and secretions from the respiratory tract; however, it can spread illness through droplets and contamination of objects.

KEY FACT

Tactile fremitus is increased in pneumonia if it is alveolar; it is decreased in bronchoalveolar pneumonia, as bronchial mucous plugs dampen the tactile fremitus to make it softer.

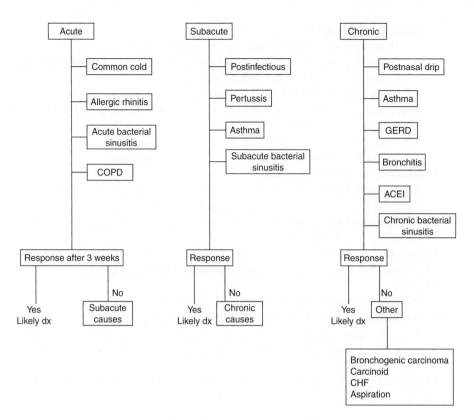

FIGURE 8.3. **Algorithm for the differential diagnosis of cough.** (Reproduced, with permission, from Le T, et al. *First Aid for the Internal Medicine Boards,* 1st ed. New York: McGraw-Hill, 2006: 555.)

SYMPTOMS

The following hallmarks of cough can help determine its etiology (see also Figure 8.3):

- Duration:
    - **Acute cough:** < 3 weeks' duration; most often seen in postnasal drip associated with the common cold (see Table 8.6).

TABLE 8.6.   Causes of Acute Cough

PREVALENCE	CAUSES OF ACUTE COUGH
Very common	Postnasal drip syndrome.
	Acute bacterial sinusitis.
	Allergic rhinitis.
	Environmental/irritant rhinitis.
Common	Pertussis.
	COPD.
Less common	Bronchogenic carcinoma.
	Asthma.
	CHF.
	Pneumonia.
	Aspiration.
	Pulmonary embolism.
	ACE inhibitors.

- **Subacute cough:** 3–8 weeks' duration.
  - Postinfectious cough is the most common cause.
  - Asthma, pertussis infection, and subacute bacterial sinusitis can also cause persistent cough in this timeframe.
- **Chronic cough:** > 8 weeks' duration (see Table 8.7).
- Postnasal drip is the most common cause of chronic cough, followed by asthma and GERD.
- Chronic bronchitis, bronchiectasis, and angiotensin-converting enzyme (ACE) inhibitor use are other common etiologies.
- **Productive vs. nonproductive:**
  - **Productive cough:** Points to an underlying inflammatory process (eg, postnasal drip, acute or chronic bronchitis, or bacterial pneumonia).
  - **Nonproductive cough:** Points to a mechanical or irritative stimulus (eg, ACE inhibitor cough).
- **Character:** A "brassy" cough may indicate major airway involvement, whereas a "barking/croupy" cough may signify laryngeal disease.
- **Timing:**
  - **Nocturnal cough:** Associated with CHF or asthma.
  - **Mealtime cough:** Associated with esophagogastric disease.
  - **Cough upon awakening:** If cough results from the pooling of secretions from postnasal drip during sleep, it points to severe bronchitis or bronchiectasis.
- **Other:** Ask about postnasal drip symptoms, GERD, asthma, and smoking history.

> **KEY FACT**
>
> Postnasal drip syndrome, asthma, and GERD account for nearly 100% of causes of chronic cough in nonsmokers with normal chest films who are not on ACE inhibitors.

Exam

- Focus on the nasal mucosa, lungs, and heart.
- If digital clubbing is present, think chronic pulmonary disease.
- Boggy nasal mucosa and cobblestoning of the posterior oropharynx may suggest postnasal drip. Wheeze or cough on forced exhalation may be present in asthma.
- Listen for crackles or rhonchi.
- Look for signs of CHF (eg, elevated JVP, peripheral edema).

TABLE 8.7. Causes of Chronic Cough

PREVALENCE	CAUSES OF CHRONIC COUGH
Common	Postnasal drip syndrome
	Asthma
	GERD
Less common	Chronic bronchitis
	Bronchiectasis
	Pertussis
Uncommon	Bronchogenic carcinoma
	ACE inhibitors
Rare (in adults)	Psychogenic cough

DIAGNOSIS/TREATMENT

Diagnosis is largely based on symptoms/duration and on the patient's response to treatment of the presumed cause.

COMPLICATIONS

Persistent and recurrent cough can lead to tussive syncope, retinal vessel rupture, persistent headache, chest wall and abdominal muscle strain (causing abdominal wall hernias or dehiscence after surgery), and rib fractures. Severe chronic cough can significantly impact quality of life, potentially restricting social activities, disrupting family life, and, in rare cases, leading to attempted suicide.

 KEY FACT

The most common causes of chronic cough are postnasal drip, asthma, and GERD.

DYSPNEA

Defined as a feeling of difficulty breathing that is disproportionate to the stimulus and thus abnormally uncomfortable. It is often described by patients as feeling "breathless" or "short of breath."

SYMPTOMS/EXAM

- Dyspnea can be caused by a multitude of conditions, necessitating a thorough history. Its **onset can provide diagnostic clues:**
  - **Sudden dyspnea** without provocation can represent pulmonary embolism, pneumothorax, or myocardial ischemia. Asthma can also present rapidly.
  - **Progressive dyspnea,** cough, and purulent sputum may represent a COPD exacerbation or pneumonia.
  - **Orthopnea:** Onset or worsening of dyspnea on becoming supine. Think heart disease or chronic lung disease.
  - **Paroxysmal nocturnal dyspnea:** Episodes of breathlessness that awaken patients from sleep. Usually points to chronic LV failure but may also be seen in chronic pulmonary disease 2° to pooling of secretions.

DIAGNOSIS/TREATMENT

- Order a CXR.
- Consider plasma brain natriuretic peptide (BNP) to determine if CHF is a possibility.
- PFTs should be among the initial studies considered.
- Consider ECG and echocardiography +/− stress testing.
- Consider testing for GERD.
- Treat the underlying condition; whatever relieves dyspnea may also help diagnose the cause.

 KEY FACT

The most common causes of chronic dyspnea are asthma, COPD, interstitial lung disease, and cardiomyopathy.

HEMOPTYSIS

The coughing up of blood that **originates below the vocal cords.** Hemoptysis can range from trivial to massive in scope, with **massive hemoptysis** defined as any amount of blood that is hemodynamically significant or impairs respiratory function. Volume may range from 100 cc to > 600 cc in a 24-hour period.

TABLE 8.8. Differential Diagnosis of Hemoptysis by Anatomic Location

AIRWAYS	PULMONARY VASCULATURE	PULMONARY PARENCHYMA	IATROGENIC
Bronchitis	LV failure.	Pneumonia.	Transbronchial lung biopsies.
Bronchogenic carcinoma	Mitral stenosis.	Inhalation of crack cocaine.	Anticoagulation.
Bronchiectasis	Pulmonary emboli. **AVMs.**	Autoimmune disease: Goodpasture syndrome; Wegener granulomatosis.	Pulmonary artery rupture from balloon-tipped catheter placement.

SYMPTOMS/EXAM

Table 8.8 outlines a differential for hemoptysis based on anatomic location, with bolded causes the most common. Other causes include aspergilloma, cystic fibrosis, lung abscess, sarcoidosis, and TB (see Table 8.9).

■ Hemoptysis can also be differentiated on the basis of **patient age:**
  ■ In patients < **40 years of age,** think bronchiectasis (if there is a history of recurrent pneumonia) or **mitral stenosis** (if a diastolic murmur is present).
  ■ In patients > **40 years of age,** consider **malignancy,** especially with a history of tobacco use, cachexia, and weight loss.
■ A URI prodrome and a benign exam in a young person may suggest bronchitis.

> **KEY FACT**
>
> Mitral stenosis is an often overlooked cause of hemoptysis, as it is associated with elevated pulmonary capillary pressure.

TABLE 8.9. Causes of Hemoptysis

Common causes of hemoptysis	Bronchiectasis.
	Lung cancer.
	Bronchitis.
	Pneumonia.
Uncommon causes of hemoptysis	Aspergilloma.
	Coagulopathy.
	CHF.
	Cystic fibrosis.
	Lung abscess.
	Pulmonary embolism.
	Sarcoidosis.
	Tuberculosis.
	Wegener granulomatosis.
	Goodpasture syndrome.
Rare causes of hemoptysis	Systemic hypertension.
	Pulmonary hypertension.
	Trauma.
	Vasculitis.
	Foreign body.
	Collagen vascular disease.
	Pulmonary atriovenous malformation.

DIAGNOSIS

■ Get a CBC with differential, UA, renal function tests, and coagulation studies.

■ Obtain a CXR.

■ Flexible bronchoscopy finds endobronchial carcinoma in 3%–6% of patients with hemoptysis and a normal CXR (see Figure 8.4).

■ If directed by the H&P, obtain sputum for cytology and acid-fast staining along with a chest CT (good for bronchiectasis, AVMs, central endobronchial lesions, and small peripheral malignancies).

■ Additional tests include ABG analysis on room air as well as ANA, ANCA, and anti–glomerular basement membrane (anti-GBM) antibody assays to assess for autoimmune disease.

TREATMENT

Treatment for hemoptysis is 2-fold: supportive care if needed and then definitive treatment:

■ **Supportive care:** Consists of bed rest, supplemental O_2, and blood products if needed. Place patient bleeding side down. Ensure ventilation with airway protection and intubate if necessary to achieve this. Avoid antitussives to allow blood clearance from airways, but consider suppression of the cough reflex if not actively bleeding.

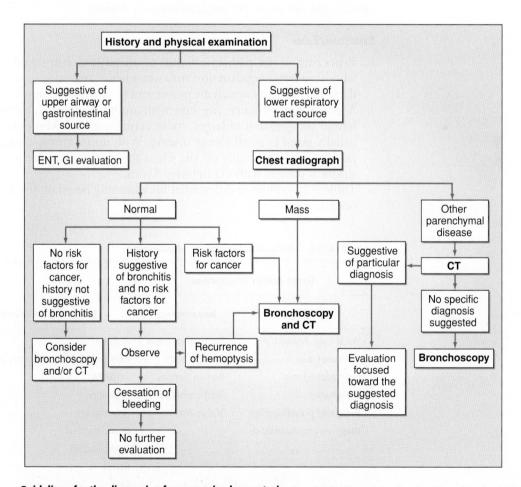

FIGURE 8.4. **Guidelines for the diagnosis of nonmassive hemoptysis.** (Reproduced, with permission, from Fauci AS, et al. *Harrison's Principles of Internal Medicine,* 17th ed. New York: McGraw-Hill, 2008, Fig. 34-2.)

- **Definitive treatment:**
  - **Nonmassive hemoptysis:** Identify and treat the specific cause.
  - **Massive hemoptysis:** A life-threatening condition; the treatment goal is to bring a rapid end to the bleeding; cases of massive hemoptysis usually require surgical involvement.
  - If the bleeding site is known, place the patient in the decubitus position, with the involved lung dependent. If bleeding is uncontrolled, urgent rigid bronchoscopy under general anesthesia allows for direct cautery or packing of bronchial lesions. A surgery consult may be necessary, but surgery is associated with high morbidity and mortality in this setting.
  - In stable patients, flexible bronchoscopy can identify the bleeding site, and angiography can embolize the involved bronchial arteries.
  - Angiography of the bronchial arteries can localize the bleeding site in > 90% of patients (< 10% of bleeds come from pulmonary arteries) and can then proceed to embolization, which is successful in > 90% of patients.

WHEEZE

A wheeze is an adventitious, "musical" lung sound produced by airflow through central and distal airways. Wheezes can be single toned or polyphonic and can occur on inspiration or expiration.

SYMPTOMS/EXAM

- Wheezing is not pathognomonic of an airway obstruction, and patients who have airway obstruction may not wheeze (eg, with severe obstruction, there may not be enough air movement to generate a sound).
- A polyphonic wheeze (ie, one with multiple notes) often indicates dynamic compression of larger, more central airways. Monophonic wheezes usually point to small airway disease. With upper airway obstruction, dyspnea on exertion usually occurs when the airway diameter is < 8 mm, and stridor is present with diameters < 5 mm.
- Table 8.10 outlines a differential for wheezing based on the location of the obstruction.

TABLE 8.10.   Differential Diagnosis of Wheezing

UPPER AIRWAY OBSTRUCTION		LOWER AIRWAY OBSTRUCTION
EXTRATHORACIC	**INTRATHORACIC**	**LOWER AIRWAY OBSTRUCTION**
Vocal cord dysfunction	Tracheal stenosis	Asthma
Postnasal drip	Foreign body	Allergic bronchopulmonary aspergillosis
Laryngeal edema	Benign tumors	(ABPA)
Malignancy	Tracheomalacia	Aspiration
Relapsing polychondritis	Malignancy	Bronchiolitis
Wegener granulomatosis		Bronchiectasis
		Cystic fibrosis
		COPD
		CHF
		Parasitic infections
		Pulmonary embolus

DIAGNOSIS/TREATMENT

- PFTs with flow volume loops (see Figure 8.2) can be used to distinguish intrathoracic from extrathoracic obstruction. Treatment choices should be based on the specific cause of the wheeze.
- Response to treatment helps confirm the diagnosis. Conversely, a lack of response should prompt the alteration of therapy (vs. looking for other potential causes).

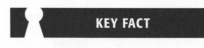

KEY FACT

"All that wheezes is not asthma."

Upper Respiratory Tract Disorders

OBSTRUCTIVE SLEEP APNEA (OSA)

A 44-year-old obese man comes to your office complaining of snoring and ↑ daytime sleepiness. His wife has reportedly witnessed apneic events while the patient sleeps. You suspect obstructive sleep apnea. What vital sign is most likely to be abnormal?

Blood pressure. Patients with obstructive sleep apnea have a 50% chance of being hypertensive.

The cessation of breathing during sleep caused by repetitive partial or complete obstruction of the airway by pharyngeal structures. Often seen in overweight patients who snore loudly and complain of daytime fatigue and sleepiness. Ultimately, clinical sequelae result from chronic sleep deprivation and recurrent oxyhemoglobin desaturation.

- **Apnea:** A temporary absence or cessation of breathing (airflow) during sleep, traditionally defined as **10 seconds** for adults.
- **Hypopnea:** Essentially "underbreathing"; breathing is present, unlike in apnea, but is slower or more shallow than normal.

SYMPTOMS/EXAM

- Patients' bed partners often complain of **loud snoring** and may witness actual apneic events. Patients often complain of **excessive sleepiness,** physically restless sleep, morning dry mouth and sore throat, personality changes, intellectual impairment, impotence, and **morning headache.**
- On exam, patients appear fatigued and often have ↑ BMI; collar size is frequently > 17 inches for men and > 16 inches for women.
- Systemic arterial **hypertension** is present in **50% of cases, and there seems to be a relationship between pulmonary hypertension and OSA.**
- Airway crowding may be present as a result of adenotonsillar hypertrophy or redundant soft tissue of the soft palate, together with an elongated uvula.

DIFFERENTIAL

If your patient complains of excessive daytime sleepiness, also consider chronic sleep deprivation, narcolepsy, alcohol use, severe restrictive lung disease, medication and drug use, periodic restless leg syndrome, schedule disorders/shift work, and chronic pain or discomfort.

DIAGNOSIS

- Polysomnography is the first-line study for diagnosis when sleep apnea is suspected, although portable monitoring is becoming more popular as a diagnostic study.

TABLE 8.11.   Interpretation of AHI Results

AHI Score	Interpretation
< 5	Normal
5–15	Mild OSA
16–30	Moderate OSA
> 30	Severe disease

- Results are reported in terms of the **apnea-hypopnea index** (AHI, or the number of episodes of apnea/hypopnea in an hour), also known as the respiratory disturbance index (RDI). Table 8.11 outlines the interpretation of AHI scores.

TREATMENT

- **Conservative measures** (for patients with an AHI < 20): Avoid EtOH, sleeping on the back, and trial intranasal steroids; encourage weight loss.
- **Continuous positive airway pressure (CPAP):** The **gold standard** for treatment; delivers constant air pressure through the nostrils to maintain a patent airway. Significantly improves quality of life and ↓ complications.
- **Aggressive treatment** (for patients with severe sleep apnea who cannot tolerate CPAP):
  - **Uvulopalatopharyngoplasty:** The most commonly performed procedure. Designed to ↑ the pharyngeal lumen by resecting redundant soft tissue.
  - **Nasal surgery:** Septal deviation repair, turbinectomy, polypectomy +/– surgical correction of craniofacial abnormalities.

COMPLICATIONS

- Patients have a 2- to 3-fold ↑ risk of motor vehicle accidents.
- **Cardiovascular complications:**
  - Contributes to difficult-to-treat systemic hypertension and probably pulmonary hypertension.
  - Significantly ↑ the risk of stroke or death from any cause; this ↑ is independent of other risk factors, including hypertension.

NASAL POLYPS

Pale, edematous masses that are covered by mucosa and are frequently encountered in patients with allergic rhinitis (see Figure 8.5). Nasal polyps arise from the sinuses (eg, the **ethmoid sinuses**) and obstruct airflow by extending into the nasal cavity.

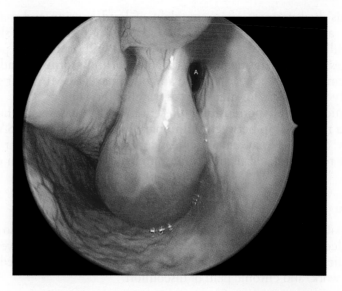

FIGURE 8.5.   Nasal polyp. (Reproduced, with permission, from Brunicardi FC, et al. *Schwartz's Principles of Surgery*, 9th ed. New York: McGraw-Hill, 2010, Fig. 18-3.)

SYMPTOMS/EXAM

- Patients may present with nasal obstruction, a diminished sense of smell, and rhinorrhea.
- Ask about a history of asthma, as up to 20%–30% of asthmatic patients with nasal polyps have a sensitivity to aspirin (and the use of aspirin in these subjects may precipitate bronchospasm).
- Polyps appear as pale, gelatinous, rounded masses in the nasal cavity and are insensitive to pain.

DIFFERENTIAL

Chronic allergic rhinitis, sinusitis, Samter triad, cystic fibrosis, Churg-Strauss syndrome, allergic fungal sinusitis.

KEY FACT

The Samter triad consists of nasal polyps, asthma, and aspirin sensitivity.

TREATMENT

- Intranasal steroids can block growth and may cause regression. Systemic corticosteroids may cause regression that can then be maintained with nasal steroids.
- Surgical removal may be necessary to relieve symptoms in severe cases (eg, those with intolerable nasal obstruction or recurrent sinusitis requiring multiple courses of antibiotics).

COMPLICATIONS

The recurrence rate can be high, and thus preventive measures (eg, controlling allergen exposure and maximizing medical therapy) are essential.

EPISTAXIS

Defined as bleeding from the nose, typically as a result of rupture of small vessels (Kiesselbach plexus) in the mucosa overlying the anterior aspect of the nasal septum.

SYMPTOMS

Bleeding can occur from the anterior nasal cavity (95% of the time) as a product of the Kiesselbach plexus or from the posterior cavity, which is a product of the sphenopalatine artery or carotid artery. With posterior bleeds, there may be associated hemoptysis or hematemesis. Because of the anatomy, a large volume of blood can be lost from posterior epistaxis.

EXAM

- If possible, conduct the exam with the patient sitting upright to prevent ingestion or aspiration of blood. Wear protective eyewear and clothing.
- With a nasal speculum, examine both sides of the nose to assess the integrity of the septum and to identify bleeding sites. Examine the posterior oropharynx for 15 seconds to look for fresh blood flowing down the back wall, which may suggest a posterior source.

DIFFERENTIAL

Nasal trauma (eg, nose picking, foreign body, forceful nose blowing), rhinitis, dry nasal mucosa, deviated septum, chronic sinusitis, inhaled steroids, cocaine use, alcohol use, antiplatelet medications, thrombocytopenia, hemophilia, leukemia, Wegener granulomatosis, nasal neoplasm, Osler-Weber-Rendu disease, von Willebrand disease, or a bleeding diathesis.

DIAGNOSIS

- Diagnose by exam as above. Obtain baseline vitals and monitor accordingly.
- Consider checking platelet count and coagulation studies.
- The diagnosis of anterior vs. posterior bleed may be difficult with large amounts of continued bleeding. The use of topical 4% cocaine or a topical decongestant plus a topical anesthetic (eg, oxymetazoline and tetracaine, respectively), applied as a spray or on a cotton strip, can halt bleeding and aid in localization.

TREATMENT

- **Anterior epistaxis:** Typically responds to continuous pressure to the nasal alae for 10 minutes.
- Have the patient sit upright and lean forward.
- Topical nasal decongestants such as a phenylephrine solution may be beneficial.
- Silver nitrate or electrocautery can cauterize the bleeding site.
- Anterior packing should be sufficient if bleeding persists.
- **Posterior epistaxis:** Likely calls for a referral. Treatment options include posterior pack placement to occlude choanae, followed by anterior packing. Endovascular embolization vs. surgical ligation of the nasal arterial supply may be necessary.

Lower Respiratory Tract Disorders

ASTHMA

A 23-year-old woman with a history of asthma previously managed by albuterol alone comes to your office complaining of a greater need for her inhaler over the past several months. She is coughing 3 days a week and has nighttime cough approximately once per week. What would be the next step in her asthma management?

This patient meets the criteria for mild persistent asthma and thus requires a controller medication. The current preferred long-term controller treatment in mild persistent asthma is a low-dose inhaled corticosteroid.

Asthma is defined as **inflammation of airways** that ↑ airway secretions and subsequent contraction of bronchial musculature. May be idiopathic or triggered by allergies or environmental factors.

- **Acute inflammation** leads to an asthma "attack."
- **Chronic inflammation** can lead to long-term narrowing and remodeling of the airways.

Asthma is more common in nonwhite populations, even after correcting for socioeconomic status. Five percent of Americans are affected, and asthma results in > 450,000 hospitalizations and 5000 deaths per year.

SYMPTOMS/EXAM

- Presents with episodic or chronic dyspnea, cough, wheezing, and chest tightness that worsens at night or in the early morning (see Table 8.12).

TABLE 8.12. Classification of Asthma Severity

STEP	GENERAL SYMPTOMS	NIGHTTIME SYMPTOMS	LUNG FUNCTION
Step 1: mild intermittent	Symptoms < 2 days per week.	≤ 2 times per month.	FEV_1 ≥ 80% predicted. Normal FEV_1 between exacerbations. FEV_1/FVC normal.
Step 2: mild persistent	Symptoms > 2 times per week but not daily. Exacerbations may affect activity.	3-4 times per month.	FEV_1 ≥ 80% predicted. FEV_1/FVC normal.
Step 3: moderate persistent	Daily symptoms. Daily use of an inhaled short-acting β_2-agonist. Exacerbations affect activity. Exacerbations ≥ 2 times per week; may last days.	> 1 time per week, but not nightly.	FEV_1 or PEF > 60% to < 80% predicted. FEV_1/FVC reduced 5%.
Step 4: severe persistent	Continual symptoms throughout the day. Limited physical activity; frequent exacerbations.	Often 7 times per week.	FEV_1 < 60% predicted. FEV_1/FVC reduced > 5%.

Adapted, with permission, from South-Paul JE, et al. *Current Diagnosis & Treatment in Family Medicine,* 2nd ed. New York: McGraw-Hill, 2008, Table 26-6.

- Precipitants may be allergens such as dust mites, cockroaches, cat dander, or pollen. Nonallergic precipitants include exercise, cold air, URIs, stress, GERD, and secondhand smoke.
- Inquire about a history of atopy (the association is more common in younger patients).
- Exam may reveal prolonged expiration, tachypnea, tachycardia, hyperresonance, accessory muscle use, and diffuse wheezes.

> **KEY FACT**
>
> Ask about this classic triad: atopy, asthma, allergic rhinitis.

DIFFERENTIAL

CHF (cardiac asthma), GERD, pulmonary embolism, Churg-Strauss syndrome, conversion disorder.

DIAGNOSIS

- Conduct spirometry (FEV_1, FVC, FEV_1/FVC) before and after the administration of a short-acting bronchodilator.
- Significant reversibility of obstruction is demonstrated by an ↑ of > 12% and at least 200 mL in FEV_1 or an ↑ of > 15% and 200 mL in FVC after bronchodilator use.
- ABGs may show a respiratory alkalosis and an ↑ in the A-a O_2 gradient; in severe exacerbations, hypoxemia develops and the $Paco_2$ normalizes.
- If nondiagnostic, consider methacholine challenge.
- ↑ $Paco_2$ and respiratory acidosis may portend fatigue and impending respiratory failure.
- Imaging may be obtained via CXR, but typically only hyperinflation can be seen.
- CBC may show eosinophilia.

TREATMENT

Options include a combination of quick-relief therapy and long-term treatment, based on asthma severity.

- **Quick-relief therapy:** Includes short-acting inhaled β_2-agonists (eg, albuterol), anticholinergics (eg, ipratropium), and glucocorticoids (eg, oral

MNEMONIC

Remember the medications for ASTHMA exacerbation:

Albuterol
Steroids
Theophylline
Humidified O_2
Magnesium
Antileukotriene

KEY FACT

Think of patients with emphysema as **"pink puffers"** because of their lack of cyanosis, use of accessory muscles, and pursed-lip breathing. Patients with chronic bronchitis are called **"blue bloaters"** because of their more marked cyanosis and fluid retention due to right heart failure.

---

prednisone). Intubation/ventilation may be necessary in cases of impending respiratory failure.
- **Long-term control therapy:** Involves use of inhaled and systemic (if necessary) corticosteroids, long-acting β_2-agonists (eg, salmeterol), leukotriene modifiers (eg, montelukast), mast cell stabilizers (eg, cromolyn), and phosphodiesterase inhibitors (eg, theophylline).

CHRONIC OBSTRUCTIVE PULMONARY DISEASE (COPD)

 A 69-year-old white woman presents to the hospital with severe COPD along with a history of multiple hospital admissions, 30-step dyspnea on exertion, weight loss, weakness, and a resting Pao_2 of 59 mmHg. Which intervention will most likely affect her survival?

Long-term O_2 supplementation is the only treatment for severe COPD that has been shown to improve survival and quality of life, ↓ dyspnea scores, and ↓ pulmonary artery pressure.

A disease state characterized by **airflow limitation** that is no longer fully reversible. COPD includes **emphysema** (destruction and enlargement of lung alveoli) and **chronic bronchitis** (chronic cough and phlegm for 3 months or more over 2 consecutive years). Chronic airflow obstruction must be present in order for the diagnosis to be made. These disease states cause destruction of lung parenchyma, leading to a decline in elastic recoil, resulting in air trapping.

COPD is the **4th leading cause of death in the United States,** and smoking is the most important risk factor. α_1-Antitrypsin deficiency is a rare genetic abnormality that leads to early-onset emphysema (1% of cases of COPD). Chronic bronchitis is frequently seen in patients in their 40s or 50s, whereas emphysema is more likely to appear in patients ≥ 60 years of age.

SYMPTOMS/EXAM

- Symptoms typically arise in patients who have smoked > 1 pack of cigarettes per day for 20 years. On exam, patients may have distant breath and heart sounds, a barrel chest, prolonged expiration, and wheezing.
- Disease-specific symptoms are as follows:
  - **Chronic bronchitis:** Presents with a productive **cough** with sputum production for at least 3 months for 2 consecutive years. Patients with chronic bronchitis have more trouble getting air in and clearing their mucus. They tend to have normal to ↑ Pco_2 and ↓ Po_2 on arterial blood gas.
  - **Emphysema:** Presents primarily with **exertional dyspnea** related to difficulty with exhaling, resulting in accessory muscle use, leading to fatigue. They tend to have ↑ Pco_2 and a normal to ↓ Po_2.

DIFFERENTIAL

Acute bronchitis, asthma, bronchiectasis, cystic fibrosis, CHF.

DIAGNOSIS

Useful diagnostic tools include CXR, spirometry, and ABG analysis.

- **CXR:** Shows flattening of the diaphragm, ↓ lung markings, and an enlarged retrosternal space (see Figure 8.6).

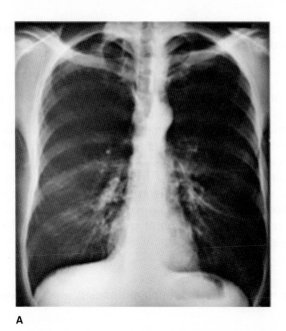
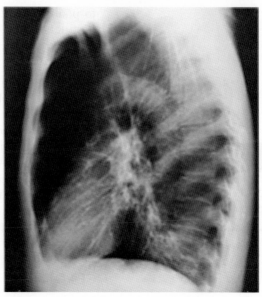

A   **B**

FIGURE 8.6.   CXR in a patient with chronic obstructive pulmonary disease. Note the flattened diaphragms, large retrosternal space, and minimal lung markings on AP (**A**) and lateral (**B**) CXR. (Reproduced, with permission, from Stobo JD, et al. *The Principles and Practice of Medicine,* 23rd ed. Stamford, CT: Appleton & Lange, 1996: 135.)

- **Spirometry:** Can detect small changes in lung function relatively easily. Symptoms of COPD usually develop when FEV_1 ↓ to < 80% predicted. A PEF rate of < 350 L/min is a sign that COPD is likely present.
- **ABGs:** Acute exacerbations reveal hypoxemia and hypercarbia with acute respiratory acidosis.

TREATMENT

- **Nonpharmacologic:** The most important intervention is **smoking cessation,** as it improves lung function initially and slows annual loss of FEV_1. Hypoxemic patients should receive **supplemental O_2.** Exercise and pulmonary rehabilitation can ↓ pulmonary symptoms and improve exercise tolerance.
- **Pharmacologic:**
  - **Inhaled anticholinergics** (eg, ipratropium): Fewer side effects and better response than inhaled β-agonists, but intermittent use of a **β-agonist inhaler** can be beneficial as an additional agent. Long-acting β-agonists may be useful as well, as they last through the night. **Tiotropium** is a long-acting anticholinergic that should be the bronchodilator of choice.
  - **Antibiotic therapy** may play a role in patients with chronic bronchitis who have ↑ volume or a purulent appearance to their sputum.
  - Inhaled **corticosteroids** can provide symptomatic relief as symptoms worsen, and oral steroid bursts during exacerbations can also ↓ symptoms.
  - **Make sure your COPD patients receive influenza and pneumococcal vaccines.**

BRONCHIECTASIS

An abnormal and permanent **dilatation of medium-sized airways** that is either focal or diffuse and is the result of repeated cycles of infection, leading to pooling of secretions in the dilated airways and thus continued bronchial destruction. It is **caused by cystic fibrosis in 50% of cases.**

SYMPTOMS/EXAM

- Presents with persistent or recurrent cough and purulent sputum production. **Hemoptysis is found in 50%–70% of cases.**
- Patients may report a history of an initial severe pneumonia episode followed by chronic cough and sputum production. However, it may also have a more insidious onset.
- Nonproductive cough may represent "dry bronchiectasis" in an upper lobe. Dyspnea and wheeze may be a sign of extensive disease or underlying COPD. Infection may ↑ sputum production and fever.
- Auscultation may reveal a combination of crackles, rhonchi, and wheeze. Clubbing of the fingernails may be present as well.

DIFFERENTIAL

COPD, asthma, bronchiolitis, allergic bronchopulmonary aspergillosis.

DIAGNOSIS

The following studies can help diagnose and/or clarify the underlying cause of bronchiectasis:

- **CXR:** Findings are fairly nonspecific, but CXR may reveal **"tram tracks,"** which are dilated airways crowded in parallel because of atelectasis. In cross-section, these produce **"ring shadows."**
- **High-resolution CT:** Offers good sensitivity for detecting bronchiectatic airways (ring shadows or tram tracks, depending on the CT plane of section).
- Sputum sample for bacterial and mycobacterial culture.
- CBC with differential.
- PFTs may show airflow **obstruction** from diffuse bronchiectasis.
- Sweat chloride levels for cystic fibrosis in cases of extensive lung involvement.
- Skin testing/serology/sputum culture for *Aspergillus* if ABPA is suggested by the history (eg, in an asthmatic person with proximal bronchiectasis).

TREATMENT

- Treatment has 4 goals: to treat/eliminate the underlying condition causing bronchiectasis, to improve clearance of secretions, to control infection, and to reverse airway obstruction.
- Administer appropriate treatment when a treatable cause is found.
- **Airway clearance techniques:** Include chest physical therapy, flutter devices (which produce oscillatory positive pressure to assist the clearance of sputum), and percussive vests. Mucolytic agents to thin secretions are controversial (eg, **DNase,** a medication that reduces mucus viscosity from DNA from degenerating neutrophils, is appropriate for cystic fibrosis but not for idiopathic bronchiectasis).
- **Antibiotics:** Used in exacerbations when there is an ↑ in sputum quantity and purulence. Empiric coverage may include amoxicillin, TMP-SMX, or quinolone with an aminoglycoside if *Pseudomonas aeruginosa* is present. Chronic cases may warrant more prolonged courses or may benefit from intermittent but regular courses of single or rotating antibiotics.
- **Bronchodilators:** Agents such as β-agonists and anticholinergics improve obstruction and aid in the clearance of secretions.
- **Surgical resection:** Currently less common with the advent of improvements in medical therapy, but may be indicated with severe focal disease.

KEY FACT

Bronchiectasis is the most common cause of hemoptysis.

KEY FACT

The most common organisms to colonize bronchiectatic lung: *Haemophilus influenzae, Staphylococcus aureus, Pseudomonas aeruginosa.*

CYSTIC FIBROSIS (CF)

The most common lethal autosomal-recessive disorder in whites, affecting 1 in every 3200 births; 1 in 25 is a carrier. It is caused by mutations affecting a sodium/chloride exchange channel (the cystic fibrosis transmembrane conductance regulator [CFTR]) that leads to multisystem dysfunction. Although CF is usually found in childhood, 7% of cases are diagnosed in adulthood, and because of improvements in therapy, > 38% of patients are now adults.

SYMPTOMS/EXAM

- Look for a history of failure to thrive, especially with recurrent infections of the airways (eg, with *Pseudomonas*).
- Suspect CF in infants with meconium ileus or intussusception.
- Patients may have a history of pancreatic insufficiency, recurrent pancreatitis, sinusitis, intestinal obstruction, chronic hepatic disease, vitamin (fat-soluble) deficiencies, male urogenital/infertility problems, or bronchiectasis. Symptoms include chronic or recurrent cough, sputum production, dyspnea, and wheezing.
- Exam may reveal digital clubbing, ↑ AP chest diameter, and apical crackles.

DIFFERENTIAL

COPD, asthma, α_1-antitrypsin deficiency, celiac disease, chronic sinusitis.

DIAGNOSIS

Because of the large number of CF mutations, 1° diagnosis is typically made on the basis of clinical criteria and laboratory analysis of sweat Cl^- values.

- **PFTs** may show a mixed obstructive and restrictive pattern.
- **ABGs** reveal hypoxemia with compensated respiratory acidosis in advanced disease.
- Sweat Cl^- concentrations > 60 mEq/L help distinguish CF from other lung diseases.
- Genotyping, measurement of nasal membrane potential difference, semen analysis, and assessment of pancreatic function aid in diagnosis.
- Sputum cultures frequently show *Staphylococcus aureus* or *Pseudomonas aeruginosa* infections.
- CXR may show hyperinflation early; other findings include peribronchial cuffing, mucous plugging, bronchiectasis (seen effectively on high-resolution CT), and ↑ interstitial markings (see Figure 8.7).

TREATMENT

- **Acute exacerbations:** Treat with bronchodilators, DNase to thin sputum, antibiotics (at least 2 with antipseudomonal coverage), and chest physical therapy.
- **Long-term therapy:**
  - Includes aerobic exercise, flutter devices, and external percussive vests to help with airway clearance.
  - Give pancreatic enzymes and the fat-soluble (A, D, E, and K) vitamins for malabsorption.
  - Nebulized DNase.
  - The only definitive treatment is double lung transplantation.

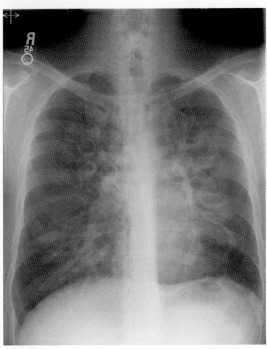

A

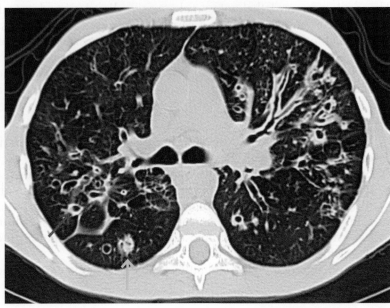

B

FIGURE 8.7. **Cystic fibrosis.** **(A)** Frontal CXR showing central cystic bronchiectasis *(arrow)* in a patient with CF. **(B)** Transaxial CT image showing cystic bronchiectasis *(red arrow)*, with some bronchi containing impacted mucus *(yellow arrow)*. (Reproduced, with permission, from USMLERx.com.)

INTERSTITIAL LUNG DISEASE (ILD)

A wide range of conditions (> 200) that are characterized by diffuse parenchymal lung involvement, often with significant morbidity and mortality. Conditions can be categorized as those that are predominantly inflammatory and fibrotic (eg, idiopathic pulmonary fibrosis) or those that are predominantly granulomatous (eg, sarcoidosis).

SYMPTOMS

- Patients may complain of onset of progressive **exertional dyspnea** or a persistent, nonproductive **cough.**
- Fatigue and weight loss are often seen. Chest pain, wheeze, and hemoptysis may be present but are less common.
- Acute presentation (days to weeks) is rare; subacute and **chronic presentations** are more common.
- Ask about smoking, occupational/environmental exposures, travel history, and a family history of lung conditions.

EXAM

- Exam may reveal tachypnea and **bibasilar end-inspiratory dry crackles** (seen in inflammatory ILD but less often in granulomatous states).
- "Inspiratory squeaks" are late inspiratory high-pitched rhonchi heard in bronchiolitis. Look at the digits for cyanosis with clubbing, which develops in late disease.

DIFFERENTIAL

- **Inflammation/fibrosis:** Think about asbestosis and other pneumoconioses, drug reaction (eg, amiodarone or chemotherapy), radiation exposure, idiopathic interstitial pneumonias, connective tissue diseases (eg, RA, SLE), ulcerative colitis/Crohn disease, heritable diseases (eg, neurofibromatosis, tuberous sclerosis).

- **Granulomatous disease:** Hypersensitivity pneumonitis, sarcoidosis, eosinophilic granulomatosis, Wegener granulomatosis, Churg-Strauss syndrome.

DIAGNOSIS

- **Labs:** Can help confirm suspected connective tissue disorders.
- **Imaging:**
  - **CXR:** Most often nonspecific. May show reticular or nodular opacities and volume loss, but often correlates poorly with the clinical or histopathologic stage of the disease. However, **honeycombing** may represent the pathologic findings of small cystic spaces and progressive fibrosis, signaling a poor prognosis.
  - **High-resolution CT:** Allows for early detection and confirmation of suspected ILD. Also serves to gauge the extent and distribution of the disease and in some cases may effectively characterize the condition and prevent the need for biopsy.
- **PFTs:** Typically show a restrictive pattern, with a ↓ TLC, FRC, and RV. The FEV_1/FVC ratio is usually normal or ↑. DL_{CO} is commonly ↓.
- **ABGs:** May be normal or reveal hypoxemia and respiratory alkalosis.
- **Lung biopsy:** The most effective way of confirming the diagnosis and assessing disease activity; can be transbronchial with fiberoptic bronchoscopy or open.

TREATMENT

Disease specific. The goals of treatment include permanent removal of the offending agent when known and suppression of the inflammatory process to limit further lung damage.

- O_2 for hypoxemia ($PaO_2 < 55$ mmHg) at rest and/or with exercise.
- **Glucocorticoids,** although there is a lack of evidence documenting their survival benefit.
- **Immunosuppressive agents** such as cyclophosphamide and azathioprine (variable success in some conditions).
- Consider lung transplantation if the ILD is severe and not responding to treatment.

ACUTE RESPIRATORY DISTRESS SYNDROME (ARDS)

Acute respiratory failure accompanied by refractory hypoxemia caused by diffuse alveolar capillary damage, leading to ↓ lung compliance and noncardiogenic pulmonary edema. ARDS may progress to extrapulmonary multisystem organ failure.

SYMPTOMS/EXAM

Presents with an acute onset (12–48 hours) of tachycardia, dyspnea, fever, cyanosis, ↑ work of breathing, and hypoxia refractory to O_2 therapy in the setting of a systemic disorder (sepsis, brain trauma) or direct lung injury (pneumonia, tuberculosis, diffuse alveolar hemorrhage, or aspiration).

DIFFERENTIAL

Pneumonia, *Pneumocystis jiroveci* pneumonia (previously *Pneumocystis carinii* pneumonia), multisystem organ failure, sepsis, toxic shock syndrome.

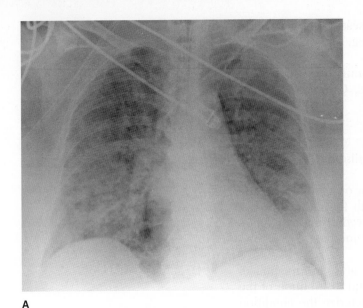

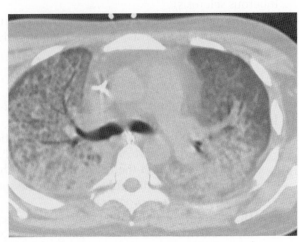

A   B

FIGURE 8.8.   Acute respiratory distress syndrome. (A) Frontal CXR showing patchy areas of airspace consolidation in a patient with ARDS. (B) Transaxial CT showing ground-glass opacity anteriorly and consolidations dependently in a patient with exudative-phase ARDS. (Reproduced, with permission, from Fauci AS, et al. *Harrison's Principles of Internal Medicine,* 17th ed. New York: McGraw-Hill, 2008, Figs. 262-2 and 262-4.)

DIAGNOSIS

- Clinically: Acute onset of respiratory distress.
- Swan-Ganz wedge pressure of < 18 mmHg, without evidence of cardiac origin.
- PaO_2-to-FiO_2 ratio ≤ 200.
- Diffuse infiltrates on CXR (see Figure 8.8).

TREATMENT

- Treat the underlying cause of ARDS.
- High FiO_2.
- Providing adequate sedation and analgesia allows patients to tolerate mechanical ventilation and to maintain a low oxygen consumption state.
- Low tidal volume strategy (protective lung strategy).

PLEURAL EFFUSION

Defined as an excess quantity of fluid in the pleural space caused either by ↑ pleural fluid formation or ↓ removal by the lymphatic system. The fluid may be **transudative** or **exudative** (see Table 8.13).

TABLE 8.13.   Pleural Effusion Classification

	PLEURAL-TO-SERUM PROTEIN (RATIO)	PLEURAL-TO-SERUM LDH (RATIO)	PLASMA LDH
Transudative	< 0.5, and	< 0.6, and	< 200
Exudative	> 0.5, or	> 0.6, or	> 200

- **Transudative effusion:** ↑ production of pleural fluid due to ↑ hydrostatic or ↓ oncotic pressures. Found in CHF, pulmonary embolism, cirrhosis, and nephrotic syndrome.
- **Exudative effusion:** ↑ production due to abnormal capillary permeability or ↓ lymphatic clearance of fluid. Found in malignancy, pneumonia, TB, pulmonary embolism, pancreatitis, esophageal rupture, collagen vascular disease, and chylothorax.

SYMPTOMS/EXAM

- Patients may experience dyspnea with large effusions. They may also complain of pleuritic pain and have symptoms of pneumonia such as productive cough, fever, and signs of consolidation.
- On exam, dullness to percussion, decreased fremitus, and ↓ breath sounds may be found on the affected side. Patients may show symptoms of their underlying disease process (cancer, pneumonia, CHF, cirrhosis).

DIAGNOSIS

- **CXR:** On upright PA and lateral films, blunting of costophrenic angles may be present with effusions > 250 mL. Decubitus films can differentiate pleural fluid from pleural scarring and can help determine if the fluid is loculated (see Figure 8.9).
- Obtain fluid via thoracentesis and send for protein, glucose, LDH, cell count, Gram stain, and culture. Also obtain pH, fungal and mycobacterial cultures, and cytology. In appropriate settings, look for pleural fluid amylase, triglycerides, cholesterol, and hematocrit. Grossly purulent fluid represents empyema.
- **Hemothorax:** A pleural hematocrit-to-peripheral hematocrit ratio > 0.5.
- **Pancreatitis, pancreatic pseudocyst, adenocarcinoma of lung, or esophageal rupture:** ↑ pleural fluid amylase.
- **Malignancy:** Cytology is only 50%–60% sensitive for detection.
- Pleural biopsy can help diagnose TB or cancer.

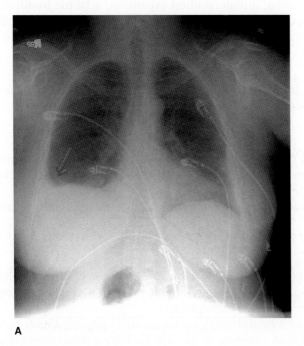
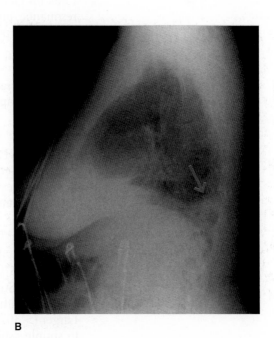

A   **B**

FIGURE 8.9.   Pleural effusion. PA (A) and lateral (B) CXRs show blunting of the right costophrenic sulcus *(arrows)*. (Reproduced, with permission, from USMLERx.com.)

TREATMENT

- **Transudative effusion:** Treat the underlying cause, and consider therapeutic thoracentesis if symptomatic. No further workup is required.
- **Exudative effusion:**
    - **Parapneumonic:** Give appropriate antibiotics for infections; insert a chest tube for drainage if complicated (eg, if pH < 7.2 **or** glucose < 60 mg/dL) or if empyema is present.
    - **Malignant:** Treat the underlying malignancy; repeat thoracentesis or chest tube insertion for symptom relief. Pleurodesis can ↓ reaccumulation of fluid.
    - **Hemothorax:** Rapid drainage via a large-bore chest tube to prevent fibrothorax.
    - **Tuberculous:** Usually resolves with treatment of TB.

KEY FACT

Any untreated pleural effusion can become infected, leading to empyema. Loculations also occur over time, requiring VATS drainage or surgical decortication.

PNEUMOTHORAX

The presence of air in the pleural space. Can be **spontaneous** (occurring without prior trauma to the thorax), **traumatic** (caused by penetrating or nonpenetrating chest injuries), **iatrogenic,** or **tension** (pressure in the pleural space is ⊕ throughout the respiratory cycle, as in mechanical ventilation or resuscitative efforts). In tension pneumothorax, ventilation is severely compromised and venous return can be ↓, reducing cardiac output and leading to a medical emergency. There are 2 types of spontaneous pneumothorax:

- **1°:** Occurs in individuals without clinically apparent lung disease (typically in tall, thin males 10–30 years of age, with smoking frequently a factor).
- **2°:** Found in patients with underlying lung disease such as COPD, asthma, CF, TB, *P jiroveci*, and ILD.

SYMPTOMS/EXAM

- Patients may complain of acute onset of unilateral chest pain and dyspnea. Exam may be normal in mild cases.
- Look for tachycardia, unilateral chest expansion, ↓ tactile fremitus, hyperresonance, and diminished breath sounds. Think tension pneumothorax if cyanosis, hypotension, and mediastinal or tracheal shift are present.

DIFFERENTIAL

Costochondritis, rib fracture, pulmonary embolism, infectious pneumonia, viral pleuritis, empyema, MI.

DIAGNOSIS

- On upright PA CXR, look for a thin visceral pleural line on expiration. In difficult or equivocal cases with a high degree of clinical suspicion, CT may be necessary (see Figure 8.10).
- ABGs, if obtained, may show hypoxemia and acute respiratory alkalosis.

TREATMENT

- Depends on the severity and nature of underlying disease.
- Small (< 15% of a hemithorax), stable pneumothoraces may resolve spontaneously. Supplemental O_2 may hasten resolution. Treat the associated pain with either NSAIDs or morphine.
- Larger (> 30% of a hemithorax), spontaneous 1° pneumothoraces respond to simple aspiration drainage of pleural air with a small-bore catheter or a larger small-bore chest tube with a 1-way valve. Follow patients with a daily CXR. Recurrent pneumothoraces will require pleurodesis.

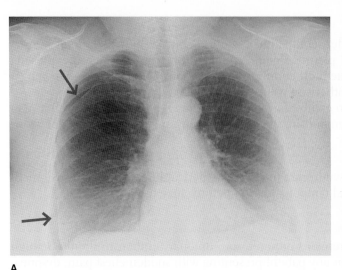
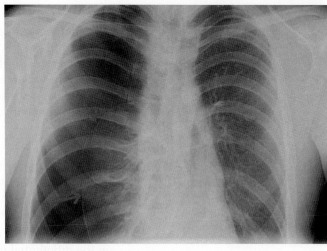

A   B

FIGURE 8.10. **Pneumothorax.** (A) Small right pneumothorax. (B) Right tension pneumothorax, with collapse of the right lung and shifting of mediastinal structures to the left. Arrows denote pleural reflections. (Reproduced, with permission, from USMLERx.com.)

- 2° **spontaneous pneumothorax,** large pneumothorax, tension pneumothorax, or those with severe symptoms should have a chest tube placed under water-seal drainage. Suction should be applied until the lung expands, and the chest tube should then be removed after cessation of the air leak.
- Thoracoscopy or open thoracotomy may be necessary in recurrences of spontaneous pneumothorax, bilateral pneumothorax, and failure of tube thoracostomy. Surgery allows for the resection of blebs as well as for pleurodesis by mechanical abrasion and insufflation of talc.

PULMONARY EMBOLISM

 A 66-year-old man presents with increasing shortness of breath over the last 24 hours. He has no cough, fever, hemoptysis, or history of lung disease. He denies any calf pain or swelling. There is no past history of cancer or thromboembolic disease. He just returned from a long flight to Europe. His physical exam is remarkable for a heart rate of 107 bpm. You suspect pulmonary embolism. What would be the next step to confirm your suspicion?

Obtain a D-dimer and imaging (a helical CT if the kidneys are normal), given his history of immobilization, lack of an alternative diagnosis, and heart rate.

An obstruction of the pulmonary vasculature that most commonly results from a deep venous thrombosis (DVT) that has embolized. Rarely, other substances can cause an obstruction, such as air, fat, and amniotic fluid. Symptoms can range from mild to complete circulatory collapse and death. Risk factors include **hypercoagulable states,** as in certain cancers; recent trauma; immobility (eg, postsurgery or long flights); pregnancy; and coagulation disorders such as factor V Leiden mutation and protein C, protein S, or antithrombin III deficiencies. **Venous stasis** and **endothelial damage** also predispose to DVT formation.

KEY FACT

If there is clinical suspicion of tension pneumothorax, initiate immediate needle thoracostomy with a 14- to 16-gauge needle in the second intercostal space at the midclavicular line. In an unstable patient, do not wait for x-ray confirmation. Tension pneumothorax will lead to decreased venous return, causing hypotension and then circulatory collapse.

KEY FACT

The risk factors for DVT/pulmonary embolism are contained in the Virchow triad: venous stasis, endothelial damage, and hypercoagulable states.

SYMPTOMS/EXAM

- Patients most often complain of acute dyspnea. With peripheral pulmonary embolism, pleuritic pain, cough, or hemoptysis may be present. Tachycardia is the most common sign on exam. Patients may often appear anxious but are otherwise well.
- Patients may also exhibit low-grade fever, JVD, or a loud P2. With a massive pulmonary embolism, syncope, hypotension, or cyanosis may be seen.

DIFFERENTIAL

MI/acute coronary syndrome, pneumonia, pericarditis, CHF, pleuritis, pneumothorax, pericardial tamponade, rib fracture, anxiety.

DIAGNOSIS

Accurate diagnosis remains difficult, so pulmonary embolism should be high on the differential for any patient presenting with sudden chest pain, dyspnea, and tachycardia in the setting of a normal CXR. Diagnostic modalities are as follows (see also Figure 8.11):

- **D-dimer:** Elevated in > 90% of patients with pulmonary embolism, but not specific, and elevations are also seen in patients with MI, sepsis, and most systemic illnesses. Its high ⊖ predictive value can help exclude pulmonary embolism. The test should not be used alone.

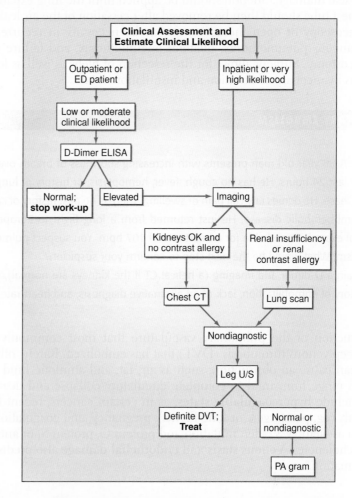

FIGURE 8.11. **Systematic approach to the diagnosis of pulmonary embolism.** (Reproduced, with permission, from Kasper DL, et al. *Harrison's Principles of Internal Medicine,* 16th ed. New York: McGraw-Hill, 2005: 1563.)

- **ABGs:** In pulmonary embolism, both P_{O_2} and P_{CO_2} will often $\downarrow$. Respiratory alkalosis and an $\uparrow$ A-a O_2 gradient may also be seen.
- **ECG:** Frequently reveals sinus tachycardia; less often shows a new-onset atrial fibrillation/flutter or an **S1Q3T3** pattern (an S wave in lead I, a Q wave in lead III, and an inverted T in III). T-wave inversion in leads V_1–V_4 reflects RV strain.
- **CXR:** A normal CXR in a dyspneic patient may suggest pulmonary embolism. **Westermark sign** (an area of lucency related to the abrupt tapering of the pulmonary vessel from the embolus, leading to vasoconstriction in the affected lobe), **Hampton hump** (a peripheral wedged-shaped density from the pulmonary infarct), pleural effusion, or atelectasis may be present.
- **Lower extremity ultrasound:** In suspected cases of pulmonary embolism, a finding of DVT establishes the need for treatment and may thus make invasive pulmonary angiography unnecessary (see Figure 8.11). Of all patients with pulmonary embolism, > 50% will not have evidence of DVT with imaging, and workup for pulmonary embolism should continue if there is a high clinical suspicion with a $\ominus$ ultrasound.
- **V/Q scan:** May show segmental regions of V/Q mismatch; results are expressed as normal-low, intermediate, and high probability for pulmonary embolism.
- **Spiral CT with contrast:** Effective for the diagnosis of large central pulmonary embolisms. Can detect peripheral thrombi up to 5th-order branches. In patients without pulmonary embolism, lung parenchymal images may reveal other diagnoses that may explain the presenting symptoms.
- **Pulmonary angiography:** The **gold standard,** but largely replaced by newer CT technology, given its invasive nature and risk.

TREATMENT

Options for management include anticoagulation to prevent further embolism, clot lysis with thrombolytic agents, and surgical removal of the clot.

- **Unfractionated heparin:** Administered IV. A weight-based nomogram for loading and maintenance improves the time needed to achieve adequate anticoagulation and $\downarrow$ bleeding risk. Drawbacks include the need for hospitalization and the risk of thrombocytopenia from heparin.
- **Low-molecular-weight heparin:** Suitable for lower-risk patients in place of unfractionated heparin. Can be used at home without the need for monitoring.
- **Warfarin:** Started promptly to achieve long-term anticoagulation; INR should be 2–3 before stopping heparin. Treatment duration is typically 6 months for a first episode when there is a reversible risk factor; 12 months after a first-episode idiopathic thrombus; and 6–12 months to indefinitely in those with recurrent disease or nonreversible risk factors.
- **IVC filters:** May be useful in patients who have failed anticoagulation or those who cannot be safely anticoagulated. Filters are associated with a higher risk of recurrent DVT.
- **Thrombolytic agents:** Reserved for patients with documented large central pulmonary embolism and hemodynamic instability.
- **Embolectomy:** Rarely performed, and usually a "last-ditch" effort to save a patient.

PULMONARY ARTERY HYPERTENSION (PAH)

An abnormal elevation in pulmonary artery pressure; defined as a resting pulmonary artery mean pressure of > 25 or > 30 with exercise. It can occur in isolation (idiopathic or 1° pulmonary hypertension) or may be 2° to a range of disorders, including connective tissue disease, advanced parenchymal lung disease, obstructive sleep apnea, congenital heart disease, advanced liver disease, HIV, chronic thromboembolic disease, and drugs. It is generally seen as a marker of advanced disease. 1° pulmonary hypertension is rare and occurs mostly in young to middle-aged women.

SYMPTOMS/EXAM

- Difficult to recognize in the early stages because symptoms and signs may be attributed to underlying disease. Patients may complain of dyspnea initially on exertion and then at rest. Dull, substernal chest pain may be present. Fatigue and syncope on exertion may occur.
- You may hear narrow splitting of S2, with a loud P2 best heard at the apex on auscultation. In advanced cases, tricuspid and pulmonary valve insufficiency and signs of right heart failure and cor pulmonale can be seen.

DIFFERENTIAL

LV systolic failure, LV diastolic dysfunction, causes of 2° pulmonary hypertension (see above).

DIAGNOSIS

- **Echocardiography:** May be the first test suggesting the presence of PAH. Most commonly reveals enlargement of the right ventricle and atrium, with tricuspid regurgitation. Allows for the estimation of pulmonary artery pressure as well as the evaluation of LV function, valvular disorders, and congenital heart disease.
- **Blood chemistries:** In cases of suspected pulmonary hypertension, CBC, a comprehensive metabolic panel, and coagulation studies may be obtained. Polycythemia may point to chronic severe hypoxemia. Abnormal LFTs may suggest underlying hepatic disease. Look for connective tissue diseases with targeted testing such as ANA, ESR, and RF. HIV testing should be considered for all patients.
- **ABGs:** May show hypoxemia with respiratory alkalosis.
- **ECG:** Look for RVH, rightward axis, RV strain, and right atrial enlargement.
- **CXR:** Reveals cardiomegaly with enlarged central pulmonary arteries. May show evidence of parenchymal lung disease such as COPD.
- **V/Q scan vs. CT:** CT is commonly employed to look for underlying pulmonary parenchymal disease as a cause for PAH.
- **Overnight oximetry:** Conduct in all patients to determine if hypoxemia worsens with sleep and requires treatment with supplemental O_2.
- **Sleep study:** Conduct in patients with symptoms consistent with sleep-disordered breathing, as this may potentially reverse PAH.
- **Right heart catheterization:** Can definitively measure pulmonary artery pressure, cardiac output, and pulmonary vascular resistance as well as left-to-right shunts and evidence of left heart dysfunction.

TREATMENT

Treatment is disease specific in 2° causes of PAH. Early detection is vital to disrupting the self-perpetuating cycle that can lead to rapid clinic progression.

- **Hypoxemic COPD:** Supplemental O_2 can slow progression.
- **High risk for thromboembolism:** Permanent anticoagulation in patients with chronic thomboembolic disease as a cause of their PAH.
- Vasodilatory agents (eg, calcium channel blockers, hydralazine, nitroglycerin) have yielded disappointing results in the treatment of PAH.

- **1° PAH:** Continuous long-term IV infusion of prostacyclin (via a portable pump) has improved survival.
- **PDE5 inhibitors** (sildenafil, tadalafil, vardenafil): Prolong vasodilatory effect of nitrous oxide, thereby improving pulmonary hemodynamics and exercise capacity in patients with idiopathic, hereditary, congenital, and HIV-related PAH.
- Bilateral lung transplantation may be necessary after failure of medical therapy.

SOLITARY PULMONARY NODULE

You are evaluating a 48-year-old man who requires a CXR for a physical exam through his work. He is otherwise healthy and denies a history of smoking. His CXR is clear with the exception of a 1-cm lesion with some central calcification in the left upper lobe. His PPD is negative. He has no prior chest films for comparison. What is your next step?

The patient has a solitary pulmonary nodule. Given its size and appearance, it is more likely to be benign, but because of his age and smoking history, you decide to obtain a CT scan. On CT the lesion has a benign appearance, so you decide on close observation of the lesion, with serial CT scan every 3–6 months for the next 2 years.

Defined as a solitary mass < 3 cm in diameter, surrounded by normal lung tissue and not associated with atelectasis, infiltrates, or adenopathy. Historically referred to as **"coin lesions."** Often found incidentally when a CXR is obtained for a different purpose. Lesions > 3 cm are pulmonary masses and are much more likely to be malignant (see Table 8.14).

SYMPTOMS/EXAM

- Patients are often asymptomatic but may have lung symptoms such as cough, hemoptysis, and dyspnea. Age, smoking history, environmental/infectious exposures, residence/travel, cancer history, and previous lung disease should be elicited.
- On exam, lungs may be entirely clear. A localized wheeze may indicate an endobronchial tumor. Look for clubbing and hypoxemia, and check for lymphadenopathy (if localized to the supraclavicular/scalene nodes, it raises concern for cancer; generalized lymphadenopathy suggests lymphoma or an infectious etiology).

TABLE 8.14. Pulmonary Nodule Classification

CHARACTERISTICS	LIKELY BENIGN	LIKELY MALIGNANT
Nodule	Very fast or no growth on serial imaging 2 years apart. Diffuse, central, or laminar "popcorn" calcification pattern.	> 2.5 cm. Spiculation. Upper lobe location.
Patient	Lifelong nonsmoker. < 30 years of age. No history of malignancy.	Smoking history. > 30 years of age. Prior diagnosis of cancer.

DIFFERENTIAL

- **Benign:** Infectious granulomas, viral infections (measles, CMV), *P jiroveci* pneumonia, lung abscess, hamartoma, chondroma, pulmonary infarct, AVM, sarcoidosis, pulmonary amyloidosis.
- **Malignant:** Bronchogenic carcinoma, bronchial carcinoid tumors, metastatic tumors (colorectal, breast, renal cell, testicular, malignant melanoma, sarcoma).

DIAGNOSIS

- Typically found incidentally on CXR. Figure 8.12 shows a diagnostic algorithm. Lesions with > 1 malignant feature should be further evaluated with CT.
- Benign patterns on imaging include a **"bull's eye"** pattern of granulomas, a **"popcorn"** pattern of hamartomas, and a diffuse, dense central core of calcification. Lesions lacking calcium or having a stippled appearance or eccentric location raise more concern for malignancy.
- **Serial CXRs:** A **comparison** of serial CXRs can check for the stability of the lesion. No change in lesion size in 2 years indicates that the lesion is likely benign. The larger the lesion, the more likely it is to be malignant (although lesions < 1 cm have a 15% chance of malignancy).
- **Chest CT:** Best for further evaluating solitary pulmonary nodules, giving a

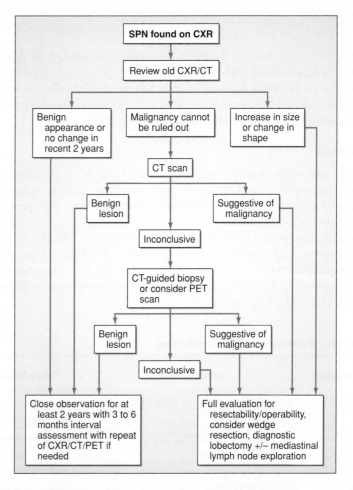

FIGURE 8.12.   **Evaluation of the solitary pulmonary nodule.** (Reproduced, with permission, from Fauci AS, et al. *Harrison's Principles of Internal Medicine,* 17th ed. New York: McGraw-Hill, 2008, Fig. 85-2.)

better indication of size, calcification pattern, and nodule density. IV contrast can further aid diagnosis and can assess for mediastinal adenopathy.

- **PET scans:** Can be used to better evaluate indeterminate lesions; sensitivity and specificity are 85%–95% and 75%–85%, respectively.

TREATMENT

- Patients with solitary pulmonary nodules who are felt to be low risk (eg, nonsmoking patients, those < 30 years of age, and those with smaller lesions with a more benign appearance on radiography) can be followed with serial CTs every 3 months for 1 year and then yearly.
- Patients who are felt to be at higher risk for cancer (eg, patients with a history of cigarette smoking; those ≥ 30 years of age; and those with larger lesions, lack of calcification, chest symptoms, interval growth of a lesion, or a ⊕ PET scan) require a histologic diagnosis either via resection, or, for those with higher preoperative risk, via biopsy by video-assisted thoracoscopy or transthoracic fine-needle biopsy.

SARCOIDOSIS

> A 47-year-old African-American woman presents with a several-week history of fatigue and malaise. She complains of low-grade fevers, shortness of breath with exertion, and cough. Her exam is unremarkable. Her CXR shows bilateral hilar adenopathy, and her PPD is negative. What condition may explain her symptoms, and what is the next step in diagnosis?
>
> You suspect sarcoidosis and refer her for bronchoscopy for biopsy of her lesions.

Defined as a chronic, idiopathic multisystem disease distinguished by accumulation of T cells and mononuclear phagocytes in affected organs, along with noncaseating granulomas and disturbance in normal tissue architecture. The lung is the most commonly affected organ, with skin, eye, liver, and lymph node involvement also common. The disorder can be acute, subacute and self-limiting, or a chronic waxing and waning disease occurring over many years. In the United States, blacks are affected more than 10 times as often as whites.

SYMPTOMS/EXAM

- Patients may be asymptomatic. However, they may also complain of fatigue, malaise, weight loss, and fever. Commonly, patients present with symptoms based on the involved organ. For the lungs, this may include exertional dyspnea; dry, nonproductive cough; and vague chest pain.
- Exam findings are usually normal but may sometimes include crackles. Lymphadenopathy may be present.

DIFFERENTIAL

TB, lymphoma, histoplasmosis, coccidioidomycosis, idiopathic pulmonary fibrosis, pneumoconiosis, syphilis, HIV, berylliosis.

DIAGNOSIS

- A diagnosis of exclusion. Diagnosed when clinical presentation and radiographic studies suggest the diagnosis and granulomatous inflammation is detected in an involved organ. Biopsy is necessary to exclude infection or malignancy.

- The H&P should focus on occupational and environmental exposures and on organs that are commonly affected, such as the lung, skin, eyes, and lymph nodes.
- CXR may show **bilateral hilar adenopathy,** but this is a nonspecific finding. In general, an abnormal CXR with a normal exam should make you think sarcoidosis. PFTs show a restrictive or mixed restrictive-obstructive pattern (if granuloma is obstructing airways), with a $\downarrow \mathrm{DL_{CO}}$.
- **Fiberoptic bronchoscopy with transbronchial biopsy** most commonly makes the diagnosis, showing a "sarcoid granuloma," which is a **well-formed noncaseating epithelioid cell** granuloma surrounded by a rim of fibroblasts and lymphocytes.
- Other tests supportive of (but not sufficient for) diagnosis include ACE level and gallium scan.
- Get PFTs, ECG, ophthalmologic evaluation, CBC, a complete metabolic panel, tuberculin skin test, urinalysis, chest radiograph, and 24-hour urine calcium at baseline.
- On follow-up, periodic screening for other organ involvement is appropriate, along with specialist referral as indicated.

TREATMENT

Systemic corticosteroids as first-line therapy; methotrexate as a first alternative.

LUNG CANCER

The leading cause of cancer death in the United States, with a 5-year survival rate of 15%. The various histologic types of bronchogenic carcinoma include **squamous cell carcinoma, adenocarcinoma, large cell carcinoma,** and **small cell carcinoma.** For purposes of staging and treatment, small cell lung cancer (SCLC) is separated from the 3 other subtypes (labeled together as non–small cell lung cancer [NSCLC]).

- Adenocarcinoma is the most common lung cancer, the most common lung cancer in women, and peripherally located.
- Squamous cell carcinoma starts centrally, may be cavitary, and is associated with hypercalcemia.

SYMPTOMS/EXAM

Major risk factor is tobacco use. Other risk factors include radon and asbestos exposure.

- Up to 15% of patients may be asymptomatic. Symptoms, when present, are a reflection of tumor location.
- With **central tumors,** patients may complain of cough, hemoptysis, wheeze and stridor, dyspnea, and fever/productive cough if postobstructive pneumonitis is present.
- **Peripheral** tumor growth may cause pleuritic chest pain, cough, and dyspnea.
- **Regional** spread of tumor may cause tracheal obstructive symptoms, dysphagia (from esophageal compression), or hoarseness; hemidiaphragm elevation with dyspnea; or Horner syndrome (ptosis, miosis, and anhidrosis on the unilateral side of face) from nerve compressions.
- Malignant effusions can lead to dyspnea.
- **Extrathoracic** metastatic disease is common and can affect nearly every organ system.

KEY FACT

Squamous **c**ell carcinoma and **s**mall **c**ell carcinomas start **c**entrally (think "sssssss"), whereas adenocarcinomas are more peripheral in origin. Large-cell carcinomas can present centrally or peripherally.

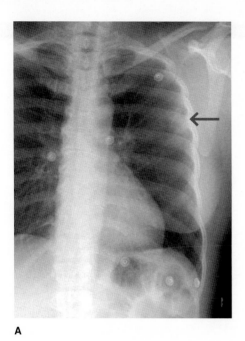
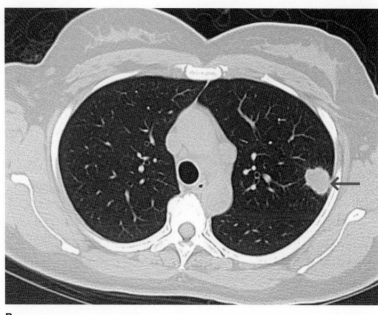

A   B

FIGURE 8.13.   **Lung cancer.** Lung cancer (*arrows*) on (**A**) frontal CXR and (**B**) transaxial CT. (Reproduced, with permission, from USMLERx.com.)

- **Paraneoplastic syndromes** can lead to anorexia, cachexia, weight loss, fever, and suppressed immunity, whereas **endocrine syndromes** can lead to symptoms related to hypercalcemia, hypophosphatemia, and hyponatremia.

DIAGNOSIS

- Screening of high-risk individuals with sputum cytology and CXR has not been shown to improve survival rate. Trials aimed at exploring screening with chest CT are currently underway. When the history/exam and screening tests suggest lung cancer, tissue diagnosis is necessary.
- A biopsy can be performed with fiberoptic bronchoscopy, mediastinoscopy, surgical resection, percutaneous biopsy of an enlarged lymph node or pleural lesion, FNA under CT guidance, or cytology of a malignant pleural effusion (see Figure 8.13).

TREATMENT

Based on diagnosis and staging:

- SCLC shows early hematogenous spread and an aggressive course and is rarely amenable to resection. With limited disease, thoracic radiation may improve survival.
- NSCLC is slower to spread and more likely to be cured with early resection. Higher stages require multimodality therapy with chemotherapy and radiation.
- **Palliative therapy** can take many forms and may assist in relieving symptoms, whether it is photoresection with laser, external beam radiation, resection of brain metastases, or aggressive pain control in advanced disease. Referral to a palliative care specialist is recommended in advanced disease, along with appropriate referral to hospice programs.

NOTES

CHAPTER 9

Nephrology

Kerry Kay, MD, MPH

Diagnostic Testing

The first steps in the evaluation of kidney disease are the measurement of serum creatinine and the urinalysis (UA). Additional laboratory tests and imaging can also assist in the diagnosis and treatment of disease. Table 9.1 summarizes the various types of diagnostic tests available in the evaluation of kidney disease and their indications. Table 9.2 reviews urinary casts as part of the UA.

TABLE 9.1. **Types and Uses of Diagnostic Tests**

DIAGNOSTIC TEST	TYPES	MEASUREMENTS	INDICATIONS
Serum creatinine		Produced in skeletal muscle metabolism and filtered by the kidney. Elevated in renal dysfunction. Higher in muscular people and lower in elderly and pregnant women. Can be elevated by medications such as ACE inhibitors, ARBs, cimetidine, trimethoprim, aminoglycosides.	First step in evaluating kidney disease. Monitor kidney function. Used in determination of BUN-to-creatinine ratio, fractional excreation of sodium or urea.
UA	Random specimen, midstream collection ("clean catch"), first morning collection, bladder catheterization.	Dipstick testing: specific gravity, pH, protein, hemoglobin, glucose, ketones, bilirubin, nitrite, leukocyte esterase. Microscopy: crystals, cells, casts, infecting organisms, and oval fatty bodies.	First test in patients with kidney disease along with serum creatinine. Screening in patients with family history of kidney disease. Other indications: infection, dehydration, diabetic ketoacidosis, proteinuria, hematuria, rhabodmyolysis, nephrolithasis.
Urine culture	Midstream clean catch, bladder catheterization, suprapubic aspiration.	> 100,000 colony-forming units/mL of one type of bacteria indicates infection in a midstream, clean catch specimen. Growth of several types of bacteria indicates contamination. Susceptibility testing may guide antibiotic therapy.	Infection. Usually ordered with urinalysis.
24-hour urine collection		Urine protein, creatinine, electrolytes, urine volume.	Quantitative testing for proteinuria. Kidney function monitoring for patients with known kidney disease. Early detection of kidney damage in the form of proteinuria. Diabetic nephropathy. Preeclampsia. Nephrotic syndrome. Multiple myeloma.

TABLE 9.1. Types and Uses of Diagnostic Tests *(continued)*

DIAGNOSTIC TEST	TYPES	MEASUREMENTS	INDICATIONS
Spot urine protein-to-creatinine ratio		Determines ratio of urine protein to creatinine of one urine sample.	Increasingly popular way to measure proteinuria; evidence shows correlation between 24-hour urine collection and spot urine protein creatinine. Proteinuria: > 3.0 mg/mg considered nephrotic range proteinuria; ratio < 0.2 is normal. Preeclampsia: > 0.2 mg/mg.
Renal ultrasound (Figures 9.1A, B)	Can include Doppler ultrasound of renal arteries and veins.	Measures thickness of renal cortex, echogenicity of kidneys, distention of urinary collecting system, kidney size, comparison of bilateral kidneys.	Hydronephrosis. Renal failure of unknown etiology. Renal abscess. Urinary calculus. Identifying and characterizing renal cysts or masses. Part of evaluation of malignancy in patients > 50 years of age and with hematuria. Localizing kidney for percutaneous procedures. Renal artery stenosis, arterial or venous thrombosis, embolus.
Intravenous pyelogram (IVP) (Figure 9.2)	X-ray of the kidneys, ureters, and bladder before and after administration of IV contrast; less frequently used because of advances in CT technology.	Characterizes structural disorders.	Obstruction such as nephrolithiasis, BPH. Tumors such as renal cell carcinoma (RCC). Polycystic kidney disease. Medullary sponge kidney. Papillary necrosis.
Computed tomography (CT)	Noncontrast and contrast-enhanced CT.	Visualizes anatomy, obstruction, infection, size, growths in the kidneys and the collecting system.	Noncontrast helical CT scan is the gold standard for detecting renal stones (95% sensitivity and 98% specificity in acute flank pain). Identifying abnormalities found on ultrasound or IVP; eg, simple vs. complex cysts. Evaluating/staging RCC. Part of evaluation for malignancy in patients > 50 years of age with hematuria.
Magnetic resonance imaging (MRI) (Figure 9.3)		Similar to CT scan but superior in soft tissue contrast, which improves detection and characterization of renal lesions.	100% sensitive and 96%–98% specific for renal artery stenosis; has decreased the role of renal artery angiography. Differentiation of benign lesions from malignant lesions in patients who cannot undergo CT. Evaluating/staging RCC.

(continues)

TABLE 9.1.   Types and Uses of Diagnostic Tests *(continued)*

DIAGNOSTIC TEST	TYPES	MEASUREMENTS	INDICATIONS
Voiding cystourethrography (VCUG)	Administration of contrast material into the bladder, followed by serial radiographs of the pelvis and abdomen during voiding.	Detects abnormalities of the bladder and urethra, vesicoureteral reflux, urine extravasation in bladder ruptures, obstructions or strictures of the urethra.	Children with UTI to evaluate for vesicoureteral reflux. Bladder obstruction. Bladder rupture.
Retrograde urethrogram	Insertion of catheter into the fossa navicularis of the distal penile urethra and injection of contrast under fluoroscopy.	Detects abnormalities of the anterior urethra, such as stricture or traumatic injury.	Suspected anterior urethral stricture or traumatic injury.
Renal biopsy[a,b]			Diagnosing unexplained acute or chronic kidney disease. Guiding future treatment in established disease. Acute nephritic syndrome. Determining renal involvement in systemic diseases; eg, SLE, Goodpasture syndrome, Wegener granulomatosis.

[a]Contraindications to kidney biopsy: The finding of kidneys < 9 cm indicates irreversible changes; multiple bilateral cysts; renal neoplasm; uncorrectable bleeding disorders; severe uncontrolled hypertension; pyelonephritis or abscess.

[b]Complications of kidney biopsy: Bleeding into collecting system, below renal capsule, or into perinephric space. Pain due to obstruction of ureter by a blood clot or renal capsular stretching due to a hematoma. Infection. AV fistulas. "Page kidney," or chronic hypertension with persistent activation of renin-angiotensin system from a large subcapsular hematoma. Consider postprocedure observation for 24 hours, since 90% of complications occur within this time.

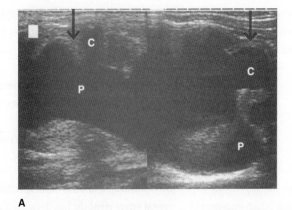
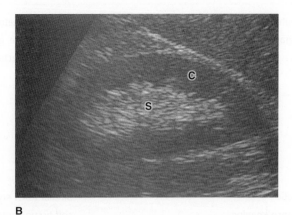

A   **B**

FIGURE 9.1.   Renal ultrasound. (**A**) Severe hydronephrosis. Renal pelvices are dilated (P). Renal calyces (C). Arrows show severely thinned renal cortices. (**B**) Normal renal ultrasound.

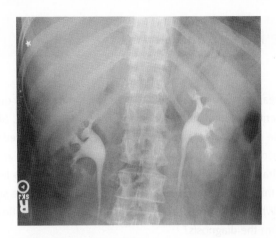

FIGURE 9.2. **Normal intravenous pyelogram.** (Reproduced, with permission, from Chen MYM, Pope Jr TL, Ott DJ. *Basic Radiology.* New York: McGraw-Hill, 2004.)

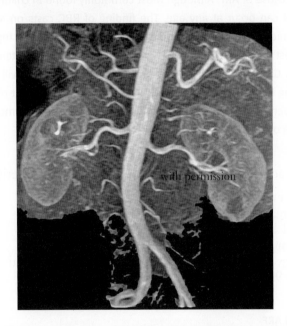

FIGURE 9.3. **Magnetic resonance angiography of the abdominal aorta with normal bilateral renal arteries.**

TABLE 9.2. **Significance of Specific Urinary Casts**

Type	Significance
Hyaline casts	Concentrated urine, febrile disease, after strenuous exercise, in the course of diuretic therapy (not indicative of renal disease).
RBC casts	Glomerulonephritis.
WBC casts	Pyelonephritis, interstitial nephritis (indicative of infection or inflammation).
Renal epithelial cell casts	Acute tubular necrosis, interstitial nephritis.
Muddy granular casts	Nonspecific; can represent acute tubular necrosis.
Broad, waxy casts	Chronic renal failure (indicative of stasis in enlarged collecting tubules).

(Adapted, with permission, from Tierney LM, et al. *Current Medical Diagnosis & Treatment,* 45th ed. New York: McGraw-Hill, 2006, Table 22-1.)

Acute Renal Failure (ARF)

 A 25-year-old woman presents to your clinic with a 2-day onset of fatigue, ↓ appetite, swollen feet, and scant, cola-colored urine. She reports an episode of sore throat and fever 2 weeks ago that resolved without treatment. On physical examination, her blood pressure is elevated at 165/102, she appears dehydrated, and you note periorbital edema. She has 3+ lower extremity edema to her thighs. UA shows blood and protein. RBC casts are seen on microscopic exam. What is the most likely diagnosis and what additional laboratory tests can confirm the diagnosis?

This presentation is consistent with poststreptococcal glomerulonephritis (PSGN), one cause of ARF. Although most commonly found in children 2–6 years of age, PSGN can occur at any age. The finding of RBC casts on microscopy is pathognomonic for glomerulonephritis. Additional confirmatory tests include a rapid strep test and/or throat culture, which may be ⊖ by presentation. ASO titer would be ⊕. C3 complement level is low. BUN and creatinine will be elevated, demonstrating the acute renal failure. It is not known if treatment of the primary infection prevents PSGN. Treatment of PSGN is symptomatic, with more than 95% of patients recovering completely in 3–4 weeks.

> **KEY FACT**
>
> Oliguria is defined as < 400 mL urine output in 24 hours and anuria as < 100 mL urine output in 24 hours in adults. A urine output of < 0.5 mL/kg/hr in children or < 1 mL/kg/hr in infants is considered oliguria.

Also known as acute kidney injury. Defined by the following criteria:

- ↑ in serum creatinine 0.5 mg/dL above baseline.
- 50% ↑ in creatinine above baseline.
- 50% GFR ↓ below baseline.
- Necessity for acute renal replacement therapy.
- The etiology of ARF is categorized as prerenal, intrarenal, and postrenal (see Tables 9.3 through 9.5).

TABLE 9.3. Clinical Presentation and Diagnosis of Prerenal ARF

CAUSES AND SUGGESTIVE CLINICAL FEATURES	UA AND OTHER CONFIRMATORY TESTS
Volume depletion: History of vomiting, diarrhea, ↓ PO intake, diuretic use, hemorrhage, burns.	Hyaline casts on microscopy (see Table 9.2).
Symptoms: Thirst, hypotension, tachycardia, dry mucous membranes.	$Fe_{Na} < 1\%$.
Low-output states: History of CHF, cirrhosis, severe valvular disease, hepatorenal syndrome, sepsis, shock.	$Fe_{Urea} < 35\%$.
Symptoms: Pulmonary edema, ↑ JVP, ascites.	BUN-to-creatinine ratio > 20:1.
Medications: NSAIDs, ACEIs, ARBs.	Urine specific gravity > 1.020.
	Urine osmolality > 500 mOsm/kg.
	$U_{Na} < 10$ mmol/L.
	Rapid resolution of ARF with restoration of renal perfusion, such as with fluid bolus or, in the case of CHF, diuresis.

TABLE 9.4. Clinical Presentation and Diagnosis of Intrarenal ARF

CAUSES AND SUGGESTIVE CLINICAL FEATURES	UA AND OTHER CONFIRMATORY TESTS
TUBULAR	
Acute tubular necrosis (ATN):	Muddy granular casts (see Figure 9.4, Table 9.2).
90% of intrarenal ARF is due to ATN.	Renal epithelial cell casts (see Table 9.2).
Tubular injury is caused by ischemia or nephrotoxins.	$Fe_{Na} > 1\%$.
Ischemic:	$Fe_{Urea} > 35\%$.
Prolonged prerenal failure, hemorrhage, hypotension, sepsis.	Urine Osm < 350 mOsm/kg
Toxic:	(failure to concentrate urine, even in oliguria).
Nephrotoxic drugs and substances (see Table 9.6),	$U_{Na} > 30$ mmol/L.
rhabdomyolysis, tumor lysis, multiple myeloma, contrast	In rhabdomyolysis: Cola-colored urine, heme-$\oplus$ urine dipstick with
nephropathy.	no RBCs on microscopy, $\uparrow$ serum creatine kinase, myoglobin.
	In tumor lysis: $\uparrow$ calcium and uric acid.
	In multiple myeloma: SPEP/UPEP.
INTERSTITIAL	
Acute interstitial nephritis (AIN):	WBC casts (see Figure 9.5, Table 9.2), WBCs on urine microscopy.
Due to allergic reaction to drug (see Table 9.6):	Urine eosinophils.
Symptoms: Fever, rash, or arthralgias.	Interstitial inflammation on renal biopsy. Treatment includes
Due to infection:	withdrawal or eradication of the offending agent and
Pyelonephritis, HIV, CMV, EBV, HBV, HCV.	corticosteroids.
Due to autoimmune disorders:	
Wegener granulomatosis, sarcoidosis, SLE, Sjögren syndrome.	
GLOMERULAR	
Glomerulonephritis/vasculitis:	Finding of RBC casts on urine microscopy is pathognomonic (see
Symptoms: Hypertension, hematuria, edema, oliguria.	Table 9.2).
Post infectious (PIGN):	Urine microscopy can also show:
Poststreptococcal glomerulonephritis (PSGN): 2–3 weeks after	Granular casts, RBCs and WBCs, dysmorphic red cells, hematuria,
streptococcal pharyngitis or skin infection.	proteinuria (see Table 9.2).
Endocarditis:	$\oplus$ blood cultures and vegetations on echocardiogram for
Symptoms: Fever, new heart murmur.	endocarditis.
Risk factors: Abnormal heart valve, IV drug use, recent dental	Consider the additional tests:
procedure.	ASO titers (PSGN), complement levels (low in SLE, PIGN/PSGN,
Other:	MPGN, cryoglobulinemia).
Goodpasture syndrome.	ANA, anti-dsDNA, anti-Smith antibodies (SLE).
Wegener granulomatosis.	Cryoglobulins, RPR, HCV, HBV, HIV (MPGN).
Churg-Strauss syndrome.	c-ANCA, anti-PR3 (Wegener granulomatosis).
Polyarteritis nodosa (PAN).	p-ANCA, anti-MPO (Churg-Strauss syndrome, PAN).
SLE.	Anti-GBM (Goodpasture syndrome).
IgA nephropathy.	Renal biopsy for definitive diagnosis.
Cryoglobulinemia.	
Membranoproliferative glomerulonephritis (MPGN).	
Henoch-Schönlein purpura.	
Medications: Gold, penicillamine.	

(continues)

TABLE 9.4.   Clinical Presentation and Diagnosis of Intrarenal ARF *(continued)*

CAUSES AND SUGGESTIVE CLINICAL FEATURES	UA AND OTHER CONFIRMATORY TESTS
VASCULAR	

CAUSES AND SUGGESTIVE CLINICAL FEATURES	UA AND OTHER CONFIRMATORY TESTS
Microvascular:	UA may be normal or RBCs may be seen; mild proteinuria or, rarely,
Hemolytic-uremic syndrome (HUS).	RBC casts or granular casts (see Table 9.2).
E coli O157:H7.	In HUS/TTP: Anemia, thrombocytopenia, schistocytes on blood
Thrombotic thrombocytopenic purpura (TTP):	smear, ↑ LDH, ↑ bilirubin, ↓ haptoglobin, stool culture, renal
Symptoms: Neurological symptoms, fever, renal failure,	failure.
petechiae, jaundice.	In DIC: Anemia, schistocytes, ↑ D-dimer, ↑ fibrinogen, ↑ PT, PTT,
Disseminated intravascular coagulation (DIC):	↓ platelets.
Sepsis, shock, malignancy, obstetric complications, placental	In preeclampsia: BP > 140/90, proteinuria > 300 mg, ↑ LFTs, low
abruption, amniotic fluid embolus, eclampsia.	platelets.
Symptoms: Bleeding, petechiae.	
Preeclampsia.	
Symptoms: Headache, RUQ pain, pulmonary edema, scotomata.	
Macrovascular:	
Renal artery thrombosis:	
History of atrial fibrillation, aortic dissection, recent MI; most	Mild proteinuria and occasional RBCs; ↑ LDH.
often in elderly.	Renal arteriogram.
Symptoms: Flank or abdominal pain, sudden-onset hypertension.	↓ antithrombin III.
Renal vein thrombosis:	
Seen in patients with nephrotic syndrome; pulmonary embolism.	Proteinuria and hematuria.
Symptoms: Flank pain, anasarca.	IVC and renal vein imaging, ultrasound, or CT scan showing ↑ in
	renal size.
Atheroembolism:	
Age usually > 50 years; often in ICU patients; recent surgery/	Eosinophilia, low complement levels, skin biopsy, renal biopsy.
procedure (angiography), administration of thrombolytics.	
Symptoms: Acute arrhythmia, hypertension, edema, rash (livedo	
reticularis, subcutaneous nodules, palpable purpura).	

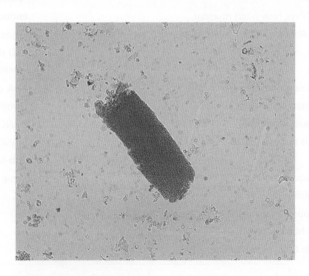

FIGURE 9.4.   Muddy brown cast. (Reproduced, with permission, from Le T, et al. *First Aid for the Internal Medicine Boards,* 1st ed. New York: McGraw-Hill, 2006: 451.)

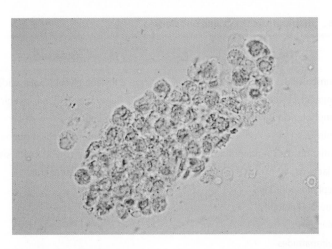

FIGURE 9.5. **White blood cell cast.** (Reproduced, with permission, from Knoop KJ, et al. *Atlas of Emergency Medicine*, 2nd ed. New York: McGraw-Hill, 2002: 676.)

EXAM/DIAGNOSIS

- Review history and medications; focus the physical exam on clinical volume status, including orthostatic changes, intake, and output.
- Obtain UA with microscopy. See Table 9.2 for the significance of various urinary casts in ARF.
- If the patient is oliguric and **not** using diuretics, determine the fractional excretion of sodium (Fe_{Na}):

$$Fe_{Na} = [(urine_{Na} \times plasma_{Cr}) / (plasma_{Na} \times urine_{Cr})] \times 100$$

A value < 1% suggests prerenal ARF. A value > 1% suggests acute tubular necrosis.

- If the patient is oliguric and **is** using diuretics, determine the fractional excretion of urea (Fe_{Urea}):

$$\text{Fractional excretion of urea} = [(urine_{Urea} \times plasma_{Cr}) / (urine_{Cr} \times plasma_{Urea})] \times 100\%$$

A value < 35% suggests prerenal ARF. A value > 50% suggests acute tubular necrosis.

TABLE 9.5.   Clinical Presentation and Diagnosis of Postrenal ARF

CAUSES/SUGGESTIVE CLINICAL FEATURES	UA/OTHER CONFIRMATORY TESTS
Urethral obstruction:	Frequently normal UA.
Prostatic hypertrophy.	Possible hematuria.
Urethral stricture.	Postvoid residual > 100 mL.
Bladder, pelvic or retroperitoneal neoplasm.	Hydronephrosis on renal ultrasound, IVP, retrograde
Calculi.	or anterograde pyelography, CT.
Crystals, myeloma light chains.	Other testing: PSA, SPEP, UPEP.
Neurogenic bladder.	
Anticholinergics, narcotics causing urinary retention.	
Symptoms: Lower urinary tract symptoms, abdominal or flank pain, palpable	
bladder, enlarged prostate, oliguria/anuria.	

TABLE 9.6.   Nephrotoxic Drugs and Substances

DRUGS	SUBSTANCES
Antimicrobials:	Ethylene glycol (oxalic acid)
Aminoglycosides	Heavy metals (lead, arsenic)
Amphotericin B	Hemoglobin
Antivirals	Myeloma light chain deposition
Antiparasitics (pentamidine)	Myoglobin (rhabdomyolysis)
β-lactams	Radiocontrast agents
Cephalosporins	Uric acid
Fluoroquinolones	Cocaine
Rifampin	
Sulfonamides	
ACEIs	
Anti-inflammatories:	
NSAIDs	
COX-2 inhibitors	
Other:	
Phenytoin	
Allopurinol	
Cimetidine	
Furosemide	
Thiazide diuretics	
Lithium chemotherapeutics	

MNEMONIC

Indications for emergent dialysis:

AEIOU

Acidosis
Electrolytes (hyperkalemia)
Ingestions
Overload (pulmonary edema)
Uremia

- Renal ultrasound to rule out obstruction.
- See Tables 9.3 through 9.5 for the clinical features and diagnostic tests.

TREATMENT

- Identify and treat the underlying cause.
- Ensure renal perfusion by maintaining adequate intravascular volume.
- Refer for dialysis in accordance with the **AEIOU** mnemonic.
- Eliminate further exposure to nephrotoxic drugs and substances (Table 9.6).
- Monitor and correct electrolyte abnormalities and urine output.
- Seek a urology consult for postrenal etiologies.

Chronic Kidney Disease (CKD)

CKD is clinically defined in the following 2 ways:

- Kidney damage for ≥ 3 months. Damage identified by abnormal kidney structure on imaging studies or by abnormal kidney function on blood tests or UA.
- A GFR < 60 mL/min +/– evidence of kidney damage for ≥ 3 months.
- Divided into 5 stages. See Table 9.7.
- Kidney failure, or end-stage renal disease (ESRD), is defined as a GFR < 15 mL/min and/or a requirement for renal replacement therapy in the form of dialysis or transplantation.

TABLE 9.7.   Stages of Chronic Kidney Disease

STAGE	DESCRIPTION	GFR (mL/min/1.73m²)
1	Kidney damage with normal or ↑ GFR	≥ 90
2	Mild reduction in GFR	60–89
3	Moderate reduction in GFR	30–59
4	Severe reduction in GFR	15–29
5	Kidney failure	< 15 or dialysis

EXAM

Screening for CKD is recommended for high-risk patients—eg, those with diabetes, family history, hypertension, recurrent UTIs, urinary obstruction, or systemic disease that can affect the kidneys.

- Screen all patients > 60 years of age.
- Screening methods include the following:
  - Serum creatinine to calculate GFR.
  - UA for proteinuria.
  - Renal imaging in patients with a history of urinary obstruction, recurrent UTIs, vesicoureteral reflux, family history of polycystic kidney disease.

SIGNS AND SYMPTOMS

Patients in stage 1–3 CKD are usually asymptomatic. Symptoms typically manifest in stages 4–5 when GFR ↓ to < 30 mL/min. Signs and symptoms are those associated with complications of CKD: hyperkalemia (cardiac arrhythmia), anemia (fatigue), renal bone disease, hypocalcemia (tetany, muscle spasms), volume overload (hypertension, pulmonary edema, extremity edema), uremia (pericarditis, restless leg syndrome, anorexia, nausea, vomiting, dry skin, pruritus, fatigue, platelet dysfunction).

DIAGNOSIS

To specify the cause of CKD, evaluate the following factors:

- Patient history, serum creatinine, GFR, UA and microscopy, and renal imaging.
- Spot urine protein-to-creatinine ratio or 24-hour protein collection to quantify proteinuria. If etiology is not clear, further workup may be indicated to evaluate for causes of kidney disease, such as hepatitis B and C, syphilis, HIV, collagen vascular diseases, and multiple myeloma.
- Biopsy is indicated if cause cannot be determined or if result would change treatment.

TREATMENT

- The following measures have been proven to **slow the progression of CKD:**
  - **Reduction of proteinuria with ACEIs/ARBs:** Beneficial for both diabetic and nondiabetic nephropathy.
  - **Treatment of hypertension:** Treat hypertension to < 130/80 if normal urine protein; treat to < 125/75 if proteinuria > 1 g/24 hours.
  - Glycemic control in diabetic patients—HbA$_{1c}$ goal < 7%.

KEY FACT

Diabetes and hypertension are the 2 main causes of chronic kidney disease.

- Avoidance of nephrotoxins.
- Treatment methods that **may prove beneficial** include lipid lowering to an LDL target < 100 mg/dL, treatment of anemia, protein restriction, and smoking cessation.
- Patients with stage 3–4 CKD should be periodically monitored with the following lab studies:
  - Hemoglobin/hematocrit
  - RBC indices
  - Reticulocyte count
  - Iron studies
  - Fecal occult blood test
  - Serum electrolytes
  - Calcium, phosphorus, and PTH
  - Serum albumin and total protein

REFERRALS

- Refer to surgeon for permanent vascular access or peritoneal dialysis catheter 6 months before anticipated date of dialysis.
- Refer to nephrologist for renal transplantation.
- Early nephrology referral has been shown to decrease morbidity and mortality.

COMPLICATIONS

- Complications can be treated as follows:
  - **Anemia:** Erythropoietin (EPO) and repletion of iron stores.
  - **Hyperkalemia:** Dietary restrictions, sodium polystyrene, and diuretics.
  - **Acidosis:** Dialysis, sodium bicarbonate.
  - **Renal osteodystrophy:** Phosphate binders, dietary restriction, calcium supplement, calcitriol.
  - **Volume overload:** Diuretics, volume restriction, dialysis.
  - **Uremia:** Dialysis.
- Dialysis-related complications:
  - **Vascular catheter–related infections** (*S aureus*, coagulase-⊖ *Staphylococcus*): Treat empirically with an IV first-generation cephalosporin and consider vancomycin coverage for MRSA. Tailor antibiotics to blood culture results from the catheter and a peripheral site. Consider removal of the catheter for fungal infections, sepsis, endocarditis, or persistent bacteremia.
  - **Peritoneal catheter–related infections** (*S aureus, S epidermidis*, enteric gram-⊖ rods): Often treated with infusion of antibiotics into the peritoneum. Add IV antibiotics in severe cases and consider catheter removal.
  - **AV fistula thrombosis:** Treatment options include intravascular clot removal and thrombolytics.

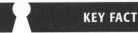

KEY FACT

Cardiovascular disease is still the most common cause of death in CKD, with risk and mortality increasing in proportion to the ↓ in GFR.

Nephrotic Syndrome

A 50-year-old man with a history of chronic lower back pain comes in with 1 week of ↑ lower extremity edema and decreased urine output. The patient denies any shortness of breath or orthopnea. The patient has used ibuprofen 800 mg 3 times/day for the last year. He denies alcohol use. He reports that over the past week, in addition to his lower extremity edema, his urine output has been dark and foamy. On physical examination, his blood pressure is 135/80 and he has 3+ edema in his bilateral lower extremities up to his sacrum. He has no rales on exam, jugular venous distention, or ascites. His blood and urine tests reveal the following:

Na = 136 mEq/L
K = 4.4 mEq/L
Cl = 107 mEq/L
CO_2 = 24 mEq/L
BUN = 32 mg/dL
Creatinine = 2.1 mg/dL
Albumin = 1.7 g/dL
UA shows 4+ protein

What would you see under urine microscopy?

The patient has nephrotic syndrome from NSAID use, which is defined as proteinuria > 3 g/day. Other causes include 1° kidney diseases, systemic diseases, and medications. Classically, microscopy shows oval fat bodies and fatty casts. Under polarized light microscopy, the oval fat bodies and fatty casts have a "Maltese cross" appearance. Additional laboratory findings include ↑ lipids and ↓ serum albumin.

Nephrotic syndrome is characterized by significant proteinuria resulting from **noninflammatory** injury to the glomeruli, hypoalbuminemia (< 2.5g/dL), edema, and hyperlipidemia. Nephrotic-range proteinuria is ≥ 3 g/day. May be 1°/idiopathic or 2° to a variety of disorders.

- **1° or idiopathic causes:**
  - **Minimal-change disease:** More common in children. May be preceded by URI or immunization. Characterized by sudden onset with heavy proteinuria. Normal on light microscopy. Fusion of foot processes of epithelial cells on electron microscopy. Responds to steroids but often relapses. Renal failure is uncommon.
  - **Focal segmental glomerulosclerosis (FSGS):** More common in African Americans. Also seen in sickle cell disease, hypertension, diabetes, IV drug use, and HIV. Associated with a higher frequency of renal failure than minimal-change disease. Treated with steroids, cyclosporin A, and cyclophosphamide.
  - **Membranous nephropathy:** More common in whites, aged 30–50 years. Seen in HBV, HCV, syphilis, malaria, gold and penicillamine use, and SLE. Approximately 25% of cases are associated with neoplasm. Presents with proteinuria with occasional microhematuria and hypercoagulability (renal vein thrombosis). Slowly progressive to renal failure. Spontaneous remission rate is 25%. Treated with steroids, cyclosporin, cyclophosphamide, and chlorambucil.
  - **Membranoproliferative glomerulonephritis (MPGN):** Can present with nephritic or nephrotic features. Associated with infection, autoimmune disease, HCV, and cryoglobulins. Low C3. Treated with observation (non-nephrotic with stable renal function) or steroids, plasmapheresis, or interferon-α. Associated with a 50% mortality rate or progression to ESRD within 5 years of renal biopsy.

- **2° causes:**
  - **Diabetic nephropathy:** The leading cause of ESRD in the United States. Onset is 5–10 years after diagnosis for type 1 DM but is more variable in type 2 DM. Biopsy shows Kimmelstiel-Wilson nodules. Treated with tight glycemic control, BP control (ie, < 130/80), and lipid control (ie, LDL < 100 mg/dL). ACEIs are first-line agents in type 1 DM; ACEIs or ARBs are used in type 2.
  - **Other etiologies:** Malignancy (classically, lymphoma or myeloma), infections (HIV, HBV, HCV, syphilis, leprosy, malaria), SLE, amyloidosis, sickle cell disease, preeclampsia, drugs (gold, NSAIDs, penicillamine, IV drug use), insect bites, and poison ivy.

SYMPTOMS/EXAM

Loss of appetite, fatigue and malaise, edema, dyspnea from pleural effusions, ascites, weight gain, muscle wasting, frothy urine, opportunistic infections, and clotting disorders. Patients with nephrotic disease are also at ↑ risk for venous thrombosis and pulmonary embolism.

DIFFERENTIAL/DIAGNOSIS

See Table 9.8 for a comparison of nephrotic and nephritic syndromes. Relevant lab tests include the following:

- **UA and microscopy:** Reveals proteinuria. Oval fat bodies or Maltese cross may be seen under polarized light. Waxy and fatty casts.
- **24-hour urine collection:** Quantifies proteinuria. Spot urine sampling for protein-to-creatinine ratio can approximate 24-hour protein excretion.
- Serum albumin. Low in nephrotic syndrome.
- Additional labs to determine 2° causes: HbA_{1c}, SPEP/UPEP, complement levels, ASO titers, ANA, anti-dsDNA, and serologies for HBV, HCV, HIV, and syphilis.
- Consider renal biopsy if etiology is unclear.

TABLE 9.8.   Comparison of Nephrotic and Nephritic Syndromes

	NEPHROTIC SYNDROME	NEPHRITIC SYNDROME
Findings	Proteinuria > 3 g/day.	Proteinuria < 3 g/day.
	Edema.	Edema.
	Hyperlipidemia and lipiduria.	Hematuria.
	Hypoalbuminemia (serum albumin < 3 g/dL).	Hypertension.
	Hypercoagulability.	ARF for days to weeks.
	Fatty and waxy casts.	Oliguria.
	Oval fat bodies and Maltese crosses.	RBC casts, WBC casts.
		Dysmorphic RBCs.
1° or idiopathic	Minimal-change disease.	PSGN (can present as nephrotic syndrome).
	FSGS.	IgA nephropathy.
	Membranous nephropathy.	
	MPGN (can present as nephritic syndrome).	
2°	Diabetic nephropathy.	SLE (can present as nephrotic syndrome).
	Malignancy (lymphoma or myeloma).	Goodpasture syndrome.
	Infectious (eg, HIV, HBV/HCV, syphilis).	ANCA-related vasculitis (Wegener granulomatosis, microscopic polyarteritis
	Amyloidosis.	nodosa, Churg-Strauss syndrome).

TREATMENT

- Control peripheral edema with loop diuretics.
- Maintain good nutrition; limit salt.
- Administer ACEIs/ARBs to slow proteinuria.
- Institute lipid-lowering therapy with a target LDL generally < 100 mg/dL.
- Treat the underlying disease.

Nephritic Disease

Typically consists of proteinuria (< 3 g/day), hematuria, hypertension, renal insufficiency, and edema due to **inflammatory** changes in the glomeruli. May be 1°/idiopathic or 2° to a variety of disorders.

- **1° or idiopathic causes:**
  - **Poststreptococcal glomerulonephritis (PSGN):** The leading cause of acute nephritic syndrome. Classically seen 2–3 weeks after pharyngitis or skin infection and can present with nephritic or nephrotic features. Diagnosed via elevated ASO titers and anti-DNase B antibodies, along with low complement levels. Treatment is supportive, and renal failure typically resolves within 4 weeks, with only 5% of cases requiring acute renal replacement therapy.
  - **IgA nephropathy (Berger):** More common among Asians and Hispanics; men > women; and patients in their teens to 20s. Presents with episodic hematuria +/− proteinuria, usually within 24 hours of a URI. Treat with ACEIs. Consider fish oil if proteinuria is < 3 g/day or steroids if > 3 g/day. Approximately 20% of cases progress to renal failure within 20 years.
  - **Hereditary (Alport):** X-linked transmission, so seen only in males; family history of hematuria; associated with sensorineural deafness and ocular abnormalities.
- **2° causes:**
  - **SLE:** Lupus nephritis can be the presenting feature. Diagnosed by anti-dsDNA and anti-Smith antibodies, along with low complement levels. Eight to 15% of SLE patients progress to ESRD. Treat with steroids.
  - **Goodpasture syndrome:** A constellation of glomerulonephritis, pulmonary hemorrhage, and anti-GBM antibodies that can present with rapidly progressive glomerulonephritis (RPGN). Circulating antibodies to type IV collagen. Diagnosed via anti-GBM antibodies. Urgent treatments include plasmapheresis, steroids, and cyclophosphamide.
  - **ANCA-related vasculitis:** Includes Wegener granulomatosis, microscopic polyarteritis nodosa, and Churg-Strauss syndrome. Can present with RPGN. Diagnosed via c-ANCA, p-ANCA, antimyeloperoxidase (MPO) antibodies, anti-proteinase 3 (anti-PR3), and renal biopsy. Urgent treatments include plasmapheresis, steroids, and cyclophosphamide.
  - Other causes: Henoch-Schönlein purpura, hypersensitivity vasculitis, cryoglobulinemia, drugs (gold, penicillamine).

SYMPTOMS/EXAM

Approximately 50% of cases are asymptomatic. Look for loss of appetite, fatigue and malaise, peripheral and periorbital edema, hypertension, oliguria and dark urine (hematuria).

DIFFERENTIAL

Table 9.8 distinguishes nephritic disease from nephrotic syndrome.

DIAGNOSIS

- **UA and microscopy:** RBC casts, dysmorphic RBCs, and WBCs. RBC casts are pathognomonic of glomerulonephritis.
- **Twenty-four-hour protein collection or spot urine protein-to-creatinine ratio** determines proteinuria.
- Obtain additional labs as indicated (complement levels, ASO titer, anti-DNase antibodies, anti-GBM antibodies, dsDNA, ANA, ESR, c-ANCA, p-ANCA).
- Renal ultrasound.
- Renal biopsy if diagnosis is unclear after workup.

TREATMENT

- Treatment principles are the same as for nephrotic syndrome.
- Treat the underlying disease.

Hematuria

The American Urological Association defines microscopic hematuria as ≥ 3 RBCs per high-power microscopic field in urinary sediment, from 2 of 3 properly collected UA specimens. Blood in the urine may be gross or microscopic.

- Red urine is not always due to RBCs from the urinary tract. Other causes include the following:
    - Medications: Phenazopyridine, nitrofurantoin, cascara, methyldopa, phenacetin, phenindoine, phenolphthalein, phenothizine, senna.
    - Myoglobin in the urine.
    - Porphyria.
    - Beets, rhubarb, food coloring.
    - Contamination from vaginal or GI bleeding.

KEY FACT

The most common causes of hematuria are UTI, prostatitis, and urinary calculi (Figure 9.6).

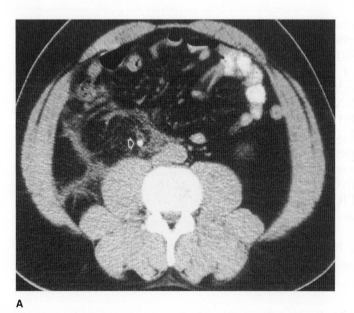

A

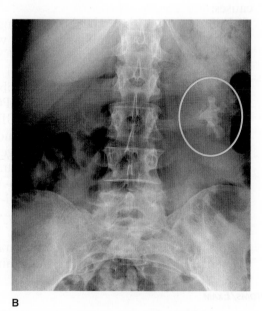

B

FIGURE 9.6.   Urinary calculi. (A) A transaxial image from a CT scan without IV contrast showing a right ureteral calculus *(arrowhead)*, with surrounding inflammatory changes of the retroperitoneal fat. (B) Prone abdominal radiograph showing right staghorn *(oval)* or struvite (Mg-NH$_4$-PO$_4$) stone filling the collecting system of the right kidney.

- Causes of hematuria are characterized as glomerular or nonglomerular:
  - **Glomerular:**
    - Glomerulonephritis (see section on nephritic disease).
    - Alport syndrome (see section on nephritic disease).
    - Thin basement membrane nephropathy (benign familial hematuria).
  - **Nonglomerular** (categorized as renal or nonrenal):
    - **Renal:** Malignancy, vascular disease (malignant hypertension, AVM, nutcracker syndrome [left renal vein compression between the abdominal aorta and superior mesenteric artery], renal vein thrombosis, papillary necrosis), infection (pyelonephritis, TB, CMV, EBV), hereditary disease (polycystic kidney disease, medullary sponge kidney).
    - **Nonrenal:** Malignancy (prostatic, ureteral, bladder), infection (prostatitis, cystitis), BPH, nephrolithiasis, endometriosis, coagulopathy (bleeding disorders or medication-induced disease), trauma (Foley catheter), vigorous exercise, *Schistosoma haematobium* (consider if from endemic areas of Africa, India, Middle East).

SYMPTOMS/EXAM

- **Gross hematuria:** Red or brown color change of urine.
- **Microscopic hematuria:** Urine microscopy showing ≥ 3 RBCs per high-power field in centrifuged urine. Often asymptomatic and discovered on urine dipstick or on UA obtained for other purposes.
- A focused history can help guide further evaluation and should include the following factors:
  - **Recent symptoms:** URIs may point toward PSGN or IgA nephropathy. Look for urinary tract symptoms that may suggest infectious or obstructive processes as well as flank pain radiating to the groin.
  - **Other:** Look for symptoms that predispose to glomerular disease, such as joint pain and rash in connective tissue disorder; edema in glomerular disease; and risk factors for endocarditis. Ask about recent vigorous exercise or traumas; ask about travel to areas where schistosomiasis is endemic. Determine if there is a family history of renal diseases or sickle cell trait/disease. Review medications, including use of NSAIDs and anticoagulants, although anticoagulants do not cause hematuria without trauma.

DIAGNOSIS

Rule out benign causes of hematuria, such as menstruation, vigorous exercise, sexual activity, trauma, or infection. If history suggests a benign cause, repeat UA 48 hours after cessation of activity. Treat patients with a UTI and repeat UA 6 weeks after treatment.

- **Gross hematuria:** Centrifuge urine.
  - **Red sediment:** Indicates hematuria.
  - **Red supernatant:**
    - **Heme-⊕ dipstick:** Indicates myoglobinuria or hemoglobinuria.
    - **Heme-⊖ dipstick:** Phenazopyridine, beets, porphyria, etc.

Patients < 50 years of age with gross hematuria require ultrasound or CT of abdomen and pelvis. All patients > 50 or < 50 but with risk factors (see below) require cystoscopy.
- **Microscopic hematuria:**
  - UA and microscopy to determine the number and morphology of RBCs, crystals, and casts.

- Electrolytes, kidney function, blood counts, and coagulation.
- Differentiate between **glomerular and nonglomerular causes:**
  - **Glomerular causes:** See sections on ARF and Nephritic Disease.
  - **Nonglomerular causes:**
    - In low-risk patients without risk factors, workup includes urine cytology and renal ultrasound.
    - Patients with gross hematuria or associated risk factors (see below) should obtain upper tract imaging (CT or IVP), lower tract imaging (cystoscopy), and urine cytology.
- Risk factors for significant disease with microscopic hematuria:
  - Smoking history.
  - Occupational exposure to benzenes, aromatic amines.
  - Age > 40 years.
  - History of gross hematuria.
  - History of urologic disorder or disease.
  - History of irritative voiding symptoms.
  - History of UTI.
  - History of pelvic irradiation.
  - Analgesic abuse.
- If workup ⊖, UA, blood pressure, and urine cytology should be obtained at 6, 12, 24, and 36 months. If ⊖ for 3 years, further urologic testing is not needed.
- If during this 36-month interval, gross hematuria, abnormal cytology, or irritative voiding symptoms without infection are present, a complete evaluation should be repeated.

TREATMENT

- Directed at the underlying cause.
- Persistent, unexplained hematuria is most likely due to a mild glomerulopathy or nephrolithiasis.

Sodium and Water Disorders

HYPONATREMIA

A 63-year-old woman with a history of hypertension presents with insidious onset of fatigue, nausea, and vomiting for 1 week. Her medications include aspirin 81 mg, hydrochlorothiazide 25 mg, and a multivitamin. On physical examination, the patient is tired but is in no acute distress. Her blood pressure is 111/72 supine and 90/62 standing. Her mucous membranes are dry, and she is noted to have decreased skin turgor. The rest of the examination is unremarkable. Laboratory tests reveal the following:

Na = 122 mEq/L
K = 3.4 mEq/L
Cl = 75 mEq/L
Total CO_2 = 22 mEq/L

BUN = 42 mg/dL

Creatinine = 1.5 mg/dL

Serum osmolality = 265

Fe_{Urea} = < 35%

What is the primary cause of the patient's hyponatremia?

The primary cause of the patient's hyponatremia is most likely the hydrochlorothiazide she is taking. Hyponatremia is a side effect of this drug and can come on insidiously, so periodic monitoring of electrolytes is recommended when a patient is on a thiazide diuretic. The patient's hyponatremia is worsened by both her hypovolemia and her acute renal failure. Her hypovolemia is evident from her orthostasis, dry mucous membranes, and poor skin turgor. The patient's creatinine is likely elevated for an elderly patient and her BUN-to-creatinine ratio is > 20, also suggesting hypovolemia. In the setting of diuretic use, the Fe_{Na} is not a reliable measure of prerenal acute renal failure; instead, the Fe_{Urea} < 35% should be used.

Defined as a plasma sodium (Na^+) level < 135 mEq/L. Figure 9.7 outlines an algorithm for the differential diagnosis of hyponatremia.

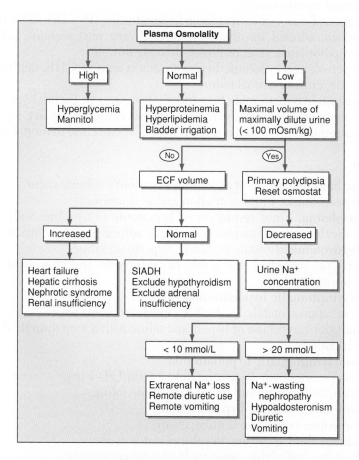

FIGURE 9.7. **Evaluation and differential diagnosis of hyponatremia.** Algorithm depicting clinical approach to hyponatremia. ECF, extracellular fluid; SIADH, syndrome of inappropriate antidiuretic hormone secretion. (Reproduced, with permission, from Kasper DL, et al., *Harrison's Principles of Internal Medicine,* 16th ed. New York: McGraw-Hill, 2005: 256.)

SYMPTOMS/EXAM

- Symptoms and signs relate to the rate and severity of the decline in Na^+.
- Clinical presentation ranges from asymptomatic to nausea, vomiting, confusion, lethargy, seizures, or coma.

DIAGNOSIS

- Obtain a thorough history to determine symptoms and identify potential causes of hyponatremia (see Figure 9.7).
- **Determine tonicity:** Plasma osmolality $(P_{osm}) = (2 \times Na^+) + (BUN / 2.8) + (glucose / 18)$. (Normal tonicity of plasma is 280–300).
- There are 3 types of hyponatremia based on tonicity: hypotonic, hypertonic, and normotonic.
- For hypotonic hyponatremia ($P_{osm} < 280$), first determine volume status:
  - Perform a clinical exam to look for volume overload (elevated JVP, S3 gallop, ascites, edema), euvolemia, or volume depletion (dry mucous membranes, flat JVP).
  - A urine $Na^+ < 10$ or a $Fe_{Na} < 1\%$ (reliable only when the patient is oliguric and not taking diuretics) is found in hypovolemic hypotonic hyponatremia 2° to extrarenal fluid losses, such as from the GI tract, skin, or hemorrhage.
  - A urine $Na^+ > 20$ suggests renal fluid loss as a cause of hypovolemic hypotonic hyponatremia, such as with diuretics, sodium wasting, and adrenal insufficiency.
  - Causes of euvolemic hypotonic hyponatremia (P_{osm} 280–300): hypothyroidism, adrenal insufficiency, SIADH (see next section), polydipsia, beer potomania, reset osmostat, thiazide diuretics.
  - Hypervolemic hypotonic hyponatremia is seen in CHF, nephrotic syndrome, cirrhosis, renal failure.
- Normotonic hyponatremia (P_{osm} 280–300) is seen in pseudohyponatremia where hyperproteinemia and hyperlipidemia cause lab artifact. Hypertonic hyponatremia ($P_{osm} > 300$) is seen in hyperglycemia and mannitol infusion.

TREATMENT

- Initiate fluid management according to patient's volume status.
  - **Hypervolemia:** Fluid restriction and/or diuretics.
  - **Euvolemia:** Fluid restriction or hypertonic (3%) saline with caution. Demeclocycline if patient is unable to adhere to water restriction.
  - **Hypovolemia:** Isotonic or, rarely, hypertonic saline.
- Correct Na^+ according to the patient's symptoms and rapidity of onset of the abnormality.
- **Acute symptomatic hyponatremia:**
  - ↑ Na^+ approximately 2 mEq/L/hr until symptoms resolve.
  - Consider careful use of hypertonic saline with a loop diuretic if volume overloaded.
- **Chronic symptomatic hyponatremia:**
  - ↑ Na^+ more slowly (approximately 1 mEq/L/1–2 hr).
  - Again, consider careful use of hypertonic saline.
- **Chronic asymptomatic hyponatremia:**
  - Immediate correction is unnecessary.
  - Manage fluid according to volume status as above.
  - Treat the underlying cause for long-term correction.

KEY FACT

To prevent central pontine myelinolysis, do not ↑ $Na^+ > 12$ mEq/L over a 24-hour period.

SYNDROME OF INAPPROPRIATE SECRETION OF ADH (SIADH)

A 58-year-old man comes in and reports feeling tired and weak for the last several weeks. On further questioning, you learn that he has a 60-pack-year smoking history and has had increasing shortness of breath and hemoptysis for the last month. On physical examination, you find that the patient appears tired but is in no acute distress. His vitals are significant for an O_2 saturation of 92% on room air. He has decreased breath sounds on the left base. The patient has no evidence of volume overload and no jugular venous distention, ascites, or lower extremity edema. His initial laboratory tests are as follows:

Na = 119 mEq/L
K = 3.9 mEq/L
Cl = 75 mEq/L
CO_2 = 22 mEq/L
BUN = 28 mg/dL
Creatinine = 1.2 mg/dL
Osmolality = 254 mOsm/L
Urine Na = 48 mEq/L
Urine osmolality = 553 mOsm/kg

What is the cause of the patient's hyponatremia?

SIADH, which is seen in cases of pulmonary and CNS processes, medications, and postoperative states. In SIADH, the elevated level of antidiuretic hormones leads to ↑ reabsorption of water, leading to a concentrated urine and hence a high urine osmolality. It is the excess free-water absorption that causes hyponatremia and a low serum osmolality.

SIADH occurs when antidiuretic hormone (ADH) is secreted independent of the body's need to conserve water, leading to inappropriate water retention in the presence of Na^+ loss. May result from a variety of disorders.

- **CNS disorders:**
    - **Head trauma:** SAH, subdural hematoma.
    - **Infection:** Meningitis, encephalitis, brain abscess.
    - **Other:** Neoplasm, CVA, MS.
- **Pulmonary disorders:** Small cell lung cancer, pneumonia, lung abscess, TB, pneumothorax.
- **Medications:** SSRIs, TCAs, carbamazepine, haloperidol, chlorpromazine, chlorpropamide, theophylline, amiodarone.
- **Other:** Malignant neoplasia.

SYMPTOMS/EXAM

The symptoms of SIADH are the result of hyponatremia and the underlying cause of the disorder.

DIAGNOSIS

- Euvolemic hyponatremia.
- P_{osm} < 280 mOsm/kg.
- Urine osmolality > 100 mOsm/kg; urine Na^+ > 20 mEq/L.
- Low uric acid and BUN due to serum dilution and ↑ renal losses.
- SIADH is a diagnosis of exclusion.

KEY FACT

Small cell lung cancer is the malignancy most commonly associated with SIADH.

TREATMENT

- As with other causes of hyponatermia, treatment of SIADH depends on the severity of the hyponatremia and the the presence of symptoms.
- Asymptomatic patients can be treated with water restriction of 1 L/day.
- In patients with severe symptoms such as seizures or mental status changes, treat aggressively, but cautiously with hypertonic saline and loop diuretics.
- Correction of hyponatremia should not exceed a rate of 0.5 mEq/L/hr. Too rapid a rate of correction risks inducing central pontine myelinolysis.
- Demeclocycline for chronic SIADH.

HYPERNATREMIA

An 86-year-old female nursing home resident with baseline dementia presents with a seizure. She had been diagnosed with pneumonia 2 days ago and started on azithromycin. Her caretaker notes that her intake has decreased over the last 2 days and she has become more somnolent. She is febrile at 38.9°C (102°F). Her blood pressure is 138/74 and her pulse is 104. On physical examination, she is somnolent, but her neurologic exam is nonfocal. Her mucous membranes are dry and she has poor skin turgor. Her cardiac exam is notable for tachycardia. Her laboratory examination reveals the following:

Na = 154 mEq/L
K = 3.2 mEq/L
Cl = 107 mEq/L
CO_2 = 22 mEq/L
BUN = 68 mg/dL
Creatinine = 2 mg/dL
Urine Na = 8 mEq/L
Urine osmolality = 680 mOsm/kg

A CT scan of the head shows no acute intracranial process.

What is the cause of her hypernatremia?

Hypernatremia in the elderly is most commonly due to the combination of inadequate fluid intake and increased fluid losses. In this case, the patient has increased insensible losses from her fever and is unable to replenish her free-water losses, resulting in hypernatremia. This can be exacerbated in the elderly because of impairments in the thirst mechanism and renal concentrating ability.

Hypernatremia is defined as a plasma Na^+ level > 145 mEq/L. It is grouped into 4 broad categories according to the underlying mechanism:

- **Inadequate intake and ↑ water loss** (U_{osm} > 600 mOsm/kg):
  - Most common cause.
  - ↑ insensible or GI losses (↑ sweating, burns, diarrhea).
  - Barriers to accessible fluids or inadequate replacement. Seen in elderly or institutionalized patients who lack access to free water.
- **↑ renal loss (polyuria):**
  - **Diabetes insipidus** (U_{osm} < 600 mOsm/kg): A defect in the secretion or action of ADH. Presents with hypernatremia with copious dilute urine (see the Endocrinology chapter).
  - **Postobstructive or post-ATN diuresis.**

- Osmotic diuresis in diabetes.
- Diuretic use.
- **1° hypodipsia:** Destruction of the hypothalamic thirst center due to neoplasm, vascular disease, granulomatous disease, or trauma.
- **Excess Na$^+$ retention** (rare): Due to accidental or intentional ingestion/infusion of hypertonic solution.

KEY FACT

Hypernatremia is almost always due to free-water deficits.

SYMPTOMS/EXAM

- Volume depletion: Dry mucous membranes, hypotension, and low urine output.
- CNS symptoms: Lethargy, weakness, irritability, confusion, seizures, and coma.

DIAGNOSIS

- Review the patient's weight, blood pressure, intake and output, and types of IV fluid.
- Check urine osmolality.
- Low urine osmality (< 250 mOsm/kg) with polyuria suggests diabetes insipidus.
- High urine osmolality (> 500 mOsm/kg) with low urine output suggests extrarenal loss.
- High urine osmolality (> 500 mOsm/kg) with high urine output suggests osmotic diuresis, post-ATN, postobstructive, or diuretic use.

TREATMENT

- As with hyponatremia, treatment depends on the presence of symptoms and the rapidity of onset of the abnormality.
- Acute hypernatremia that lasts < 24 hours should be corrected within 24 hours.
- If the hypernatremia is chronic or of unknown duration, the correction should occur over 48 hours because too rapid a correction of hypernatremia can cause cerebral edema. Correct the serum sodium at a rate of 1–2 mEq/L/hr. Do not ↓ Na$^+$ > 12 mEq/L per 24-hour period.
- **Calculate the free-water deficit:**

$$\text{Water deficit} = [(\text{plasma sodium} - 140) / 140] \times \text{TBW}$$

- Hypovolemic patients with unstable vital signs should be treated initially with isotonic normal saline. Once stabilization has occurred, the free-water deficit can be repleted by 5% dextrose in water, quarter, or half isotonic normal saline.
- Correct 50% of the calculated free-water deficit in the first 12–24 hours, with the remainder corrected in the next 24–48 hours.

KEY FACT

In patients who are hypotensive and volume depleted, use isotonic saline initially and switch to hypotonic saline once tissue perfusion is adequate.

Potassium Disorders

HYPERKALEMIA

A 60-year-old woman with a history of chronic renal failure on dialysis, hypertension, and diabetes presents with malaise, nausea, and ↓ appetite after missing her last dialysis appointment. On physical examination, you find an ill-appearing female in no apparent distress. On respiratory exam, you hear rales halfway up both lung fields but no ↓ breath sounds or rhonchi. Her jugular venous distention is elevated at 15 cm, and you hear an S3 gallop. She has 2+ edema to her knees bilaterally, which, she reports, is ↑ from usual. Her initial laboratory results are as follows:

Na = 143 mEq/L
K = 7.6 mEq/L
Cl = 107 mEq/L
CO_2 = 16 mEq/L
BUN = 62 mg/dL
Creatinine = 7.4 mg/dL

How would you treat her hyperkalemia?

The patient's chronic kidney disease means that her kidneys are unable to excrete potassium and that she relies on dialysis to lower her potassium to safe levels. A stat ECG showing peaked T waves or widening QRS intervals would be concerning for impending cardiac arrhythmia due to hyperkalemia. Options for immediate but transient ↓ in potassium levels include β-agonists such as albuterol or insulin (given with glucose), both of which will drive potassium into cells. Calcium gluconate can temporarily stabilize the myocardium and prevent progression to arrhythmia. Potassium exchange resins, such as sodium polystyrene sulfonate (Kayexalate), potassium-wasting diuretics such as furosemide, and dialysis are the only ways to permanently remove the potassium from the body.

Serum potassium > 5.5 mEq/L. Causes of hyperkalemia include the following:

- **High K+ intake:** From supplements or diet (rarely occurs without baseline renal dysfunction).
- **Extracellular K+ shift** (↓ cellular entry or ↑ release):
  - Metabolic acidosis.
  - Insulin deficiency and hyperglycemia such as in diabetic ketoacidosis.
  - Tissue damage from rhabdomyolysis, trauma, or burns, or release during tumor lysis syndrome.
  - β-adrenergic blockade.
- **Impaired renal excretion:**
  - Renal failure.
  - Decreased renal perfusion, as seen with severe CHF or volume depletion.
  - Type IV renal tubular acidosis.
  - Hypoaldosteronism.
  - Adrenal insufficiency.
- **Medications:** ACE inhibitors, ARBs, NSAIDs, spironolactone.

SYMPTOMS/EXAM

May be asymptomatic or may present with symptoms ranging from muscle weakness to ventricular fibrillation (VF).

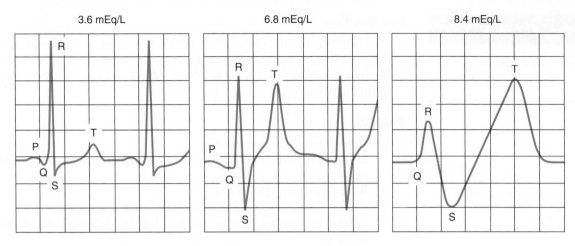

3.6 mEq/L   6.8 mEq/L   8.4 mEq/L

F I G U R E   9 . 8 .   **Electrocardiographic effects of hyperkalemia.** (Reproduced, with permission, from Morgan GE Jr, et al. *Clinical Anesthesiology,* 4th ed. New York: McGraw-Hill, 2006, Fig. 28-6.)

DIAGNOSIS

- Review the history, medications, and exam, focusing on chest pain, palpitations, muscle weakness, flaccid paralysis, and ileus.
- Obtain basic labs, including electrolytes, BUN, and creatinine.
- Consider additional labs as indicated by the history—eg, CK for rhabdomyolysis; LDH, uric acid, phosphorus, and calcium for tumor lysis syndrome; U_{osm} and U_{K^+} to calculate the transtubular K^+ gradient in hypoaldosteronism.
- ECG findings may be used as an indicator of severity. Figure 9.8 shows characteristically progressive changes that occur with increasing serum potassium levels.
  - **Mild:** Normal or peaked T waves.
  - **Moderate:** QRS prolongation or flattened P waves.
  - **Severe:** VF.

TREATMENT

- IV calcium gluconate to stabilize the myocardium.
- ↑ K^+ entry into cells with insulin and glucose, β_2-adrenergic agonists (inhaled albuterol), and $NaHCO_3$.
- For long-term elimination, use sodium polystyrene sulfonate (cation-exchange resin), loop diuretics, and dialysis.

HYPOKALEMIA

Defined as potassium level < 3.5 mEq/L. Causes include the following:

- Low K^+ intake.
- ↑ GI loss: diarrhea, vomiting.
- Intracellular K^+ shift, such as in metabolic alkalosis or use of β-agonist.
- ↑ renal excretion, as with loop and thiazide diuretics, excess mineralocorticoids (hyperaldosteronism, Cushing, European black licorice ingestion), congenital (Bartter, Gitelman, Liddle, 17-α-hydroxylase deficiency), hyperglycemia (osmotic diuresis), hypomagnesemia, and renal tubular acidosis.

KEY FACT

Patients with hypokalemia are often also hypomagnesemic. The hypokalemia cannot be corrected unless the magnesium level is corrected. Treat both at the same time.

Symptoms/Exam

- Symptoms generally occur when serum potassium is < 2.5–3.0 mEq/L.
- Muscle weakness, fatigue, cramps, constipation, ileus. Severe symptoms include flaccid paralysis, hyporeflexia, tetany, rhabdomyolysis, and cardiac arrhythmias.

Diagnosis

- 24-hour urine collection for K^+:
  - **Extrarenal causes (GI losses, low intake, intracellular shifts):** < 25 mEq/day.
  - **Renal causes:** > 25 mEq/day.
- Spot urine for K^+ (more easily obtained, but less accurate):
  - **Extrarenal causes (GI losses, low intake, intracellular shifts):** < 20 mEq/day.
  - **Renal excretion:** > 40 mEq/day.
- ECG may show U waves, T-wave flattening, arrhythmias (PSVT, PVC, PAC, ventricular fibrillation, atrial fibrillation), ST depressions.
- See the Endocrinology chapter for evaluation of adrenal abnormalities.

Treatment

- Replete K^+, usually as KCl.
- Oral route is preferred but may cause abdominal pain. Take with food.
- If repleting through a peripheral IV, rate should not exceed 10 mEq/L/hr. With a central line, rate can be up to 20 mEq/L/hr. IV site may burn.
- K^+-sparing diuretics in patients with chronic urinary K^+ loss.

Acid-Base Disorders

Acid-base disorders are changes in serum pH that result from a change in either arterial PCO_2 or serum HCO_3^-. There are 4 types (see sections below): metabolic acidosis, metabolic alkalosis, respiratory acidosis, and respiratory alkalosis.

In a healthy person:

- pH = 7.40
- PCO_2 = 40 mmHg
- PO_2 = 100 mmHg
- HCO_3^- = 24 mEq/L

In a metabolic acid-base disorder, the primary change is in HCO_3^-. In a respiratory acid-base disorder, the primary change is in PCO_2. In all acid-base disorders, the body compensates to return serum pH to 7.40. In metabolic disorders, the compensation is respiratory. In respiratory disorders, the compensation is metabolic (Table 9.9).

METABOLIC ACIDOSIS

A 17-year-old girl with a history of type 1 diabetes is admitted to the ER with persistent vomiting. She reports that she has not been taking her insulin regularly for the past few days. On physical examination, she is

TABLE 9.9.   **Changes and Compensatory Mechanisms Seen in Acid-Base Disorders**

DISORDER	pH	[H+]	[HCO₃-]	PCO₂	COMPENSATION
Metabolic acidosis	↓	↑	↓↓	↓	Respiratory alkalosis (ie, hyperventilation)
Metabolic alkalosis	↑	↓	↑↑	↑	Respiratory acidosis (ie, hypoventilation)
Respiratory acidosis	↓	↑	↑	↑↑	Metabolic alkalosis (renal HCO₃- reabsorption)
Respiratory alkalosis	↑	↓	↓	↓↓	Metabolic acidosis (renal HCO₃- excretion)

tachycardic and tachypneic, but her blood pressure is stable. You find her to be in mild respiratory distress, with dry mucous membranes and fruity breath. Her laboratory values are as follows:

Na = 136 mEq/L

K = 5.4 mEq/L

Cl = 107 mEq/L

CO_2 = 14 mEq/L

BUN = 28 mg/L

Creatinine = 1.2 mg/L

Glucose = 397 mg/dL

ABG shows pH of 7.1.

UA shows 3+ glucose and is ⊕ for ketones.

What is the underlying acid-base disorder?

Anion-gap metabolic acidosis due to diabetic ketoacidosis (DKA). The anion gap is 15. Patients in DKA have ketones in both serum and urine. Exhaled acetone, a ketoacid, gives the patient her fruity breath. The ↑ serum sugar leads to osmotic diuresis, causing hypovolemia. Acidemia causes hyperkalemia as the body attempts to normalize pH by exchange of H+ intracellularly and K+ extracellularly. The tachypnea is a compensatory respiratory alkalosis to the primary process of metabolic acidosis. Management of DKA includes fluids, insulin, and close attention to electrolytes, especially potassium, which usually is severely depleted. Once urine output is verified, potassium is included in the patient's IV fluids.

Metabolic acidosis is defined by a serum pH < 7.35 due to a ↓ in extracellular HCO_3^-. It is caused by either a gain in acid or a loss of HCO_3^-. There are 2 categories of metabolic acidosis: anion-gap (AG) metabolic acidosis and non-AG (hyperchloremic) metabolic acidosis.

- **AG metabolic acidosis:** Production of endogenous or addition of exogenous acids.
  - The anion gap is calculated as follows:

$$AG = (Na^+) - [(Cl^-) + (HCO_3^-)]$$

- Normal AG is 6–10.
  - Calculate the osmolar gap to assess for toxin ingestion.
  - Osmolar gap = measured Osm – calculated Osm.

↑ AG suggests an AG metabolic acidosis, even if plasma HCO_3^- is normal.

Hypoalbuminemia causes a ↓ in the anion gap. Remember to adjust for hypoalbuminemia. For every 1-g/dL decline in serum albumin, anion gap ↓ by 2.5 mEq/L.

Causes of AG metabolic acidosis:

MUDPILERS

Methanol ingestion
Uremia
Diabetic ketoacidosis
Paraldehyde ingestion
INH overdose
Lactic acidosis
Ethylene glycol ingestion
Rhabdomyolysis
Salicylate ingestion

- Calculated serum osmoles = $(2 \times Na) + (BUN / 2.8) + (glucose / 18) + (ETOH / 4.6)$.
  - Osmolar gap > 10 in ethanol, methanol, ethylene glycol ingestion.
  - Osmolar gap < 10 in paraldehyde or salicylate ingestion.
- Causes of AG metabolic acidosis include (see Mnemonic MUDPILERS):
  - Lactic acidosis (tissue hypoxia, shock, hypovolemia, dehydration, sepsis).
  - Ketoacidosis (diabetes mellitus, ethanol, starvation).
  - Uremia.
  - Ingestion (paraldehyde, methanol, salicylate, ethylene glycol).
- **Non-AG (hyperchloremic) metabolic acidosis:** Loss of bicarbonate.
- Calculate the urine AG to distinguish between renal and extrarenal losses of bicarbonate:

$$U_{AG} = U_{Na} + U_K - U_{Cl}$$

  - $U_{AG} < 0$ suggests GI loss of bicarbonate, such as from diarrhea.
  - $U_{AG} > 0$ suggests renal causes such as renal failure, renal tubular acidosis.

SYMPTOMS/EXAM

- Depend on the underlying cause:
  - Dehydration and fruity breath in diabetic ketoacidosis.
  - Tachypnea in salicylate intoxication.
  - Ataxia, confusion, seizures, coma in ethylene glycol intoxication.
- Patient can be asymptomatic or have nonspecific signs such as fatigue, anorexia, confusion, tachycardia, tachypnea, dehydration.

DIAGNOSIS

- Calculate AG or urine AG as above.
- Labs: Evaluate via renal function, serum lactate, serum or urine ketones, salicylates.
- Calculate osmolar gap to rule out ingestion of alcohol (ethanol, methanol, ethylene glycol).

TREATMENT

- Treat the underlying cause.
- Bicarbonate therapy is controversial and, if used, is generally reserved for severe acidosis (arterial pH < 7.10–7.15).

METABOLIC ALKALOSIS

Defined as an ↑ in plasma bicarbonate concentration: serum pH > 7.45. **Causes:** Divided into **chloride-responsive** and **chloride-unresponsive** forms.

- **Chloride responsive** (urine chloride [U_{Cl^-}] < 15 mEq/L):
  - Vomiting
  - Diuretics (after discontinuation)
  - Nasogastric suction
  - Stool losses
  - Posthypercapnic alkalosis
  - Cystic fibrosis

- **Chloride unresponsive** ($U_{Cl^-} > 15$ mEq/L):
    - Diuretics (current use)
    - Hyperaldosteronism
    - Cushing syndrome
    - Exogenous mineralocorticoids or glucocorticoids
    - Renovascular hypertension
    - Hypomagnesemia, hypokalemia
    - Liddle syndrome
    - Bartter syndrome
    - Gitelman syndrome

DIAGNOSIS/TREATMENT

- $\uparrow$ serum bicarbonate in chemistry panel.
- Measure U_{Cl^-} concentration.
- Treat chloride-responsive metabolic alkalosis with NaCl infusion.
- The presence of hypertension suggests primary hyperaldosteronism, Cushing syndrome, exogenous meneralocorticoids or glucocorticoids, or Liddle syndrome.
- Treat the underlying cause.

RESPIRATORY ACIDOSIS

Defined as an $\uparrow$ in PCO_2 (hypercapnia) due to $\downarrow$ alveolar ventilation. Serum pH < 7.35. **Causes:**

- **Central:** Drugs (opiates, anesthetics, sedatives), stroke, infection.
- **Airway:** Obstruction (obstructive sleep apnea), asthma, COPD.
- **Parenchyma:** Pneumonia or bronchitis, pulmonary edema, ARDS, barotrauma.
- **Neuromuscular:** Spinal cord injury, kyphoscoliosis, poliomyelitis, Guillain-Barré syndrome, myasthenia gravis, MS, severe hypokalemia or hypophosphatemia.

SYMPTOMS/EXAM

- **CNS symptoms:** Headache, blurred vision, restlessness, anxiety.
- **CO_2 narcosis:** Tremors, asterixis, myoclonus, delirium, somnolence, seizures.

DIAGNOSIS/TREATMENT

- Arterial pH < 7.40 and $PCO_2 > 40$ mmHg.
- Process can be acute or chronic. Change in pH depends on chronicity:
    - Acute respiratory acidosis: HCO_3^- increases by 0.1 for every mmHg PCO_2 increases.
    - Chronic respiratory acidosis: HCO_3^- increases by 0.35 for every mmHg the PCO_2 increases.
- Distinguish intrinsic pulmonary disease from extrapulmonary disease using the alveolar-arterial (A-a) oxygen gradient:
    - $\text{A-a}\,(O_2) = (Fi_{O_2}\% / 100) \times (P_{atm} - 47\text{ mmHg}) - (Pa_{CO_2} / 0.8) - Pa_{O_2}$, where:
        - Fi_{O_2} room air $= 21\%$.
        - Atmospheric pressure $= 760$ mmHg at sea level.
        - Water vapor pressure pH_2O (mmHg) $= 47$ mmHg at 37°C (98.6°F).
        - Respiratory quotient RQ (VCO_2/VO_2) $= 0.8$ (usual).

- A normal A-a gradient is 10–20 mmHg.
  - An A-a gradient > 20 suggests intrinsic pulmonary disease causing impaired gas exchange.
- Initiate mechanical ventilation if necessary while correcting the underlying disorder.

RESPIRATORY ALKALOSIS

Defined as ↑ alveolar ventilation leading to a ↓ in PCO_2 (hypocapnia). **Causes:**

- Hypoxemia
- Anxiety
- Salicylates
- Pain
- Sepsis
- Hepatic failure
- Congestive heart failure
- Pulmonary embolus
- Pneumonia
- Hyperthyroidism
- CNS lesions (stroke or neoplastic)
- Pregnancy (progesterone)

SYMPTOMS/EXAM

- Anxiety, tachypnea.
- **CNS symptoms:** Lightheadedness, altered mental status.
- Acute hypocapnea can cause intracellular shifts, leading to hypocalcemia, in turn leading to paresthesias, circumoral numbness, and carpopedal spasms.

DIAGNOSIS/TREATMENT

- Arterial pH > 7.40 and PCO_2 < 40 mmHg.
- As with respiratory acidosis, respiratory alkalosis can be acute or chronic. Change in pH depends on chronicity:
  - Acute respiratory alkalosis: HCO_3^- decreases by 0.22 for every mmHg PCO_2 decreases.
  - Chronic respiratory alkalosis: HCO_3^- decreases by 0.5 for every mmHg PCO_2 decreases.
- Use the A-a oxygen gradient as above.
- Correct the underlying disorder.

MIXED ACID-BASE DISORDERS

Defined as 2 or more independent acid-base disorders existing at the same time. **Examples:**

- A patient with DKA (metabolic acidosis) who develops pneumonia (respiratory acidosis).
- The "triple ripple": A patient overdoses on salicylates and has profuse vomiting caused by AG metabolic acidosis (salicylates) and metabolic alkalosis (vomiting) with respiratory alkalosis (salicylates directly stimulate the respiratory center).

DIAGNOSIS

- Identify the most prominent disorder by determining the greatest change in HCO_3^- or PCO_2.
- Apply the formula for expected compensation. If compensation is not appropriate, a coexisting disorder is present.

Other Urinary Tract Disorders

RHABDOMYOLYSIS

Defined as a breakdown of skeletal muscle fibers, leading to the release of muscle contents into the bloodstream. Causes include immobilization (such as elderly fall victims), crush injury, overexertion, infections, drugs, and toxins (such as statins and colchicine).

SYMPTOMS

Myalgias, red to brown urine due to myoglobinuria.

DIAGNOSIS

- ↑ in serum CK levels; may be > 100,000 IU/L.
- Urine dipstick ⊕ for blood, but urine sediment with no RBCs (indicates that myoglobin is present and not hemoglobin).

COMPLICATIONS

- Hyperkalemia from muscle breakdown, causing cardiac arrhythmia or cardiac arrest.
- Early hypocalcemia, but with hypercalcemia during the recovery phase.
- Metabolic acidosis.
- Acute renal failure from myoglobin precipitation, leading to tubular obstruction.

TREATMENT

- Goal is to prevent renal failure.
- IV hydration to ensure renal perfusion (up to 12 L of fluid can be sequestered in necrotic muscle) and to flush out obstructing casts.
- Maintain urine output of 300 mL/hr until myoglobinuria is resolved.
- Alkalinize urine to pH > 6.5 to decrease toxicity of myoglobin to tubules.
- Use of mannitol and sodium bicarbonate is controversial.

NEPHROLITHIASIS

 A 47-year-old man presents to the ER with acute onset of dysuria and severe left flank pain radiating to the groin. Duration has been 1 hour. You find him in discomfort, unable to find a comfortable position. On physical examination, you find exquisite left costovertebral angle tenderness with no peritoneal signs. UA shows 3+ blood with no nitrites and leukocyte esterase. A chemistry panel shows normal renal function. What imaging would you use for diagnosis?

A noncontrast helical CT scan. This presentation is consistent with nephrolithiasis, and noncontrast helical CT scan is the gold standard for detection of renal stones.

SYMPTOMS/EXAM

- Presents with colicky flank pain +/− radiation to the groin.
- Urinary frequency, urgency, and dysuria.
- Microscopic or gross hematuria.
- Male-to-female ratio is 3:1.

DIAGNOSIS

- **Collect and analyze the stone!** Type of stone may change treatment.
- **Labs:**
  - UA: Hematuria.
  - BUN, creatinine: Elevated only with bilateral obstruction.
  - Plasma calcium, phosphorus, and uric acid.
  - PTH for hyperparathyroidism if calcium is high-normal or elevated.
  - For recurrent nephrolithiasis, 24-hour urine collection (to assess volume, pH, Na^+, calcium, oxalate, phosphorus, citrate, uric acid, cysteine, and creatinine).
- **Imaging:** CT scan is the gold standard for nephrolithiasis. Plain-film radiography can show radiopaque stones (calcium oxalate and calcium phosphate), but less radiopaque stones (uric acid, cysteine, and magnesium ammonium phosphate [struvite]) may go undetected.

KEY FACT

The majority of kidney stones are calcium oxalate. The ureterovesical junction is the most common site of renal stone impaction.

TREATMENT

- Treat with pain control and IV fluids.
- ↑ urine volume through daily ingestion of 2.5–3.0 L of fluid.
- Stones smaller than 5–6 mm usually pass without intervention.
- With infection of obstruction, urologic consult is needed for emergent decompression of the upper urinary tract.
- Minimally invasive surgical techniques include extracorporeal shock wave lithotripsy, percutaneous nephrostolithotomy, rigid and flexible ureterorenoscopy.
- After a first stone, bloodwork for electrolytes, calcium, phosphorus, uric acid, and parathyroid hormone is indicated.
- Strain urine to collect stone.
- Additional treatment depends on the type of stone:
  - **Calcium:** ↓ protein intake. Treat with thiazides in hypercalciuria and potassium citrate if normocalciuria. Calcium restriction has not been shown to reduce recurrences. May form more calcium oxalate stones and worsen osteoporosis.
  - **Uric acid:** Moderate protein intake. Consider potassium citrate. 2° to gout or increased cell turnover, as in leukemia or myeloproliferative disease. Stones are radiolucent. Urine alkalinization with potassium citrate or potassium bicarbonate. Allopurinol for patients with ↑ urinary uric acid levels.
  - **Cysteine:** Diagnostic of cysteinuria (a rare heritable disorder of cysteine transport in the proximal tubule). Urine alkalinization with potassium citrate or potassium bicarbonate.
  - **Magnesium ammonium phosphate (struvite):** Caused by UTI with urea-producing bacteria such as *Proteus* or *Klebsiella*. Can develop into a staghorn calculus involving the entire renal pelvis and calyces. Initiation of appropriate antimicrobial therapy can slow progress, but surgical intervention is generally required.

POLYCYSTIC KIDNEY DISEASE

A hereditary disorder, most commonly of autosomal-dominant inheritance, involving renal cyst formation, with possible progression to renal failure. Hemorrhage into cysts may also occur, causing hematuria.

SYMPTOMS

- Flank and abdominal pain, hematuria, hypertension.
- With advanced disease, kidneys can be enlarged and palpable.

DIAGNOSIS

Imaging by CT or ultrasound.

TREATMENT

- Blood pressure control.
- Aspiration of cysts may help with pain from hemorrhage or compression.
- Nephrectomy if severe pain from kidney enlargement or recurrent UTIs.
- Dialysis or kidney transplantation.

NOTES

CHAPTER 10

Dermatology

Michael Mendoza, MD, MPH

Diagnosis of Dermatologic Disease

TERMINOLOGY

Skin lesions may be characterized as primary (ie, caused by a primary disease process; see Table 10.1) or as secondary (changes resulting from a variety of factors; see Table 10.2). They may also be distinguished by their configuration (Table 10.3) as well as by their distribution (eg, localized or generalized).

DIAGNOSTIC TECHNIQUES

Key diagnostic techniques include the following:

- **KOH prep:** Used to diagnose fungal infection. With a blade, scrape scale onto a glass slide, and add KOH (must be heated if not preserved with DMSO). KOH dissolves keratin but not hyphae walls. Look for branching structures (Figure 10.1).
- **Tzanck smear:** Used to test for HSV or VZV. Rupture the vesicle, place fluid on a glass slide and stain with Giemsa or Wright stain. Presence of multinucleated giant cells identifies herpesvirus infection (Figure 10.2).
- **Wood's lamp:** Emits UV light ("black light") at 366 nm. Can be used to diagnose tinea capitis, tinea versicolor, erythrasma, vitiligo, melasma, and porphyria.

TABLE 10.1. Descriptions of Primary Dermatological Lesions

Lesion	Description	Examples
Macule	Any circumscribed color change in the skin that is nonpalpable and < 1cm.	Vitiligo, café au lait.
Papule	A solid, elevated area < 1 cm in diameter. Top may be pointed, rounded, or flat.	Acne, warts.
Plaque	A solid, elevated circumscribed area > 1 cm in diameter, usually flat topped.	Psoriasis.
Vesicle	A circumscribed, elevated lesion < 1 cm in diameter containing clear fluid.	Blisters of HSV/VZV.
Bulla	A circumscribed, elevated lesion > 1 cm in diameter containing clear fluid.	Bullous erythema multiforme, bullous pemphigoid.
Pustule	A vesicle containing a purulent exudate.	Acne, folliculitis.
Nodule	A deep-seated mass with indistinct borders that elevates the overlying epidermis.	Tumors, cysts.
Wheal	A circumscribed, elevated, flat-topped, firm elevation of skin resulting from tense edema of the papillary dermis.	Urticaria.

TABLE 10.2.   Descriptions of Secondary Dermatological Lesions

2° CHANGE	DESCRIPTION	EXAMPLES
Scale	Dry, thin plates of keratinized epidermal cells (stratum corneum).	Psoriasis, ichthyosis.
Lichenification	Thickening of skin, with exaggerated skin markings resulting from chronic rubbing of the skin.	Atopic dermatitis, lichen planus.
Erosion and oozing	A moist, circumscribed, slightly depressed area representing a blister base with the roof of the blister removed.	Burns; bullous erythema multiforme.
Crusts	Dried exudate of plasma on the surface of the skin following acute dermatitis.	Impetigo, contact dermatitis.
Fissures	A linear erosion.	Angular cheilitis.
Scars	A flat, raised, or depressed area of fibrotic tissue.	Acne scars, burn scars.
Atrophy	Depression of the skin surface caused by thinning of one or more layers of skin.	Lichen sclerosus et atrophicus.
Color	The lesion should be described as red, pink, yellow, brown, tan, or blue. Particular attention should be paid to blanching; failure to blanch suggests bleeding into the dermis (petechiae).	

BIOPSY PROCEDURES

- **Shave biopsy:** Performed by shaving tangentially to the skin with a blade. Indicated for elevated (exophytic) lesions.
- **Punch biopsy:** Performed by exerting rotational torque with a punch biopsy tool. No closure required for lesions ≤ 3 mm in diameter. Indicated for obtaining full-thickness skin specimens.
- **Excisional biopsy:** Best performed with an elliptical incision to prevent "dog ears." Indicated for the diagnosis of suspected malignancy and complete excision of lesions.

TABLE 10.3.   Differential of Dermatologic Lesions by Configuration

CONFIGURATION	EXAMPLES
Annular (circular)	Annular lesions present in granuloma annulare; urticaria and dermatophyte infections.
Linear (straight lines)	Linear papules present in lichen striatus, incontinentia pigmenti, and scabies.
Grouped	Grouped vesicles occur in herpes simplex or zoster.
Discrete	Discrete are independent of each other.

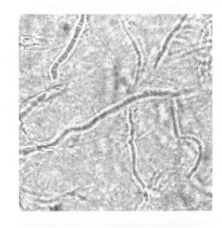

FIGURE 10.1.   KOH preparation. (Reproduced, with permission, from Wolff K, Johnson RA. *Fitzpatrick's Color Atlas & Synopsis of Clinical Dermatology*, 6th ed. New York: McGraw-Hill, 2009, Fig. 25-1.)

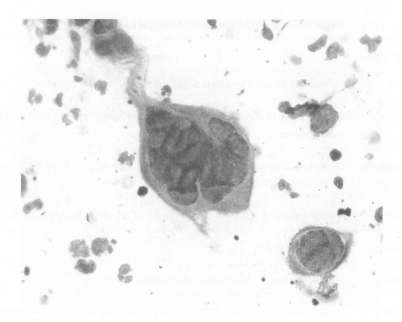

FIGURE 10.2. **Tzanck smear.** (Reproduced, with permission, from Wolff K, Johnson RA. *Fitzpatrick's Color Atlas & Synopsis of Clinical Dermatology,* 6th ed. New York: McGraw-Hill, 2009, Fig. 27-7.)

KEY FACT

With recalcitrant acne in female patients, look for hirsutism and irregular menses, which may point to congenital adrenal hyperplasia, polycystic ovarian syndrome, or Cushing disease.

KEY FACT

Steroid creams used on the face can cause dermatitis resembling rosacea.

KEY FACT

Isotretinoin is teratogenic, so advise women to use a reliable method of birth control. Side effects include dry skin, cheilitis, hypertriglyceridemia, transaminitis (therefore, LFTs must be followed), and depression.

Common Skin Disorders

COMMON PEDIATRIC SKIN DISORDERS

Table 10.4 outlines the presentation, diagnosis, and treatment of common viral and bacterial causes of rash in infants and children (Figure 10.3).

ACNE

Defined as chronic inflammation and blockage of the pilosebaceous units with ↑ production of sebum and colonization of *Propionibacterium acnes*. Exacerbated by medications such as glucocorticoids; anabolic steroids; lithium; isoniazid (INH); some OCPs; cyclosporine; vitamins B_2, B_6, and B_{12}; and iodides.

SYMPTOMS/EXAM

Noninflammatory comedones ("blackheads" and "whiteheads") and/or inflammatory papules, pustules, and cysts (see Figure 10.4).

TREATMENT

- **First line:** Topical benzoyl peroxide; topical antibiotics (eg, clindamycin), topical retinoids.
- **Second line:** Oral antibiotics—eg, doxycycline 100 mg BID.
- **Third line:** Isotretinoin (Accutane), a retinoid that is anti-inflammatory. OCPs can also be switched to a less androgenic variety and spironolactone. (Don't forget to check K^+!)

ROSACEA

Chronic inflammatory facial dermatitis of adults characterized by papules and pustules on a background of telangiectasias.

SYMPTOMS/EXAM

- The earliest symptom is **flushing,** followed by erythema, telangiectasias, papules, pustules, and, rarely, lymphedema. Distribution is on the cheeks, nose, forehead, and chin.
- Triggered by **hot liquids, spicy food, alcohol, sun,** and **heat.**
- No comedones are seen (compared with acne vulgaris).

DIFFERENTIAL

- Acne vulgaris, contact dermatitis, photosensitive eruptions, seborrheic dermatitis, SLE.
- Steroid creams used on the face can mimic rosacea.

TREATMENT

- Avoid exacerbating factors.
- **Topical treatment: Metronidazole** gel or cream; sodium sulfacetamide lotion, topical antibiotics, topical azelaic acid.
- **Oral treatment:** Low-dose doxycycline × 2–3 months. Appropriate in the presence of ocular involvement or if topical therapy is not effective.
- **Severe disease:** Isotretinoin.

COMPLICATIONS

Rhinophyma occurs primarily in middle-aged men with long-standing disease (Figure 10.5). Blepharitis and conjunctivitis are also potential complications.

ATOPIC DERMATITIS

A chronic inflammatory skin disease that is considered familial, with allergic features. It often occurs in patients with other atopic disorders, such as **asthma** and **allergic rhinitis.** Typically begins in infancy; 50% incidence in the first year of life and an additional 30% between the ages of 1 and 5. Thought to be immune related, with roughly 85% of patients having ↑ IgE.

SYMPTOMS/EXAM

- Acute lesions can include vesicles (Figure 10.6). Skin lesions in older individuals with more chronic disease are characterized by **lichenification** as well as by excoriated and fibrotic papules.
- The **flexural** areas (neck, antecubital fossae, and popliteal fossae) are most commonly involved; other common sites include the face, wrists, and forearms.
- Other physical findings that support the diagnosis include xerosis (dry skin), infraorbital skin folds (Dennie-Morgan lines), periorbital darkening, hyperlinear palms (accentuation of fine palmar skin lines), keratosis pilaris (follicular accentuation that is usually present on the extensor surfaces of the upper arms), and anterior subcapsular cataracts and keratoconus.

TABLE 10.4. **Common Causes of Rash in the Pediatric Population**

DISEASE	USUAL AGE	PRODROME	MORPHOLOGY/DISTRIBUTION
Measles (rubeola virus) (Figure 10.3A)	Infants to young adults.	High fever, symptoms of URI, conjunctivitis.	Erythematous macules and papules become confluent. Begins on the face and moves centrifugally.
Rubella (rubella virus) (Figure 10.3B)	Adolescents/ young adults.	Absent or low-grade fever, malaise, upper respiratory symptoms.	Rose-pink maculopapules; not confluent. Begins on the face and moves downward rapidly.
Erythema infectiosum (parvovirus B19) (Figure 10.3C)	3–12 years.	Usually none.	Slapped cheeks; reticular erythema or maculopapular rash. Usually affects the arms and legs, but may be generalized.
Enteroviral exanthems (coxsackievirus, echovirus, other enteroviruses) (Figure 10.3D)	Young children.	Fever (occasionally).	Extremely variable; may be maculopapular, petechial, purpuric, or vesicular. Usually generalized, but may be acral.
Hand-foot-mouth syndrome (several coxsackieviruses) (Figure 10.3E)	Young children.	Fever (occasionally), sore mouth.	Gray-white vesicles 3–7 mm in size on normal or erythematous base. Hands and feet are most commonly affected, but may affect the diaper area and is occasionally generalized.
Adenovirus exanthems (adenoviruses) (no image)	Young children.	Fever; symptoms of URI.	Rubelliform, morbilliform, roseola-like rash. Generalized.
Chickenpox (VZV) (Figure 10.3F)	1–14 years.	Fever, headache, and malaise 48 hours before exanthem.	Macules and papules rapidly become vesicles on an erythematous base, followed by crusts. Often begins on the scalp or face; more profuse on the trunk than on extremities.
Roseola (may be linked to HHV-6) (Figure 10.3G)	< 3 years.	High fever for 3–5 days before exanthem.	Maculopapular rash in rosettes appears **after** fever declines. Affects trunk and neck but may be generalized. Lasts hours to days.
Kawasaki disease (Figure 10.3H)	< 5 years.	High fever, irritability.	Polymorphous—papular, vesicobullous, or morbilliform; erythema with desquamation. Generalized, often with perineal accentuation and desquamation.
Scarlet fever (group A streptococcus) (Figure 10.3I)	School age.	Acute onset, with fever, sore throat.	Diffuse erythema with sandpaper texture. Facial flushing with circumoral pallor; linear erythema in skin folds.
Staphylococcal scalded skin syndrome (*S aureus* epidermolytic toxin) (Figure 10.3J)	< 5 years.	None.	Abrupt onset, with tender erythroderma. Eruption with intensification in the neck, face, axillae, and groin.
Henoch-Schönlein purpura (Figure 10.3K)	4–7 years.	Possibly abdominal pain.	Palpable purpuric or petechial rash. Begins on the malleoli and extends to the buttocks.

Associated Findings	Diagnosis	Special Management
Koplik spots, "toxic" appearance, photophobia, cough, adenopathy, high fever.	Usually clinical; acute/convalescent hemagglutinin (HAI) serologic test.	Report to public health; give immunoglobulin within 6 days of exposure.
Postauricular and occipital adenopathy; headache, malaise, mild pruritus.	Rubella IgM or acute/convalescent HAI serologic test.	Report to public health; check for exposure to pregnant women.
Waxes/wanes for several weeks; occasionally presents with arthritis, headache, and malaise.	Usually clinical; acute/convalescent serologic test.	Carries the potential complication of aplastic crisis.
Low-grade fever, occasional myocarditis, aseptic meningitis, pleurodynia.	Usually clinical; viral throat culture; rectal swabs in selected cases.	In the presence of petechiae or purpura, meningococcemia must be considered.
Oral ulcers, occasional fever, adenopathy.	Same as for enteroviral exanthems.	
Fever; symptoms of URI; occasionally pneumonia.	Viral isolation or acute/convalescent seroconversion.	
Pruritus, fever, oral and genital lesions, occasional malaise.	Usually clinical; Tzanck preparation or direct immunofluorescence.	Antihistamines for itching; aspirin is contraindicated (Reye syndrome).
Cervical and postauricular adenopathy.	Clinical.	
Conjunctivitis, cheilitis, glossitis, peripheral edema, adenopathy, strawberry tongue.	Clinical.	Admit to the hospital for IVIG and salicylates.
Exudative pharyngitis, palatal petechiae, abdominal pain.	Throat cultures.	IM penicillin or oral erythromycin.
Fever, conjunctivitis, rhinitis.	Clinical: culture of *S aureus* from systemic site (not skin).	Neonate; if blistering is present, hospitalize for IV antibiotics and fluid/electrolyte therapy.
Arthralgia, nausea, vomiting, diarrhea, GI bleeding.	Clinical.	Consider Rocky Mountain spotted fever or meningococcemia; steroids for severe cases.

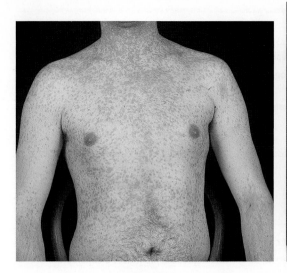

FIGURE 10.3A. **Measles.** (Reproduced, with permission, from Fauci AS, et al. *Harrison's Principles of Internal Medicine*, 17th ed. New York: McGraw-Hill, 2008, Fig. 185-3.)

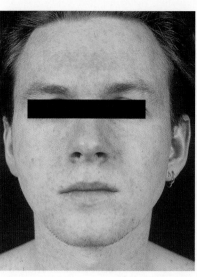

FIGURE 10.3B. **Rubella.** (Reproduced, with permission, from Wolff K, Johnson RA. *Fitzpatrick's Color Atlas & Synopsis of Clinical Dermatology,* 6th ed. New York: McGraw-Hill, 2009, Fig. 27-21.)

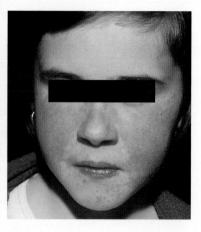

FIGURE 10.3C. **Erythema infectiosum.** (Reproduced, with permission, from Wolff K, Johnson RA. *Fitzpatrick's Color Atlas & Synopsis of Clinical Dermatology,* 6th ed. New York: McGraw-Hill, 2009, Fig. 27-24A.)

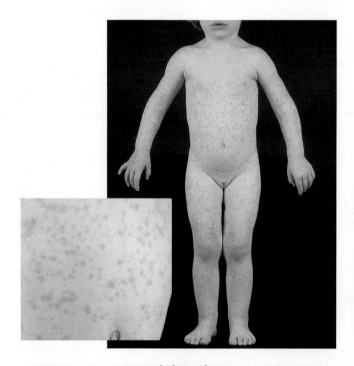

FIGURE 10.3D. **Enteroviral exanthems.** (Reproduced, with permission, from Wolff K, Johnson RA. *Fitzpatrick's Color Atlas & Synopsis of Clinical Dermatology,* 6th ed. New York: McGraw-Hill, 2009, Fig. 27-19.)

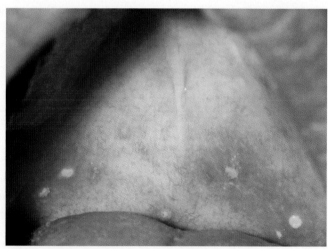

FIGURE 10.3E. **Hand-foot-mouth syndrome.** (Reproduced, with permission, from Wolff K, Johnson RA. *Fitzpatrick's Color Atlas & Synopsis of Clinical Dermatology,* 6th ed. New York: McGraw-Hill, 2009, Fig. 27-20.)

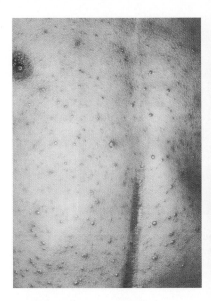

FIGURE 10.3F.   Chickenpox. (Reproduced, with permission, from Fauci AS, et al. *Harrison's Principles of Internal Medicine*, 17th ed. New York: McGraw-Hill, 2008, Fig. 173-1.)

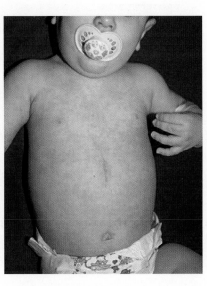

FIGURE 10.3G.   Roseola. (Reproduced, with permission, from Wolff K, et al. *Fitzpatrick's Dermatology in General Medicine,* 7th ed. New York: McGraw-Hill, 2008, Fig. 192-14.)

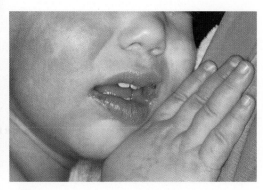

FIGURE 10.3H.   Kawasaki disease. (Reproduced, with permission, from Wolff K, Johnson RA. *Fitzpatrick's Color Atlas & Synopsis of Clinical Dermatology,* 6th ed. New York: McGraw-Hill, 2009, Fig. 14-44.)

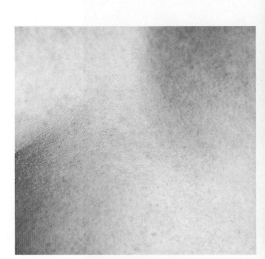

FIGURE 10.3I.   Scarlet fever. (Reproduced, with permission, from Fauci AS, et al. *Harrison's Principles of Internal Medicine*, 17th ed. New York: McGraw-Hill, 2008, Fig. 130-2.)

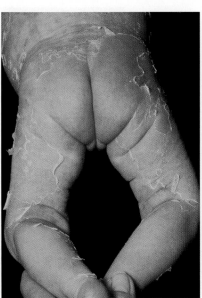

FIGURE 10.3J.   Staphylococcal scalded skin syndrome. (Reproduced, with permission, from Wolff K, et al. *Fitzpatrick's Dermatology in General Medicine,* 7th ed. New York: McGraw-Hill, 2008, Fig. 178-5.)

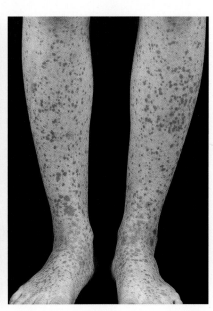

FIGURE 10.3K.   Henoch-Schönlein purpura. (Reproduced, with permission, from Wolff K, Johnson RA. *Fitzpatrick's Color Atlas & Synopsis of Clinical Dermatology,* 6th ed. New York: McGraw-Hill, 2009, Fig. 14-35.)

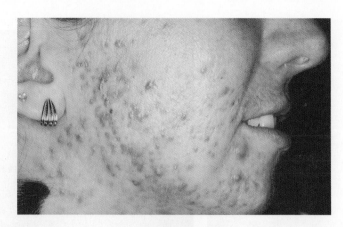

FIGURE 10.4. **Severe inflammatory acne with pustules and comedones.** (Courtesy of Kalman Watsky, MD, as published in Kasper DL, et al. *Harrison's Principles of Internal Medicine,* 16th ed. New York: McGraw-Hill, 2005: 295.)

Differential

Contact dermatitis, seborrheic dermatitis, drug reactions, psoriasis (axillary, gluteal, or groin lesions are more characteristic of psoriasis).

Diagnosis

Diagnosed visually. Pruritus, a chronic recurring course, a ⊕ family history of atopy, and early age of onset are all suggestive of the diagnosis.

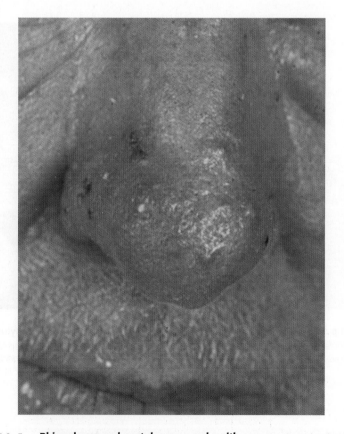

FIGURE 10.5. **Rhinophyma and pustules on a male with rosacea.** (Reproduced, with permission, from Wolff K, Johnson RA. *Fitzpatrick's Color Atlas & Synopsis of Clinical Dermatology,* 6th ed. Online Picture Gallery. New York: McGraw-Hill, 2009, Fig. 1e-R5.)

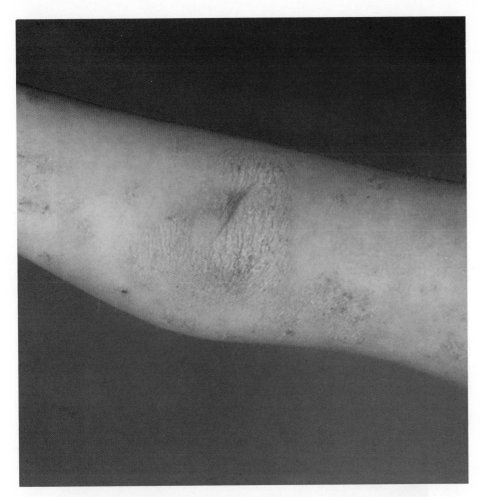

FIGURE 10.6. Atopic dermatitis in the antecubital region of a child. (Reproduced, with permission, from Wolff K, Johnson RA. *Fitzpatrick's Color Atlas & Synopsis of Clinical Dermatology,* 6th ed. Online Picture Gallery. New York: McGraw-Hill, 2009, Fig. 2e-Ad12.)

TREATMENT

- **Skin hydration with lotions and emollients.** Bleach in bath water may improve infected atopic eczema in children.
- Eliminate exacerbating factors, including excessive bathing, low-humidity environments, emotional stress, xerosis (dry skin), rapid temperature changes, and exposure to solvents and detergents.
- Topical corticosteroids or topical calcineurin inhibitors (tacrolimus/pime-crolimus) are appropriate for patients with inflamed skin; antihistamines can be given for pruritus.
- Antibiotics for bacterial superinfection.
- UVB or PUVA light therapy in difficult cases.

DYSHIDROTIC ECZEMA (POMPHOLYX)

- An intensely pruritic, chronic recurrent dermatitis, typically involving the palms and soles (Figure 10.7).
- **Sx/Exam:** Starts as an episode of intense itching, followed by the formation of small vesicles. Desquamation occurs over 1–2 weeks, leaving fissures and erosions. Recurrences may be seen.

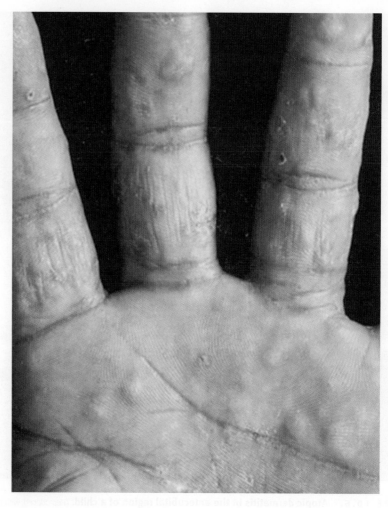

FIGURE 10.7. Dyshidrotic eczema. (Reproduced, with permission, from Fauci AS, et al. *Harrison's Principles of Internal Medicine*, 17th ed. New York: McGraw-Hill, 2008, Fig. 10-5.)

- **DDx:** Tinea, contact dermatitis.
- **Tx:** Treated with medium- to high-potency topical corticosteroids in mild cases and with a short course of systemic steroids in severe cases. Recalcitrant cases may respond to PUVA or UVA.

DISCOID (NUMMULAR) ECZEMA

- Intensely pruritic dermatitis of unknown etiology.
- **Sx/Exam:** Presents with nummular (coin-shaped) papules, scaling, crusting, and serous oozing. Lesions can be singular or multiple (up to 50) and are generally 2–10 cm in diameter and circular in shape. Distribution is over the trunk and lower extremities (the head is spared; see Figure 10.8).
- **DDx:** Tinea corporis; xerotic dermatitis.
- **Tx:** Treat with a short course of medium- to high-potency topical steroids. Systemic corticosteroids may be needed for more severe cases, but important to watch for rebound disease when using oral steroids. Avoid irritants (if identifiable).

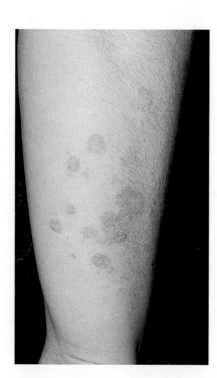

FIGURE 10.8. Nummular eczema. (Reproduced, with permission, from Wolff K, Johnson RA. *Fitzpatrick's Color Atlas & Synopsis of Clinical Dermatology*, 6th ed. New York: McGraw-Hill, 2009, Fig. 2-24.)

SEBORRHEIC DERMATITIS

A chronic inflammatory eruption hypothesized to be caused by *Malassezia furfur* yeast (formerly *Pityrosporum ovale*) colonization. Known as "cradle cap" in infants.

SYMPTOMS/EXAM

- Presents with dry or **greasy,** salmon-colored scales on an erythematous base.
- Primarily affects the scalp, **postauricular region,** central facial area (especially the **eyebrows** and **nasolabial folds**), and flexural areas (Figure 10.9).
- Crust and fissures can develop and can become superinfected.

DIFFERENTIAL

Atopic or contact dermatitis, psoriasis (seborrheic dermatitis is usually more "pinkish-red" compared with the deep red of psoriasis), impetigo, rosacea.

KEY FACT

Parkinson disease, stroke, and acutely ill patients can present with seborrheic dermatitis. If severe and recalcitrant, seborrheic dermatitis can also be a presenting symptom in patients with HIV.

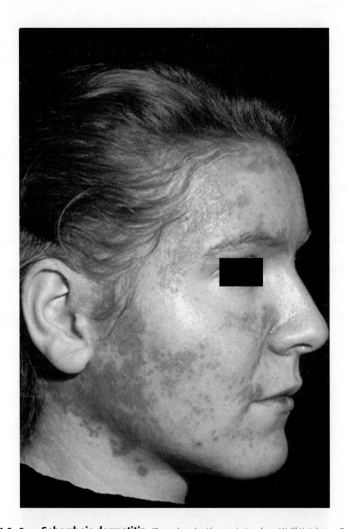

FIGURE 10.9. Seborrheic dermatitis. (Reproduced, with permission, from Wolff K, Johnson RA. *Fitzpatrick's Color Atlas & Synopsis of Clinical Dermatology,* 6th ed. Online Picture Gallery. New York: McGraw-Hill, 2009, Fig. 2e-Sd10.)

TREATMENT

- **Scalp:** Treat with shampoos containing coal tar, zinc pyrithione, selenium sulfide, or 2% ketoconazole (Nizoral).
- **Face, intertriginous areas:** Topical steroids +/– topical antifungal cream, calcineurin inhibitors. Use steroids on the face as short-term treatment only!
- Treat infants with emollients and 1% hydrocortisone ointment or an antifungal/hydrocortisone combination.

PSORIASIS

A chronic, noninfectious, immune-mediated inflammatory dermatosis. Roughly 2% of the population is affected, with a bimodal distribution (peaks at 22 and 55 years of age). Early onset predicts a more serious disease course. Triggered by environmental factors such as infection, stress, trauma, and drugs (β-blockers, lithium). HLA-Cw6 is the most commonly associated HLA-type.

SYMPTOMS/EXAM

- Presents with well-demarcated erythematous plaques covered by **waxy, silvery-white scales** (Figure 10.10). Characterized by bilateral involvement of the extensor surfaces, scalp, palms, and soles. Sometimes pruritic.
- **Nail pitting** is seen in half of cases.
- A severe form is seen in **HIV** infection.
- **Koebner phenomenon** is a form of the disease that occurs at sites of trauma.
- **Guttate psoriasis** generally follows a **streptococcal** infection (eg, strep throat) and presents with an acute symmetrical eruption of "droplike" lesions on the trunk and limbs.
- Auspitz sign is bleeding on removal of a scale.

TREATMENT

- **Topical treatment:** Potent topical corticosteroids, a vitamin D analog (calcipotriene), topical retinoids.
- **Systemic treatment:** Phototherapy (UVB), photochemotherapy (PUVA), oral retinoids, methotrexate, cyclosporine, biologicals (efalizumab, infliximab).
- Penicillin VK or erythromycin is used to treat strep throat in guttate psoriasis.

KEY FACT

Systemic corticosteroids are contraindicated in psoriasis because of severe rebound disease with medication withdrawal.

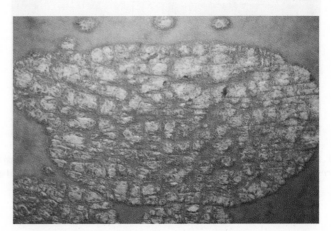

FIGURE 10.10. Psoriasis. (Reproduced, with permission, from Fauci AS, et al. *Harrison's Principles of Internal Medicine,* 17th ed. New York: McGraw-Hill, 2008, Fig. 52-7.)

COMPLICATIONS

Psoriatic arthritis (affects 5% of patients, asymmetric oligoarthritis, classically "sausage digit" presentation); sacroiliitis.

PITYRIASIS ROSEA

An acute, self-limited disorder characterized by scaly oval papules and plaques. **Often seasonal** (peaking in the spring and fall). Generally found in adolescents and young adults in response to a viral infection (**HHV-6** and **HHV-7** have been implicated). **Affects females more often than males.**

SYMPTOMS/EXAM

- Presents as a generalized rash preceded by the appearance of a 2- to 5-cm **herald patch.** Days later, many smaller plaques appear on the trunk, arms, and thighs (Figure 10.11).
- Plaques are oval and pink, with a delicate peripheral "**collarette of scale,**" and are often distributed parallel to the lines of the ribs, creating the characteristic "**Christmas tree**" distribution.
- Sometimes accompanied by pruritus.

DIFFERENTIAL

Guttate psoriasis, pityriasis versicolor, scabies, 2° syphilis.

TREATMENT

Spontaneous resolution usually occurs in 1–2 months. Moderate-potency steroids may be given for itching.

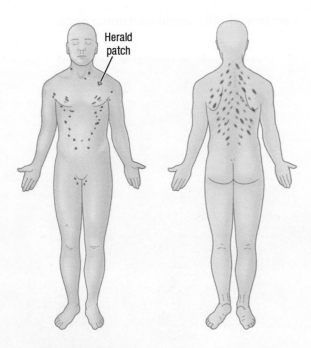

Herald
patch

FIGURE 10.11. **Distribution of pityriasis rosea.** (Reproduced, with permission, from Wolff K, Johnson RA. *Fitzpatrick's Color Atlas & Synopsis of Clinical Dermatology,* 6th ed. New York: McGraw-Hill, 2009, Fig. 7-1.)

LICHEN PLANUS

An eruption characterized by **purple, polygonal, papular, pruritic papules** affecting the flexor surfaces, mucous membranes, and genitalia. Its cause is unknown but is thought to be immune related. Roughly two-thirds of cases occur in patients 30–60 years of age. Prevalence is less than 1%, with no racial preference.

SYMPTOMS/EXAM

- The rash starts symmetrically on the limbs, especially the wrists, and may spread to become generalized within 4 weeks, but may also progress more slowly.
- Typical lesions are itchy, flat-topped polygonal papules a few millimeters in diameter (Figure 10.12). They classically show a surface network of delicate white lines (Wickham striae).
- Papules are initially red but become violaceous. Papules can flatten or become hypertrophic. Although 50% of cases clear within 9 months, the condition often recurs.
- Associated with chronic **HBV, HCV,** and **HIV.**
- **Nail involvement in 10%–15%.**

DIFFERENTIAL

Psoriasis, guttate psoriasis, pityriasis rosea, scabies.

TREATMENT

- The disease is usually self-limited.
- Moderate- to high-potency topical steroids are indicated for symptomatic treatment.
- Oral lesions are treated with steroid-containing paste.

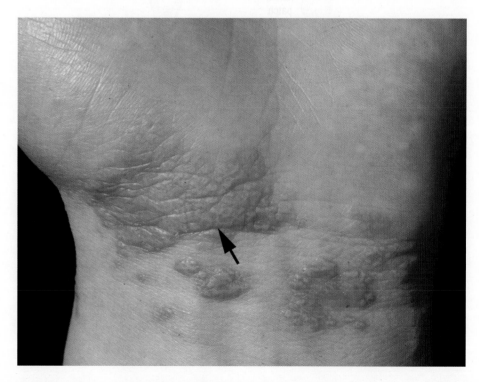

FIGURE 10.12. Lesions of lichen planus. (Reproduced, with permission, from Wolff K, Johnson RA. *Fitzpatrick's Color Atlas & Synopsis of Clinical Dermatology*, 6th ed. New York: McGraw-Hill, 2009, Fig. 7-4A.)

CONTACT DERMATITIS

Any dermatitis that results from direct contact between skin and a substance. The 2 variants are allergen and irritant. **Irritants are responsible for 80% of cases.**

Irritant Contact Dermatitis

- In irritant dermatitis, the trigger substance leads to breakdown of the normal epidermal barrier, causing the possibility of physical, chemical, or mechanical irritation.
- A reaction can be initiated by common irritants, such as daily-use products (eg, soap), or may result from one-time exposure to an allergen (eg, bleach, alkali). Patients with compromised skin barriers (eg, those with atopic dermatitis) are at higher risk.
- Sx/Exam:
  - Presents with erythema, fissures, and pruritus. In severe cases, bullae can develop.
  - Often affects the hands, especially the web spaces, but may also involve the face and eyelids.
- **Dx:** Patch testing can distinguish irritant contact from allergic contact dermatitis.
- **Tx:**
  - Avoid triggers; restore the normal epidermal barrier; use emollients. More severe cases can be treated with topical corticosteroids.
  - Systemic steroids are generally not helpful without irritant removal.

Allergic Contact Dermatitis

- In allergic dermatitis, a trigger substance induces a **delayed type IV immune response** in affected individuals. The first step takes 12–14 days to complete, and on reexposure to an allergen, dermatitis occurs in 12–48 hours.

KEY FACT

Laundry detergent is only infrequently a cause of allergic contact dermatitis.

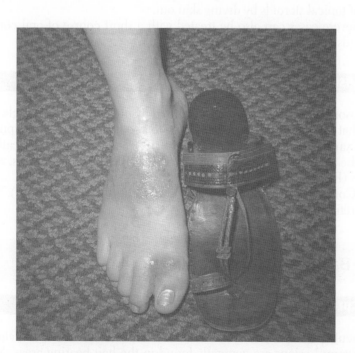

FIGURE 10.13. Contact dermatitis. (Reproduced, with permission, from Hurwitz RM. *Pathology of the Skin: Atlas of Clinical-Pathological Correlation.* Stamford, CT: Appleton & Lange, 1991: 3.)

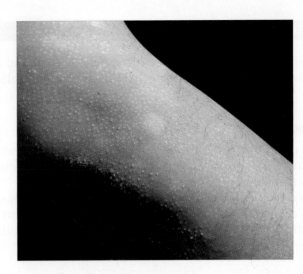

FIGURE 10.14. **Keratosis pilaris.** Keratosis pilaris in a patient with concurrent ichthyosis vulgaris. (Reproduced, with permission, from Wolff K, et al. *Fitzpatrick's Dermatology in General Medicine,* 7th ed. New York: McGraw-Hill, 2008, Fig. 85-1.)

Patients with venous stasis dermatitis can often have contact dermatitis superimposed without clinical signs or symptoms. These patients typically fail to respond to conservative treatment of their stasis ulcers and may develop an allergic reaction to the treatment regimens.

- The most common plant allergen is oleoresin urushiol (found in poison ivy, poison oak, poison sumac, and mango skin). Other common allergens include nickel, formaldehyde, perfume, latex, and medications.
- **Sx/Exam:** Presents with an intensely pruritic rash that is papular and erythematous, with indistinct margins. The rash can be linear (as in poison ivy) or can reflect the pattern of exposure to the allergen (eg, rings, clothing, footwear; see Figure 10.13).
- **Tx:**
  - **Avoid allergens.**
  - Mild cases may be treated with medium- to high-potency topical steroids.
  - With more severe oozing, wet-dry compresses may facilitate application of topical steroids by drying skin out.
  - Severe cases can also be treated with a short course of oral corticosteroids.

KERATOSIS PILARIS

- **Autosomal dominant** condition caused by plugging of the follicle by keratin that has failed to exfoliate, leading to a red or skin-colored papule.
- **Sx/Exam:** Usually asymptomatic, but can cause pruritus. Typically found on the lateral face, trunk, upper and lower extremities, thighs, and buttocks (Figure 10.14).
- **Tx:** Conservative treatment (exfoliation, lactic acid preparations). Try topical tretinoin for recalcitrant cases.

Bacterial Infections

FOLLICULITIS

- An acute pustular infection of hair follicles, usually due to *S aureus*.
- **Sx/Exam:** Lesions are generally found in the hair-bearing areas. Men can get sycosis barbae in the beard area (Figure 10.15).

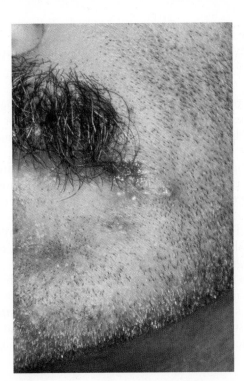

FIGURE 10.15.   Folliculitis in the beard area, with impetigo at the corner of the mouth.
(Reproduced, with permission, from Wolff K, et al. *Fitzpatrick's Color Atlas & Synopsis of Clinical Dermatology,* 5th ed. New York: McGraw-Hill, 2005: 980.)

- **DDx:** Furuncles, carbuncles.
- **Dx:** If possible, obtain a swab to identify the causative organism.
- **Tx:**
    - **Acute infections:** Systemic and topical antibiotics (usually empiric for *Staphylococcus*).
    - **Chronic infections:** Carrier sites (eg, the nose) must be treated with topical mupirocin (Bactroban). Successive courses of systemic antibiotics may also be needed.
    - **Hygiene** is key to treatment, along with weight loss and control of diabetes.
- **Cx:** Patients can get a gram-⊖ folliculitis (*Pseudomonas*) following prolonged treatment with isoretinoin.

CELLULITIS

A bacterial infection of the skin, with some extension into the subcutaneous tissues. Seventy percent of patients are men. Additional risk factors include leg ulcers, trauma, intertrigo, tinea pedis, venous insufficiency, obesity, and a history of cellulitis.

SYMPTOMS/EXAM

- Presents with systemic symptoms such as fever, chills, and myalgias as well as rubor, calor, tumor, and dolor. Most commonly affects the extremities (73% of cases affect the lower extremities) but can involve any area of the body.
- Margins are generally not well demarcated (compared with erysipelas, which has distinct margins).
- Regional lymphadenopathy is common, and lymphangitis can be present.
- Abscess may be seen, as well as macular erythema that is largely confluent.

DIFFERENTIAL

DVT, contact dermatitis, drug and foreign body reactions, insect stings.

DIAGNOSIS

- Pathogens associated with cellulitis include the following:
  - Cellulitis associated with furuncles, carbuncles, or abscesses is usually caused by *S aureus*. Methicillin-resistant *S aureus* (MRSA) can be seen.
  - Cellulitis that is diffuse or unassociated with a defined portal is most commonly caused by streptococcal species. β-hemolytic streptococci, including groups A, B, and, less often, C and G, are common causative agents.
  - Facial cellulitis is associated with *H influenzae* in children.
  - Cellulitis following puncture wounds is most often caused by *Pseudomonas aeruginosa*.
  - Exposure to fresh water or seawater is associated with *Aeromonas hydrophila* and *Vibrio* spp.
  - Animal bites point to *Pasteurella multocida* and *Erysipelothrix*.
- Cultures are usually not helpful, establishing the diagnosis in only 50% of cases, and generally do not result in a change of management (antibiotics).

TREATMENT

- The guidelines set forth in 2005 by the Infectious Diseases Society of America suggest a penicillinase-resistant semisynthetic penicillin or a first-generation cephalosporin (A–I) unless streptococci or staphylococci resistant to these agents are common in the community.
- For penicillin-allergic patients, options include clindamycin or vancomycin.

COMPLICATIONS

Necrotizing fasciitis, gas gangrene (Figure 10.16).

IMPETIGO

A superficial skin infection due to **staphylococci** and/or **streptococci (group A)**. Affects men and women in all age groups. Lesions are classically found on the face.

SYMPTOMS/EXAM

- 1° lesions are thin-walled vesicles/pustules that easily rupture (Figure 10.17).
- Lesions spread rapidly and become crusted and are classically described as "**honey crusted.**"

DIFFERENTIAL

HSV, fungal infection.

TREATMENT

- Removal of crusts via saline soaks and topical mupirocin.
- Systemic antibiotics (empirically directed against staph or strep) are appropriate for more severe cases.

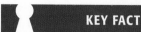

KEY FACT

Bullous impetigo is usually caused by *S aureus,* exfoliative toxins A and B.

KEY FACT

Recurrent impetigo suggests nasal carriage of *S aureus.* Treat with intranasal mupirocin.

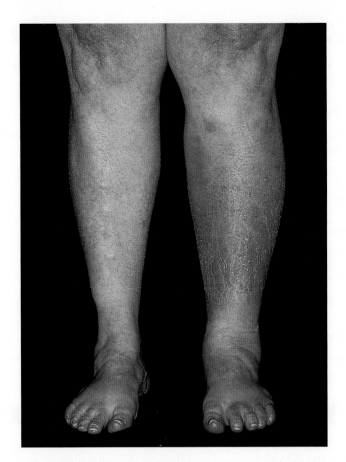

FIGURE 10.16. Cellulitis of the lower extremity. (Courtesy of Frank Birinyi, MD, as published in Knoop KJ, et al. *Atlas of Emergency Medicine,* 2nd ed. New York: McGraw-Hill, 2002: 348.)

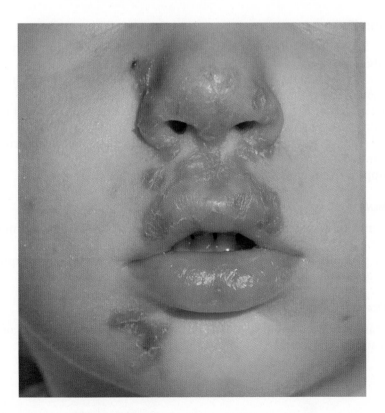

FIGURE 10.17. Lesions of impetigo. (Reproduced, with permission, from Wolff K, Johnson RA. *Fitzpatrick's Color Atlas & Synopsis of Clinical Dermatology,* 6th ed. New York: McGraw-Hill, 2009, Fig. 24-11.)

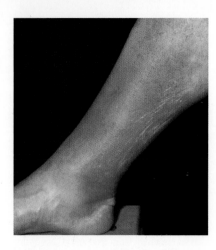

FIGURE 10.18. **Erysipelas.** Note the well-demarcated borders of erysipelas compared with general cellulitis. (Reproduced, with permission, from Wolff K, et al. *Fitzpatrick's Dermatology in General Medicine,* 7th ed. New York: McGraw-Hill, 2008, Fig. 179-1.)

ERYSIPELAS

An acute inflammation of the dermis by **Group A β-hemolytic streptococci.** Elderly and immunocompromised patients are at higher risk.

SYMPTOMS/EXAM

- Presents with well-demarcated erythema, edema, and tenderness (a type of cellulitis), typically affecting the face and lower legs (Figure 10.18).
- Patients are generally systemically ill, presenting with fever, chills, and malaise.
- Lesions can rapidly advance.

DIFFERENTIAL

Angioedema; allergic contact dermatitis.

TREATMENT

Treat with IV antibiotics directed against *Streptococcus*.

COMPLICATIONS

Guttate psoriasis or acute glomerulonephritis can follow streptococcal infection.

ANTHRAX

Caused by *Bacillus anthracis*, a gram-⊕, spore-forming aerobic rod; transmitted through the skin or mucous membranes, by inhalation of or contact with contaminated soil, by animals, or through biologic warfare. Two toxins—edema toxin and lethal toxin—are involved.

SYMPTOMS/EXAM

- Has 3 manifestations: cutaneous (95% of cases), GI, and pulmonary (**woolsorter's disease**).
- Presents as a nonspecific illness (fever, malaise, nausea and vomiting). Then, over 2–7 days, characteristic lesions develop.
- The 1° lesion is a small, erythematous macule that evolves into a papule with vesicles, significant erythema, and edema.
- In 1–3 days, the papule ulcerates, leaving the characteristic **necrotic eschar.** No pain or tenderness is seen at this point.
- **Suppurative regional adenopathy** can develop.

TREATMENT

- Treat with IV penicillin G. Oral tetracycline may be effective for mild disease.
- For penicillin-allergic patients, aminoglycosides, macrolides, or quinolones are second-line therapy.

COMPLICATIONS

Most cases resolve without sequelae, but 10%–20% of untreated cases of cutaneous anthrax are fatal.

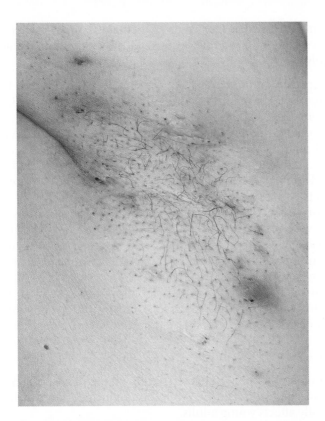

FIGURE 10.19.   Hidradenitis suppurativa. Note the bulging and depressed scars and draining sinus in the axillae. (Reproduced, with permission, from Wolff K, Johnson RA. *Fitzpatrick's Color Atlas & Synopsis of Clinical Dermatology,* 6th ed. New York: McGraw-Hill, 2009, Fig. 1-15.)

HIDRADENITIS SUPPURATIVA

- A chronic, suppurative cutaneous process that results from occlusion of follicles and secondary inflammation of the apocrine glands.
- Females are affected more often than males; it is more prevalent in obese women.
- Part of the "follicular occlusion triad" that consists of acne conglobata, hidradenitis suppurativa and dissecting cellulitis of the scalp.
- Sx/Exam:
    - Presents with recurrent deep boils for > 6 months in flexural sites (Figure 10.19).
    - Commonly affects the axillae, groin, vulva, and perineal or perianal areas, sparing the face (hence its proposed name, acne inversa). Lesions tend to recur.
- **Tx:** Treatment is often challenging. Topical antibiotics, antiandrogens, oral antibiotics, Accutane, and surgical excision are all used, typically with limited results.

> **KEY FACT**
>
> Perianal hidradenitis suppurativa and Crohn disease are similar and may be linked.

Mycotic Infections

TINEA (DERMATOPHYTES)

The most common type of fungal infection of the skin and nails. Often called "ringworm." The appearance of tinea is variegated, depending on location, but commonly it is seen as localized, erythematous, scaly lesions that form as pustules or vesicles with satellite lesions. Tinea is differentiated according to the site involved:

- **Tinea capitis ("cradle cap"):** Occurs primarily in children. Differentiate from seborrheic dermatitis in adults. Treat with griseofulvin. Consider terbinafine and itraconazole.
- **Tinea pedis ("athlete's foot"):** Chronic cases can usually be treated with a topical antifungal cream for 4 weeks. Interdigital tinea pedis, which is often macerated in appearance (Figure 10.20), may require only 1 week of therapy. Resistant cases may require oral medication (beware of cost and side effects).
- **Tinea corporis ("ringworm"):** Lesions typically have sharply demarcated margins, with scaling (Figure 10.21). Treat with daily antifungal creams. Cases associated with contact sports (eg, wrestling), called tinea corporis gladiatorum, generally respond better to oral antifungals (griseofulvin) and restriction from activity for 10–15 days.
- **Tinea cruris ("jock itch"):** Much more common in men. Obesity and sweaty physical activity are risk factors. Treat with topical antifungals. Use of talc or desiccant powders can help prevent recurrence.

Tinea Versicolor

A chronic fungal infection characterized by pigmentary changes. Caused by overgrowth of *Malassezia furfur*. More common in humid or tropical locations. Typically affects young adults.

SYMPTOMS/EXAM

- In fair-skinned people, presents with brown or pinkish superficially scaly macules and patches that may be oval or round. Typically involves the trunk and proximal parts of the limbs.
- In darker-skinned people, hypopigmentation is seen (Figure 10.22).
- Wood's lamp (+) for pale yellow fluorescence.

DIFFERENTIAL

Vitiligo, tinea corporis.

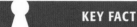

KEY FACT

Tinea pedis is the most common cause of cellulitis in otherwise healthy patients.

KEY FACT

Dermatophytid (id reaction) is a hypersensitivity reaction to a tinea infection on a distant body site (eg, a patient with tinea pedis develops pruritic vesicles on the back).

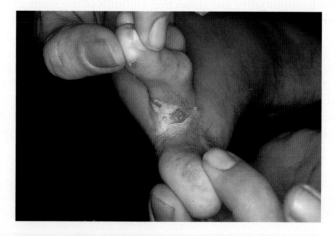

FIGURE 10.20. Interdigital tinea pedis. (Reproduced, with permission, from Orkin M, et al. *Dermatology.* Originally published by Appleton & Lange. Copyright © 1991 by the McGraw-Hill Companies, Inc.)

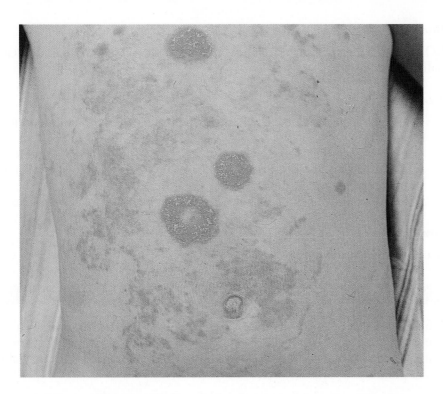

FIGURE 10.21. Tinea corporis. Note the sharply demarcated margins with scale. (Reproduced, with permission, from Wolff K, et al. *Fitzpatrick's Color Atlas & Synopsis of Clinical Dermatology,* 5th ed. New York: McGraw-Hill, 2005: 702.)

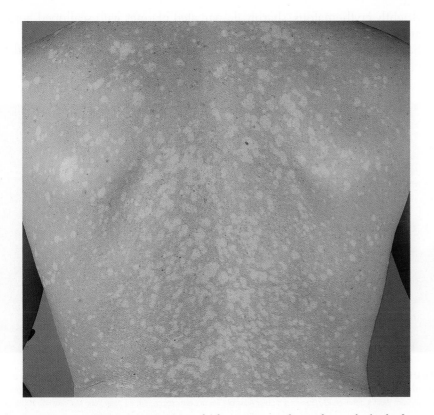

FIGURE 10.22. Tinea versicolor. Note the hypopigmented macules on the back of a tanned individual. (Reproduced, with permission, from Wolff K, Johnson RA. *Fitzpatrick's Color Atlas of Clinical Dermatology,* 6th ed. New York: McGraw-Hill, 2009, Fig. 13-13.)

DIAGNOSIS

KOH scraping reveals hyphae and budding spores ("**spaghetti and meat-balls**" appearance).

TREATMENT

- Topical antifungal (clotrimazole or miconazole); selenium sulfide lotion; ketoconazole shampoo.
- A single dose of ketoconazole at a dosage of 400 mg leads to short-term cure in 90% of cases. Most helpful to have the patient work up a sweat an hour after taking medication.
- Systemic antifungals (itraconazole) × 7 days can be used for resistant cases.

COMPLICATIONS

Recurrence is common.

CANDIDIASIS/INTERTRIGO

A fungal infection that favors moist areas, with the intertriginous areas most commonly involved. Risk factors include DM, obesity, sweating, heat, maceration, and systemic and topical steroid use. Antibiotics and OCPs may also be contributory.

SYMPTOMS/EXAM

- Initial vesiculopustules enlarge and rupture, becoming eroded and confluent.
- Brightly erythematous, sharply demarcated plaques with scalloped borders are seen (Figure 10.23).
- Satellite lesions (pustular lesions at the periphery) may coalesce and become part of a larger lesion.

KEY FACT

Diaper rash may be candidal diaper dermatitis. Look for satellite lesions.

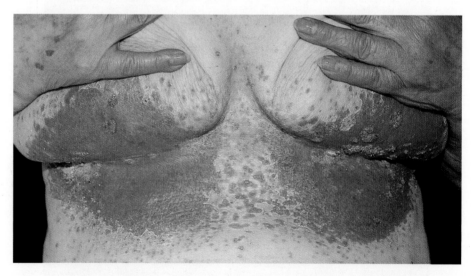

FIGURE 10.23.   Cutaneous candidiasis/intertrigo. Small peripheral satellite papules and pustules coalesce to create a large eroded area in the submammary region. (Reproduced, with permission, from Wolff K, Johnson RA. *Fitzpatrick's Color Atlas of Clinical Dermatology,* 6th ed. New York: McGraw-Hill, 2009, Fig. 25-23.)

DIAGNOSIS

KOH scraping shows pseudohyphae and yeast forms.

TREATMENT

Keep affected areas dry; treat with topical antifungals (powders or creams).

Viral Infections

MOLLUSCUM CONTAGIOSUM

Discrete, pearly-pink, umbilical papules commonly involving the trunk, face, and neck, but may occur anywhere. Caused by a DNA poxvirus. Occurs mostly in children and young adults, and more common in immunodeficient patients. Spread by direct contact (eg, sexual contact, towels).

SYMPTOMS/EXAM

- Presents with dome-shaped papules a few millimeters in size, with central umbilication or puncta (Figure 10.24).
- Lesions are usually multiple and occur in groups.
- Intracytoplasmic inclusion bodies called Henderson-Paterson bodies are present.

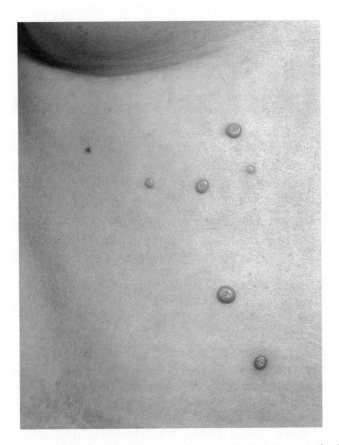

FIGURE 10.24.   **Molluscum contagiosum on the chest of a female.** Note the discrete, solid papules with central umbilication. (Reproduced, with permission, from Wolff K, et al. *Fitzpatrick's Dermatology in General Medicine,* 7th ed. New York: McGraw-Hill, 2008, Fig. 195-12A.)

DIFFERENTIAL

Viral warts, skin tags.

TREATMENT

- The disease is self-limited.
- In adults or older children, lesions can be removed via expression with forceps, with curettage under local anesthesia, or with cryosurgery.
- Most therapies are off-label.
- Topical imiquimod, liquid nitrogen, cantharone, salicylic acid, tea tree oil, or no therapy.

COMPLICATIONS

Infection can be especially severe in immunosuppressed patients.

VIRAL EXANTHEM

- A rash associated with general features of a viral illness (myalgias, arthralgias, sore throat). Primarily seen in children and adolescents.
- **Sx/Exam:** The rash is erythematous and maculopapular, with a blotchy appearance, generally affecting the trunk and limbs. The viral cause is generally not identified.
- **DDx:** Chickenpox, measles, rubella, fifth disease, coxsackievirus (hand-foot-mouth disease).
- **Tx:** Treat with emollients or cooling agents (calamine).

Parasitic Infections

SCABIES

A 14-year-old boy presents to your office with a pruritic, crusting rash on his feet of 2 weeks' duration. Topical corticosteroids have failed to improve his condition. How would you proceed?

The skin should be scraped and examined under the microscope for characteristic mites. Treatment is usually begun with permethrin. Clothing and household contacts need to be treated as well.

Caused by skin infection by the mite *Sarcoptes scabiei* (Figure 10.25). The female mite burrows into the skin to lay eggs. The infection is highly contagious and spreads through prolonged contact with an infected host.

SYMPTOMS/EXAM

- Presents with small pruritic papules, pustules, and burrows (Figure 10.26). Lesions are intensely pruritic, especially at night.
- Infection usually spares the face and scalp and is classically located in the web spaces of the hands (Figure 10.27). It is also common in the axillae, antecubital fossa, gluteal crease, feet, genitalia, nipples, and waistband (Figure 10.28).
- Itching and rash are due to a type IV hypersensitivity reaction to the mite, eggs, and feces, and cause a 2–4-week delay between infection and onset of symptoms.
- Excoriations and crusts develop secondary to scratching.

KEY FACT

Infectious mononucleosis treated with amoxicillin can cause a rash similar to a viral exanthem.

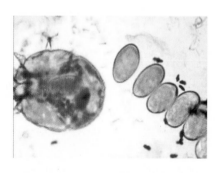

FIGURE 10.25. Microscopic appearance of scabies *(Sarcoptes scabiei).*
(Reproduced, with permission, from Wolff K, et al. *Fitzpatrick's Dermatology in General Medicine,* 7th ed. New York: McGraw-Hill, 2008, Fig. 208-5.)

KEY FACT

The symptoms of scabies may persist for weeks to months despite effective treatment.

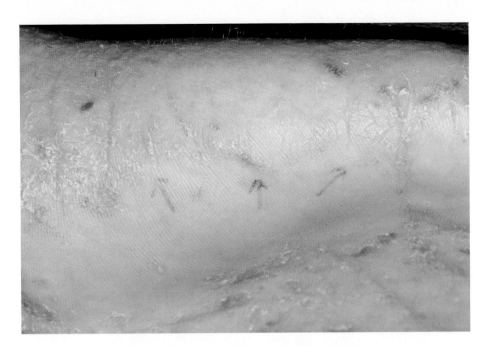

FIGURE 10.26. **Linear burrows of infection caused by scabies.** (Reproduced, with permission, from Wolff K, Johnson RA. *Fitzpatrick's Color Atlas of Clinical Dermatology*, 6th ed. New York: McGraw-Hill, 2009, Fig. 28-18.)

DIAGNOSIS

■ Examine skin scrapings with microscopy to identify mites, ova, and fecal pellets called scybala (Figure 10.29).
■ The diagnosis should be confirmed with a skin scraping and viewed under a low-power microscope.

TREATMENT

■ Apply permethrin 5% below the neck. Leave on for 8 hours and shower off. May be repeated in 1 week.
■ Wash clothes and linens in hot water.
■ STDs should be excluded.
■ Consider treating family members who sleep in the same room.

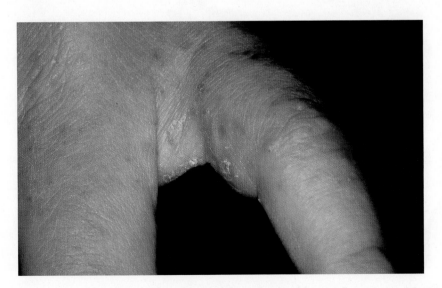

FIGURE 10.27. **Burrows of scabies mite in the web spaces of the hands.** (Reproduced, with permission, from Wolff K, Johnson RA. *Fitzpatrick's Color Atlas of Clinical Dermatology*, 6th ed. New York: McGraw-Hill, 2009, Fig. 28-16.)

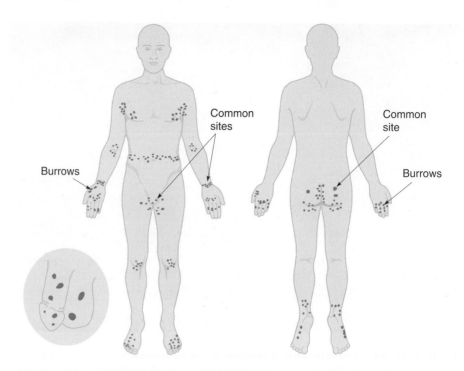

FIGURE 10.28. **Common sites of scabies infection.** (Reproduced, with permission, from Wolff K, Johnson RA. *Fitzpatrick's Color Atlas of Clinical Dermatology*, 6th ed. New York: McGraw-Hill, 2009, Fig. 28-1.)

PEDICULOSIS

Skin infection by lice. Lice do not transmit disease; their main effect is embarrassment. The female louse lays eggs (nits) at the base of the hair that adhere to the hair shaft as it grows. Lice do not jump or fly and are not passed by pets. Head and body lice are interchangeable; genital lice ("crabs") are another species.

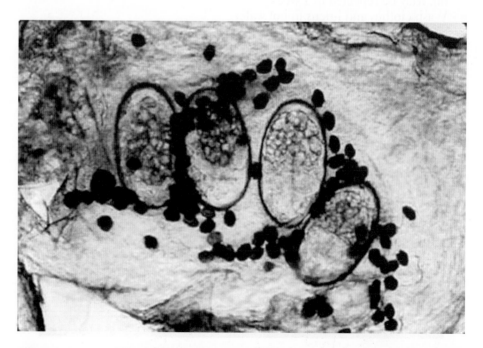

FIGURE 10.29. **Eggs and fecal pellets of the scabies mite found in skin scrapings under light microscopy.** (Courtesy of A Hoke, as published in Tierney LM, et al. *Current Medical Diagnosis & Treatment*, 45th ed. New York: McGraw-Hill, 2006.)

SYMPTOMS/EXAM

- Transmitted by direct contact or by fomites. May affect the head, body, or genital region.
- Patients may be asymptomatic or may present with pruritus resulting from allergy to lice saliva.
- Lice are visible to the naked eye and are 3–4 mm in size.

DIAGNOSIS

Diagnosed by direct visualization on exam.

TREATMENT

Permethrin 1% cream rinse is available OTC. Shampoo hair and towel dry. Apply permethrin cream and rinse in 10 minutes. Treatment may be repeated in 7–10 days.

Immunologic and Autoimmune Disease

BLISTERING DISEASES

Pemphigus vulgaris and bullous pemphigoid are among the most common autoimmune blistering disorders. Table 10.5 outlines the presentation of both.

TABLE 10.5. Bullous Pemphigoid vs. Pemphigus Vulgaris

	BULLOUS PEMPHIGOID	PEMPHIGUS VULGARIS
Site of blistering	Subepidermal.	Intraepidermal.
Epidemiology	Affects patients aged > 60 years; the most common blistering disorder.	Affects patients aged 40–60 years.
Pruritus	Prominent.	Not prominent.
Nikolsky sign (superficial separation of skin with lateral pressure)	⊖	⊕
Frequency of oral mucosal lesions	Affect a minority of patients (< 30%).	Affect > 50% of patients.
Character of blisters and bullae	Intact, tense (Figure 10.30).	Rupture easily; flaccid (Figure 10.31).
Complications	Few complications.	Superinfection; high mortality from sepsis if untreated; ocular involvement dictates a referral.
Subtypes		Drug induced (penicillamine and ACEIs), paraneoplastic.

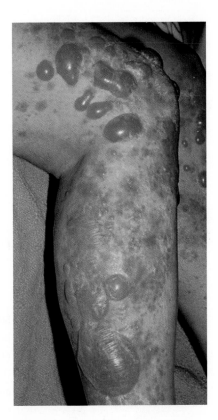

FIGURE 10.30. Bullous pemphigoid. (Reproduced, with permission, from Wolff K, et al. *Fitzpatrick's Dermatology in General Medicine,* 7th ed. New York: McGraw-Hill, 2008, Fig. 54-4.)

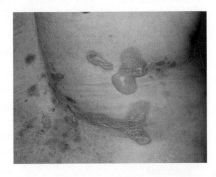

FIGURE 10.31. Pemphigus vulgaris. (Reproduced, with permission, from Wolff K, et al. *Fitzpatrick's Dermatology in General Medicine,* 7th ed. New York: McGraw-Hill, 2008, Fig. 52-3.)

TABLE 10.6. Immunologic Mechanisms of Cutaneous Drug Reactions

MECHANISM	EXAMPLES
Type I: Classic immediate hypersensitivity	Urticaria, angioedema, anaphylaxis.
Type III: Immune complex	Leukocytoclastic vasculitis, serum sickness, urticaria, angioedema.
Type IV: Delayed hypersensitivity	Contact dermatitis, exanthematous reactions, photoallergic reactions.
Systemic infection impairing immune response	Mononucleosis, ampicillin-induced rash, HIV, sulfonamide-induced toxic epidermal necrolysis.
Unknown immunologic mechanisms	Lichenoid reactions, fixed drug eruptions.

Cutaneous Drug Reactions

Mechanisms of dermatologic drug reactions may be immunologic (Table 10.6) or nonimmunologic. Examples of nonimmunologic drug reactions include cutaneous phototoxicity with tetracycline use or the itching and erythema caused by mast cell mediator release in response to NSAIDs or radiographic contrast. Table 10.7 outlines the etiologies and clinical presentation of severe cutaneous drug reactions.

TABLE 10.7. Differential Diagnosis of Severe Drug Reactions

DIAGNOSIS	MUCOSAL LESION	TYPICAL SKIN LESION	FREQUENT SYMPTOMS AND SIGNS	OTHER UNRELATED CAUSES	DRUGS MOST OFTEN IMPLICATED
Stevens-Johnson syndrome	Erosions are usually at 2 or more sites.	Small blisters on dusky purpuric macules or atypical targets (Figure 10.32). Rare areas of confluence may be seen. Involves detachment of 10% or less of body surface area (BSA).	Some 10%–30% present with fever.	Postinfectious erythema multiforme major (acute dermatitis characterized by distinctive, fixed-target lesions [Figure 10.33]; caused by HSV or *Mycoplasma*).	Sulfa drugs, phenytoin, carbamazepine, lamotrigine, allopurinol.
Toxic epidermal necrolysis	Same as above.	Individual lesions like those of Stevens-Johnson syndrome (Figure 10.34). ⊕ Nikolsky sign; large sheet of necrotic epidermis. Involves > 30% of BSA.	Fever is nearly universal. "Acute skin failure" and leukopenia are also seen.	Viral infections, immunization, chemicals, *Mycoplasma* pneumonia.	Same as above.
Anticonvulsant hypersensitivity syndrome	Infrequent.	Severe exanthems (may become purpuric); exfoliative dermatitis.	Some 30%–50% of cases present with fever, lymphadenopathy, hepatitis, nephritis, carditis, eosinophilia, and atypical lymphocytes.	Cutaneous lymphoma.	Anticonvulsants.

TABLE 10.7.   Differential Diagnosis of Severe Drug Reactions *(continued)*

DIAGNOSIS	MUCOSAL LESION	TYPICAL SKIN LESION	FREQUENT SYMPTOMS AND SIGNS	OTHER UNRELATED CAUSES	DRUGS MOST OFTEN IMPLICATED
Serum sickness	Absent.	Morbilliform lesions, sometimes with urticaria.	Fever, arthralgias.	Infection.	
Anticoagulant-induced necrosis	Infrequent.	Erythema; then purpura and necrosis, especially of fatty areas.	Pain in affected areas.	DIG.	Warfarin.
Angioedema	Often involved.	Urticaria or swelling of the face.	Respiratory distress or cardiovascular collapse.	Insect stings, foods.	NSAIDs, ACEIs, penicillin.

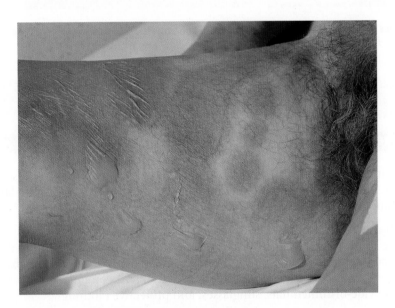

FIGURE 10.32.   Lesions of Stevens-Johnson syndrome. (Reproduced, with permission, from Wolff K, et al. *Fitzpatrick's Color Atlas & Synopsis of Clinical Dermatology,* 5th ed. New York: McGraw-Hill, 2005: 145.)

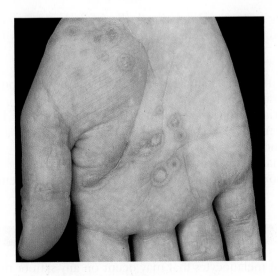

FIGURE 10.33.   Lesions of erythema multiforme. (Reproduced, with permission, from Wolff K, et al. *Fitzpatrick's Dermatology in General Medicine,* 7th ed. New York: McGraw-Hill, 2008, Fig. 38-2.)

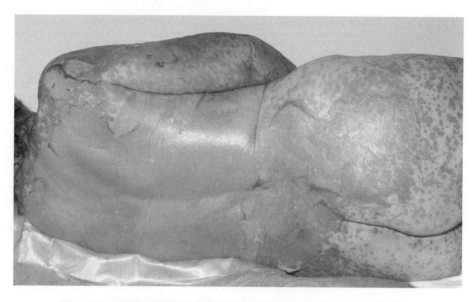

FIGURE 10.34. Lesions of toxic epidermal necrolysis. (Reproduced, with permission, from Wolff K, et al. *Fitzpatrick's Color Atlas & Synopsis of Clinical Dermatology*, 5th ed. New York: McGraw-Hill, 2005: 147.)

Cutaneous Oncology

1° PREVENTION OF SKIN CANCER

UVA and UVB both lead to photoaging; UVB more commonly causes skin cancer. The following recommendations are for 1° prevention of skin damage and cancer:

- Minimize sun exposure during peak UV midday hours (10–4 P.M.).
- Use sunscreen with at least SPF 15. Physical sunscreens (eg, titanium dioxide or zinc oxide) deflect or block the sun's rays. Chemical sunscreens absorb or filter UV rays. Broadband sunscreens may contain a combination of both.
- Use wide-brimmed hats, sunglasses, and protective clothing.

ATYPICAL NEVI

- Nevi sharing features of melanoma. Typically large (> 6 mm), hyperpigmented, and asymmetric, with irregular "fuzzy" borders ("fried egg" appearance).
- Sx/Exam:
  - Lesions may occur anywhere on the body but are more common in sun-exposed areas (eg, the back).
  - Have variable appearance, but usually show the **ABCDE** appearance (see mnemonic).
- **DDx:** Melanoma.
- **Tx:** Excisional biopsy only if melanoma is suspected.
- **Complications:** The incidence of melanoma is ↑ in patients with atypical nevi.

MELANOMA

A malignancy of melanocytes that may occur on any skin or mucosal surface. It is the 7th most common cancer in the United States, with the incidence doubling every 10 years. Superficial spreading melanoma (which makes up

70% of cases) tends to stay "superficial" and has a better prognosis than nodular melanoma (15%), which tends to grow downward. *CDKN2A* is a gene associated with familiar melanoma. Risk factors are expressed in the mnemonic **MMRISK.**

SYMPTOMS/EXAM

Presents with a changing mole (see Figure 10.35 and the mnemonic **ABCDE**) that may enlarge suddenly, begin to bleed, begin to itch, or become painful. May occur anywhere on the body, but more common in sun-exposed areas.

DIFFERENTIAL

Atypical nevi; seborrheic keratosis.

DIAGNOSIS

- Clinical exam and excisional biopsy.
- Tumor thickness (Breslow classification) and lymph node spread are the most important prognostic factors.
- No staging workup is necessary if the lesion is < 1 mm in thickness, which is considered low risk.

TREATMENT

- Excision with appropriate borders.
- Sentinel lymph node dissection for melanomas > 1 mm thick to determine if adjuvant therapy is needed.
- Close follow-up.

COMPLICATIONS

Metastasis. Five-year survival rates with lymph node involvement and distant metastasis are 30% and 10%, respectively.

BASAL CELL CARCINOMA (BCC)

- The most common skin cancer (80%); occurs in sun-exposed areas, especially the central face and ears.

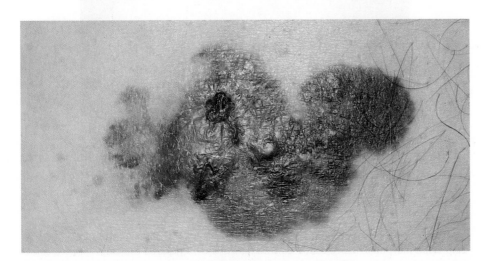

FIGURE 10.35. Superficial spreading melanoma. A highly characteristic lesion with an irregular pigmented pattern and scalloped borders. (Reproduced, with permission, from Wolff K, et al. *Fitzpatrick's Color Atlas & Synopsis of Clinical Dermatology,*5th ed. New York: McGraw-Hill, 2005: 318.)

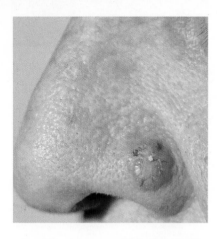

FIGURE 10.36. Nodular basal cell carcinoma. A smooth, pearly nodule with telangiectasias. (Reproduced, with permission, from Wolff K, et al. *Fitzpatrick's Color Atlas & Synopsis of Clinical Dermatology,* 5th ed. New York: McGraw-Hill, 2005: 283.)

KEY FACT

The central face and ears are high-risk areas of ↑ recurrence and metastatic potential for basal cell carcinoma.

- **Sx/Exam:** Presents with a shiny, "pearly" papule with an umbilicated center and telangiectasias (Figure 10.36).
- **DDx:** Molluscum contagiosum, keratoses.
- **Dx:** Shave biopsy.
- **Tx:** Excision or destruction (electrodesiccation and curettage) of the lesion. Patient education for sun avoidance is key to further prevention. Mohs micrographic surgery is often indicated for BCC on the head and neck, and for large BCC or recurring BCC.
- **Complications:** Metastatic spread. Occurs in < 0.1% of patients.

ACTINIC KERATOSIS

- A superficial keratotic lesion that is a precursor of SCC. Prevention by avoidance of sun exposure is key.
- **Sx/Exam:** Presents as a discrete, reddish-pink keratotic lesion, usually with a white scale, that feels "rough" (Figure 10.37). Found in sun-exposed areas, mostly on the face and dorsal hands.
- **Dx:** Biopsy is not indicated. Diagnosed by clinical presentation on the basis of location and rough feel.
- **Tx:** Cryotherapy, topical 5-FU, topical imiquimod, photodynamic therapy.

SQUAMOUS CELL CARCINOMA (SCC)

- Represents 20% of all skin cancers. May arise within actinic keratoses, within HPV-induced lesions, and within burn and radiation scars. SCC is more common than BCC in immunocompromised individuals.

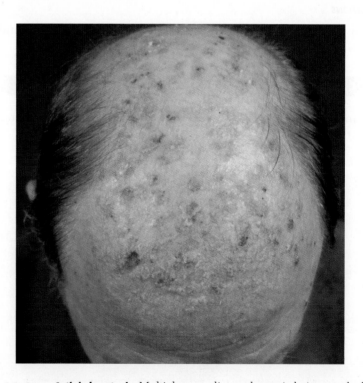

FIGURE 10.37. Actinic keratosis. Multiple premalignant keratotic lesions on the bald scalp of this individual. (Reproduced, with permission, from Wolff K, et al. *Fitzpatrick's Color Atlas & Synopsis of Clinical Dermatology,* 5th ed. New York: McGraw-Hill, 2005: 263.)

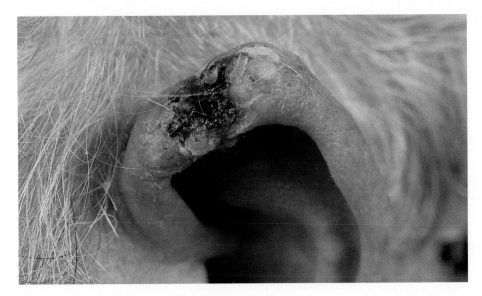

FIGURE 10.38. **Squamous cell carcinoma.** A hyperkeratotic nodule with ulceration. (Reproduced, with permission, from Wolff K, et al. *Fitzpatrick's Color Atlas & Synopsis of Clinical Dermatology,* 5th ed. New York: McGraw-Hill, 2005: 279.)

- **Sx/Exam:** Presents with a hyperkeratotic lesion with crusting and ulceration (Figure 10.38). May occur anywhere, but most commonly seen in sun-exposed areas.
- **Tx:** Surgical excision with clear margins.
- **Cx:** Has a higher rate of metastasis than BCC. The 5-year recurrence rate is 8%, and the metastatic rate is 5%.

KEY FACT

SCC is more common and more aggressive in immunosuppressed patients, or transplant patients.

CUTANEOUS T-CELL LYMPHOMA

- **A T-cell lymphoma that begins in the skin;** the most common type is mycosis fungoides. Most often affects patients > 50 years of age. Twice as common in men and more common in African Americans.
- **Sx/Exam:** Presents with pruritic, eczematous patches and plaques distributed over non–sun-exposed areas of skin. Tumors develop later in the disease course.
- **Cx:** Sézary syndrome is the leukemic form of T-cell lymphoma. Without treatment, patients succumb to opportunistic infections.

Miscellaneous Dermatologic Disorders

KELOID

- A hypertrophic scar; more common in African Americans.
- **Tx:** Intralesional corticosteroid injections. Surgical excision is **not** recommended, as lesions can recur larger than before.

DISORDERS AFFECTING THE HAIR

Table 10.8 outlines dermatologic disorders of the hair.

TABLE 10.8. Dermatologic Disorders Affecting the Hair

DISORDER	HISTORY/EXAM	TREATMENT
Androgenic alopecia	Hereditary; affects individuals 12–70 years of age; presents with gradual progression of hair loss over the temple and crown area.	Topical minoxidil; finasteride.
Alopecia areata	Nonscarring autoimmune alopecia characterized by well-demarcated patches of hair loss.	Local steroid injection; topical steroids.
Telogen effluvium	Diffuse loss of scalp, axillary, and pubic hair occurring 2–4 months after an inciting event (psychological stressors, major surgery, childbirth, crash diets, endocrine disorders).	Treat the underlying cause.
Traction alopecia	Alopecia occurring in high-tension hair styles (tight braids, ponytails). May be permanent.	Change in hair style.

MELASMA

- Splotchy hyperpigmented macules that affect sun-exposed areas of skin, most commonly on the face (Figure 10.39). The cause is thought to be hormonally mediated.
- More common in women and darker-skinned persons (especially Hispanics).
- **Tx:** Topical therapy (hydroquinone cream) and strict sunscreen application. Hydroquinone has been associated with ochronosis and must be used cautiously and for a maximal 3-month duration. Can be chronic, but if associated with pregnancy, it will usually regress within a year. If patients fail to respond, refer to a dermatologist for chemical peel or bleaching agents.

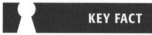

KEY FACT

Melasma occurs in 75% of pregnancies.

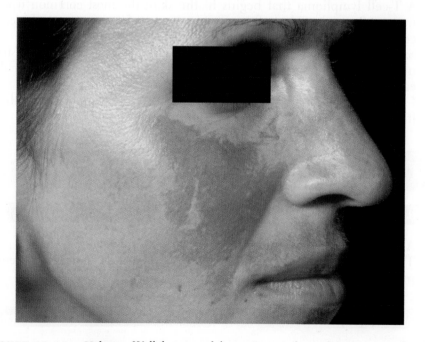

FIGURE 10.39. Melasma. Well-demarcated, hyperpigmented macules are seen on the cheek, nose, and upper lip. (Reproduced, with permission, from Wolff K, Johnson RA. *Fitzpatrick's Color Atlas & Synopsis of Clinical Dermatology*, 6th ed. New York: McGraw-Hill, 2009, Fig. 13-8.)

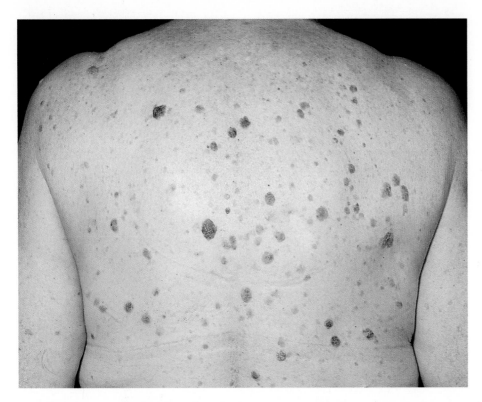

FIGURE 10.40. **Seborrheic keratosis.** Multiple seborrheic keratoses with a "stuck-on" appearance are seen on the back. (Reproduced, with permission, from Wolff K, Johnson RA. *Fitzpatrick's Color Atlas & Synopsis of Clinical Dermatology,* 6th ed. New York: McGraw-Hill, 2009, Fig. 9-41.)

SEBORRHEIC KERATOSIS

- The most common benign epidermal growth.
- **Sx/Exam:** Usually asymptomatic; has a classic "stuck-on" appearance (Figure 10.40).
- **Tx:** No treatment is necessary, but growths can be frozen or curetted if bothersome.

NOTES

CHAPTER 11

Neurology

Magdalen Edmunds, MD, MPH

Headache

MIGRAINE HEADACHE

Migraines are divided into **2 categories:** those **without aura** (formerly known as common migraine) and those **with aura** (also known as classic migraine). Migraines typically present among patients 10–30 years of age.

SYMPTOMS/EXAM

- **Migraine without aura (common migraine):** Described as recurrent headaches lasting 4–72 hours. To diagnose, at least 2 of the following characteristics must be present: **unilateral** distribution, **pulsatile** quality, severity limiting daily activities, and exacerbation by physical activity. One of the following characteristics must also be present: **nausea** or **vomiting, photosensitivity,** and sensitivity to noise or smell.
- **Migraine with aura (classic migraine):** Classic migraines present with symptoms similar to those of the common migraine, but the **headache is preceded by an aura.** An aura is a reversible symptom indicative of focal cerebral dysfunction. Examples of auras include: gradual onset and spread of scotomas, scintillations, and/or hemianopic field defects; unilateral paresthesias or numbness; unilateral weakness; and speech disturbance. Symptoms may "march" from one area to another.
- It is not uncommon to have aura symptoms with gradual onset and no subsequent headache.
- The neurologic exam is generally normal.
- Women taking oral contraceptives (OCPs) who have migraines should use OCP options that do not contain estrogen because of the ↑ stroke risk.

DIFFERENTIAL

Other forms of headache, intracranial mass, temporal (giant cell) arteritis, sinusitis, subarachnoid hemorrhage, pseudotumor cerebri, transient ischemic attack (TIA).

DIAGNOSIS

Based on symptoms, a ⊕ family history, and lack of neurologic findings.

TREATMENT

- **Acute attacks:** NSAIDs, acetaminophen, triptans, ergotamines, narcotic analgesics, antiemetics.
- **Prophylaxis:** β-blockers, calcium channel blockers, tricyclic antidepressants (TCAs), anticonvulsants, methysergide. Avoidance or mitigation of triggers such as stress, missed meals, menses, and sleep deprivation.

COMPLICATIONS

- Associated risk of rebound headaches with frequent analgesic use.
- Migraine is a risk factor for stroke.

KEY FACT

Migraines are more common in women than in men.

TENSION HEADACHE

The most common type of recurring headache other than migraine.

- **Sx/Exam:**
    - Presents as a bilateral headache with pain in the frontal and occipital regions in a **bandlike distribution.** Headaches are exacerbated by stress, fatigue, glare, or noise.
    - Often involves contraction of the scalp and posterior neck muscles, with a normal neurologic exam.
- **Dx:** Based on the history and lack of neurologic findings.
- **Tx:**
    - **Acute headache:** Aspirin, NSAIDs, ergotamines.
    - **Prophylaxis:** TCAs, SSRIs, β-blockers, relaxation techniques.
- **Cx:** Risk of rebound headaches with frequent analgesic use.

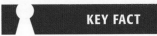

> **KEY FACT**
>
> Tension headaches are the most common type of headache.

CLUSTER HEADACHE

Occurs most often in middle-aged men.

- **Sx/Exam:**
    - Described as a recurrent, **unilateral,** excruciating **periorbital** headache that lasts from 15 minutes to 3 hours. Headaches are nonpulsatile and constant, frequently occurring at night.
    - Look for Horner syndrome, **ipsilateral conjunctival injection, lacrimation,** and nasal congestion (Figure 11.1).
    - Cluster headaches classically take place in groups over days to weeks, occurring at the same time of day and in the same location.
    - The neurologic exam is usually normal.
- **DDx:** Migraine, glaucoma, sinusitis, uveitis, trigeminal neuralgia.

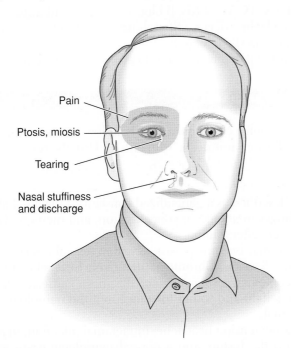

FIGURE 11.1.   Symptoms of cluster headache. (Reproduced, with permission, from Simon RP, et al. *Clinical Neurology,* 7th ed. New York: McGraw-Hill, 2009, Fig. 2-14.)

- **Dx:**
  - Based on the history and lack of neurologic findings. Often there is no family history of headache.
  - Consider a head CT or MRI for new headache onset after 30 years of age.
- **Tx:**
  - **Acute attack:** 100% O_2, triptans, ergotamines, intranasal lidocaine, butorphanol.
  - **Prophylaxis:** Avoid triggers such as alcohol, stress, and medications causing vasodilation. To prevent acute recurrence, a prednisone burst and taper may be helpful. For long-term prevention, consider ergotamines, valproate, calcium channel blockers, lithium, and methysergide.
- **Cx:** Horner syndrome. The severity of pain has driven some to suicide.

REBOUND HEADACHE

Described as a chronic or nearly daily headache associated with **frequent use of medication for acute head pain.**

- **Sx/Exam:**
  - Presents with bilateral head pain in a bandlike distribution around the head, neck, and scalp.
  - Muscle contraction, tenderness, and photosensitivity are also seen. The neurologic exam is normal.
- **Dx:** Based on the history and lack of neurologic findings.
- **Tx:**
  - Discontinue the analgesics causing the rebound headaches.
  - **Acute attack:** Consider treating headaches during withdrawal with triptans, prednisone, or ergotamines.
  - **Prophylaxis:** TCAs, SSRIs, β-blockers, anticonvulsants.
  - Avoid headache triggers. Stretching, aerobic exercise, and relaxation techniques may be of benefit.
- **Cx:** One-third of patients relapse into analgesic overuse pattern.

POSTTRAUMATIC HEADACHE

This type of headache commonly occurs following minor head injuries or hyperextension-flexion injuries ("whiplash"). Usually resolves in weeks to months.

- **Sx/Exam:**
  - Usually described as a generalized constant headache that is associated with changes in attention, concentration, and memory. Onset tends to be < 2 weeks after trauma.
  - Symptoms may become persistent within several weeks of injury. Acute cases last < 8 weeks. Chronic posttraumatic headache lasts > 8 weeks.
  - Some people may also experience dizziness, nausea, irritability, insomnia, and ↓ light and sound tolerance, but the neurologic exam is typically normal.
- **DDx:** Migraine; tension headache; intracranial infection, mass, or bleed.
- **Dx:** Based on the history and a normal neurologic exam with a normal head CT and LP (if performed).
- **Tx:**
  - Supportive care; pain management.
  - Antiemetics and TCAs may be of benefit.
- **Cx:** ↓ patient functionality.

TEMPORAL ARTERITIS (GIANT CELL ARTERITIS)

A 52-year-old woman is seen in the clinic because she is feeling "tired and achy all over." She has a headache "by my right eye" and blurred vision. She states that "my arms wear out so fast I can't comb my hair." She also complains of jaw ache when she chews. As you examine her, she reports pain when you palpate her scalp. How do you proceed?

This patient needs to be started on prednisone immediately because her symptoms and exam are concerning for temporal arteritis. After starting prednisone, a temporal artery biopsy should be arranged.

A treatable neurologic emergency characterized by subacute inflammation of the external carotid arterial system and vertebral arteries. It is most common in **women > 50 years of age.**

SYMPTOMS/EXAM

- Patients often describe a **new** temporal or diffuse headache that may be associated with **transient visual loss, scalp tenderness, jaw claudication. Polymyalgia rheumatica (PMR)** may also be present. Symptoms include fever, myalgia, malaise, anorexia, anemia, weight loss, tenderness, and stiffness in the shoulders and hips. 50% of people with temporal arteritis have PMR.
- On exam, look for temporal arteries that may be dilated, tender, thickened, and nonpulsatile.
- More rare findings are a funduscopic exam that reveals a pale optic disc on the affected side or cranial neuropathies.

DIFFERENTIAL

Glaucoma, uveitis, rheumatoid arthritis (RA), trigeminal neuralgia, retinal embolism, Takayasu arteritis.

DIAGNOSIS

- Diagnosis is guided by the history and exam. History may reveal coexisting PMR.
- Biopsy of affected temporal arteries shows vasculitis with mononuclear cell infiltration or granulomatous inflammation.
- An ESR > 50 mm/hr is common (although rare cases may show a normal ESR). Normochromic, normocytic anemia with thrombocytosis is also common.

TREATMENT

Prednisone 60 mg daily for 1–2 months, with slow taper, and monitoring of symptoms and ESR. Aspirin ↓ the risk of stroke or visual loss.

COMPLICATIONS

Fifty percent of untreated patients may suffer permanent visual loss, with one-half experiencing bilateral loss. Temporal arteritis is also associated with ↑ risk of cranial neuropathy, TIA, stroke, and thoracic aortic aneurysm.

KEY FACT

"A sed rate over 50 in a patient over 50"—temporal arteritis.

BENIGN INTRACRANIAL HYPERTENSION (PSEUDOTUMOR CEREBRI)

 An obese 37-year-old woman presents with headaches that worsen with lifting heavy objects and "ringing of the ears." She has also noted blurry vision. Exam shows limited abduction of her left eye, and funduscopy reveals optic disc swelling and hard exudates. How do you proceed?

To evaluate concern for ↑ ICP, a CT scan and LP must be done. These tests will confirm your suspicion of pseudotumor cerebri.

A disorder consisting of **headache, ↑ ICP, and papilledema** unexplained by any other identifiable cause. The disorder is usually idiopathic and typically affects obese, hirsute-appearing young women.

SYMPTOMS/EXAM

- Presents with diffuse headaches that may worsen on straining. Often associated with visual loss or diplopia, transient visual obscurations, pulsatile tinnitus, limited abduction of 1 or both eyes, and ↓ level of consciousness.
- A funduscopic exam shows papilledema (Figure 11.2). Visual function testing reveals an ↑ physiologic blind spot. Severe cases have constricted visual fields and ↓ acuity.

DIFFERENTIAL

Intracranial mass or bleed, hydrocephalus, dural venous thrombosis, migraine, glaucoma. Associated causative factors include hypervitaminosis A, hypoparathyroidism, Addison disease, and medications (eg, corticosteroids, tetracycline, OCPs).

DIAGNOSIS

- Findings include papilledema with possible abducens nerve palsy.
- Head CT or MRI may be normal or may show **small ventricles** or **empty sella.**

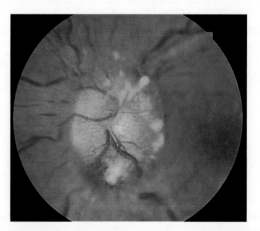

FIGURE 11.2.   Papilledema. Papilledema means optic disc edema from raised intracranial pressure. This obese young woman with pseudotumor cerebri was misdiagnosed as a migraineur until fundus examination was performed, showing optic disc elevation, hemorrhages, and cotton-wool spots. (Reproduced, with permission, from Fauci AS, et al. *Harrison's Principles of Internal Medicine,* 17th ed. New York: McGraw-Hill, 2008, Fig. 29-12.)

- LP shows elevated opening pressure with a normal CSF profile.
- CT angiography or magnetic resonance venogram shows no dural sinus thrombosis.

TREATMENT

- Start acetazolamide +/− a diuretic.
- Discontinue contributing medications or excessive vitamin A.
- Repeated LPs or lumboperitoneal shunting may be necessary for refractory cases. Weight reduction.

COMPLICATIONS

Optic atrophy; permanent visual loss.

INTRACRANIAL ARTERIOVENOUS MALFORMATION (AVM)

Congenital abnormal connections between arterioles and venules without intervening capillaries. Usually discovered when the malformation or related aneurysm hemorrhages. Most are supratentorial and are found by 40 years of age.

SYMPTOMS/EXAM

- Presents with persistent generalized or stereotyped unilateral headaches or seizure.
- The neurologic exam is usually normal, without hemorrhage. Abnormal mental state, signs of meningeal irritation, seizure, signs of ↑ ICP, hemiparesis or paralysis, aphasia, and ↓ sensation may be associated with hemorrhage.
- AVMs account for about 10% of subarachnoid hemorrhages.
- Found most commonly in men between the 2nd and 4th decades of life.
- **Tx:** See section on subarachnoid hemorrhage below. If AVM has not bled, it is controversial whether to treat the malformation.

DIFFERENTIAL

Migraines, cluster headaches, intracranial mass, epilepsy, stroke, subarachnoid hemorrhage, cerebral aneurysm, amyloid angiopathy.

DIAGNOSIS

- Obtain an MRI/MRA. EEG for patients with seizure; head CT if hemorrhage is suspected.
- Perform an LP to examine CSF for blood if hemorrhage is suspected and CT is not diagnostic.
- Arteriography if hemorrhage, aneurysm, or AVM is detected (Figure 11.3) or if the source remains unclear.

TREATMENT

- Stop any anticoagulant or antiplatelet medications.
- Anticonvulsants for seizure activity but not for prophylaxis.
- Neurosurgery for hemorrhage in patients with a reasonable life expectancy and an accessible lesion. Embolization or radiation of surgically inaccessible lesions.

COMPLICATIONS

Headaches, hemorrhage, focal neurologic deficits, seizures, hydrocephalus.

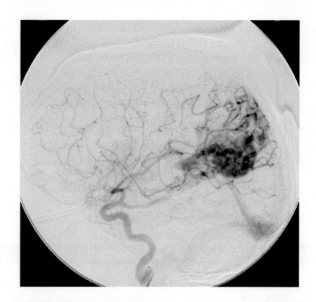

FIGURE 11.3. Arteriovenous malformation. (Reproduced, with permission, from Ropper A, Brown RH. *Adams and Victor's Principles of Neurology,* 9th ed. New York: McGraw-Hill, 2009, Fig. 34-26B.)

DIAGNOSIS OF DANGEROUS CAUSES OF HEADACHE

Table 11.1 summarizes signs of underlying organic causes of headaches in the absence of other diagnostic features.

TABLE 11.1. Presentation of Dangerous Causes of Headaches

SYMPTOM	POSSIBLE CAUSE
Sudden onset of "the worst headache of my life."	Subarachnoid hemorrhage.
Neck stiffness with severe headache.	Bacterial meningitis.
Sudden ↓ level of consciousness.	Intracranial bleed, intracranial mass.
Progressively worsening headache.	Intracranial mass.
Daily headaches that awaken the patient from sleep or are severe on arising in the morning.	Intracranial mass with ↑ ICP. (Migraine is the most common cause of morning headache.)
Onset of headaches after 30 years of age.	Intracranial mass.
Progressive visual, motor, or balance disturbance, or cognitive changes.	Intracranial mass, vascular lesion.
Onset of headache after age 50 years of age.	Temporal arteritis, intracranial mass.

Cerebrovascular Disease

ISCHEMIC STROKE

An ischemic CVA is defined as a sudden brain dysfunction with neurologic deficits **lasting > 24 hours** caused by occlusion of a vessel supplying the brain. A lacunar infarct is strongly associated with poorly controlled hypertension or diabetes.

SYMPTOMS/EXAM

- Patients present with abrupt onset of focal or multifocal neurologic symptoms that correlate with the area of the brain supplied by the affected arteries.
- Motor weakness, sensory deficits, ↓ reflexes, and mental status changes can occur.
- On cardiovascular exam, an arrhythmia or carotid or abdominal artery bruits may be appreciated as a potential source of the stroke.
- Lacunar infarct syndromes include clumsy hand dysarthria, pure motor hemiparesis, pure hemisensory loss, and ataxic hemiparesis.
- Table 11.2 outlines the presentation of common stroke syndromes.

DIFFERENTIAL

Seizure, complicated migraine, subdural hematoma, dural sinus thrombosis, Bell palsy, MS, intracranial mass, CNS infection, CNS inflammation, CNS arteritis.

DIAGNOSIS

- **Noncontrast CT:**
  - Done to ensure that the symptoms are not due to a hemorrhage.
  - Ischemic lesions do not usually appear during the first 24–48 hours after stroke. Lesions appear hypodense (dark) and ↑ in density with evolution.
  - Lacunar infarcts may not be seen or may appear as small hypodense lesions.
- **MRI:** Shows ischemic changes within hours of the event as well as small infarcts missed by CT. MRI also offers better visualization of the posterior fossa (Figure 11.4).

KEY FACT

Eighty-five percent of strokes are ischemic, but you must rule out hemorrhage as the cause first.

KEY FACT

The risk of stroke doubles for each decade > 55 years of age.

TABLE 11.2. Key Stroke Syndromes

LEFT (DOMINANT) HEMISPHERE	RIGHT (NONDOMINANT) HEMISPHERE	BRAIN STEM	CEREBELLUM
Left gaze preference.	Right gaze preference.	Hemiparesis or quadriparesis.	Gait ataxia.
Aphasia.	Neglect (of the left side).	Sensory loss in hemibody or all limbs.	Truncal ataxia.
Right visual field deficit.	Left visual field deficit.	Ipsilateral face and contralateral body symptoms.	Ipsilateral limb ataxia.
Right hemiparesis.	Left hemiparesis.	Disconjugate gaze.	
Right hemisensory loss.	Left hemisensory loss.	Dysphagia, ↓ consciousness.	

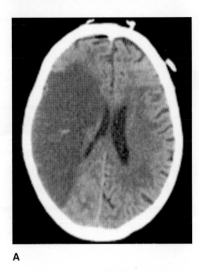
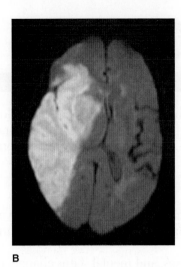
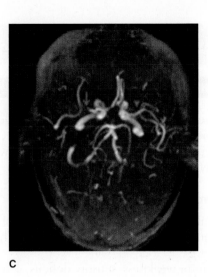

A   B   C

FIGURE 11.4. **Acute ischemic stroke.** Acute left hemiparesis in a 62-year-old woman. **(A)** Noncontrast transaxial head CT with loss of gray and white matter differentiation and asymmetrically decreased size of the right lateral ventricle in a right MCA distribution (indicating mass effect). **(B)** Transaxial diffusion-weighted MRI with reduced diffusion in the same distribution, consistent with an acute infarct. **(C)** Maximum-intensity projection of a transaxial time-of-flight MRA shows the cause: an abrupt occlusion of the proximal right MCA *(arrow)*. Compare with the normal left MCA *(arrowhead)*. (Reproduced, with permission, from USMLERx.com.)

- **Carotid and transcranial ultrasound or MRA plus ECG and echocardiogram with bubble study:** To assess for a cardioembolic source. Cardiac monitoring for arrhythmia.
- **Cerebral angiography:** The "gold standard" of cerebrovascular imaging. Shows the site and severity of occlusive disease. Also shows intracranial artery dissection if present. However, CT angiography and MRA are currently more favorably used.
- **Hypercoagulable workup:** Appropriate if the patient is < 55 years of age or has associated signs, symptoms, or risk factors. Consider sickle cell disease in a child.

TREATMENT

- **Stabilize the patient:**
  - Assess the airway.
  - Avoid hypotonic IV fluids to prevent worsening cerebral edema.
  - Bed rest to avoid orthostatic hypotension.
- **IV thrombolytic therapy:**
  - Potential tissue plasminogen activator (tPA) candidates can receive tPA within 3–4.5 hours of initiation of stroke symptoms. Most inclusion and exclusion criteria focus on the risk of bleeding. Head CT must show no hemorrhage, and bleeding disorders must be ruled out.
  - If the patient is outside of the IV tPA window, may be a candidate for intra-arterial thrombolysis or mechanical embolectomy.
  - If the patient is not a candidate for thrombolytic therapy, start antiplatelet therapy.
- **Antiplatelet therapy:** Give aspirin and/or clopidogrel or ASA/dipyridamole (Aggrenox).
- **Anticoagulation:**
  - Rule out coagulopathy.
  - Check a head CT for intracranial hemorrhage.
  - Heparin is relatively contraindicated in large infarcts with mass effect or hemorrhagic conversion.
  - Warfarin may be given on an outpatient basis for atrial fibrillation-related stroke.

- Transient monocular blindness (amaurosis fugax) requires ophthalmologic evaluation.
- Treat hypertension **only in a hypertensive emergency.**
- Discontinue any contributing hormone or oral contraceptive medications.
- **Carotid endarterectomy:** For 2° prevention if ipsilateral carotid artery stenosis is > 70%.
- **Speech, occupational and physical therapy;** swallow study before diet is started.

COMPLICATIONS

Cerebral edema with mass effect, hemorrhagic transformation, MI, aspiration pneumonia, disability, DVT, depression, death.

> **KEY FACT**
>
> Stroke is the third leading cause of death in the United States.

INTRACEREBRAL HEMORRHAGE (ICH)

> A 60-year-old man who is frequently seen in the emergency department for alcohol intoxication is brought in by EMS after being found down. His blood pressure in the field is 205/110. When you examine him, you note that his speech is slurred and the left side of his face is drooping. How do you proceed?
>
> Concern for ICH is high and a noncontrast CT of the head with CBC, chemistry panel, and coagulation studies are important first steps in evaluating this patient.

Defined as a rupture or aneurysm of an intracerebral artery that causes direct pressure on part of the brain and ↑ ICP. **Hypertensive ICH is the most common subtype and evolves rapidly.** Can rupture into ventricles, potentially causing life-threatening transtentorial herniation. Risk factors include **male gender, age > 55 years, high alcohol intake,** anticoagulation, and uncontrolled DM.

> **KEY FACT**
>
> Hypertensive ICH evolves rapidly.

SYMPTOMS/EXAM

- Presents with sudden severe headache, nausea, vomiting, and ↓ level of consciousness.
- Rapid onset of focal neurologic symptoms is seen.
- Meningeal irritation is possible and may lead to stiff neck (nuchal rigidity), leg pain, and low back pain. Papilledema may also be seen.

DIFFERENTIAL

Ischemic stroke, subarachnoid hemorrhage, seizure, subdural or epidural hematoma, dural sinus thrombosis, intracranial mass, CNS infection, CNS inflammation.

DIAGNOSIS

- CT shows immediate **high-density (bright) lesions in the brain parenchyma** (Figure 11.5).
- In the presence of ventricle enlargement, consider neurosurgical ventriculostomy. Large cerebellar hemorrhages are rapidly fatal.
- Check bleeding times, platelet count, toxicology screen, and chem 12.

TREATMENT

- **Neurosurgery:** Appropriate for any contributing treatable AVM, aneurysm, or excisable tumor, or for decompression of superficial intracerebral hema-

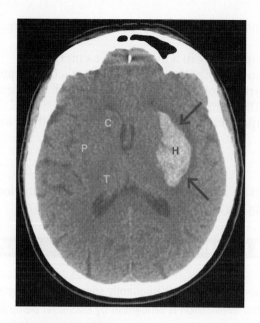

FIGURE 11.5. Intracerebral hemorrhage. Transaxial image from a noncontrast head CT shows an intraparenchymal hemorrhage (H) and surrounding edema (*arrows*) centered in the left putamen, a common location for hypertensive hemorrhage. C, P, and T denote the normal contralateral caudate, putamen, and thalamus. (Reproduced, with permission, from Fauci AS, et al. *Harrison's Principles of Internal Medicine,* 17th ed. New York: McGraw-Hill, 2008, Fig. 364-17.)

tomas. These measures can be lifesaving if the cerebellar hemorrhage is large. Patients with small aneurysms as the cause of ICH may benefit from endovascular coil treatment over surgical clipping.
- Treat ↑ ICP with mannitol, hyperventilation, and cooling blankets.
- Supportive care; speech and physical therapy. Conduct a swallow study before diet is started.

COMPLICATIONS

Permanent disability; mortality.

SUBARACHNOID HEMORRHAGE (SAH)

Defined as an acute bleed into the subarachnoid space. The most common causes are trauma or rupture of an aneurysm, an AVM, and a neoplasm. The classic description of the headache by the patient is **"the worst headache of my life."**

SYMPTOMS/EXAM

- Presents with sudden severe headache and nuchal rigidity.
- Kernig sign (passive extension of a flexed knee produces pain and resistance) and Brudzinski sign (passive flexion of the neck causes flexion of the hips and knees) may be ⊕. Also associated with ↓ level of consciousness.
- Nausea, vomiting, confusion, and irritability may be seen. Photophobia and visual disturbances are common.
- Focal neurologic deficits may be present, including cranial nerve palsies. Seizure is possible.
- Papilledema may be found on funduscopy.

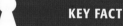

KEY FACT

Most nontraumatic SAHs are due to rupture of a saccular aneurysm.

DIFFERENTIAL

Meningitis, ICH, ischemic stroke, migraine, hypertensive emergency, TIA, temporal arteritis.

DIAGNOSIS

■ **Head CT:** May show **hemorrhage** into the subarachnoid space (Figure 11.6).
■ **LP:** If the CT is normal but SAH is still suspected, obtain an LP to examine CSF for xanthochromia (yellowish color of CSF) or blood.
■ Cerebral arteriography can show the source when the patient is stable.
■ A history of Ehlers-Danlos syndrome, Marfan syndrome, or polycystic kidney disease may be associated with an SAH.

TREATMENT

■ **Stabilize the patient:** Give IV osmotic agents or diuretics for suspected herniation.
■ **Neurosurgery consult:** Appropriate for any contributing treatable AVM, aneurysm, or excisable tumor. Endovascular coiling is the current treatment recommendation.

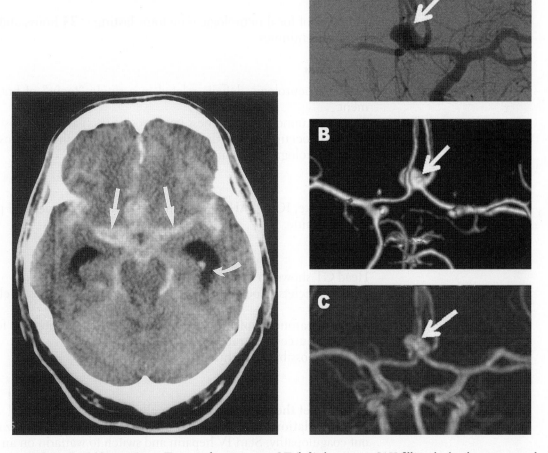

FIGURE 11.6. Subarachnoid hemorrhage. Transaxial noncontrast CT (left) showing an SAH filling the basilar cisterns and sylvian fissures (*straight arrows*). The curved arrow shows the dilated temporal horns of the lateral ventricles/hydrocephalus. Coned-down images (right) from a catheter angiogram (**A**), a CT angiogram (**B**), and an MRA (**C**) show a saccular aneurysm arising from the anterior communicating artery (*arrow*). (Left image reproduced, with permission, from Tintinalli JE, et al. *Tintinalli's Emergency Medicine: A Comprehensive Study Guide,* 6th ed. New York: McGraw-Hill, 2004, Fig. 237-4. Right image reproduced, with permission, from Doherty GM. *Current Diagnosis & Treatment: Surgery,* 13th ed. New York: McGraw-Hill, 2010, Fig. 36-6.)

- Seizure prophylaxis is no longer recommended.
- **Treat hypertension:** Gradually treat mean arterial BP > 130 mmHg but maintain SBP > 120 mmHg.
- Give analgesics and antiemetics. Advise patient to avoid exertion or straining.
- Recommend bed rest and smoking cessation.

COMPLICATIONS

Rebleeding, stroke.

TRANSIENT ISCHEMIC ATTACK (TIA)

A 69-year-old man who takes "water pills" but "misses one here and there" presents to the ER with sudden right-sided arm and leg weakness and slurred speech. As his head CT is being arranged, he begins to regain function of his right arm and leg. When his CT is done, he clearly states, "I feel much better now. Can I go?" His head CT is normal. How do you proceed? When evaluating a TIA, studies and tests should be performed as if the patient has had a CVA. This man is at ↑ risk for having a stroke in the future, and the TIA presents an opportunity to ↓ that risk.

Abrupt onset of focal neurologic symptoms **lasting < 24 hours** and often lasting only 5–20 minutes.

SYMPTOMS/EXAM

- Multiple neurologic deficits related to a single "focus" of brain involvement.
- Transient monocular blindness (amaurosis fugax) and other visual disturbances can occur. Vertigo, diplopia, ataxia, and dysarthria are possible.
- Focal neurologic symptoms resolve within 24 hours.

DIFFERENTIAL

Ischemic stroke, ICH, SAH, seizure, hypoglycemia, syncope, Bell palsy, complicated migraine.

DIAGNOSIS

- Head CT shows no acute changes.
- Check platelets, blood glucose, cholesterol, homocysteine level, and RPR for syphilis.
- Check a carotid duplex ultrasound and an echocardiogram for possible embolic sources or carotid stenosis.
- ECG for possible arrhythmia.

TREATMENT

- **Antiplatelet therapy:** Aspirin and/or clopidogrel.
- **Anticoagulation:** For cases with a cardiac source of embolization. Rule out coagulopathy. Start IV heparin and switch to warfarin on an outpatient basis.
- **Carotid endarterectomy:** For carotid stenosis > 70% on the side of the source.
- **Treat contributing factors:** Arrhythmias, hyperlipidemia, hypertension, hyperviscosity, DM, arteritis. Recommend smoking cessation.

COMPLICATIONS

Recurrent symptoms; risk for stroke.

Cerebral Lobe Dysfunctions

APHASIAS

Acquired language disorders. Major aphasias are described as follows:

- **Broca aphasia:** Speech that is **nonfluent, effortful,** sparse, and monotone. Also associated with impaired naming, repetition, and writing. **Comprehension is generally preserved,** and the patient is often aware of the deficit. Right hemiparesis and depression are common.
- **Wernicke aphasia: Fluent, possibly excessive** speech, with frequent paraphasias (substituting one word or phrase for another) and normal articulation. Patients may also have **impaired comprehension** of reading and speech as well as deficits in reading, writing, naming, and repetition. A right visual field cut may be present.
- **Global aphasia:** Involves impairment of all language functions, often accompanied by lethargy, right hemiparesis, hemisensory loss, apraxia, and visual field deficits.

MNEMONIC

Wernicke aphasia is **W**ord salad.

Broca aphasia speech is **B**roken and effortful.

DIFFERENTIAL

Dementia, postconcussive syndrome, MS, partial status epilepticus.

DIAGNOSIS

Diagnosis is based on neuropsychiatric evaluation and the clinical exam, including language functions such as repetition, spontaneous speech, comprehension, and naming.

TREATMENT

Supportive care; speech therapy. Psychological support may be necessary.

COMPLICATIONS

Those with deficits of comprehension (eg, Wernicke aphasia) have a poorer prognosis for functional improvement or recovery than do those with deficits of expression.

AGNOSIA

Impaired recognition of familiar people or objects despite preservation of intelligence, attention, and perception. May involve visual, auditory, and/or tactile modalities. Subtypes are as follows:

- **Visual agnosia:** Inability to recognize familiar objects; often associated with right visual deficit. Impairment may be limited to identification or discrimination of **faces** of known people (prosopagnosia), **colors** (color agnosia), known **objects** (object agnosia), or a whole item despite recognition of the parts (simultagnosia).
- **Auditory agnosia:** Inability to recognize familiar sounds despite intact hearing. Impairment may be limited to words, environmental sounds, or music.
- **Astereognosia:** Inability to identify objects through tactile stimulation despite intact sensation of touch. Patients may be able to describe and draw

an object and name it from its image in the drawing yet not recognize it through touch.

DIFFERENTIAL

Dementia, mental retardation, postconcussive syndrome, Parkinson disease.

DIAGNOSIS

- Based on the exam, including language functions such as repetition, spontaneous speech, comprehension, and naming.
- MRI to examine for a possible underlying cause.

TREATMENT

Supportive care. Treat any underlying condition.

DYSARTHRIA

Poor articulation of appropriate words (slurred speech).

- **Sx/Exam:** Hoarseness and/or drooling may be seen. Reading comprehension and writing abilities remain intact.
- **DDx:** Developmental disability, postconcussive syndrome, dementia.
- **Dx:**
  - Based on the clinical exam, including normal language functions such as repetition, spontaneous speech, comprehension, and naming.
  - Head CT or MRI for any underlying cause.
- **Tx:** Speech and language therapy.

AMNESIAS

Severe disturbance of retained memory, with intact attention and language functions. Visuospatial functions are generally intact. These disturbances include the following:

- **Transient global amnesia** is described as a paroxysmal, **transient loss of recent memory,** with preserved immediate recall and remote memory. Usually involves impaired ability to retain new information. Often caused by an emotional or physically stressful incident that occurred shortly before symptoms began. The patient may be confused and anxious, but **personal identity is retained.** Focal neurologic signs are absent. Typically lasts 30 minutes to 24 hours.
- **Wernicke syndrome** is a significant impairment of short-term memory, with inability to form new memories and impaired remote memory. Caused by a deficiency in thiamine (vitamin B_1). Usually associated with heavy, long-term alcohol use. Patients have **apathy** and **lack of insight** into the disorder but are alert and responsive. Confabulation is common. Associated with peripheral neuropathy, hypothermia, nystagmus, and gait ataxia.

DIFFERENTIAL

Seizure, TIA, conversion disorder, delirium, dementia, organic brain syndrome, malingering.

DIAGNOSIS

- Based on the history and on the finding of anterograde amnesia with loss of recent memory. Otherwise neurologically normal in transient global amnesia. Peripheral neuropathy, nystagmus, and gait ataxia are present in Korsakoff syndrome.
- Brain imaging to examine for an underlying condition.

TREATMENT

- **Transient global amnesia:** Reassurance; neurology consult.
- **Korsakoff syndrome:** Give thiamine before glucose to avoid precipitating Wernicke encephalopathy leading to ataxia, ophthalmoplegia, nystagmus, and confusion. Recommend a recovery program for alcoholic patients.

COMPLICATIONS

Korsakoff syndrome can lead to persistent vertical nystagmus, gait ataxia, and learning impairments.

KEY FACT

Transient global amnesia typically occurs in patients > 40 years of age.

Seizure

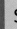

A mother brings her 8-year-old boy to the clinic because his teachers complain that he "daydreams too much" and has 20-second "staring spells" during which he stays still and does not react to anything that is said. He is doing well in school and has many friends. His exam is unremarkable. How do you proceed?

The description of the child indicates appropriate development, so you suspect absence seizures. An EEG is an appropriate diagnostic measure as well as educational material for the parent and school.

Defined as a sudden change in neurologic function resulting from an abnormal, excessive, synchronous discharge of cortical neurons.

FOCAL (PARTIAL) SEIZURE

In **simple partial seizures,** patients preserve consciousness but may be aphasic. In **complex partial seizures,** consciousness is altered. The patient tends to experience amnesia for the event, and automatisms may be present. Focal seizures are further categorized according to location:

- **Temporal lobe seizure:**
  - The **most common** seizure type in **adults.**
  - The seizure presents with unresponsive, quiet staring for 1–3 minutes and often is accompanied by an **aura** (eg, sensation of a particular smell, dizziness, nausea, or déjà vu).
  - Oral or ipsilateral manual automatisms may be present. Contralateral dystonic posturing of the arm and hand is common.
  - Postictal lethargy and confusion may last several minutes.
- **Frontal lobe seizure:**
  - Usually lasts 15–40 seconds without an aura or a postictal state.
  - Commonly occurs during sleep.

- If the motor cortex is involved, rhythmic unilateral clonic activity may occur and spread across the body. Asymmetric tonic posturing is common with involvement of the supplemental motor area.
- **Occipital lobe seizure:**
  - Commonly begins with a visual aura that can range from spots or lights to formed visual hallucinations that are usually stereotyped from seizure to seizure.
  - May spread to the temporal lobe or the motor cortex.

DIFFERENTIAL

Syncope, orthostatic hypotension, hypoglycemia, hypoxia, migraine, TIA, panic attack, psychogenic seizure, narcolepsy, tics.

DIAGNOSIS

- Obtain a detailed history of the event, prodromal symptoms, witnessed seizures, and postictal state. Evaluate for risk factors—eg, head trauma, stroke, tumor, AVM, or a family history of seizures. The threshold of people with a seizure history can be lowered by triggers like sleep deprivation, stress, illness, medications, flickering lights, or stimuli.
- Check a CBC, a complete metabolic profile, and a toxicology screen as well as calcium, magnesium, alcohol, and ammonia levels.
- EEG and video EEG monitoring.
- MRI to elucidate the underlying cause.

TREATMENT

- **Acute seizure:** Stabilize patients and protect them from harm. Administer lorazepam IV or IM; diazepam IV or per rectum in gel form; or midazolam IV or sublingually. Give glucose if the patient is hypoglycemic. Treat severe hypertension. Correct any metabolic causes.
- **Single, isolated seizure episode:** In the absence of risk factors, ongoing antiepileptic therapy is usually deferred. The recurrence rate is about 20%, and recurrences usually occur within 1 year.

COMPLICATIONS

- May progress to a generalized tonic-clonic seizure.
- Falls and injuries.
- Patients are at risk for depression, anxiety, and psychosis.
- Side effects and drug interactions associated with antiepileptic medications.

GENERALIZED SEIZURE

Generalized seizures involve the whole brain and are categorized as follows:

- **Tonic-clonic (grand mal):**
  - No aura occurs. The tonic phase gradually progresses to a clonic phase, with each lasting about 30 seconds.
  - **Incontinence or tongue biting** may occur during the seizure.
  - The postictal state includes coarse breathing, with gradual awakening over several minutes. Postictal acidosis with $\downarrow HCO_3$, $\uparrow CK$, and $\uparrow$ prolactin occurs within 30 minutes after a seizure.
- **Absence (petit mal):**
  - Sudden-onset **staring spells,** usually **lasting about 10 seconds,** with immediate recovery. Those lasting 20–30 seconds may also have simple automatisms.

- **Eye fluttering** or altered postural tone is common and may occur many times per day.
    - EEG shows **generalized spike-and-wave** discharges.
    - Usually seen in neurologically normal **children 4–14 years of age.**
- **Myoclonic:**
    - Brief, **sharp muscle jerks** with no impairment of consciousness.
    - Movements may be symmetric, asymmetric, or multifocal.
    - EEG shows a **generalized polyspike-and-wave discharge.**
- **Tonic:**
    - Brief, sudden, bilateral, and symmetric tonic posturing, with brief impairment of consciousness and rapid recovery.
    - EEG shows **sudden, diffuse low-voltage β waves** or background attenuation.
    - Usually seen in neurologically abnormal patients.

DIFFERENTIAL

Syncope, psychogenic seizure, hypoglycemia, hypoxia, TIA, complex migraine, orthostatic hypotension, tics.

DIAGNOSIS

- Obtain a detailed history of witnessed seizures that may be induced by sleep deprivation, stress, illness, medications, flickering lights, or stimuli. Look for a history of symptoms of prodrome, seizure, and/or postictal state. Evaluate for risk factors such as head trauma, stroke, tumor, AVM, or a family history of seizures.
- Check a CBC, a complete metabolic profile, and a toxicology screen as well as calcium, magnesium, alcohol, and ammonia levels.
- EEG and video EEG monitoring.
- MRI to determine the underlying cause.

TREATMENT

The same as for focal (partial) seizures above.

FEBRILE SEIZURE

- **Sx/Exam:** A brief (< 15 minutes) tonic-clonic seizure that is associated with fever. No known neurologic cause and there may be a genetic predisposition. Usually occurs before 6 years of age. Commonly caused by a spike in temperature associated with viral or bacterial illness.
- **DDx:** Meningitis, encephalitis, syncope, status epilepticus, migraine.
- **Dx:** Usually based on history and physical exam. Laboratory or imaging studies usually not indicated. If the seizure has atypical features, a neurologic workup, including labs, head imaging, and EEG, may be indicated.
- **Tx:** Supportive care, antipyretics, airway management.

STATUS EPILEPTICUS

A neurologic emergency consisting of continuous seizure activity lasting > 10 minutes or repetitive seizures lasting > 30 minutes, without a return to a baseline neurologic level between seizures.

DIFFERENTIAL

Syncope, TIA, intracranial infection, migraine, hypoglycemia, Bell palsy, psychogenic seizure.

KEY FACT

Absence seizures primarily affect patients 4–14 years of age.

KEY FACT

Most patients with > 3 seizure-free years on medication will not have recurrences.

KEY FACT

Atypical features of febrile seizure are those that localize, last > 15 minutes, or happen more than once during an illness or > 24 hours after the onset of fever.

DIAGNOSIS

A clinical diagnosis in cases of sustained overt convulsions. An EEG may be needed for more subtle findings.

TREATMENT

- Stabilize the patient and give 4 mg IV of lorazepam; if patient continues to seize, may repeat. If not responsive to lorazepam, administer a loading dose and infusion of **fosphenytoin,** with continuous ECG monitoring. Consider intubation.
- If the patient continues seizing after 30 minutes, the seizure is considered refractory. The patient should be sedated with midazolam and propofol as well as intubated vs. a loading dose and infusion of phenobarbital.

COMPLICATIONS

Respiratory failure, rhabdomyolysis, hyperthermia, neuronal cell damage.

EPILEPSY

Consists of a history of ≥ 2 unprovoked seizures due to underlying brain disease.

- **Sx/Exam:** History of recurrent seizures.
- **Dx:** Diagnosed by a history of recurrent, unprovoked seizures with documentation of seizure focus or an underlying brain lesion or disease.
- **Tx:**
  - Medication choice depends on seizure type. Generalized seizures should be treated with valproic acid; absence seizures with ethosuximide; and partial seizures with carbamazepine or phenytoin.
  - Antiepileptics are teratogenic. Perform a pregnancy test before starting any antiepileptic medication and offer OCPs to young women.
  - Surgery to remove seizure foci is possible in many patients.
  - Ketogenic diets and vagal nerve stimulators are sometimes recommended.

KEY FACT

Most cases of epilepsy start before 20 years of age.

Syncope

A 75-year-old man comes to your clinic after falling when he got up at night to urinate. He denies any loss of consciousness and reports his vision going black before he fell to the ground. What will your next steps be?

In a case of syncope, cardiac causes are always a concern, and this patient warrants a workup if he hasn't had one recently. In elderly patients, medications should also be considered as a cause. However, his syncope was most likely caused by a vasovagal response during micturition.

Episodic loss of consciousness and postural tone, with spontaneous recovery. Can occur with any global ↓ in cerebral perfusion. Incidence ↑ with age. **Vasovagal syncope is the most common subtype.** Other types of syncope include orthostatic, neurogenic, and cardiogenic. Cardiogenic syncope carries a worse prognosis.

Symptoms/Exam

- Loss of consciousness, with loss of postural tone and spontaneous recovery.
- Preceded by nausea, faintness, blurred vision, diaphoresis, vertigo, paresthesias, or pallor.
- **No postevent confusion.**
- Exam is likely unremarkable at the time of evaluation.

Differential

Stroke, TIA, seizure, hypoglycemia, benign paroxysmal positional vertigo (BPPV).

Diagnosis

- Check medications, activities, and position at the time of the event.
- Check for orthostatic BP changes.
- Tilt-table testing and the Valsalva maneuver are diagnostic for an orthostatic source.
- ECG for arrhythmia; echocardiogram for cardiac outlet obstruction.

Treatment

Treat the underlying cause. Avoid precipitating factors and medications.

KEY FACT

The most common form of syncope is vasovagal.

KEY FACT

Syncope has no postevent confusion.

Peripheral Polyneuropathies

GUILLAIN-BARRÉ SYNDROME (ACUTE IDIOPATHIC POLYNEUROPATHY)

A 41-year-old man comes to your office complaining of ↓ feeling and strength in both legs after he became acutely ill following dinner a few days ago. He also complains of "tingling" in his feet and some difficulty walking. Exam reveals ↓ lower extremity muscle strength with a lack of DTRs. The patient states that his arms now feel weaker as well. How do you proceed?

You admit the patient to the hospital for monitoring of Guillain-Barré syndrome that progresses to require ventilation.

Symmetric, progressive ascending muscle weakness that usually **starts in the legs** and may be **acute or subacute.** The condition is life-threatening if respiratory or swallowing muscles are involved. Can follow minor respiratory or GI illness, inoculation, or surgical procedures. Carries a poorer prognosis when it follows *Campylobacter jejuni* infection. It is unknown why certain people develop the disease and others do not.

Symptoms/Exam

- The hallmark is **lack of DTRs.** Progressive weakness of ≥ 2 limbs typically begins with the proximal lower extremities.
- Shortness of breath, constipation, facial weakness, dysphagia, ophthalmoplegia, dysarthria, and sensory disturbances are commonly seen.
- Also associated with disturbances in BP, heart rate, and pulmonary function.
- Symptom progression halts in < 2–3 weeks.

KEY FACT

Guillain-Barré syndrome after a *C jejuni* infection is often severe.

KEY FACT

Corticosteroids can worsen Guillain-Barré symptoms.

DIFFERENTIAL

Chronic inflammatory demyelinating polyneuropathy, HIV infection, transverse myelitis, intraspinal mass, porphyria, toxic neuropathy, poliomyelitis, botulism, tick paralysis, periodic paralysis syndrome.

DIAGNOSIS

- CSF shows ↑ protein but a normal cell count, although sometimes this is not found in the first week.
- Electrophysiologic studies can show marked **slowing of motor and sensory conduction velocity,** consistent with denervation and axonal loss.

TREATMENT

- Plasmapheresis or IVIG may improve recovery time and ↓ residual neurologic effects.
- IVIG is preferable in children and in cases involving cardiovascular instability. Steroids can worsen Guillain-Barré symptoms.
- Symptomatic treatment. Severe cases should be monitored in the ICU.

COMPLICATIONS

May have mild residual deficits. Relapse is possible years later. Fatal in 5% of cases.

CHRONIC INFLAMMATORY DEMYELINATING POLYNEUROPATHY (CIDP)

- **Sx/Exam:** Presents with **relapsing or persistent ascending muscle weakness,** beginning in the legs, **without improvement** after 6 months. DTRs are absent. Paresthesias can develop, and fatigue is common.
- **Dx:** Diagnosed using electrophysiologic studies to assess for demyelinating neuropathy with axonal degeneration. CSF protein is ↑ with a normal cell count.
- **Tx:** Often responds to long-term corticosteroids. Consider a trial of azathioprine or cyclophosphamide if the patient is unresponsive to corticosteroids.

DIABETIC NEUROPATHY

- **Sx/Exam: Polyneuropathy** is the most common. Patients experience numbness and tingling in a **stocking/glove distribution. Autonomic neuropathy** affects the internal organs and is associated with digestive, urinary, sexual, and visual changes.
- **DDx:** Spinal cord tumor, inflammatory neuropathy, vitamin B_{12} deficiency, herpes zoster.
- **Dx:** Symptoms and neurologic exam. Basic labs tests to rule out other causes. Consider EMG and MRI.
- **Tx:** Improved glycemic control, foot care, regular ophthalmologic exams, smoking cessation. **Medications:** TCAs, gabapentin, capsaicin cream.

Brachial Plexus Disorders

Usually a unilateral sensorimotor deficit traceable to 1 or more cords of the brachial plexus. Most cases have no apparent cause. May be due to trauma, radiation, infection, electrical injury, compression, or infiltration. There are multiple subtypes:

- **Whole plexus lesion:** The entire arm is paralyzed, with sensory loss complete past a line drawn from the shoulder to the middle third of the upper arm.
- **Upper brachial plexus paralysis:** Loss of shoulder abduction and elbow flexion. The affected arm is held internally rotated at the shoulder, with the elbow extended and the forearm pronated. Sensory loss occurs over a small area of the deltoid muscle. Also known as **Erb palsy** or "waiter's tip."
- **Lower brachial plexus paralysis:** Paralysis and wasting of the small muscles of the hand and of the long finger flexors and extensors, leading to **Klumpke palsy,** also known as "claw hand" deformity. Sensory loss is found on the ulnar border of the hand and the inner forearm. Horner syndrome is possible.
- **Lateral cord lesion:** Weakness of flexion and pronation of the forearm.
- **Medial cord lesion:** Combined median and ulnar nerve deficit. ↓ or absent hand sensation and finger flexor function are seen with atrophy of intrinsic hand muscles.
- **Posterior cord lesion:** Weakness of the deltoid muscle and extensors of the elbow, wrist, and fingers. Sensory loss is seen on the outer side of the arm.
- **Brachial neuritis:** Acute onset of excruciating and generally unilateral shoulder pain followed days later by weakness of the shoulder and parascapular muscles. Numbness may also be seen.

DIFFERENTIAL

Cervical radiculopathy, polymyalgia rheumatica, vertebral artery dissection.

DIAGNOSIS

- Electrophysiologic testing of the affected muscles.
- AP and axillary lateral shoulder radiography for concerns of related fracture.
- MRI may reveal infiltrative processes.

TREATMENT

- Physical/occupational therapy. Bracing prevents contractures.
- Possible surgery, with nerve grafting and muscle or tendon transfers.
- Corticosteroids for brachial neuritis.

COMPLICATIONS

Incomplete recovery. Chronic shoulder pain is possible in brachial neuritis.

Mononeuropathies

MEDIAN NERVE ENTRAPMENT (CARPAL TUNNEL SYNDROME)

Loss or impairment of superficial sensation in the palmar aspect of the thumb, the index finger, and often the radial half of the third finger.

SYMPTOMS/EXAM

- Presents with pain and paresthesias in the same distribution. **Symptoms ↑ at night.**
- Also characterized by thenar muscle weakness and atrophy. Abductor pollicis brevis and opponens pollicis muscle weakness is seen.

- Patients have a tendency to "flick" and wiggle the fingers in attempts to relieve **paresthesias.**
- **Tinel** and **Phalen signs** may be ⊕.

DIAGNOSIS

- Based on the history and exam. Check for a history of repetitive hand movements.
- Electrophysiologic studies can show slowing of sensory or motor conduction velocity at the wrist.
- Check for underlying conditions such as pregnancy, hyperparathyroidism, diabetes, amyloidosis, RA, sarcoidosis, acromegaly, or recent or poorly healed fractures.

TREATMENT

- Treat with NSAIDs, rest, vitamin B_6, nocturnal wrist splinting, and possible surgical decompression. Local corticosteroid injections can sometimes provide temporary relief.
- Treat any underlying conditions.

OTHER PERIPHERAL MONONEUROPATHIES

- **Sx/Exam:** Findings are outlined in Table 11.3.
- **Dx:**
    - Diagnosed through clinical findings and EMG studies.
    - Spinal MRI imaging if spinal involvement is a concern; MRI of the affected area if symptoms are severe.

T A B L E 1 1 . 3 . Selected Peripheral Mononeuropathy Symptoms

NERVE	SYMPTOMS
Long thoracic nerve	Inability to raise the arm; **winging of the scapula** medial border with resistance against the outstretched arm.
Axillary nerve	**Paralysis of arm abduction;** atrophy of the deltoid muscle; ↓ sensation over the outer shoulder.
Radial nerve	**"Wrist drop":** Paralysis of elbow extension; supination of the forearm; extension of the wrist and fingers; extension and abduction of the thumb in the plane of the palm; flexion of the elbow with the forearm between pronation and supination.
Ulnar nerve	**"Claw hand" deformity:** Small hand muscle atrophy with finger hyperextension at the metacarpophalangeal joints and flexion at the interphalangeal joints. Sensory loss over the fifth finger and the ulnar aspect of the fourth finger and palm.
Lateral cutaneous nerve of the thigh	Paresthesias and ↓ sensation over the anterolateral aspect of the thigh from the inguinal ligament to above the knee.
Femoral nerve	Weakness of knee extension; atrophy of the quadriceps muscle; inability to fixate the knee. **No patellar reflex.**
Sciatic nerve	Lower leg pain and weakness. Weakness of knee flexion, foot eversion, and dorsiflexion. Absent ankle jerk; ↓ sensation over lateral shin, dorsal and distal foot, heel, sole, and toes. (In contrast, **sciatica** is associated with pain over the lumbosacral area and lateral leg; gluteal muscle weakness; and ↓ sensation over the posterior thigh, the posterior and lateral leg, and the sole.)

- Tx:
  - Treatment is symptomatic; supportive treatment for mild cases.
  - Treat the underlying cause.
  - Surgery for severe cases or threatened paralysis of affected musculature.

Chronic Progressive Upper and Lower Motor Degeneration

AMYOTROPHIC LATERAL SCLEROSIS (ALS)

 A 58-year-old right-handed man notices left calf "stiffness" that causes him to trip frequently. Over several months, right arm muscle cramping and twitching have led to difficulty buttoning his shirt. He presents to your office with new difficulty swallowing and slurred speech. Exam reveals weakness and muscle atrophy in his extremities and hyperreflexia and fasciculations in the left lower extremity. An overactive gag reflex is present. What additional studies do you order?

EMG and nerve conduction velocity studies to confirm ALS.

A devastating neurodegenerative disease, with **degeneration of lower and corticospinal motor neurons.** Most cases are sporadic.

Symptoms/Exam

- Presents with difficulty swallowing, chewing, coughing, breathing, and speaking (bulbar involvement).
- Vague sensory complaints and weight loss are common.
- **Upper and lower motor neuron (UMN/LMN) signs** in the bulbar region and upper and/or lower extremities include spasticity, hyperreflexia, atrophy, weakness or paralysis, fasciculations, hypotonia, and extensor plantar reflexes. Extraocular and sphincter muscles are generally spared. No sensory deficits.

Differential

Progressive bulbar palsy (bulbar involvement), pseudobulbar palsy (UMN bulbar symptoms), progressive spinal muscular atrophy (primarily LMN deficit in the limbs), 1° lateral sclerosis (purely a UMN deficit in the limbs), poliomyelitis, MS, cervical myelopathy.

Diagnosis

- Definitive diagnosis requires the presence of UMN and LMN signs in the bulbar region and in at least 2 other regions: cervical, thoracic, or lumbosacral, or 3 spinal regions.
- EMG findings of diffuse degenerative signs with normal or near-normal nerve conduction (except in severe atrophy) are highly suggestive. Further workup is needed to eliminate other potential causes.

Treatment

- Riluzole ↓ presynaptic glutamate release and may slow symptom progression.

> **KEY FACT**
>
> ALS has progressive UMN and LMN signs.

- Symptomatic and supportive care. Anticholinergics ↓ drooling and saliva pooling.
- Spasticity may be improved with baclofen or diazepam.
- Physical therapy to ↓ contractures; braces or walker to promote mobility.

COMPLICATIONS

Progressive and fatal, usually within 3–5 years of onset.

Demyelinating Diseases

MULTIPLE SCLEROSIS (MS)

A 29-year-old woman has fatigue and some right-sided "clumsiness." These symptoms wane over weeks. Months later, she notices blurry vision and decides to get new glasses. However, new-onset left-hand numbness and a "tingling" sensation around her trunk prompt her to visit your clinic first, where she is found to have focal areas of ↓ sensation. What are your next steps? New-onset neurologic symptoms in a young woman are concerning for intracranial or spinal cord lesions. An MRI finds 3 small periventricular white matter lesions. Further symptoms and subsequent tests over time confirm MS.

A chronic **multifocal demyelinating** neurologic disorder that involves different parts of the CNS at various points in time. There is a female-to-male ratio of 2:1. Prevalence ↑ with further distance from the equator. The disease takes **4 forms**: relapsing and remitting, 1° progressive, 2° progressive, and progressive relapsing (Table 11.4). Most cases are relapsing and remitting.

SYMPTOMS

- Presents with focal limb weakness, numbness, paresthesias, a bandlike sensation around the trunk or a limb, and ataxia.
- Diplopia, dysarthria, intention tremor, and bladder dysfunction are also seen.
- **Optic neuritis** (sudden loss or blurring of vision in 1 eye) is the presenting symptom in 25% of cases.
- Symptoms are transient, lasting days to weeks. May present as spastic paraparesis and sensory deficit.

KEY FACT

The incidence of MS is highest among whites.

KEY FACT

MS is the most common acquired neurologic disability in young adults.

TABLE 11.4. Types of Multiple Sclerosis

TYPE	FEATURES
Relapsing and remitting.	Relapses followed by incomplete remissions. During relapses, symptoms can grow more severe.
1° progressive.	Gradual, steady progression of symptoms from initial presentation.
2° progressive.	Gradual progression of symptoms and disability over time following a period of relapsing-remitting disease.
Progressive relapsing.	Gradual symptom progression over time accompanied by acute attacks of worse symptoms.

EXAM

Lhermitte sign (an electric shock–like sensation down the spine with flexing of the neck) may be ⊕, with paresthesias in the trunk and limbs with neck flexion. Focal areas of sensory deficit and weakness or an afferent papillary defect may be seen.

DIFFERENTIAL

ALS, Bell palsy, brain or spinal cord infection, HIV, trauma, sarcoidosis, stroke, syphilis, SLE, Lyme disease, TIA, trigeminal neuralgia.

DIAGNOSIS

- Generally diagnosed on the basis of > 1 CNS lesion.
- MRI is the most sensitive study and shows white matter lesions (Figure 11.7).
- Visual evoked potentials show prolonged responses, and CSF is ⊕ for **oligoclonal bands.**

TREATMENT

- Disease-modifying therapy includes interferon-β_{1b} or -β_{1a}, glatiramer acetate.
- Symptomatic therapy with corticosteroids.
- Canes, braces, walkers, wheelchairs, and assistance with daily functions.

COMPLICATIONS

Relapsing and remitting courses may progress to a chronic progressive form. Residual impairment of color vision and depth perception is common, as is chronic disability.

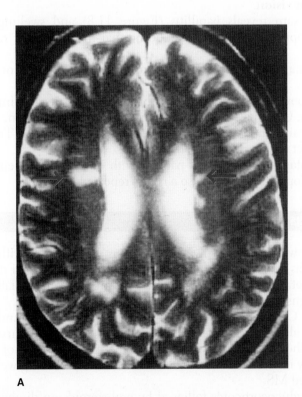
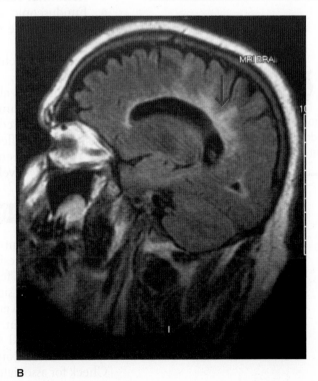

A **B**

FIGURE 11.7. Multiple sclerosis. Transaxial T_2-weighted MRI **(A)** and sagittal FLAIR image **(B)** showing multiple MS plaques *(arrows)* in the periventricular matter oriented radially from the corpus callosum ("Dawson fingers"). (Images A and B reproduced, with permission, from Ropper AH, Samuels MA. *Adams & Victor's Principles of Neurology,* 9th ed. New York: McGraw-Hill, 2009, Fig. 36-1.)

ACUTE DISSEMINATED ENCEPHALOMYELITIS (ADEM)

Defined as an inflammatory demyelinating disease with a pathologic presentation similar to MS, but usually monophasic. Most often develops 2–4 weeks after a febrile illness in a child < 12 years of age. Rarely develops after vaccination, but when it does, it is most often associated with the measles, mumps, and rubella vaccine.

- **Sx/Exam:** History of preceding illness or immunization. Altered consciousness, headache, ataxia, meningeal signs, seizure, fever.
- **DDx:** MS, transverse myelitis, optic neuritis, acute cerebellar ataxia, Miller-Fisher variant of Guillain-Barré syndrome.
- **Dx:** T_2 MRI cortical lesions, elevated CSF myelin basic protein (oligoclonal bands are not usually seen), WBCs, and RBCs, and elevated platelets of ESR can be seen.
- **Tx:** High-dose steroids or IVIG.
- **Cx:** Epilepsy, mental retardation, language and motor deficits, bladder and bowel function problems.

OPTIC NEURITIS

Partial or total vision loss from optic nerve demyelination. Roughly one-half of all patients develop multiple sclerosis (MS).

- **Sx/Exam:**
  - Presents with **eye pain** that may be preceded by loss of vision for 1–2 days.
  - An **afferent pupillary defect** is seen (↓ direct response seen with a swinging flashlight test).
  - **Abnormal color vision.**
  - Funduscopic exam reveals papillitis (Figure 11.8) and swelling or edema of the optic nerve head (may be normal in retrobulbar optic neuritis).
- **DDx:** Uveitis, retinal artery or vein occlusion, retinal detachment or hematoma.
- **Dx:** Findings as above. Most cases are **retrobulbar with a normal initial funduscopic exam.** CSF may show pleocytosis and ↑ IgG production.
- **Tx:** IV methylprednisolone for 3 days, followed by oral prednisone. Treatment does not affect long-term vision outcomes.
- **Cx:** A high percentage (40%–70%) of patients with isolated optic neuritis subsequently develop MS. There is also a risk of repeated attacks.

TRANSVERSE MYELITIS

- **Sx/Exam:** Presents with rapidly evolving paraparesis or paraplegia with ascending paresthesias, sensory loss, sphincter dysfunction, and loss of deep sensation in the feet. On exam, a sensory level on the trunk and bilateral extensor plantar signs are present.
- **Dx:** Diagnosed via CSF showing a moderate level of lymphocytes and an ↑ in total protein, although this may not be found early in the course of the disease. MRI shows focal demyelination in the expected level of the spinal cord. History may include infectious illness in the preceding weeks. Check for associated MS.
- **Tx:** Treat with IV glucocorticoids followed by oral steroids on discharge. Plasmapheresis is considered a second-line agent.

KEY FACT

Optic neuritis is a common presenting symptom of MS.

KEY FACT

In retrobulbar optic neuritis initial exam: "The doctor sees nothing and the patient sees nothing."

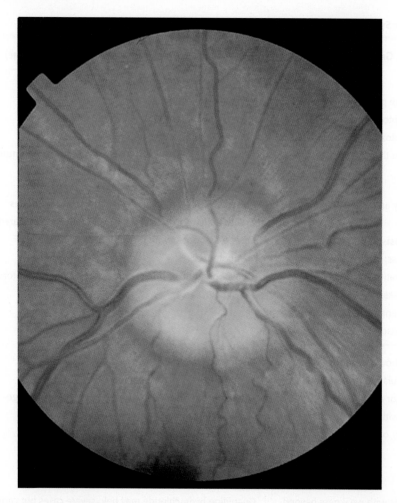

FIGURE 11.8.   Papillitis. Optic nerve head edema. Vascular congestion, elevation of the nerve head, and blurred disk margins are characteristically seen in papilledema, papillitis, and compressive lesions of the optic nerve. (Reproduced, with permission, from Tintinalli JE, et al. *Tintinalli's Emergency Medicine: A Comprehensive Study Guide,* 6th ed. New York: McGraw-Hill, 2004, Fig. 238-22.)

Neuromuscular Disorders

 KEY FACT

The hallmark of myasthenia gravis is muscle weakness that worsens with activity and improves with rest.

MYASTHENIA GRAVIS VS. MYASTHENIC SYNDROME

A 32-year-old woman develops continuous "double vision." She attributes it to stress, but a vacation yields minimal improvement. Weeks later, her problem worsens, and she becomes increasingly tired during the day, especially in the late afternoon to evening. She visits your office, where an exam reveals ptosis and voice hoarseness. What further evaluation should be conducted, and what is the diagnosis?

A ⊕ Tensilon test and ↑ serum acetylcholine receptor antibodies confirm myasthenia gravis.

Table 11.5 distinguishes the clinical presentation of myasthenia gravis from that of myasthenic syndrome.

 KEY FACT

Lambert-Eaton syndrome is associated with small cell lung cancer.

TABLE 11.5.   Myasthenia Gravis vs. Myasthenic Syndrome

DISEASE	MYASTHENIA GRAVIS	MYASTHENIC SYNDROME (LAMBERT-EATON SYNDROME)
General	An **autoimmune disease.** Antibodies are usually against the postsynaptic muscle membrane acetylcholine receptors. Associated with **thymoma,** thyrotoxicosis, SLE, and RA. **Women are affected** more often than men.	Generally **a paraneoplastic syndrome.** Frequently associated with **SLE.** Involves an immune-modulated defective release of acetylcholine in the neuromuscular junction. Associated with **small cell lung cancer** and **autoimmune diseases** such as pernicious anemia.
Symptoms/exam	**Symptoms worsen with activity** and fluctuate during the day. Involves slow progression of **ptosis; diplopia; altered tone of speech;** limb weakness; and difficulty with chewing, swallowing, or respiration. Relapses and remissions for weeks. Myasthenic crisis consists of absent gag reflex, limpness of the body, and ↑ respiratory muscle weakness.	Presents with proximal limb **weakness that improves with activity.** Extraocular muscles are generally spared. May be associated with dry mouth, constipation, and impotence. ↑ environmental or body temperatures worsen symptoms.
Diagnosis	Electrophysiologic testing may show ↓ **response** of muscle to repetitive motor nerve stimulation. High serum acetylcholine receptor antibody levels are found in 80%–90% of those with generalized disease. **Edrophonium** (the Tensilon test) or neostigmine improves symptoms.	Confirmed electrophysiologically by ↑ **response** to repetitive nerve stimulation. Serum **autoantibodies to the P/Q subtype of voltage-gated calcium channels** are highly sensitive and specific to this syndrome.
Treatment	Acetylcholinesterase inhibitors. Thymectomy for younger patients with weakness beyond the extraocular muscles. Corticosteroids initially worsen weakness. Azathioprine, plasmapheresis, IVIG, mycophenolate mofetil.	Plasmapheresis, corticosteroids, azathioprine, or IVIG. Guanidine hydrochloride may help severe cases but carries the risk of renal failure and bone marrow suppression. Treat the underlying condition.
Complications	Respiratory complications can be fatal.	Worsens over time. Respiratory compromise may result.

Muscular Disorders

MUSCULAR DYSTROPHIES

- **Sx/Exam:** Present with progressive muscle weakness and muscle wasting. Age at onset and distribution of symptoms depend on type (Table 11.6).
- **Dx:** Diagnosed by muscle biopsy histology, which distinguishes different types of muscular dystrophy. EMG reveals myopathic findings and/or myotonia.
- **Tx:** No specific treatment is available. Physical therapy can prevent or improve contractures or deformities. Surgical intervention may be necessary.

KEY FACT

The most common muscular dystrophy is Duchenne.

TABLE 11.6. Presentation of Common Muscular Dystrophies

Type	Age at Onset	Mode of Inheritance	Distribution and Symptoms	Prognosis	Serum CK
Duchenne	1–5	X-linked recessive.	Affects the pelvic and shoulder girdle muscles and then the extremities and respiratory muscles. Presents with muscular pseudohypertrophy. Also associated with mental retardation, deformities, and contractures.	Rapid progression. Fatal 15 years after onset.	Markedly ↑
Becker	5–25	X-linked recessive.	Affects the pelvic and then the shoulder girdle muscles.	Slow progression.	↑
Limb-girdle	10–30	Autosomal recessive; dominant, X linked or sporadic.	Affects the pelvic or shoulder girdle muscles; then progresses to other muscles. Presents with calf hypertrophy.	Variable. May be severe in midlife.	Mildly ↑
Facioscapulohumeral	Any	Autosomal dominant.	Affects the face and shoulder girdle muscles; then progresses to the pelvic muscles and lower extremities.	Slow progression; minor disability.	Can be normal
Myotonic	Any	Autosomal dominant.	Weakness and myotonia (ie, "spasming") of facial, sternocleidomastoid, and distal extremity muscles. Associated with baldness, cataracts, gonadal atrophy, cardiac abnormalities, mental retardation, and endocrinopathy.	Variable.	Normal or mildly ↑

INFLAMMATORY MYOPATHIES

Defined as muscle fiber destruction and inflammatory infiltration of muscles. Associated with some **autoimmune disorders,** including SLE, Sjögren syndrome, scleroderma, and RA. Peak incidence is in the **5th and 6th decades. More women are affected** than men. Subtypes are as follows:

- Polymyositis:
    - Presents with muscle pain, weakness, and atrophy, especially of the proximal limb muscles. Begins with leg weakness that progresses to arm weakness. Dysphagia and respiratory difficulties are also seen.
    - Raynaud phenomenon, malaise, arthralgias, low-grade fever, and weight loss are common.
- Dermatomyositis:
    - Presentation similar to polymyositis, but with a **heliotrope rash,** which is an erythematous rash appearing over the eyelids, around the eyes, or on the extensor surfaces of the joints.
    - Erythema over the face, neck, shoulders, and upper chest, leading to **"shawl sign."**
    - **Gottron sign** consists of scaly patches over the dorsa of the proximal hand joints, periungual erythema, and nail bed capillary dilation (Figure 11.9).
    - Skin or muscle **calcinosis** is common.

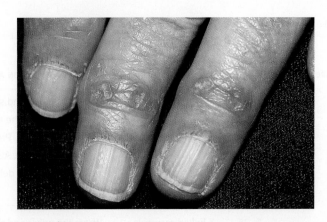

FIGURE 11.9. **Gottron sign.** Gottron papules, nail fold telangiectasias, and dystrophic cuticles in dermatomyositis. (Reproduced, with permission, from Wolff K, et al. *Fitzpatrick's Dermatology in General Medicine,* 7th ed. New York: McGraw-Hill, 2008, Fig. 157-5.)

> **KEY FACT**
>
> Dermatomyositis is associated with lung, breast, ovarian, and GI cancers.

> **KEY FACT**
>
> Muscle biopsy is the gold standard for diagnosis of polymyositis and dermatomyositis.

- **Inclusion body myositis:** Painless proximal weakness of the lower extremities and then the upper extremities, especially the quadriceps and finger flexors. Has a progressive course, with early loss of patellar reflexes.

DIFFERENTIAL

Myasthenic syndrome, myasthenia gravis, MS, ALS, polymyalgia rheumatica, trichinosis, hypothyroidism, HIV myopathy.

DIAGNOSIS

- Muscle biopsy shows necrosis of muscle fibers and inflammatory cell infiltration, with distinctions made for polymyositis vs. dermatomyositis.
- Labs show ↑ serum CK and aldolase.
- EMG reveals short, low-amplitude, polyphasic motor unit potentials, possibly with abnormal spontaneous activity.
- Antinuclear antibodies are likely present.

TREATMENT

- Anti-inflammatory drugs. Prednisone should be initiated and then lowered as serum muscle enzyme levels ↓. Consider a trial of methotrexate and azathioprine as second-line agents.
- Physical therapy to preserve function.
- For inclusion body myositis, immunosuppressive therapy is preferred.

COMPLICATIONS

Approximately 25% of patients with dermatomyositis have an occult malignancy. Patients with respiratory muscle involvement can have hypercapnia and respiratory failure. Severe muscle inflammation can precipitate rhabdomyolysis, causing renal failure.

Metabolic Myopathies

CONGENITAL METABOLIC MYOPATHIES

Described as muscle pain and cramps due to insufficient energy production related to hereditary defects in glycogen (eg, glycogen storage diseases), lipid, adenine nucleotide, or mitochondrial metabolism.

SYMPTOMS/EXAM

- **Glycotic/glycogenolytic disorders:**
    - Presents with muscle pain, cramps, stiffness, and/or swelling with high-intensity exercise. Patients are easily fatigued with exertion. There are multiple types. Presentation age ranges from birth to 20–30 years.
    - Recurrent myoglobinuria (cola-colored urine that is heme ⊕ and ⊖ for RBCs) may occur.
- **Disorders of lipid metabolism:**
    - Muscle pain or tightness and/or myoglobinuria induced by prolonged exercise or prolonged fasting, infection, exposure to cold, general anesthesia, or a low-carbohydrate, high-fat diet. Predominantly present within the first few years of life.
    - Recurrent episodes of hypoketotic hypoglycemia may occur.
    - Hypertrophic or dilated cardiomyopathy and fatty liver may occur.
- **Mitochondrial myopathies:** Muscle weakness, poor endurance, and/or exertional myoglobinuria.

DIFFERENTIAL

Muscular dystrophy, myasthenia gravis, MS, infection.

DIAGNOSIS

- Check chem 12 and LFTs. Determine serum levels of lactate, CK, pyruvate, LDH, uric acid, carnitine, ketones, ammonia, and myoglobin.
- Check urine ketones, dicarboxylic acid, and myoglobin excretion at rest and with exercise.
- EMG for cases with fixed weakness (vs. intermittent for most cases).
- Obtain muscle biopsy after blood and urine testing.
- **Glycotic/glycogenolytic disorders:** CK may be elevated at rest.
- **Disorders of lipid metabolism:**
    - ↓ carnitine concentrations may be found in plasma and tissue, as may an ↑ ratio of serum free fatty acids to ketones. ↑ urine dicarboxylic acid level may be found.
    - Hypoketosis with hypoglycemia.
- **Mitochondrial myopathies:**
    - Elevated serum lactate and pyruvate levels.
    - Ragged red fibers on muscle biopsy.

TREATMENT

- Reduction in intense or prolonged physical activity.
- Treatment of myoglobinuria as needed.
- Avoidance of skipped meals; dietary changes, depending on the disorder.

COMPLICATIONS

- Rhabdomyolysis can occur with severe myoglobinuria.
- Progressive symptoms may lead to respiratory failure in some cases.

ENDOCRINE MYOPATHIES

- **Sx/Exam:** Present with proximal muscle pain and weakness.
- **Dx:** Diagnosed by the symptoms and exam outlined above in the setting of an **endocrinopathy** such as hypo- or hyperthyroidism, hypo- or hyperparathyroidism, hypo- or hyperadrenalism, hypopituitarism, or acromegaly with no other source.
- **Tx:** Treat the underlying endocrine disorder.

ALCOHOLIC MYOPATHIES

- **Sx/Exam:** Muscle pain, swelling, proximal limb weakness, and possible dysphagia develop after acute or chronic heavy drinking. Weakness may be focal or asymmetric.
- **Dx:** ↑ serum CK; myoglobinuria. Associated with a history of heavy alcohol use.
- **Tx:** Potassium and phosphorus correction. Recommend nutrition counseling and alcohol cessation.

DRUG-INDUCED MYOPATHIES

- **Sx/Exam:** Present with symmetric proximal muscle weakness, myalgia, and fatigue.
- **Dx:** ↑ serum CK; myopathic EMG findings. Look for a history of contributory medications such as potassium-depleting drugs, corticosteroids, chloroquine, clofibrate, bretylium, colchicine, HMG-CoA reductase inhibitors (eg, statins), aminocaproic acid, cocaine, or zidovudine.
- **Tx:** Discontinuation of the implicated drug.
- **Cx:** Severe rhabdomyolysis leads to myoglobinuric renal failure.

Vertigo

The perception of movement of the body or the environment when no movement occurs. May be central or peripheral.

CENTRAL VERTIGO

SYMPTOMS/EXAM

The illusion of movement of the body or environment in conjunction with nausea, vomiting, or gait ataxia.

- Associated with vertical, unidirectional, or multidirectional nystagmus that may be different in the 2 eyes.
- **No extinguishing of symptoms or symptom latency occurs with provocative maneuvers** such as the Dix-Hallpike (or Nylen-Bárány) maneuver.
- Diplopia, dysarthria, facial motor or sensory asymmetry, ↓ gag reflex, and asymmetry of tongue protrusion are possible.
- Other motor or sensory deficits, hyperreflexia, extensor plantar responses, or limb ataxia may be present.

DIFFERENTIAL

Stroke, intracerebral hemorrhage, Ménière disease, orthostatic hypotension, drug toxicity, TIA, postconcussion syndrome, MS.

DIAGNOSIS

Diagnosed by the exam results shown above. A plain head CT can reveal the source, with MRI showing smaller lesions and infarcts as well as a better view of the posterior fossa.

TREATMENT

Patients should be referred to a neurologist or neurosurgeon.

KEY FACT

Central vertigo symptoms are not ↓ or abolished with provocative maneuvers.

COMPLICATIONS

Possible surgical complications; continued symptoms if the lesion is untreatable.

PERIPHERAL VERTIGO

SYMPTOMS/EXAM

Presents in the same manner as central vertigo, but symptoms are generally intermittent and more severe or distressing.

- **Hearing loss or tinnitus** is common.
- **Unidirectional or rotational nystagmus** (not vertical) may be present. Eyes drift toward the affected side.
- Provocative maneuvers such as the Dix-Hallpike (or Nylen-Bárány) maneuver elicit symptoms and nystagmus with symptom latency and extinguishment on repetition.

DIFFERENTIAL

- BPPV, labyrinthitis, Ménière disease (recurrent episodes of vertigo, nausea, vomiting, tinnitus, and hearing loss), drug toxicity.
- Side effects of anticonvulsants, antibiotics, hypnotics, analgesics, or alcohol.

DIAGNOSIS

- Provocation of symptoms with the Dix-Hallpike (or Nylen-Bárány) maneuver.
- Obtain a fasting chem 12, ESR, TSH, RPR, and CBC to look for underlying contributing conditions.

TREATMENT

- Meclizine for BPPV. Correct any underlying metabolic disorders.
- Discontinue or taper contributing medications.
- Offer education on desensitization exercises and canalith repositioning procedures.

Movement Disorders

ATAXIAS

Incoordination and irregularity of voluntary movement. Categorized as follows:

- **Vestibular ataxia:** Ataxia with unilateral nystagmus that ↑ with gaze away from the affected side. Romberg sign is ⊕, and patients fall toward the affected side.
- **Cerebellar ataxia:**
  - Presents with hypotonia and irregularities in the rate, amplitude, and force of voluntary movements. Terminal dysmetria, "overshooting," and terminal intention tremor are seen.
  - Complex movements are performed as a series of individual movements.
  - Nystagmus, gaze pareses, and defective saccadic and pursuit movement are possible.

- **Proprioceptive ataxia:**
  - Symmetrically affects the legs and gait, with limited or no arm involvement.
  - Involves impairment of vibratory sense, joint position sense, and proprioception.
  - Also associated with numbness or tingling in the legs.
  - Improved balance is achieved with use of a cane or other support or by watching one's own feet while walking. Symptoms worsen when the patient's eyes are closed.
  - Romberg sign is ⊕, and patients exhibit a wide-based, high-stepping gait and poor heel-to-toe walking.

DIFFERENTIAL

Vertigo, sensory deficit, toxins.

DIAGNOSIS

Based on exam findings. Neuroimaging for suspected cerebellar causes.

TREATMENT

Supportive treatment; treat any underlying conditions.

Friedreich Ataxia

An idiopathic **progressive spinocerebellar disorder** beginning at 4–20 years of age. The most common hereditary ataxia. Typically **autosomal recessive,** with an expanded GAA trinucleotide repeat on chromosome 9 in the frataxin gene. Associated progressive **kyphoscoliosis** can lead to **restrictive lung disease** and **cardiomyopathy.**

SYMPTOMS/EXAM

- **Progressive mixed sensory and cerebellar gait ataxia** involves all limbs within 2 years of onset.
- Extensor plantar responses occur within 5 years.
- ↓ knee and ankle reflexes are seen, along with cerebellar dysarthria and impaired leg and joint position and vibratory senses. Weakness of the legs and arms tends to be found late in the course of the disease.
- **Pes cavus** and kyphoscoliosis are common, and nystagmus, paresthesias, tremors, vertigo, spasticity, and ↓ vision and hearing are also seen.

DIFFERENTIAL

Vitamin E deficiency, ataxia-telangiectasia, Refsum disease, abetalipoproteinemia, spinocerebellar ataxia.

DIAGNOSIS

- Diagnosis is guided by the clinical history and exam.
- Sensory nerve action potentials are absent or ↓.
- MRI reveals cervical spinal cord atrophy and minimal cerebellar atrophy; chest and spine x-rays show kyphoscoliosis.
- Echocardiography reveals associated ventricular hypertrophy.

TREATMENT

Supportive care and treatment of associated cardiac and endocrine disorders. Orthopedic procedures can assist with foot deformities.

KEY FACT

Friedreich ataxia is the most prevalent inherited ataxia.

COMPLICATIONS

Disability, with inability to walk unassisted, may occur within 5 years of onset. Patients are typically bedridden 10–20 years after onset. The average life span is 35 years.

Ataxia-Telangiectasia

An inherited **autosomal-recessive** disorder characterized by **cerebellar ataxia,** progressive pancerebellar degeneration, variable **immunodeficiency,** impaired organ maturation, predisposition to malignancy, and **ocular and cutaneous telangiectasia.** Onset is in infancy, and the disease is usually fatal in adolescence.

SYMPTOMS/EXAM

- Presents with nystagmus, cerebellar dysarthria, with gait, **limb, and trunk ataxia.** Loss of vibration and position sense, **choreoathetosis,** areflexia, and disorders of eye movement are seen.
- **Telangiectasias** appear during the teen years, first on the eyes (**oculocutaneous**) and then on sun-exposed areas of the skin (Figure 11.10).
- Mental deficiency appears in the second decade.
- Recurrent upper and lower respiratory tract infections are seen, as are progeria-like skin and hair changes, hypogonadism, and insulin resistance.

DIFFERENTIAL

Refsum disease, Niemann-Pick disease, Friedreich ataxia, cerebral palsy, familial spinocerebellar atrophies, cerebellar tumor.

DIAGNOSIS

- Guided by the history and exam.
- Look for ↑ levels of AFP and CEA and/or chromosomal abnormalities such as inversions and translocations in chromosomes 7 and 14.

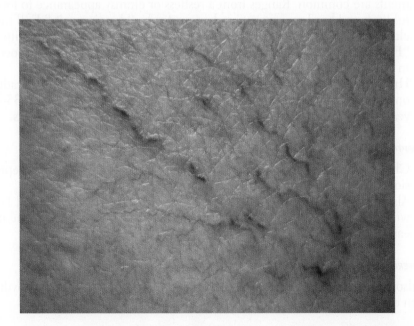

FIGURE 11.10. Blanching dilated superficial capillaries representing telangiectasia.

(Reproduced, with permission, from Wolff K, et al. *Fitzpatrick's Dermatology in General Medicine,* 7th ed. New York: McGraw-Hill, 2008, Fig. 4-34.)

- IgA is ↓ or absent; IgG is ↓ or normal; IgM is ↑ or normal; and IgE is ↓ or absent.
- Low lymphocyte count; poor skin test response to common antigens.

TREATMENT

- Avoid all x-rays because of patients' abnormal cellular sensitivity to ionizing radiation.
- Supportive care; antibiotics for any bacterial infections.

COMPLICATIONS

Death usually occurs in adolescence. Associated with a risk of leukemia and lymphoma.

Acute Cerebellar Ataxia

- **Sx/Exam:** Acute onset of usually truncal ataxia a few weeks after viral illness. May also be associated with dysmetria and nystagmus. Varicella, EBV, HSV-1, and coxsackievirus are the most commonly involved viruses.
- **DDx:** Meningitis, encephalitis, ADEM, toxin ingestion, CVA, brain tumor, neuroblastoma, hereditary ataxias.
- **Dx:** Brain CT to rule out tumor; LP if patient is febrile or has meningitic signs; screen for toxins, including alcohol; consider urinary catecholamines if concerned for neuroblastoma.
- **Tx:** Supportive care; symptoms usually self-resolve within 2–3 weeks. Approximately 10% of patients have long-term neurologic deficits.

CHOREA

Clinically distinguished as follows:

- **Chorea:** Rapid, irregular, involuntary, and purposeless movement that goes from one body part to another. **Facial grimacing** and tongue movements are common. Ranges from a restless or clumsy appearance to forceful limb and head movements and an unsteady, **"dancing gait."** Full muscle strength is preserved, and attempted muscle contraction is intermittent. **"Explosive speech"** has irregular volume and tempo. No symptoms occur in sleep.
- **Huntington disease:** An **autosomal-dominant** disorder, with gradual onset and progression of **chorea** and **dementia,** usually starting at 35–50 years of age. Chromosome 4 shows excess **CAG trinucleotide repeats.**

SYMPTOMS/EXAM

- Chorea, dystonia, tics, inhibitory pauses in voluntary movements, depression, and psychosis are common features.
- Also associated with irritability, moodiness, antisocial behavior, and later with dementia. Fidgetiness and restlessness may be seen early in the disease.

DIFFERENTIAL

Wilson disease, drug-induced tardive dyskinesia, Parkinson disease, Sydenham chorea, stroke, subdural hematoma, SLE.

DIAGNOSIS

- Clinical suspicion is confirmed with genetic studies of the **HD (huntingtin) gene.** A family history usually elicits similar cases.
- A head CT shows cerebral and caudate nucleus atrophy (Figure 11.11).

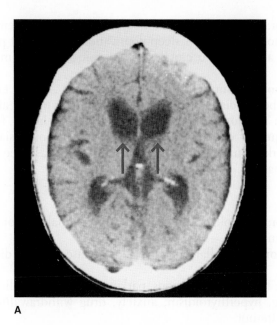 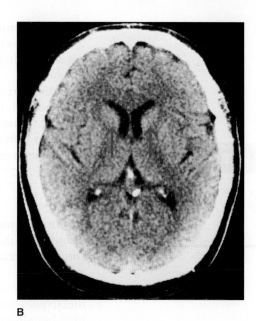

A   B

FIGURE 11.11. **Cerebral and caudate nucleus atrophy in Huntington disease.** (A) Noncontrast transaxial CT image in a 54-year-old patient with Huntington disease shows atrophy of the caudate nuclei *(arrows)* and diffuse cerebral atrophy with ex vacuo dilation of the lateral ventricles. Compare with a normal 54-year-old subject **(B)** *(arrows on caudate nuclei).* (Reproduced, with permission, from Ropper A, Brown RH. *Adams and Victor's Principles of Neurology,* 9th ed. New York: McGraw-Hill, 2009, Fig. 39-4.)

TREATMENT

- Supportive treatment. Dopamine receptor blockers for chorea symptoms; SSRIs to reduce aggression.
- Offer genetic counseling to family members.

COMPLICATIONS

- Usually fatal 10–20 years after clinical onset.

ATHETOSIS

Slow, **sinuous, writhing movements** that may be generalized or restricted to one area of the body. Symptoms are ↑ by emotional stress and voluntary activity and are not present during sleep. In some cases, symptoms occur only during specific activities, such as speaking or writing.

DIFFERENTIAL

Huntington disease, Wilson disease, Parkinson disease, cerebral palsy, Sydenhams chorea, drug toxicity, SLE, stroke.

DIAGNOSIS

Diagnosis is guided by the history and exam. Check for underlying conditions or causes such as polycythemia vera or thyrotoxicosis in chorea.

TREATMENT

Treat any underlying disease. Supportive care.

TREMOR

Rhythmic oscillatory movement characterized by the action taken during symptoms. Categorized as follows:

- **Postural tremor:** Tremor with sustained posture of an extremity. Symptoms ↑ with emotional stress or sleep deprivation and are not present during sleep. They also ↑ with use of TCAs, valproic acid, lithium, and bronchodilators.
- **Intention tremor:** Tremor during movement that ↑ as a target is approached. May be associated with cerebellar signs. No tremor at rest.
- **Resting tremor:** Tremor at rest. May affect the fingers, hands, forearms, or feet. Has a **frequency of 4–6 Hz.** Associated with hypokinesia or rigidity when due to parkinsonism (for more on Parkinson disease, see the Geriatric Medicine chapter).

KEY FACT

Postural tremor is usually an exaggeration of normal physiologic tremor.

DIFFERENTIAL

- **Postural tremor:** Physiologic tremor, benign essential tremor, cerebellar disorders, Wilson disease.
- **Intention tremor:** Cerebellar or brain stem disease, Wilson disease, drug toxicity.
- **Resting tremor:** Basal ganglia lesions, parkinsonism, Wilson disease, heavy metal poisoning, hyperthyroidism, anxiety, drug withdrawal/toxicity, benign hereditary tremor.

DIAGNOSIS

Diagnosis is guided by the history and exam. In intention tremor, MRI may show a lesion of the superior cerebellar peduncle.

TREATMENT

Treat any underlying condition. β-blockers or anticonvulsants may reduce benign essential tremor. Severe intention tremor may be treated with thalamus stereotactic surgery or high-frequency stimulation via an implanted device.

CREUTZFELDT-JAKOB DISEASE

A **prion disease** characterized by **rapidly progressive dementia** in association with **diffuse myoclonic jerks.** Also known as subacute spongiform encephalopathy.

KEY FACT

The dementia of Creutzfeldt-Jakob disease has rapid onset and progression.

SYMPTOMS/EXAM

- Presents with rapidly progressive dementia, with late akinetic mutism and coma.
- Anxiety, **personality change,** depression, emotional lability, delusions, and hallucinations are also seen.
- Motor symptoms include myoclonus, cerebellar ataxia, rigidity, bradykinesia, tremor, chorea, and dystonia.

DIFFERENTIAL

Alzheimer disease, Parkinson disease, progressive supranuclear palsy, intracerebral mass, hydrocephalus, multi-infarct dementia.

DIAGNOSIS

- Definitive diagnosis is by immunodetection of the prion in brain tissue on biopsy.
- Brain MRI T_2-weighted and diffusion-weighted images show hyperintense signals in the basal ganglia.
- EEG may show periodic sharp waves or spikes. CSF protein may be ↑.

TREATMENT

Treatment is supportive.

COMPLICATIONS

Fatal within several months of diagnosis.

TICS

Repetitive, stereotyped movements or vocalizations.

- **Sx/Exam:** May present as blinking, sniffing, stretching of the neck or mouth, or touching something repetitively. Voluntary suppression may produce anxiety, whereas performing the tic may relieve tension. Symptoms ↑ with emotional stress and ↓ with voluntary activity. No symptoms occur during sleep.
- **DDx:** Tourette syndrome, encephalitis, chorea, Huntington disease, Wilson disease, seizure, tardive dyskinesia, tuberous sclerosis.
- **Dx:** Based on the history and exam.
- **Tx:** Benzodiazepines or clonidine may be helpful. Antipsychotic medications such as haloperidol may be used for severe cases. Injected botulinum toxin can alleviate symptoms.

RESTLESS LEGS SYNDROME

Leg "restlessness," along with crawling, itching, or stretching sensations in the calves, relieved by movement.

- **Sx/Exam:** Symptoms worsen when the patient lies down at night or sits while at rest. Sleep may be disturbed.
- **DDx:** Akathisia, periodic movements of legs, peripheral neuropathy.
- **Dx:** Clinical diagnosis. Check for **pregnancy, iron deficiency anemia,** uremia, or peripheral neuropathy. Family history is often ⊕. Associated with periodic limb movement disorder, leading to involuntary leg twitching or jerking every 10–60 seconds during sleep.
- **Tx:** Treat the underlying condition. Levodopa, ropinirole, pramipexole, clonazepam, propoxyphene, and clonidine are commonly used.
- **Cx:** Daytime somnolence; development of tolerance to treatment.

> **KEY FACT**
>
> Eighty percent of patients with restless legs syndrome have periodic limb movement disorder.

Sleep Disorders

NARCOLEPSY

Sudden onset of irresistible sleep throughout the day; occurs during unusual circumstances such as talking, eating. Affects men and women equally. Usually has genetic association.

- **Sx/Exam:** Cataplexy, sudden loss of muscle tone with strong emotion, no loss of consciousness. Sleep paralysis and visual or auditory hallucinations. The age of onset tends to be 15–35 years of age.
- **DDx:** OSA, seizure, syncope, excessive daytime somnolence, drug use, brain tumor.
- **Dx:** Diagnosis of exclusion, 2–6 episodes of narcolepsy a day, sleep study.
- **Tx:** Timed naps around meals, trial of stimulants, TCA, MAO-I.

NIGHT TERRORS

- **Sx/Exam:** Usually occurs in children 2–7 years of age. Arousal with fear and anxiety, tachycardia, diaphoresis. Individual is often difficult to arouse and will spontaneously go back to sleep. Non-REM sleep disorder.
- **DDx:** Sleepwalking, postictal wandering, confusional arousals.
- **Tx:** Usually self-resolves by adolescence; may be triggered by stressful events or certain medications.

(For information on obstructive sleep apnea, see the Pulmonary chapter. For information on insomnia, see the Geriatric Medicine chapter.)

Tinnitus

- **Sx/Exam:**
  - High-pitched noise in the ear that may last for several minutes or persist. When symptoms are severe, they may interfere with concentration or sleep.
  - Otologic exam may be normal.
  - Cerumen impaction is common, and head or neck carotid bruit may be present.
- **DDx:** Conductive hearing loss, palatal myoclonus, otosclerosis, otitis media, head trauma, glomus tumor, jugular venous hum, Ménière disease.
- **Dx:**
  - Guided by the history. Examine for hearing loss and obtain a complete audiographic evaluation.
  - In the presence of a pulsatile tinnitus suggestive of a vascular etiology, MRI angiography is warranted.
  - If tinnitus is asymmetric or unilateral, an MRI of the internal auditory canals is needed to check for possible acoustic tumor.
  - "Clicking" tinnitus may be due to palatal myoclonus.
- **Tx:**
  - Amplification of normal sounds or music; "white noise" to mask the symptoms.
  - Treat related sleep interference with nortriptyline 50 mg PO at night.
  - Surgical ablation of any contributing vascular anomaly or tumor.
  - Caution patients to avoid excessive noise and ototoxic medications. Recommend stress reduction.

KEY FACT

Tinnitus is strongly associated with some degree of hearing loss.

Selected Ophthalmologic and Cranial Nerve Disorders

INTERNUCLEAR OPHTHALMOPLEGIA

Defined as a disconjugate gaze, with impaired adduction and nystagmus of the abducting eye, due to a lesion of the **medial longitudinal fasciculus.** Consider **MS** if the disease is bilateral or in a young adult. Vascular disease is likely in older patients or those with unilateral involvement.

- **Sx/Exam:** The ipsilateral eye fails to adduct when the patient looks toward the opposite side (Figure 11.12). Instead of complete paralysis of adduction, there may be slow adducting saccades in the affected eye. Nystagmus is present in the unaffected eye.

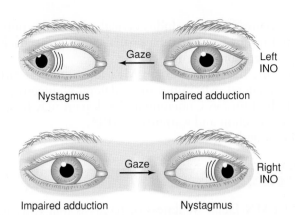

FIGURE 11.12. Eye movements in internuclear ophthalmoplegia. (Reproduced, with permission, from Simon RP, et al. *Clinical Neurology,* 7th ed. New York: McGraw-Hill, 2009, Fig. 4-17.)

- **DDx:** MS, vascular disease, brain stem encephalitis, intrinsic brain stem tumors, syringobulbia, drug toxicity, Wernicke encephalopathy, myasthenia gravis, SLE.
- **Dx:** Guided by the exam. Neuroimaging is required to look for possible etiologies.
- **Tx:** Treat any underlying cause.

NYSTAGMUS

- Rhythmic involuntary eye movement. Subtypes:
    - **Pendular nystagmus:** Involuntary rhythmic eye oscillation, with equal velocity in both directions.
    - **Jerk nystagmus:** Slow phase of rhythmic, involuntary eye movement in 1 direction and fast phase in the opposite direction. May be horizontal, vertical, or rotatory.
- **Sx/Exam:** Symptoms can occur at the extremes of gaze under normal conditions. Vertigo, hearing loss, tinnitus, or cranial nerve abnormalities are possible, depending on the cause.
- **DDx:** Associated causative factors include drug toxicity (anticonvulsants or sedatives), alcohol intoxication, brain stem disorders, lithium toxicity (vertical jerk nystagmus), BPPV, and head trauma.
- **Dx:**
    - Guided by the history and exam. Neuroimaging is appropriate for those without an identifiable cause.
    - Vertigo may be present when the cause is a vestibular lesion.
    - Hearing loss or tinnitus is associated with peripheral lesions or those of the corticospinal tract. Cranial nerve abnormalities point to a central lesion.
- **Tx:** Discontinue contributory medications. Treat any identified cause, including surgery if necessary. Neurology referral for unidentifiable causes.

KEY FACT

The direction of jerk nystagmus is named for the direction of the fast phase.

HORNER SYNDROME

Unilateral **miotic pupil** with **ipsilateral mild ptosis**, often associated with **ipsilateral anhidrosis**.

- **Sx/Exam:** Response to light and accommodation is normal. The ipsilateral conjunctiva may be acutely injected, and the ipsilateral face may be warm and hyperemic. Slow pupillary dilation is seen on the affected side.
- **DDx:** Argyll Robertson pupil (associated with late syphilis; the pupil accommodates but does not react), neuroblastoma, history of ocular trauma.

Associated causative factors include cervical cord lesion, pulmonary apical or mediastinal tumor, neck trauma or mass, cluster headache, carotid artery thrombosis, and brain stem infarct.

- **Dx:** Based on the history and exam. MRI for numbness of the ipsilateral face and contralateral extremities or ipsilateral abducens palsy; CXR for suspicion of chest tumor. Concomitant neck pain may be associated with carotid artery dissection and warrants an MRA.
- **Tx:** Treat the underlying cause.

BELL PALSY

Abrupt onset of **LMN facial weakness** or paralysis that is usually **unilateral** (Figure 11.13).

- **Sx/Exam:**
    - Symptoms progress over hours to 1–2 days. An **impaired sense of taste, hyperacusis,** and **lacrimation** are common.
    - The ipsilateral eye may be difficult to close. Pain around the ipsilateral ear is possible.
    - Patients often have difficulty eating.
    - No abnormalities are found beyond the facial nerve territory.
- **DDx:** Intracranial tumor, stroke, Ramsay Hunt syndrome, Lyme disease, sarcoidosis, AIDS, acoustic neuroma, Guillain-Barré syndrome.
- **Dx:**
    - Based on the history and exam. Nerve conduction studies can point to the prognosis.

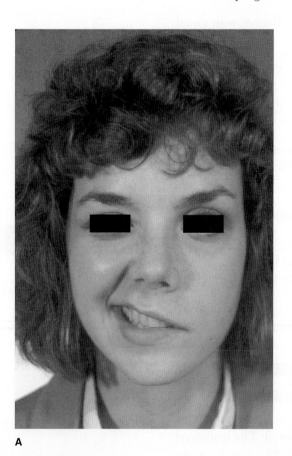 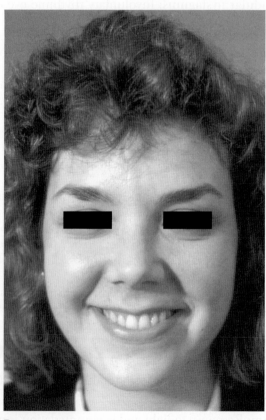

A   B

FIGURE 11.13. **Bell palsy.** (A) 28-year-old female with acute-onset left facial paralysis involving the entire left face. Treated with oral steroids. (B) Full recovery 2 months after onset. (Reproduced, with permission, from Lalwani AK. *Current Diagnosis & Treatment in Otolaryngology—Head & Neck Surgery,* 2ed. New York: McGraw-Hill, 2008, Fig. 68-1.)

- Labs or studies are needed to exclude other causes if the history or exam is not conclusive. Although the cause is usually **idiopathic,** it may be associated with **pregnancy** or **diabetes,** Lyme disease, HIV, or herpesvirus infection.
- **Tx:** Treatment with oral corticosteroids may be effective within the first few days of palsy development. In the past, acyclovir was also thought to be beneficial, but evidence now suggests that antivirals are not effective. Lubricating eye drops may be used, along with an ipsilateral eye patch, if the eye is difficult to close. Most patients have complete recovery within weeks to months without treatment.
- **Cx:** Severe pain, older age, hyperacusis, and complete palsy at diagnosis are associated with a poorer prognosis, with disfigurement affecting about 10% of patients.

KEY FACT

Bell palsy symptoms usually peak within 48 hours.

RAMSAY HUNT SYNDROME

Ipsilateral facial weakness, with herpetic eruption of the ear, palate, pharynx, or occipital scalp.

- **Sx/Exam:** May involve deafness, tinnitus, or vertigo.
- **DDx:** Bell palsy, stroke, TIA, Guillain-Barré syndrome.
- **Dx:** Based on clinical findings.
- **Tx:** Treat acutely with **acyclovir** and **corticosteroids.**
- **Cx:** Postherpetic neuralgia in the affected areas or persistent facial weakness. Fewer than one-half of patients achieve a complete recovery. For more on postherpetic neuralgia, see the Geriatric Medicine chapter.

TRIGEMINAL NEURALGIA

A 62-year-old woman presents with an intermittent dull ache on the lower right side of her face that is worsened by chewing and is not relieved by OTC analgesics. Her symptoms have been occurring for a month and are now "stabbing" and ↑ even with talking. Exam elicits pain on touching the lower right side of the patient's face. Head CT is ⊖. What is the diagnosis?
Trigeminal neuralgia.

An **idiopathic facial pain syndrome** with onset often in the 6th decade. The male-to-female incidence ratio is 2:3. If the syndrome is bilateral or diagnosed in a young female patient, consider MS as a cause.

SYMPTOMS/EXAM

- Presents as **stabbing, brief unilateral pain** in the areas of the **2nd and 3rd branches of the trigeminal nerve** (Figure 11.14). Touching the affected area, eating, or a draft of air over the face elicits the pain.
- Symptoms radiate from the corner of the mouth to the ipsilateral eye, ear, or nostril. Symptoms during sleep are rare.
- Otherwise neurologically normal.

DIFFERENTIAL

Temporal arteritis, TMJ dysfunction, atypical facial pain, glaucoma, brain stem tumor, MS, dental abscess, postherpetic neuralgia.

DIAGNOSIS

Guided by the history and exam. Head CT is ⊖. In a young patient, suspect MS and obtain evoked potential testing, an MRI, and CSF tests.

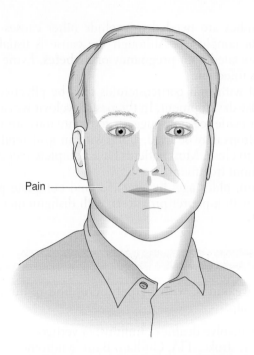

Pain

FIGURE 11.14. **Distribution of symptoms in trigeminal neuralgia.** (Reproduced, with permission, from Simon RP, et al. *Clinical Neurology,* 7th ed. New York: McGraw-Hill, 2009, Fig. 2-8.)

KEY FACT

Treatment of trigeminal neuralgia with carbamazepine is diagnostic and therapeutic.

TREATMENT

Carbamazepine and **oxcarbazepine** are first-line agents but require monitoring of cell counts and LFTs. Baclofen and gabapentin can be considered as second-line therapies.

COMPLICATIONS

Spontaneous remissions can occur for months, but some patients have progression of the disorder, with more frequent symptoms and possibly persistent low-grade pain.

SELECTED CRANIAL NERVE PALSIES

Table 11.7 compares the clinical presentations of selected cranial nerve palsies.

TABLE 11.7. Presentation of Selected Cranial Nerve Palsies

OCULOMOTOR NERVE (CN III)	TROCHLEAR NERVE (CN IV)	ABDUCENS NERVE (CN VI)
The affected eye is **deviated down and out.** Ptosis and paralysis of accommodation are seen. Diplopia is seen, except in lateral gaze toward the affected side. Pupillary function may be impaired.	The eye is elevated in forward gaze. This ↑ with adduction and is greatest with the head tilted toward the affected side. The effect ↓ with abduction and is abolished when the head is tilted away from the affected side. Downward gaze adducts the affected eye and worsens diplopia. Tilting of the head ↓ diplopia.	Adduction of the involved eye at rest. Failure of attempted abduction. Diplopia is seen on lateral gaze to the affected side. Esotropia (a cross-eyed appearance) is present.

DIFFERENTIAL

- Myasthenia gravis, trauma, thyroid ophthalmopathy.
- Be concerned for aneurysm, hemorrhage, tumor, or uncal herniation if the pupil is dilated and nonreactive. Risk factors for CN palsies include **hypertension, diabetes,** MS, sarcoidosis, atherosclerosis, tumor, ischemia, and aneurysm.

DIAGNOSIS

- Based on the clinical exam.
- CT or MRI may be needed if pupillary function is impaired, a structural lesion is suspected, the patient is > 40 years of age or has associated pain, other neurologic findings are present, or symptoms persist past several weeks.
- Conduct a Bielschowsky head-tilt test for CN IV palsy (⊕ if head tilt toward the side of the affected eye yields elevation of the affected eye and marked diplopia).

KEY FACT

In oculomotor (CN III) palsy, the affected eye is "down and out."

TREATMENT

- Treat the underlying condition.
- Surgery for severe, persistent symptoms.
- Prisms can reduce diplopia.
- May resolve spontaneously in 6–12 months. Possible surgery if symptoms persist. Alternate eye patching in young children for CN VI palsy.

Spinal Cord Disorders

SPINAL ARTERIOVENOUS MALFORMATION

SYMPTOMS/EXAM

- Presents with weakness or paralysis of one or both legs, along with numbness or paresthesias in the same distribution. An upper, lower, or mixed motor deficit is seen in the legs.
- Associated with acute, **lancinating pain** in the back or legs that **worsens with recumbency.** Hyperreflexia is seen caudal to the lesion. Sphincter function is compromised.
- Symptoms are also present in the arms with cervical lesions.
- A bruit, cutaneous angioma, or dermatomal nevus may be present over the affected area of the spine, but are rare findings.

DIFFERENTIAL

Guillain-Barré syndrome, spinal cord infarction, transverse myelitis, MS, stroke, cauda equina syndrome.

DIAGNOSIS

- Based on **selective angiography.**
- MRI of the spine or CT myelography shows one or more enlarged and tortuous draining vessels in the subarachnoid space, usually at the lower spinal cord. The spinal cord may appear enlarged in the area of the lesion.
- CSF shows high protein but little or no cellular reaction.
- Associated with **SAH** or myelopathy.

TREATMENT

Embolization of the lesion or ligation of its feeding vessels and excision of the anomalous AVM nidus.

COMPLICATIONS

Increasing gait disability can progress to the point at which the patient is bed-ridden.

CERVICAL SPONDYLOSIS

SYMPTOMS/EXAM

- Presents with limited head and neck movement with neck pain or stiffness.
- Pain in the arms, muscle atrophy, and occipital headache are also seen. Lhermitte sign is often ⊕. When flexion of the head causes a transient shooting electrical sensation down the spine, the Lhermitte sign is ⊕.
- A segmental motor or sensory deficit may be present in the arms, with UMN deficits in the legs.
- If the C5–C6 interspace is affected, may lead to hyperreflexic triceps reflex, with absent biceps and supinator reflexes.

DIFFERENTIAL

MS, motor neuron disease, subacute combined degeneration of the spinal cord, spinal mass, syringomyelia.

DIAGNOSIS

- Supportive history and exam.
- Cervical x-rays show **osteophytes** and **narrowing of the disk space** (cervical disk degeneration) and intervertebral foramina (leading to **impingement of nerve roots**).
- CSF shows ↑ protein and a normal cell count.
- MRI of the neck or CT myelogram may be needed for confirmation.

TREATMENT

↓ cervical movement and subsequent pain with a cervical collar. Surgical intervention may be needed to prevent progression or for severe or refractory pain.

COMPLICATIONS

Chronic pain or weakness.

SUBACUTE COMBINED DEGENERATION OF THE SPINAL CORD

- **Sx/Exam:**
  - Presents with distal extremity weakness and paresthesias starting in the hands.
  - Also associated with ↓ sensation, with deficits in vibratory and joint position senses.
  - Later symptoms include **spastic paraparesis** and **ataxia** due to ↓ postural sensation in the legs.
  - Extensor plantar responses are present.
  - Visual impairment with optic atrophy is seen. Psychosis is possible.
- **DDx:** MS, ALS, spinal mass, cervical spondylosis.
- **Dx:** By exam. Labs show macrocytic megaloblastic anemia and low serum vitamin B_{12} if not treated. The Schilling test is abnormal if the source is pernicious anemia.
- **Tx:** IM vitamin B_{12} injections.
- **Cx:** Progression without treatment can lead to ataxia, visual impairment, and psychosis.

CHAPTER 12

Surgery

Ryohei Otsuka, MD

TABLE 12.1.   Cardiac Risk Stratification

MAJOR	INTERMEDIATE	MINOR
MI within 6 months, with persistent ischemic symptoms.	MI > 6 months ago.	Advanced age.
Decompensated CHF.	Stable/mild angina.	Abnormal ECG.
Significant arrhythmias.	Compensated or prior CHF.	Rhythm other than sinus (eg, atrial fibrillation).
Severe valvular disease.	DM.	Poor functional capacity.
	Renal insufficiency.	History of stroke.
		Uncontrolled hypertension.

KEY FACT

The indications for coronary revascularization in the preoperative patient are no different from those in patients not facing surgery. "Prophylactic" CABG and/or angioplasty/stenting should not be done unless it is likely to ↑ survival.

KEY FACT

Check 12-lead ECG for patients undergoing vascular surgery who have at least 1 clinical risk factor and in patients undergoing intermediate-risk surgery who have CHD, peripheral arterial disease, or cerebrovascular disease.

KEY FACT

Incentive spirometry ↓ the risk of complications and should be taught to patients preoperatively.

Preoperative Evaluation

Preoperative evaluation is required before cardiac and noncardiac surgery. This consists of a focused history and physical exam centering on the cardiac and respiratory systems. The presence of comorbid conditions may necessitate additional lab, ECG, cardiac stress, PFT, or CXR testing. Nonselective imaging and lab screening tests have been shown to be of minimal value.

CARDIAC RISK EVALUATION

A preoperative cardiac risk assessment should address **3 major components:**

1. The patient's risk of a major **cardiac complication** (Table 12.1).
2. The patient's current **functional status** (Table 12.2).
3. The cardiac risk associated with the **planned procedure** (Table 12.3).

Guidelines for further cardiac evaluation and for the mitigation of cardiac risk are outlined in Figure 12.1.

PERIOPERATIVE β-BLOCKERS

Studies indicate that perioperative β-blockers ↓ cardiac complications in patients with known or suspected CAD. All studies used β_1-selective agents.

- β-blockers are recommended for the following:
  - Patients who are already taking β-blockers for angina, arrhythmia, and/or hypertension.
  - Patients undergoing vascular surgery who have cardiac ischemia on preoperative evaluation.

TABLE 12.2.   Functional Status Assessment

EXCELLENT (> 7 METs)[a]	MODERATE (4–7 METs)	POOR (< 4 METs)
Squash.	Cycling.	Vacuuming.
Jogging (10-minute mile).	Climbing a flight of stairs.	Activities of daily living (eg, eating, dressing, bathing).
Scrubbing floors.	Golf (without cart).	
Singles tennis.	Walking 4 mph.	Walking 2 mph.
	Yardwork (eg, raking leaves, weeding, pushing a power mower).	Writing.

[a]MET = metabolic equivalent, a unit used to estimate the (energy) oxygen consumption during physical activity. 1 MET = oxygen consumption of a 70-kg, 40-year-old man in a resting state.

TABLE 12.3. Degree of Cardiac Risk Associated with Surgical Procedures[a]

Low: "ABCDE-TURP"	Intermediate: "CHOPIN"	High: "EVA"
Ambulatory procedures	**C**arotid endarterectomy	**E**mergency major procedures
Breast procedures	**H**ead procedures	**V**ascular procedures
Cataract procedures	**O**rthopedic procedures	**A**nticipated prolonged surgical procedures
Dermatologic procedures	**P**rostatectomy	associated with large fluid shifts or blood loss
Endoscopic procedures	**I**ntraperitoneal and intrathoracic procedures	
Trans**U**rethral **R**esection of the **P**rostate	**N**eck procedures	

[a]Cardiac risk is stratified as follows: low risk = < 1%; intermediate risk = < 5%; high risk = > 5%.

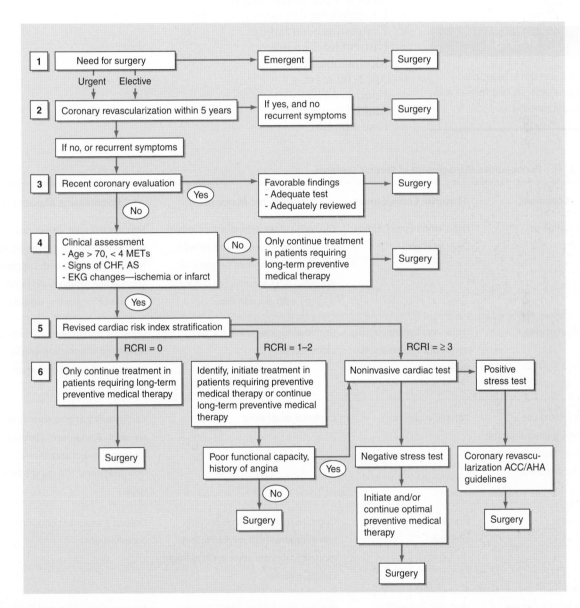

FIGURE 12.1. Algorithm for cardiac risk assessment. (Reproduced, with permission, from Fauci AS, et al. *Harrison's Principles of Internal Medicine*, 17th ed. New York: McGraw-Hill, 2008, Fig. 8-2.)

KEY FACT

PFTs and ABGs are not routinely ordered and should be obtained only if you would do so even if the patient were not undergoing surgery.

KEY FACT

Poor glycemic control is associated with a higher incidence of infection and delayed wound healing.

- Don't use β-blockers for patients with high-grade conduction system disease.
- The target is a resting heart rate of 60 bpm.
- β-blockers should continue intraoperatively and postoperatively so that a heart rate of 60–65 bpm is maintained.

PULMONARY RISK EVALUATION

The risk factors for perioperative pulmonary complications include the following:

- Surgery on the chest or abdomen.
- Neck or intracranial surgery.
- Chronic lung disease.
- Congestive heart failure.
- Current tobacco use.
- Morbid obesity.
- Age > 60 years.
- Prior stroke.
- Altered mental status.
- Low albumin.

TABLE 12.4. Perioperative Management of Chronic Diseases

Condition	Potential Complications	Preoperative Management	Postoperative Management
DM, on insulin as outpatient	Hypo- and hyperglycemia; DKA; infection.	Give 50% of usual long-acting insulin the morning of surgery (exception: glargine, which should be given at the usual dose the evening before surgery) with glucose drip.	Strongly consider insulin drip titrating to normoglycemia; otherwise, restart long-acting insulin with supplemental short-acting insulin (with rapid titration of long-acting insulin).
DM, not on insulin	Hypo- and hyperglycemia; nonketotic hyperosmolar state.	Omit oral hypoglycemic the day before surgery.	Consider insulin drip; use regularly scheduled short-acting insulin if needed and restart oral agent when possible.
Chronic steroid use (especially greater than the equivalent of prednisone 20 mg for 3 weeks)	Adrenal crisis (rare).	Continue usual dose.	Can usually just give chronic dose; consider "stress-dose" steroids for longer/major surgeries—hydrocortisone 100 mg q 8 hr × 2–3 days.
Liver disease	Mortality, hemorrhage, infection.	Optimize treatment of underlying complications; high morbidity and mortality rates are seen in Child-Pugh Class C patients.	Optimize treatment of underlying complications.
Chronic kidney disease	Mortality, hemorrhage, electrolyte disturbance, infection.	Monitor electrolytes; check bleeding time if uremia; assess for anemia/consider erythropoietin for elective surgery.	Monitor electrolytes and fluid volume.

Perioperative Management

Table 12.4 outlines the perioperative management of common chronic diseases. Table 12.5 discusses indications for perioperative prophylaxis.

PERIOPERATIVE MANAGEMENT OF ANTICOAGULATION

- **Aspirin** can be continued for patients with a high risk of perioperative vascular complications. If discontinued, it should be stopped 7 days before surgery. Resume approximately 24 hours after surgery.
- **Warfarin** should be stopped 4–5 days before surgery and replaced with heparin. Unfractionated heparin is stopped 5 hours before surgery, and low-molecular-weight heparin (LMWH) is stopped 12–24 hours before surgery. Unfractionated heparin or LMWH with warfarin therapy may be restarted postoperatively once hemostasis has been achieved.
- **Clopidogrel** should be stopped 7–10 days before surgery.
- **NSAIDs** should be stopped at least 3 days before surgery unless benefits exceed risks (ie, severe arthritis).

KEY FACT

Low-risk patients who are < 40 years of age, have no risk factors, and require general anesthesia for < 30 minutes do not need DVT prophylaxis.

KEY FACT

Sucralfate and H_2 receptor blockers both reduce the likelihood of GI bleeding by 50%, but they have known disadvantages such as ↓ absorption of medications and a possible ↑ risk of nosocomial pneumonia.

TABLE 12.5. Indications for Perioperative Prophylaxis

CONDITION	AT-RISK GROUPS	RECOMMENDATIONS
Bacterial endocarditis	Patients with prosthetic valves, previous infective endocarditis, valvulopathy following heart transplantation, or complex CHD.[a]	**Dental** (involving gingival tissue, dental periapical regions, or perforating the oral mucosa) **and respiratory tract procedures:** PO amoxicillin, IV ampicillin, PO cephalexin, or PO/IV clindamycin 30–60 minutes before the procedure. Prophylaxis is **NOT** recommended for bronchoscopy, genitourinary/GI tract procedures.
DVT	All surgical patients are at risk for DVT, especially those undergoing major surgery, those having orthopedic surgery, and those > 40 years of age or with additional DVT risk factors.	**"Minidose" heparin:** Usually 5000 U SQ BID–TID. **Low-molecular-weight heparin:** Enoxaparin 30 mg BID or 40 mg QD. Thromboembolic disease stockings (TEDs). Sequential compression devices. **Warfarin:** Dose adjusted; for very-high-risk patients only.
GI bleeding (2° to stress-induced gastric mucosal disease)	At especially high risk for GI bleeding are patients with coagulopathy, those with respiratory failure requiring mechanical ventilation, and those with a history of GI ulcer/bleeding.	H_2 receptor blockers, PPIs, sucralfate.
Constipation	All postoperative patients on narcotic pain medications.	Docusate sodium (eg, Colace), senna.

[a]**Congenital heart disease (CHD)** only in the following conditions: unrepaired cyanotic CHD, completely repaired CHD with prosthetic material or device, and repaired CHD with residual defects to the site of a prosthetic patch or prosthetic device.

Postoperative Care

Recovery from surgery can be divided into 3 phases:

- The **immediate** postoperative phase.
- An **intermediate** postoperative phase encompassing the hospitalization period.
- A **convalescent** phase.

IMMEDIATE POSTOPERATIVE PERIOD

The principal causes of complications and death following major surgery are acute cardiac, pulmonary, and fluid derangements. Monitor postoperative patients until cardiopulmonary and neurologic function has returned to baseline.

INTERMEDIATE POSTOPERATIVE PERIOD

During the time from complete recovery from anesthesia until discharge from the hospital, the patient must recover basic bodily functions and become self-sufficient. Measures with which to achieve these goals are outlined in Table 12.6.

Postoperative Fever

- Most early postoperative fever is caused by the inflammatory response to surgery and resolves spontaneously.
- The timing of fever after surgery is the key to generating DDx of postoperative fever (Table 12.7).

Pain Management

Postoperative pain serves no practical function and can give rise to a range of complications, including the following:

> **KEY FACT**
>
> Malignant hyperthermia is a rare disorder caused by general anesthesia. It usually develops within 30 minutes of starting anesthesia inhalation.

> **KEY FACT**
>
> Two important infectious causes of fever in the first 36 hours after laparotomy are (1) intraperitoneal leakage from injury to bowel and (2) invasive soft tissue infection caused by either β-hemolytic streptococci or clostridial species (most commonly, *Clostridium perfringens*).

TABLE 12.6. Management of the Intermediate Postoperative Period

SYSTEM	MANAGEMENT
Fluid/electrolyte	Careful monitoring of volume status/electrolytes. Postoperative fluid replacement includes maintenance fluid, losses from drains, third-space losses (eg, tissue edema, ileus), extra needs (eg, burns, fever).
Pulmonary	Deep breathing exercises/incentive spirometry. Adequate pain control. Early mobilization. Early recognition and treatment of cardiac failure.
GI	Early feeding has been effective in most cases. Patients receiving opioid pain medication may need stool softener and/or laxative. Consider an NG tube if patients have marked ileus.
NG tube	Low intermittent suction, frequent irrigation, addition of potassium to replace GI fluid loss.
Infection	Routine postoperative antimicrobial use should be discouraged, as it is costly and is associated with ↑ rates of microbial drug resistance and incidence of *C diff*.

TABLE 12.7.   **Postoperative Fever and Etiology**

Timing After Surgery	Common Etiology
Immediate fever (within hours of surgery)	Medications, blood products, trauma before or from surgery, or prior infection.
Acute fever (in the first week after surgery)	Nosocomical infection (**pneumonia** or **UTI** is much more common than surgical site infections [SSIs] or IV catheter infection); noninfectious causes include pancreatitis, myocardial infarction, pulmonary embolism, atelectasis, thrombophlebitis, alcohol withdrawal, and acute gout.
Subacute fever (> 1 week after surgery)	SSIs, IV catheter infection, antibiotic-associated diarrhea (most commonly, *C difficile*), DVT/PE, thrombophlebitis, drug fever (eg, β-lactams, sulfa, H_2-blockers, and heparin).
Delayed fever (> a month after surgery)	Most are from infections such as viral infections from blood products, parasitic infections. SSIs with indolent microorganisms (eg, coagulase-negative staphylococci) in high-risk patients with implanted medical devices.

- Splinting of the diaphragm, which can lead to reluctance to breathe and can result in atelectasis and pneumonia.
- Limited mobility, which can lead to venous stasis and cause DVT.
- Release of catecholamines, leading to vasospasm and hypertension, causing stroke, MI, and bleeding.
- Table 12.8 outlines options for postoperative pain management.

TABLE 12.8.   **Postoperative Pain Medications**

Route/Medication Class	Examples	Advantages	Side Effects
IV opioids	Morphine, hydromorphone, methadone.	Potent analgesia.	Respiratory depression, nausea, vomiting, altered sensorium.
IV nonopioid analgesics	Ketorolac tromethamine (an NSAID).	Analgesic and anti-inflammatory.	Potential for gastric ulcer; impaired coagulation; ↓ renal function with long-term use.
PO analgesics	Acetaminophen with codeine (T#3); hydrocodone with acetaminophen (Vicodin).	Acetaminophen acts as an antipyretic and allows patients to be "transitioned" home with adequate pain relief.	Tolerance with long-term use.
Patient-controlled analgesia	Usually morphine.	Controlled by the patient. The possibility of overdose is limited because the patient must be awake to self-administer. The maximum dose and timing are preset by the physician.	Respiratory depression, nausea, vomiting, altered sensorium, inadequate analgesia if the patient is unable to depress the button.
Continuous epidural analgesia	Morphine +/− bupivacaine (topical to the epidural space).	Intense and prolonged segmental analgesia, ↓ respiratory depression, longer pain relief, ↓ alteration of sensorium than IV opioids.	Pruritus, nausea, respiratory depression, hypotension, urinary retention (usually requires a bladder catheter).
Intercostal block	Bupivacaine.	Useful for diminishing pain following thoracic and abdominal procedures.	Risk of pneumothorax.

The final postoperative phase begins when a patient is discharged from the hospital. The following support services should be considered to ensure a smooth transition home, minimize postoperative complications, and hasten the patient's recovery from surgery:

- Visiting/home nursing agencies.
- Physical/occupational therapy.
- Rehabilitation services.
- Wound care specialists.

Wound Management

Wound healing can be thought of as a **stepwise process** proceeding from coagulation and inflammation through fibroplasia, matrix deposition, angiogenesis, epithelialization, collagen maturation, and wound contraction. There are 2 types of healing: **1st-intention (1°)** and **2nd-intention (2°) healing.** These 2 forms may be combined in **delayed 1° closure.**

- **1st-intention (1°) healing:** Occurs when tissue is cleanly incised and reapproximated and repair occurs without complication.
- **2nd-intention (2°) healing:** Occurs in open wounds through the formation of granulation tissue and eventual coverage of the defect by normal migration of epithelial cells.
- **Delayed 1° closure:** Combines 1° and 2° healing. A wound is allowed to heal open (under an occlusive dressing) for about 5 days and is then reapproximated using suture or other ligature.

ANESTHESIA

- **Topical anesthesia** (eg, LET gel, EMLA cream): Used to decrease the pain of infiltration.
- **Local anesthesia** (eg, lidocaine, lidocaine with epinephrine, bupivacaine).
- **Nerve block:** Good for fingers, toes, hands, feet, face, and mouth.

WOUND PREPARATION

Thorough wound preparation facilitates wound healing and prevents wound infection.

- **Debridement.**
- **Foreign body removal:** Retained foreign bodies are at risk for developing infection. Wound exploration +/- radiography or ultrasound (for radiolucent foreign bodies) is necessary.
- **Irrigation:** Copious irrigation is important to adequately clean wound.
- **Disinfection:** Povidone-iodine (Betadine) may be wound toxic and should not be used in an open wound.

KEY FACT

Don't use lidocaine with epinephrine for digits, genitals, nose, earlobes, or skin flaps because of the risk of vasoconstriction and necrosis.

KEY FACT

The pain of local anesthesia can be reduced by:
- Using a small needle (< 25 gauge).
- Slowing infiltration.
- Using a buffering agent (sodium bicarbonate).
- Warming the anesthetic agent to body temperature.

WOUND CLOSURE

The wound closure method is chosen, depending on the location, size, and mechanism of the wound as well as patient factors (eg, child).

- **Suturing:**
  - In healthy patients, the ideal closure for **small superficial wounds** (eg, skin lacerations) consists of fine **interrupted sutures** placed loosely and conveniently close to the wound edge.
  - **Mattress sutures** (horizontal and vertical) promote wound edge eversion and minimize tension on skin edges. These are ideal in wounds with some tension.
  - **Running subcuticular sutures** are useful for long wounds in which the tension has already been minimized by deep sutures.
  - **Deeper abdominal wounds** require closure of fascial layers (but not necessarily the peritoneum) with continuous nonabsorbable or slowly absorbable sutures.
  - Some general suture types and their relative advantages and disadvantages are listed in Table 12.9.

TABLE 12.9. Types of Sutures

SUTURE	CHARACTERISTICS	ADVANTAGES	DISADVANTAGES	EXAMPLES OF CLINICAL USE
Absorbable				
Natural				
Catgut (plain or chromic)	Made from sheep intestine.	Quickly absorbed (good for fast-healing areas).	Poor tensile strength; high tissue reactivity (both drawbacks are minimized with chromic).	OB/GYN (eg, perineal lacerations).
Synthetic (eg, Dexon, Vicryl, PDS)	Made of chemical polymers; absorbed by hydrolysis; may be monofilament or multifilament.	Strong, with predictable rates of loss in tensile strength; minimal tissue reaction.	Some have high tissue drag; coatings can reduce knot security.	Deep (dermal or buried) closures.
Nonabsorbable				
Natural				
Silk	Made of raw silk spun by silkworms; may be coated in wax.	Excellent handling.	High tissue reactivity; risk of infection.	Rarely used. Intraoral surgery.
Stainless steel wire	Made of a stainless steel alloy and comes in monofilament and multifilament.	High tensile strength.	May kink and break.	Cardiothoracic surgery; neurosurgery; orthopedics.
Synthetic (eg, nylon, Dacron, Prolene)	Generally inert; may be monofilament or multifilament.	Low tissue reactivity; high tensile strength.	High memory (requires 3–4 knot throws to hold).	Superficial (subcuticular) skin closures.

TABLE 12.10. Risk Factors for Wound Dehiscence

Host Factors	Operator Factors
Smoking	Tissue injury
Malnutrition, starvation	Poor blood supply
Steroids	Poor apposition of tissues (unclosed dead
Infection	space, unreduced fracture)
Hypoxia and hypovolemia	
Radiation	
Trauma	
Uremia	
DM	
Drugs (especially chemotherapeutic agents)	
Advanced age	

- **Staple:** A quick and strong closure, cosmetically acceptable, used for scalp, torso, and extremities.
- **Skin adhesive** ("glue"; eg, Dermabond): Minimal pain, less pain required in repair, used for low-tension wounds.

WOUND CARE

- **Antibiotic prophylaxis:** Consider antibiotics only in high-risk wounds such as heavily contaminated wounds, animal and human bites, or immunocompromised patients.
- **Tetanus prophylaxis:** Give tetanus vaccine to patients who have not had a 3-dose primary tetanus vaccination series or whose last tetanus vaccine was > 10 years ago (> 5 years ago if tetanus-prone wounds).
- **Suture removal:**
  - Face: 3–5 days.
  - Scalp: 5–7 days.
  - Trunk/arm/hand: 7–10 days.
  - Leg/foot: 10–14 days.

CAUSES OF WOUND DEHISCENCE

- **Dehiscence** is defined as undesired spontaneous separation of wound edges.
- The most common causes are **infection** and **excessively tight sutures.**
- Wound dehiscence can be caused by **host factors** and/or operator **factors** (Table 12.10).

Surgical Infections

MAJOR FACTORS

The main determinants of surgical infection are **patient-related** factors, **procedure-related** factors, and **microbial factors.**

- **Patient-related risk factors** include DM/perioperative hyperglycemia, tobacco use, remote infection at the time of surgery, obesity, malnutrition,

TABLE 12.11. Common Pathogens Causing Surgical Infections

ORGANISM	CHARACTERISTICS
Staphylococci (*S aureus*)	The most common pathogen in wound infections; associated with foreign bodies.
Streptococci	Can invade minor skin breaks and spread through connective tissue.
Klebsiella	Often invades the inner ear, enteric tissues, and lung.
Enteric organisms (Enterobacteriaceae and enterococci)	Often found with anaerobes such as peptostreptococci, *Bacteroides,* and *Clostridium.*
Clostridium	Anaerobic; often found in ischemic tissue.
Pseudomonas	Opportunistic in critically ill or immunosuppressed patients.
Fungi, yeast, and parasites	Cause abscesses.

low albumin, steroid use, prolonged preoperative hospital stay, prior site irradiation, and colonization with *Staphylococcus aureus.*

- **Procedure-related risk factors** include the presence of dead space, shaving of the site the night before procedure, improper preoperative skin preparation, improper antimicrobial prophylaxis, and implantation of foreign bodies.
- **Microbial factors:** Common pathogens are listed in Table 12.11.

MANAGEMENT OF INFECTION

- An infected surgical site **must be opened** either partially or entirely, depending on the extent of infection.
- Perform Gram stain and culture of purulent drainage.
- Administer empiric antibiotics.
- Switch to narrow-spectrum antibiotics once Gram stain and culture reveal a likely organism.

Acute Abdomen

Any sudden spontaneous nontraumatic disorder whose chief manifestation is in the abdominal area and for which urgent operation may be necessary.

SYMPTOMS

- Abdominal pain, fever, anorexia, nausea, vomiting, diarrhea, or constipation.
- **Jaundice, hematemesis, hematochezia,** or **hematuria** may also be seen.

EXAM

The following are common exam findings, however, some may be absent in specific cases:

- **General:** Rigidly motionless, pale, tachycardic, hypotensive, and hypo- or hyperthermic.
- **Abdominal examination** (see also Table 12.12):
  - **Inspection:** Tensely distended; old surgical scars.
  - **Auscultation:** Silent bowel sounds.
  - **Percussion:** Tenderness and tympany.
  - **Palpation:** Guarding, rigidity, rebound tenderness.
- **Rectal exam must be performed** in all patients with an acute abdomen.
- **Pelvic exam** in female patients.

DIFFERENTIAL

- Acute appendicitis, acute cholecystitis/cholangitis, acute pancreatitis.
- **Other:** Bowel obstruction, incarcerated hernia, ruptured ectopic pregnancy, ruptured aortic aneurysm, perforated peptic ulcer (and others).

DIAGNOSIS

- **Labs:** Leukocytosis and anemia may be seen on CBC; chem 7 may reveal ↑ BUN/creatinine and metabolic acidosis. Obtain LFTs to look for ↑ transaminases and/or hyperbilirubinemia. An ↑ lipase/amylase level may indicate acute pancreatitis. A urine pregnancy test must be performed on all females of reproductive age!
- **Imaging:**
  - Upright CXR may reveal subdiaphragmatic air (perforated viscous) or lower lung pathology that may mimic an acute abdomen.
  - **Abdominal radiograph (AXR)** may show signs of bowel obstruction or free air.

TABLE 12.12. Physical Exam Findings Associated with Acute Abdomen

CONDITION	APPEARANCE	PALPATION	AUSCULTATION
Perforated viscus	Scaphoid abdomen.	Tense; guarding and rigidity.	Diminished bowel sounds; loss of liver dullness.
Peritonitis	Motionless patient.	Guarding and rebound tenderness.	Absent bowel sounds (late).
Inflamed mass or abscess	Variable distention.	Tender to palpation; special signs (Murphy, psoas, obturator).	Variable bowel sounds.
Intestinal obstruction	Distention; visible peristalsis (late).	Diffusely tender to palpation; hernia or mass (some).	Hyperactive (early) or hypoactive (late) bowel sounds.
Paralytic ileus	Distention.	No localized tenderness.	Hypoactive bowel sounds.
Ischemic or strangulated bowel	No distention (until late).	Pain out of proportion to exam findings; rectal bleeding (some).	Variable bowel sounds.
Bleeding	Pallor, shock; distention.	Pulsatile (aneurysm) or tender (eg, ectopic pregnancy) mass; rectal bleeding.	Variable bowel sounds.

- Ultrasound is useful for evaluating the biliary tree and ruptured abdominal aortic aneurysm in unstable patients.
- A CT scan should be obtained routinely.

TREATMENT

Depends on the cause. Surgery is often required. In a patient with true acute abdomen, **urgent exploratory laparotomy** is sometimes necessary before the precise diagnosis can be made.

Appendicitis

A bacterial infection in the wall of the appendix that is due to obstruction of the proximal lumen. Can eventually lead to gangrene and perforation.

A 16-year-old boy presents to your office on a weekday afternoon with severe abdominal pain. On further history, his mother states that he vomited after dinner last night and did not eat breakfast this morning. When she dropped him off at school, he was complaining of mild periumbilical pain. By 10 A.M., he was curled up on the classroom floor, unable to move and was complaining of generalized abdominal pain. On presentation, he is febrile, tachycardic, and mildly hypotensive. Physical exam reveals abdominal guarding and tenderness at the McBurney point, with ↓ bowel sounds. CBC shows leukocytosis with a left shift. CT scan reveals an inflamed mass in the RLQ consistent with appendicitis. What should be the next step in management?

The patient should be taken to the operating room for emergent appendectomy.

ACUTE APPENDICITIS

SYMPTOMS

- Often begins with vague midabdominal pain, followed by **anorexia, nausea, vomiting,** and **low-grade fever.**
- Classically progresses to localized tenderness to palpation in the **RLQ.**

EXAM

- Temperature is only slightly ↑ (eg, 37.8°C [100.04°F]) in the absence of perforation.
- Patients with early (nonperforated) appendicitis often appear quite well.
- Abdominal tenderness with guarding and possible rebound can be seen in later stages.
- Tenderness is seen at the **McBurney point,** one-third the distance from the anterior superior iliac spine to the umbilicus.
- Patients may also have pain on flexion of the hip (**psoas sign**), pain on internal rotation of the hip (**obturator sign**), or pain on the right side when pressing on the left (**Rovsing sign**).
- **Appendicitis in pregnancy** can present with **RUQ tenderness** due to the gravid uterus.

DIFFERENTIAL

PID (especially in women 20–40 years of age), ectopic pregnancy, ovarian torsion, cholecystitis, diverticulitis, gastroenteritis, psoas abscess, right inguinal hernia, mesenteric adenitis.

DIAGNOSIS

- **Labs:** **Leukocytosis** is seen (usually > 10,000/μL). WBCs and/or RBCs may be present in urine (especially in retrocecal or pelvic appendicitis).
- **Imaging:**
  - **AXR:** **Not the choice of imaging** unless other conditions (eg, perforation, intestinal obstruction, ureteral calculus) are suspected.
  - **CT:** Most useful when the clinical presentation and/or lab findings are less than typical. A ⊕ CT scan would be an indication for surgery. Classic findings include an **enlarged appendix with wall thickening or enhancement or periappendiceal fat stranding** (Figure 12.2).
  - **RLQ ultrasound:** Less reliable than CT, but useful in pregnant women and children.

TREATMENT

- Open or laparoscopic appendectomy.
- Prophylactic preoperative antibiotics (usually a single-drug regimen using a cephalosporin).
- Antibiotics +/− percutaneous abscess drainage if surgery is contraindicated or unavailable.

COMPLICATIONS

- **Perforation:** Usually due to delay in seeking medical care. Occurs late (> 12 hours after onset of symptoms) and associated with more severe pain and a higher fever. Affects patients < 10 or > 50 years of age.

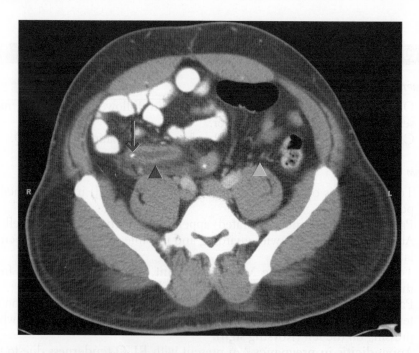

FIGURE 12.2. **Appendicitis CT scan.** An appendicolith is seen in the proximal portion of an enlarged appendix with thickened, hyperenhancing wall. Note the inflammatory changes of the periappendiceal fat *(red arrowhead)*, in distinction to the normal appearance of intra-abdominal fat shown by the yellow arrowhead. (Reproduced, with permission, from USMLERx.com.)

- **Peritonitis:** Can be localized or generalized; results from microscopic perforation of a gangrenous appendix or gross perforation into the peritoneal cavity, respectively.
- **Appendiceal abscess:** Occurs when the infection is walled off by adjacent omentum or viscera.
- **Pylephlebitis:** A suppurative thrombophlebitis of the portal venous system.

Small Bowel Obstruction (SBO)

Small bowel obstruction is the most common and surgically relevant disorder of the small intestine. Etiologies include postoperative **adhesions** (more than 50%), neoplasms, hernias, intussusception, foreign bodies, and gallstones. Obstruction can be mechanical or functional; proximal, middle, or distal; and complete or partial.

SYMPTOMS

- **Proximal (high) obstruction:** Presents with abdominal pain and vomiting.
- **Mid- or distal obstruction:** Presents with periumbilical or poorly localized abdominal cramping, along with distention and constipation/obstipation. Feculent vomitus may also be seen.
- **Dehydration** and mild fever are seen.

EXAM

- Vital signs are normal in the early stages.
- Peristalsis may be visible beneath the abdominal wall in thin patients.
- Exam reveals mild abdominal tenderness.
- Peristaltic rushes, gurgles, and **high-pitched tinkles** are sometimes audible.

DIFFERENTIAL

- **Postoperative ileus:** Gas in the colon on AXR. Only mild dilation of small bowel.
- **Large bowel obstruction:** Obstipation and colonic dilation on AXR.
- **Intestinal pseudo-obstruction:** Symptoms and signs of obstruction without evidence of obstruction. Associated with SLE, drugs, and amyloidosis.
- **Other:** Acute gastroenteritis, acute appendicitis, acute pancreatitis.

DIAGNOSIS

- **Labs:** Don't rely on labs, as these are often normal. Leukocytosis, evidence of dehydration, and/or electrolyte abnormalities may be seen. Creatine kinase and lactate are serum markers of intestinal compromise but are elevated only late in the course of disease.
- **Imaging:**
  - **AXR:** Supine and upright AXRs reveal a ladderlike pattern of dilated small bowel loops with air-fluid levels (Figure 12.3).
  - **CT:** Highly accurate in making the diagnosis and confirming the level of SBO. Also helpful in identifying the etiology.

TREATMENT

- **Partial obstruction** (gas seen in the colon on AXR): Can be managed expectantly with **NPO and an NG tube.**

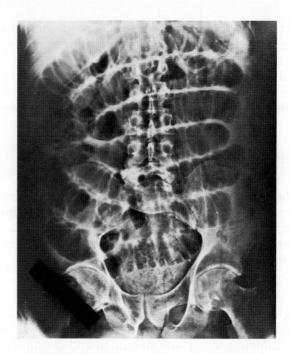

FIGURE 12.3. **Small bowel obstruction.** (Reproduced, with permission, from Doherty GM, Way LW. *Current Surgical Diagnosis & Treatment,* 12th ed. New York: McGraw-Hill, 2006: 666.)

- **Complete obstruction:**
  - Requires **operation,** in part to rule out **strangulation** (bowel dilation that impairs blood supply, which can eventually lead to necrosis, sepsis, perforation, and death).
  - Patients must be NPO and have an NG tube.
  - Treat dehydration and/or electrolyte abnormalities if present.
  - Antibiotics should be given if strangulation is suspected.

Large Bowel Obstruction (LBO)

Approximately 15% of intestinal obstructions in adults occur in the large intestine, most commonly in the **sigmoid colon.** The most common cause of LBO is **colorectal cancer;** other causes include diverticular disease, volvulus, inflammatory disorders, benign tumors, fecal impaction, and miscellaneous rare problems.

SYMPTOMS/EXAM

- Presents with abdominal cramping, constipation and/or obstipation, and vomiting. Onset can be rapid (volvulus) or insidious (cancer).
- Exam reveals abdominal distention, tympany, high-pitched "tinkles" on auscultation of bowel sounds, and tenderness to palpation +/− signs of peritonitis (rebound tenderness).

DIFFERENTIAL

SBO, paralytic ileus, pseudo-obstruction (Ogilvie syndrome).

DIAGNOSIS

- **Labs:** May be normal. Leukocytosis and electrolyte abnormalities are seen with progression of disease.

- **Imaging:**
    - **AXR:** Demonstrates a dilated colon (distinguished from the small intestine by its haustral markings, which do not cross the entire lumen of the distended colon) with air-fluid levels.
    - **CT:** The best study for identifying the exact location and etiology of the bowel obstruction.
    - **Barium enema** if volvulus is suspected, as it can be therapeutic as well as diagnostic.

TREATMENT

- Surgery almost always required.
- The patient may require a **staged operation,** consisting of an initial colonic resection and diverting colostomy, followed by a later reanastomosis.

DIVERTICULAR DISORDERS

Approximately 65% of adults in the Western world develop diverticula by 80 years of age, most commonly in the sigmoid colon. Colonic diverticula are classified as false because they consist of mucosa and submucosa that have herniated through the muscular coats. True diverticula (containing all layers of bowel) are rare in the colon.

Diverticulosis

Defined as the presence of multiple false diverticula.

- **Sx/Exam:** Usually asymptomatic. Exam reveals mild tenderness in the LLQ.
- **DDx:** Diverticulitis, colon cancer.
- **Dx:**
    - **Labs:** Fever and leukocytosis are absent in patients with diverticula (and no diverticulitis).
    - **Imaging:** Diverticuli can be visualized at colonoscopy and on CT and barium enema studies.
- **Tx:** High-fiber diet; bulking agents (psyllium); education and reassurance; surgical resection for massive hemorrhage or to rule out carcinoma.

Diverticulitis

A complication of diverticulosis that can range from mild inflammation to colonic perforation with peritonitis.

SYMPTOMS/EXAM

- Presents with acute onset of LLQ pain.
- Nausea, vomiting, or dysuria may be seen, depending on the location and extent of inflammation.
- Peritoneal signs are seen if the disease presents late (with perforation).
- Exam reveals low-grade fever, mild abdominal distention, LLQ tenderness, and a LLQ mass.

DIFFERENTIAL

Appendicitis, mesenteric ischemia, bowel obstruction, Crohn disease.

DIAGNOSIS

- **Labs:** Leukocytosis; ⊖ fecal occult blood (if present, suggests malignancy).

KEY FACT

Diverticular hemorrhage is a possible complication of diverticulosis. It is painless and usually stops spontaneously.

- Imaging:
    - **AXR:** Reveals free air in the presence of a perforation. Shows ileus and partial obstruction +/– LLQ mass.
    - **CT: The best initial study (preferably with IV contrast).** Reveals diverticuli, bowel wall thickening, and surrounding inflammation (Figure 12.4).
    - **Barium enema: Contraindicated** 2° to the possibility of barium leaking into peritoneal cavity.

TREATMENT

- **Expectant management:**
    - NPO, IV fluids.
    - Broad-spectrum antibiotics:
        - **Outpatient** (mild): Trimethoprim-sulfamethoxazole or metronidazole plus quinolone.
        - **Inpatient** (moderate to severe): IV piperacillin-tazobactam, ampicillin-sulbactam, quinolone to cover anaerobes and gram-negative rods.
    - Colonoscopy should be performed 4–6 weeks after the acute attack to exclude coexisting neoplastic disease. (Avoid colonoscopy during acute phase because of the risk of perforation.)

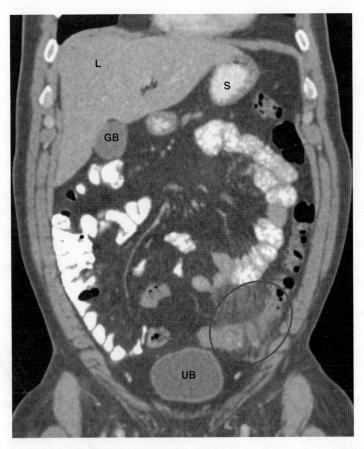

FIGURE 12.4. Acute diverticulitis. Coronal reconstruction from a contrast-enhanced CT demonstrates sigmoid diverticula with perisigmoid inflammatory "fat stranding." The area of abnormality is circled in red. (L = liver; S = stomach; GB = gallbladder; UB = urinary bladder.) (Reproduced, with permission, from USMLERx.com.)

- **Surgical management:**
  - Indicated for abscess formation, **perforation, or failure of expectant management;** may sometimes be managed with percutaneous drainage of paracolic abscesses.
  - Severe cases usually require laparotomy and **possible colectomy** (often done as a **staged operation**). Laparoscopic operations are difficult in the setting of inflammation.

SIGMOID VOLVULUS

Rotation of a segment of the intestine on an axis formed by its mesentery that leads to obstruction of the lumen and circulatory impairment of the bowel. The sigmoid is the segment most commonly involved in colonic volvulus.

SYMPTOMS/EXAM

Presents with acute abdominal pain and obstipation. Exam reveals abdominal distention.

DIFFERENTIAL

Cecal volvulus and other causes of LBO (carcinoma, benign tumors, fecal impaction, diverticular disease).

DIAGNOSIS

- **AXR:** A single, greatly distended loop of bowel that has lost its haustral markings is usually seen rising up out of the pelvis (sometimes termed **megacolon**).
- **Barium enema:** The pathognomonic finding is the **"bird's beak"** or **"ace of spades"** deformity, named for the way the barium column tapers toward the volvulus (Figure 12.5). This procedure may be therapeutic.

TREATMENT

- **Endoscopic decompression** with a flexible colonoscope or sigmoidoscope.
- **Emergent operation (partial or total colectomy):** Performed if strangulation or perforation is present or if attempts at decompression are unsuccessful.

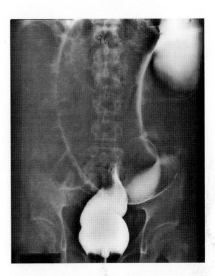

FIGURE 12.5. Sigmoid volvulus: greatly dilated sigmoid. Contrast barium enema shows stenosis known as "bird's beak" or "ace of spades" deformity. (Reproduced, with permission, from Doherty GM. *Current Diagnosis & Treatment: Surgery,* 13th ed. New York: McGraw-Hill, 2010, Fig. 30-16.)

Anorectal Disorders

A 70-year-old African-American man with a history of CAD calls your answering service on Sunday night complaining of "bright red blood in my stool" for a few days. He had a normal colonoscopy 6 months ago and has no history of weight loss or anemia. When you see him in the office on Monday morning, he has stable vital signs and no abdominal pain, and anoscopy reveals a friable internal hemorrhoid. CBC reveals a stable hemoglobin/hematocrit. What is the next step in management?

You prescribe a stool softener and advise your patient to increase his fluid intake, get regular exercise, and limit time spent on the commode.

HEMORRHOIDS

Hemorrhoidal tissues that cause bleeding, pain, or mucus are pathologic, usually occurring in the setting of ↑ intra-abdominal pressure that can occur in pregnancy, in the presence of obesity, and with lifting or straining (ie, constipation).

SYMPTOMS

- **Internal hemorrhoids:** Painless; present with bright red blood per rectum, mucous discharge, and rectal fullness or discomfort. Classification is based on the degree of prolapse:
    - **1st degree:** Hemorrhoids do not protrude through the anus.
    - **2nd degree:** Hemorrhoids prolapse but reduce spontaneously.
    - **3rd degree:** Hemorrhoids prolapse and require manual reduction.
    - **4th degree:** Hemorrhoids cannot be reduced and may strangulate.
- **External hemorrhoids:** Present with severe perianal pain and perianal mass.

EXAM

Exam reveals vascular dilation, friable mucosa, and local perineal irritation.

DIFFERENTIAL

Malignancy, diverticular disease, IBD, adenomatous polyps, procidentia.

DIAGNOSIS

- **Labs:** CBC to rule out anemia if chronic bleeding is present.
- **Anoscopy:** Allows direct visual inspection of the anal canal.

TREATMENT

- **Medical:** Best for 1st- and 2nd-degree internal hemorrhoids. Consists of dietary changes (eliminating constipating foods and increasing fiber), stool softener, exercise, and limiting toilet time.
- **Surgical:** Used when medical management fails and often indicated for 3rd- and 4th-degree hemorrhoids. The 3 classic techniques are elastic band ligation, sclerosis, and excisional hemorrhoidectomy.

COMPLICATIONS

Bleeding, pain, necrosis, and, rarely, perianal sepsis.

Thrombosed External Hemorrhoid

Acute intravascular thrombosis that develops within an external hemorrhoid, causing severe perianal pain.

SYMPTOMS/EXAM

- Presents with sudden, severe perianal pain that peaks within 48–72 hours.
- Exam reveals a purplish-black, edematous, tense subcutaneous perianal mass (Figure 12.6).

DIFFERENTIAL

Nonthrombosed external hemorrhoid, internal hemorrhoid, skin tag.

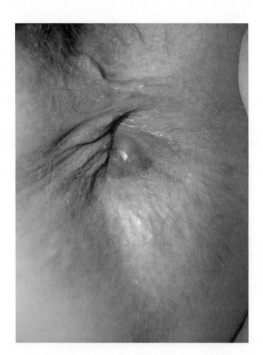

FIGURE 12.6. **External thrombosed hemorrhoid.** External hemorrhoid with a small skin break that resulted in bleeding. (Reproduced, with permission, from LeBlond RF, et al. *DeGowin's Diagnostic Examination,* 9th ed. New York: McGraw-Hill, 2009, Plate 28.)

DIAGNOSIS

Anoscopy allows direct visual inspection of the anal canal.

TREATMENT

- **< 48 hours after onset of symptoms:** Excision of the entire thrombosis, simple incision with clot expression (higher recurrence rate).
- **48–72 hours after onset of symptoms:** Warm sitz baths, high-fiber diet, stool softeners, reassurance.

ANAL FISSURE

A split in the anoderm that results from forceful dilation of the anal canal, most commonly during defecation.

SYMPTOMS/EXAM

- Presents with pain with defecation, along with blood on the tissue and stool or dripping into the toilet water (but not mixed in the stool). Constipation is common.
- Exam reveals disruption of the anoderm in the anterior or posterior midline involving the epithelium immediately distal to the dentate line.

DIFFERENTIAL

Crohn disease, anal TB, anal malignancy, abscess or fistula disease, HSV.

DIAGNOSIS

Anoscopy may reveal the classic triad of a proximal hypertrophied anal papilla above a fissure, with the sentinel pile at the anal verge.

TREATMENT

- **Medical:** Stool softeners, bulking agents, sitz baths, topical anesthetic ointment, nitroglycerin ointment, nifedipine cream.
- **Surgical:** Consider surgery for chronic (> 1 month) or chronic recurrent ulcers. Lateral internal anal sphincterectomy is the procedure of choice.

ANORECTAL ABSCESS AND FISTULA

When glands in the anorectum become infected, they can develop into an abscess and an associated fistula tract.

SYMPTOMS/EXAM

- Presents with severe, continuous throbbing anal pain.
- Anal swelling, fever, urinary retention, and sepsis may be seen.
- Exam reveals a tender perianal or rectal mass. A fistula tract may not be discovered until exam is performed under anesthesia.

DIFFERENTIAL

Crohn disease, pilonidal disease, hidradenitis suppurativa, diverticulitis, anal fissure.

DIAGNOSIS

- No imaging is necessary in uncomplicated cases.
- Sinography, transrectal ultrasound, CT, and MRI can be useful in complex or recurrent cases.

TREATMENT

Surgical drainage under general anesthesia.

PILONIDAL DISEASE

An infection of natal cleft hair follicles, which, when obstructed, become distended and rupture into the subcutaneous tissue, forming an abscess. The highest incidence is in white males 15–40 years of age, with a peak incidence in those 16–20 years of age.

SYMPTOMS/EXAM

- Presents with pain, tenderness, purulent drainage, inspissated hair, and induration near the perianal region.
- Patients are typically overweight, hirsute males who perspire profusely.
- Exam of the coccyx or sacrum reveals small pits or abscesses on or close to the midline.

DIFFERENTIAL

Abscess-fistula disease, hidradenitis suppurativa, furuncle, actinomycosis.

DIAGNOSIS

Physical exam is adequate for diagnosis.

TREATMENT

- Surgical incision, drainage, and curettage of the abscess cavity to remove hair nests and skin debris.

- Meticulous skin care, hygiene, and shaving of the surrounding area for at least 3 months after the surgical procedure.
- May require more definitive surgery (eg, excision of pits, marsupialization).

FECAL IMPACTION

May develop after excisional hemorrhoidectomy, in chronically debilitated patients, or from the use of constipating pain medications without stool softeners and fiber.

SYMPTOMS

- Diarrhea (only liquid stool is able to pass the obstructing inspissated fecal bolus).
- Pelvic pain and fullness.

EXAM

Digital rectal exam (DRE) reveals hard, dry stool that obstructs the rectum. Abdominal exam may reveal a pelvic or abdominal mass.

DIFFERENTIAL

Sigmoid malignancy or other obstructing lesion.

TREATMENT

- Digital disimpaction at the bedside.
- Treatment in the operating room, with local or regional anesthesia, may be necessary to provide pelvic floor relaxation and pain control.

PRURITUS ANI

An intense itching of the anus and perianal skin. The cause is often multifactorial and includes anorectal conditions (eg, diarrhea, fecal incontinence, hemorrhoids), infections (candidiasis, pinworms, human papillomavirus), local irritants (eg, moisture, underwear, diet, drug), dermatologic diseases (eg, psoriasis, seborrheic dermatitis), systemic disease (eg, DM, hyperbilirubinemia).

SYMPTOMS/EXAM

- **Itching and scratching** of perianal area.
- Exam may reveal skin irritation and/or a coexisting anorectal condition. DRE with anoscopy, proctoscopy, or colonoscopy may be indicated.

DIAGNOSIS

- Diagnoses by history and exam, as indicated above. History should focus on systemic disease and changes in medications, bowel habits, and diet.
- Biopsy is indicated when dermatologic neoplasm (eg, Bowen or Paget disease) is suspected.

TREATMENT

- Treat underlying disorder.
- Eliminate itch-scratch cycle.
- Avoid potential irritant food such as coffee, tea, citrus fruits, chocolate.
- Medications: Antihistamine, topical steroid (short-term use only), topical lidocaine.

TABLE 12.13. Types of Hernias

Type	Pathophysiology	Location	Characteristics
Indirect inguinal	A persistent processus vaginalis.	The groin **lateral** to the inferior epigastric vessels.	May present at birth. Can descend into the scrotum.
Direct inguinal	A defect of the transversalis fascia in Hesselbach triangle.[a]	The groin **medial** to the inferior epigastric vessels.	Most occur in middle-aged or elderly patients.
Femoral	Occurs through the femoral canal.	The upper thigh medial to the femoral vein.	Less common; usually occurs in women. Can easily become incarcerated or strangulated.
Incisional/ventral	Breakdown of fascial closure from prior surgery.	At the site of a previous surgical incision.	Often asymptomatic. May become larger on standing or with ↑ intra-abdominal pressure.
Umbilical	Occurs through the fibromuscular umbilical ring.	The umbilicus.	Repair only if it persists beyond 5 years of age.
Obturator	Occurs through the large obturator canal.	Deep structures of the pelvis/thigh (not visualized externally).	Has a female-to-male ratio of 6:1. Can present as bowel obstruction.
Epigastric	Occurs through defects in the aponeurosis of the rectus sheath.	Midline between the umbilicus and the xiphoid process.	Most commonly occurs in middle age but may also present in young children.

[a]Hesselbach triangle is defined inferiorly by the inguinal ligament, laterally by the inferior epigastric arteries, and medially by the conjoined tendon.

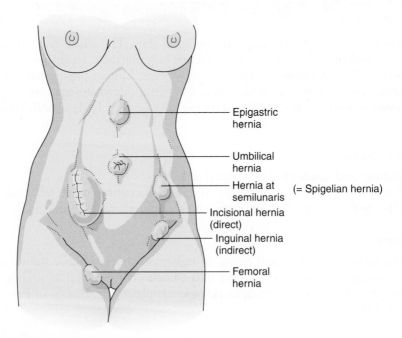

FIGURE 12.7. Hernia sites. (Reproduced, with permission, from DeCherney AH, Nathan L. *Current Diagnosis & Treatment: Obstetrics & Gynecology*, 10th ed. New York: McGraw-Hill, 2007, Fig. 2-10.)

Abdominal Wall Hernias

An abnormal protrusion of intra-abdominal tissue through a fascial defect in the abdominal wall. Approximately 75% occur in the groin, most of these being inguinal hernias (Table 12.13). Hernias can be completely reducible, incompletely reducible, or nonreducible, depending on the ability to manually push the herniated tissue back into the abdomen. Bowel strangulation is a dreaded complication that usually occurs in nonreducible hernias (Figure 12.7).

KEY FACT

Diastasis recti is a separation of the rectus abdominis muscles without a *fascial defect* and is often mistaken for an abdominal hernia. Most noticeable when patients strain or lift the head from the pillow.

Breast Cancer

A 30-year-old woman who is otherwise healthy presents to you for the first time because she wants to be tested for the "breast cancer gene." She is concerned because her 52-year-old mother was diagnosed with metastatic breast cancer at 38 years of age. What is the next step in management?

You advise her that she is likely a candidate for *BRCA1/BRCA2* mutation testing, given that she has a 1st-degree relative with premenopausal breast cancer. You refer her for genetic testing.

Breast cancer is the second deadliest cancer in women. **Risk factors** include the following:

- A ⊕ 1st-degree family history, particularly of premenopausal breast cancer.
- Mutations of *BRCA1* and *BRCA2*.
- Advanced age.
- Estrogen exposure; HRT.
- Age at menarche < 12; age at first birth > 30; age at menopause > 55.
- Alcohol use.
- A history of a benign breast biopsy.
- A history of atypical hyperplasia on breast biopsy.
- OCP use is probably **not** a risk factor in average-risk women, but may be in those with a ⊕ family history.

Screening methods include the following:

- **Breast self-examination (BSE):** Teaching BSE is not recommended; it has not been shown to have benefit.
- **Clinical breast exam (CBE):** Not standardized; has a sensitivity of approximately 50%. There is insufficient evidence to recommend for or against routine CBE alone or in combination with screening mammography.
- **Mammography:** The U.S. Preventive Services Task Force (USPSTF) recommends **biennial screening for women aged 50–74 years.** Screening before 50 years of age should be individualized, based on the context and risk. Sensitivity is 90% and is higher in older women.
- **BRCA1/BRCA2 mutation testing:** Appropriate for patients with the following:
  - A ⊕ family history of **premenopausal** breast cancer.
  - A known breast cancer.
  - Coexisting breast and ovarian cancer.
  - A family history of male breast cancer.

DIFFERENTIAL

Fibrocystic disease, fibroadenoma, abscess, adenosis, scars, mastitis.

DIAGNOSIS

- Breast cysts can be evaluated with ultrasound and then aspirated.
- Breast masses require either FNA or core needle biopsy, possibly followed by excisional biopsy.
- Any mass that is felt on exam **must** be further evaluated with biopsy, even if no abnormality is seen on mammography.
- **Algorithm:** If mass, then bilateral mammogram, then tissue sampling, then possible further workup, depending on tissue findings.

TREATMENT

Treatment for **early-stage breast cancer** is as follows:

- **Ductal carcinoma in situ (DCIS):** A premalignant condition that is high risk for becoming breast cancer. Treatment consists of excision (lumpectomy) with ⊖ margins and radiation therapy to the breast.
- **Lobular carcinoma in situ (LCIS):** A condition associated with ↑ risk of breast cancer arising elsewhere in the breast. Treatment with tamoxifen may be considered, but close follow-up and observation are usually indicated.
- **Invasive ductal or lobular carcinoma:** Lumpectomy followed by radiation therapy is equivalent to mastectomy. Mastectomy for large tumors or for patient preference.
- **Sentinel lymph node biopsy:** Indicated for invasive disease and may be indicated in certain cases of carcinoma in situ.
- **Adjuvant therapy:**
    - In general, any patient with an infiltrating ductal or lobular cancer > 1 cm or with ⊕ lymph nodes should receive adjuvant therapy.
    - Hormone therapy with tamoxifen (for 5 years) is effective only with estrogen- or progesterone-receptor-⊕ (ER- or PR-⊕) breast cancers. Where appropriate, tamoxifen ↓ the risk of recurrence by 40%.
    - Polychemotherapy ↓ the risk of recurrence by 25%.

The treatment approach for **advanced (metastatic) breast cancer** includes the following:

- **ER/PR-⊕ masses:**
    - **1st-line therapy:** For postmenopausal women, 1st-line treatment consists of an **aromatase inhibitor.** Aromatase inhibitors prevent conversion of adrenal androgens into estrogens by aromatase enzymes in muscle and fat.
    - **2nd-line hormonal therapy:** Includes megestrol acetate or tamoxifen.
- **ER/PR-⊖ masses (or progression of disease despite 1st-line treatment in hormone receptor-⊕ patients):**
    - Initial chemotherapy can be multiagent, but once patients progress after 1st-line treatment, single-agent treatment is commonly used.
    - Active chemotherapy drugs include paclitaxel, docetaxel, doxorubicin, methotrexate, vinorelbine, capecitabine, and 5-FU.
- **Patients with HER2 receptor overexpression:**
    - Overexpression of the HER2 receptor is associated with a poorer prognosis in breast cancer.
    - Trastuzumab (Herceptin) is a humanized monoclonal antibody against the HER2 receptor found on breast cancer cells.
    - Patients with HER2 overexpression show responses to trastuzumab alone or in combination with chemotherapy.

Abdominal Aortic Aneurysm (AAA)

A permanent local dilation of the abdominal aorta, defined as being > 1.5 times the normal diameter. A diameter > 3 cm is generally considered aneurysmal. AAA is a relatively common condition and most patients are asymptomatic; however, it can be fatal when it ruptures. The risk of rupture increases with the size of the aneurysm. Risk factors for AAA include smoking, hypertension, a family history of AAA, and male gender.

SYMPTOMS

- Usually **asymptomatic** until the aneurysm ruptures.
- Ruptured AAA presents with hypotension, abdominal or back pain, and a pulsatile abdominal mass. May also present with buttock, groin, testicular, or leg pain.

EXAM

Larger AAAs, can be felt as pulsatile masses.

DIAGNOSIS

Imaging:

- **Ultrasound** is the standard imaging tool for screening/monitoring and is highly sensitive and specific. One-time sonographic screening is recommended for **men 65–75 years of age** who have ever **smoked** (Figure 12.8).
- CT scan should be obtained for symptomatic patients who are stable. CT scan is also recommended for preoperative aneurysm evaluation.

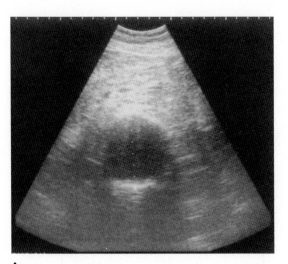

A

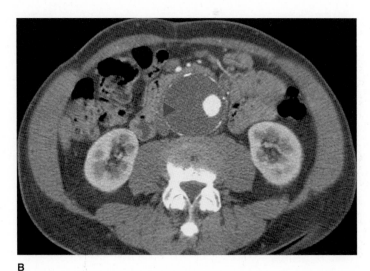

B

FIGURE 12.8.   Abdominal aortic aneurysm. (A) Bedside ultrasound image of 6.5-cm abdominal aneurysm. **(B)** Transaxial image from contrast-enhanced CT showing 5.5-cm aneurysm with extensive mural thrombus *(arrowhead)*. (Image A reproduced, with permission, from Tintinalli JE, et al. *Tintinalli's Emergency Medicine: A Comprehensive Study Guide,* 6th ed. New York: McGraw-Hill, 2004, Fig. 58-2. Image B reproduced, with permission, from Doherty GM. *Current Diagnosis & Treatment: Surgery,* 13th ed. New York: McGraw-Hill, 2010, Fig. 34-16.)

Treatment

Asymptomatic patients: Management is based on **aortic diameter.**

- Aortic diameter < **3.0 cm:** No further testing.
- Aortic diameter **3.0–4.5 cm:** Annual ultrasound.
- Aortic diameter > **4.5 cm:** Refer to vascular surgeon.
- Aortic diameter > **5.5 cm:** Repair; the primary methods of AAA repair are open and endovascular.
- Ruptured AAA: Emergent open repair or endovascular repair.

CHAPTER 13

Pediatric and Adolescent Medicine

Narges Farahi, MD

Pediatric Medicine

THE NEWBORN

The Newborn Exam

An infant's first exam is an important time to identify neonatal distress and become aware of congenital abnormalities and correctable defects. A pertinent history and physical includes:

- **History:** Include family history, maternal labs, maternal health during pregnancy and labor, outcomes of previous pregnancies, and potential toxic exposures.
- **Apgar scores:** Performed at 1 and 5 minutes; may be repeated at 10 minutes if indicated (Table 13.1). Low 5-minute Apgar scores correlate with an ↑ risk of death in the first year as well as with cerebral palsy.

EXAM

- Skin:
  - **Acrocyanosis:** Blue hands and feet are often normal, but generalized cyanosis may be a sign of a congenital heart defect and warrants immediate evaluation.
  - **Birthmarks:** Benign birthmarks include capillary hemangiomas and Mongolian spots. Some are a sign of an underlying disorder, such as café-au-lait spots (> 6 may point to neurofibromatosis type 1) and ash leaf spots (a sign of tuberous sclerosis; Figure 13.1).
- Head:
  - **Caput succedaneum:** Swelling of the scalp caused by pressure on the head against the dilating cervix. Crosses suture lines (Figure 13.2).
  - **Cephalohematoma:** Bleeding between the skull and periosteum. Does not cross suture lines. Generally benign.
  - **Subgaleal hemorrhage:** Bleeding beneath the scalp; can result in extensive blood loss. Crosses suture lines.
  - **Eyes:** An abnormal light reflex may be a sign of glaucoma, cataracts, or a tumor such as retinoblastoma.
  - **Ears:** Low-set ears may be associated with congenital anomalies. Preauricular pits may be a sign of congenital hearing loss.

TABLE 13.1. Apgar Scores

	SCORE		
SIGN	**0**	**1**	**2**
Appearance	Blue or pale	Body pink; extremities blue	Completely pink
Pulse	Absent	60–100 bpm	> 100 bpm
Grimace (reflex irritability)	No response	Grimace	Cry or cough
Activity (muscle tone)	Floppy	Some flexion	Flexion; active movement
Respirations	Absent	Slow, irregular	Good, crying

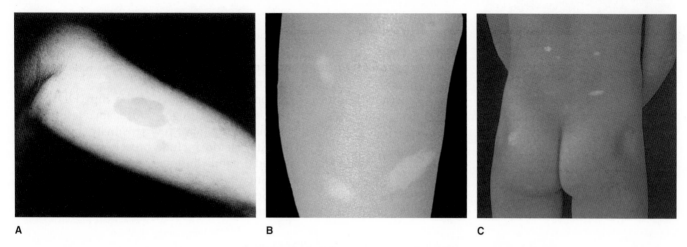

A   **B**   **C**

FIGURE 13.1.   (A) Café-au-lait spots and (B, C) ash leaf macules. (Image A reproduced, with permission, from Ropper A, Brown RH. *Adams and Victor's Principles of Neurology,* 8th ed. New York: McGraw-Hill, 2005: 869. Images B and C reproduced, with permission, from Wolff K, Johnson RA. *Fitzpatrick's Color Atlas & Synopsis of Clinical Dermatology,* 6th ed. New York: McGraw-Hill, 2009, Fig. 15-23.)

- **Nose:** Check for the patency of both nares. Since infants are obligate nose breathers, blockage of the nasal passage by abnormal tissue (choanal atresia) may lead to respiratory distress.
- **Oropharynx:** Check for cleft lip or palate. Epstein pearls at the junction of the hard and soft palates are epithelial retention cysts and are considered normal.
- **Chest:** Clavicular fractures may occur during delivery complicated by shoulder dystocia. Look for crepitus, step-offs, bruising, and tenderness.
- **Heart:** Murmurs in the immediate newborn period are common and are usually benign (see the Cardiology section below). Cyanosis, abnormal pulses, and signs of CHF are signs of heart disease.
- **Abdomen:**
  - An abnormal mass is most often associated with kidney disease (tumor, hydronephrosis, multicystic kidney disease).
  - Consider diaphragmatic hernia in an infant with scaphoid abdomen and respiratory distress.
  - Hepatosplenomegaly is associated with neonatal infection (CMV), metabolic disorders, and CHF.
- **Genitalia:** Cryptorchidism may be present in up to 3% of term male infants and generally resolves by the first birthday.

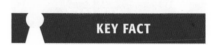

KEY FACT

More than 6 café-au-lait spots may indicate neurofibromatosis type 1.

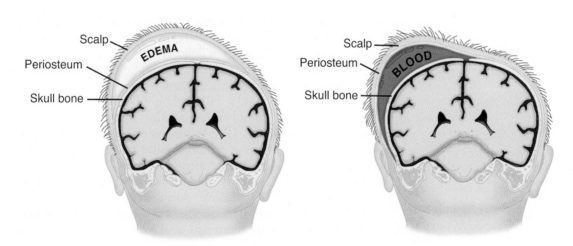

FIGURE 13.2.   (A) Caput succedaneum and (B) cephalhematoma. (Reproduced, with permission, from Cunningham FG, et al. *Williams Obstetrics*, 23rd ed. New York: McGraw-Hill, 2010, Fig. 29-12.)

- **Musculoskeletal:**
  - **Spine:** Pits or hair tufts at the base of the spine may suggest spina bifida occulta.
  - **Upper extremities:** ↓ movement and asymmetric Moro reflex may indicate a brachial plexus injury.
  - **Lower extremities:** Developmental dysplasia of the hip (DDH) presents with asymmetric skin folds in the thighs. Provocative tests including Barlow and Ortolani maneuvers have low sensitivity, but a clunk felt may represent DDH. Risk factors include breech presentation, female gender, white race, and ⊕ family history.
- **Neurologic:** Look for normal newborn reflexes, including suck, rooting, grasp, tonic neck, and Moro. Several beats of ankle clonus and the Babinski reflex are normal in newborns.

Newborn Screening and Prophylaxis

SCREENING

NEWBORN SCREENS

A group of tests performed on all newborns to identify congenital disorders in which early diagnosis can prevent long-term sequelae.

- **Hearing:**
  - Three in 1000 healthy infants have significant hearing loss.
  - Universal hearing screening helps identify most children with hearing loss.
  - Risk factors for hearing loss include congenital infection, abnormal craniofacial anatomy, and ⊕ family history.

PROPHYLAXIS

- **Hemorrhagic disease of the newborn prophylaxis:**
  - A bleeding disorder due to vitamin K deficiency in newborns.
  - IM vitamin K is given for prevention.
- **Ophthalmia neonatorum prophylaxis:** Erythromycin or tetracycline ointment prevents gonococcal and chlamydial conjunctivitis.
- **Hepatitis B prophylaxis:**
  - All pregnant women should be screened for hepatitis B during each pregnancy by checking HbSAg.
  - Children born to mothers with ⊕ HbSAg should receive hepatitis B immune globulin (HBIG) and HBV vaccine in the first 12 hours of life.
  - If the mother's HbSAg status is unknown at the time of delivery, she should be screened immediately. In all cases, the HBV vaccine should be given within 12 hours of delivery.
    - In children ≤ 2000 g, HBIG should be given within 12 hours of delivery if the test result is still unknown or ⊕.
    - In children > 2000 g, HBIG should be given as soon as the mother's test is ⊕ and should be given within 7 days.
- **Prevention of perinatal HIV transmission:** Although there are different protocols for prevention of maternal-child transmission of HIV, all protocols recommend the following measures:
  - Oral antiretrovirals for the mother during the prenatal period.
  - IV zidovudine (AZT or ZDV) during labor.
  - Scheduled cesarean if the mother has a high HIV-1 viral load.
  - Treatment of the newborn with oral AZT.

Circumcision

- **Risks:** Bleeding, infection, injury to the urethra or other surrounding structures, removal of too much skin, unsatisfactory cosmetic outcome.
- **Benefits:** Slightly ↓ the risk of penile cancer, UTIs in the first year of life, and transmission of HIV infection.
- **Contraindications:** Genital abnormalities (eg, hypospadias) or bleeding disorder.

Problems in the Neonatal Period

BIRTH TRAUMA

Complications associated with birth trauma include the following:

- **Intraventricular hemorrhage:** Risk factors include prematurity, birth trauma, and asphyxia (Figure 13.3).
- **Hypoxia:** Related to chronic intrauterine conditions such as placental insufficiency or to acute events such as cord prolapse or maternal hypoxia.
- **Fractures:** May occur with traumatic delivery. Clavicle fractures are most common.
- **Peripheral nerve injuries:** Often related to traumatic delivery but may be idiopathic. Shoulder dystocia is a risk factor for brachial plexus injury. Most brachial plexus injuries resolve spontaneously in the first year. Physical therapy may be beneficial.

NEONATAL JAUNDICE

More than one-half of newborns develop clinical jaundice in the first week of life. Risk factors include maternal diabetes, male gender, prematurity, and Asian race. Etiologies are outlined in Table 13.2.

KEY FACT

All infants born at < 32 weeks' gestation should receive a head ultrasound to look for hemorrhage.

KEY FACT

The rate of kernicterus fell sharply after the introduction of phototherapy and exchange transfusions, but recently it has risen with the ↑ in early hospital discharges.

KEY FACT

Any jaundice in the first 24 hours of life is pathologic and requires further evaluation.

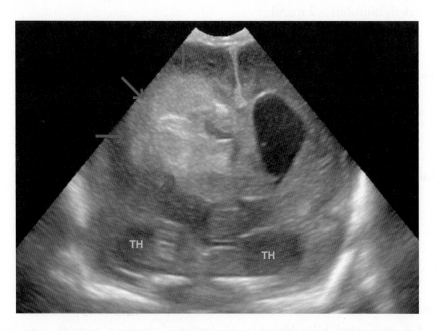

FIGURE 13.3.   Neonatal hemorrhage. Grade IV neonatal hemorrhage centered in the right germinal matrix, extending into the right lateral ventricle and parenchyma *(arrows)* and associated with hydrocephalus (note the dilated temporal horns [TH] of the lateral ventricles). (Reproduced, with permission, from USMLERx.com.)

TABLE 13.2.   **Etiologies of Unconjugated Hyperbilirubinemia**

	CAUSE	DIAGNOSIS/COMMENTS
Hemolytic	Rh and ABO incompatibility	Maternal Coombs antibody for signs of isoimmunization.
	Hereditary spherocytosis	Spherocytes on peripheral smear. Confirm with a red cell osmotic fragility test.
	G6PD deficiency	An X-linked disorder seen most commonly in African, Mediterranean, and Asian families.
Nonhemolytic	Enclosed hemorrhage (cephalohematoma)	As blood is resorbed, bilirubin levels will ↑.
	Inherited disorders of conjugation	Examples include Crigler-Najjar and Gilbert syndromes.
	Physiologic (normal)	May be due to ↑ hematocrit (even in the absence of true polycythemia) and initial lack of gut flora.
	Breast milk jaundice	Most likely related to free fatty acids in breast milk, which can ↑ enterohepatic circulation of bilirubin. Typically appears after the first week and may persist for many weeks.
	Breast-feeding jaundice	Related to dehydration while the mother's milk supply is coming in; resolves when feeding is well established.
	Infection	Congenital and acquired infections may cause jaundice.

SYMPTOMS/EXAM

- Jaundice progresses from head to toe with increasing bilirubin levels.
- **Physiologic jaundice:** Jaundice after first 24 hours, peaks at 3–5 days of life, lasts up to 1 week.
- **Pathologic jaundice:** Appears in first 24 hours, lasts > 1 week, fast rate of rise (> 5 mg/dL/day), higher bilirubin levels (> 15 mg/dL), direct (conjugated) bilirubin > 2 mg/dL.
- **Acute bilirubin encephalopathy:** Early signs include lethargy, hypotonia, and poor suck.

DIFFERENTIAL

- Unconjugated bilirubinemia (see Table 13.2).
- Conjugated bilirubinemia.
- Biliary tree disease.
- Hepatocellular disease.

DIAGNOSIS

- Total and direct bilirubin levels.
- Hematocrit.
- Mother's hematocrit.
- Mother's and infant's blood type.
- DAT (Coombs test of infant).
- LFTs and liver ultrasound for conjugated bilirubinemia.

TREATMENT

- **Unconjugated bilirubinemia:** Hydration, ↑ feeding, phototherapy, and exchange transfusion. A nomogram correlating safe bilirubin levels with age should be used to determine when to treat with phototherapy and exchange transfusion.
- **Conjugated bilirubinemia:** Treatment of underlying cause. Conjugated bilirubinemia is nontoxic (does not cause encephalopathy/kernicterus) and is not improved by phototherapy. Phototherapy causes bronzing of the skin.

- **Cx:** The long-term complication of unconjugated hyperbilirubinemia is **kernicterus**, chronic bilirubin encephalopathy. Kernicterus presents with movement disorders and deafness.

NECROTIZING ENTEROCOLITIS (NEC)

The most common life-threatening GI illness in neonates. More common among premature infants. The etiology is unknown but may be related to ischemia and infection.

- **Sx/Exam:** Abdominal distention, feeding intolerance, and blood in the stools.
- **Dx:** Radiographs may reveal pneumatosis intestinalis (intramural air; Figure 13.4).
- **Tx:** NPO, broad-spectrum antibiotics; surgery may be necessary.

NEONATAL SEPSIS

Neonatal sepsis may have **early** or **late** onset.

- **Early sepsis** (in the first week of life) is a result of vertical transmission. Risk factors include prolonged rupture of membranes (> 18 hours), maternal fever, chorioamnionitis, group B streptococcus (GBS) with inadequate treatment (< 4 hours antibiotics), and prematurity.
- **Late sepsis** (after the first week of life). Risk factors include prematurity, indwelling lines, endotracheal intubation, prior antibiotics.

SYMPTOMS/EXAM

- **Early sepsis (first week of life):**
  - Usually presents in the first 24 hours.
  - Characterized by temperature instability, respiratory distress, hypotension, and poor perfusion.
  - Common pathogens include GBS and *Escherichia coli*.
  - Pneumonia is a common cause.

MNEMONIC

Causes of neonatal jaundice:

CHIMPS

Cephalohematoma
Hemolysis
Inherited disorders
Milk
Physiologic
Sepsis

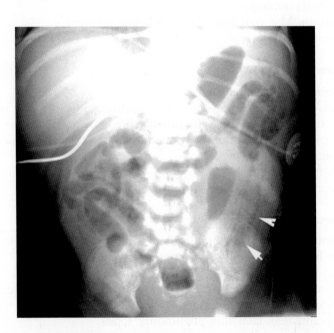

FIGURE 13.4.   Pneumatosis intestinalis. Short arrows highlight pneumatosis intestinalis on an abdominal radiograph of a patient with necrotizing enterocolitis. (Reproduced, with permission, from Brunicardi FC, et al. *Schwartz's Principles of Surgery,* 9th ed. New York: McGraw-Hill, 2010, Fig. 39-19.)

- **Late sepsis (after the first week):**
    - May present with poor feeding, temperature instability, lethargy, and apnea.
    - Causal organisms include *Staphylococcus aureus*, GBS, *Enterococcus*, *Pseudomonas*, and other gram-⊖ organisms.
    - Meningitis is more common in this period.

DIAGNOSIS

Laboratory abnormalities may include a low or high WBC count, thrombocytopenia, metabolic acidosis, hypoglycemia, and ↑ CRP.

TREATMENT

Broad-spectrum antibiotics are appropriate while awaiting culture results (blood, urine, and CSF). Ampicillin with gentamicin is a common regimen.

TOXOPLASMOSIS

- **Transmission:** Transplacental transmission during maternal primary infection. Risk factors for maternal infection include contact with cat feces and intake of undercooked meat or unpasteurized milk.
- **Signs:**
    - Classic triad: Obstructive hydrocephalus, chorioretinitis, intracranial calcification.
    - Also presents with fever, hepatosplenomegaly, anemia, hyperbilirubinemia.
- **Dx:** Toxoplasmosis serologies.
- **Tx:** Pyrimethamine plus sulfadiazine.

RUBELLA

- **Transmission:** Transplacental.
- **Signs:** Cataracts, cardiac involvement (especially PDA), "blueberry muffin rash," hearing loss.
- **Dx:** Rubella serologies.
- **Prevention:** Maternal immunization before pregnancy.
- **Tx:** None.

CYTOMEGALOVIRUS (CMV)

- **Transmission:** Transplacental.
- **Signs:** CMV is the leading cause of sensorineural hearing loss in children. Other manifestations include intrauterine growth retardation (IUGR), hepatosplenomegaly, thrombocytopenia, and CNS effects (microcephaly, chorioretinitis).
- **Dx:** Urine culture for CMV.
- **Tx:** Treatment with ganciclovir may be beneficial.

HERPES SIMPLES VIRUS (HSV)

- **Transmission:** Typically transmitted during vaginal delivery when the mother has active lesions or asymptomatic viral shedding.
- **Signs:**
    - Mucocutaneous disease: Vesicular rash, keratoconjunctivitis.
    - CNS: Encephalitis, seizures.
    - Disseminated: Hepatitis, pneumonia, sepsis.
- **Dx:** Viral culture.
- **Prevention:** Suppressive acyclovir therapy should be started at 36 weeks' gestation for pregnant women with recurrent genital herpes. Cesarean

delivery is indicated for women with active genital lesions or prodromal symptoms at the time of delivery.
- **Tx:** Acyclovir.

SYPHILIS

- **Transmission:** Transplacental.
- **Signs:**
  - **Early congenital syphilis** (age < 2 years, typically presents in the first 6 weeks): Jaundice, rash, rhinitis ("snuffles"), osteochondritis.
  - **Late congenital syphilis** (age > 2 years): Tooth and bone abnormalities, including Hutchinson's teeth, hearing impairment, mental retardation.
- **Dx:** Serologic tests in mother and infant.
- **Prevention:** Treat mother during pregnancy.
- **Tx:** Treat child with penicillin if mother is untreated or had an inadequate response to treatment, or if there are clinical signs of disease.

TRANSIENT TACHYPNEA OF THE NEWBORN (TTN)

> Shortly after the delivery of a term baby boy by cesarean section, you are called to the nursery to evaluate the infant. His respiratory rate is 55 breaths/min, and he is noted to be a bit dusky when he tries to breast-feed. His O_2 saturation is normal, but he has some mild retractions with respiratory effort. What is your management strategy?
>
> Start a sepsis workup with CBC, cultures, and CXR. If the sepsis workup appears ⊖, the most likely diagnosis is transient tachypnea of the newborn. The infant should be closely monitored and supported with O_2 as needed. Always consider congenital cardiac anomalies in a newborn with respiratory distress.

Tachypnea due to retained fetal lung fluid. Risk factors include precipitous delivery, cesarean delivery, and maternal diabetes.

- **Sx/Exam:** Respiratory distress is generally present within several hours of birth. Respiratory rate typically exceeds 60 breaths/min.
- **Dx:** CXR reveals streaky perihilar opacities and fluid in the fissures.
- **Tx:** Management is supportive; may require O_2. The syndrome typically resolves in 12–24 hours.

MECONIUM ASPIRATION SYNDROME

Aspiration of meconium results in chemical pneumonitis, mucous plugging, and inactivation of surfactant. Risk factors include low amniotic fluid volume, postdates pregnancy, IUGR, and signs of fetal distress.

- **Sx:** Signs of respiratory distress, including tachypnea, grunting, nasal flaring, and retractions.
- **Dx:** CXR shows patchy, coarse infiltrates and hyperexpansion.
- **Tx:** Resuscitation should include suction of the hypopharynx under direct visualization **if the infant is depressed.** This does not prevent many cases of meconium aspiration, as aspiration also occurs in utero. Vigorous infants do not require suctioning.

RESPIRATORY DISTRESS SYNDROME (RDS) (ALSO HYALINE MEMBRANE DISEASE)

Caused by surfactant deficiency. Greatest risk factor is prematurity. Other risk factors include maternal diabetes and cesarean delivery without labor.

- **Sx/Exam:** Poor lung compliance and atelectasis ↑ work of breathing and lead to eventual respiratory failure.
- **Dx:** CXR shows ground-glass opacities (Figure 13.5).
- **Tx:** Prevent RDS with antenatal corticosteroids to improve lung maturity. Treat with exogenous surfactant and mechanical ventilation.

CRYPTORCHIDISM

Describes testes that have not descended into the scrotum. May be unilateral or bilateral. Approximately 3% of full-term male newborns have an undescended testis at birth.

- **Tx:** By 1 year of age, 80% of all undescended testes are in the scrotum. Surgical orchidopexy is indicated if descent has not occurred by 1 year.
- **Cx:** Infertility and testicular malignancy. The risk of malignancy (although lower) persists even after placement into the scrotum.

Genetic and Congenital Disorders

CHROMOSOMAL ABNORMALITIES

- **Trisomy 21 (Down syndrome):**
  - Incidence: 1 in 600 live births; incidence ↑ with increasing maternal age.
  - Clinical features: Mental retardation, short stature, characteristic facies (epicanthal folds, midface hypoplasia), heart defects, and GI tract disorders.
  - Complications: ↑ risk of leukemia, hypothryoidism, and Alzheimer dementia.

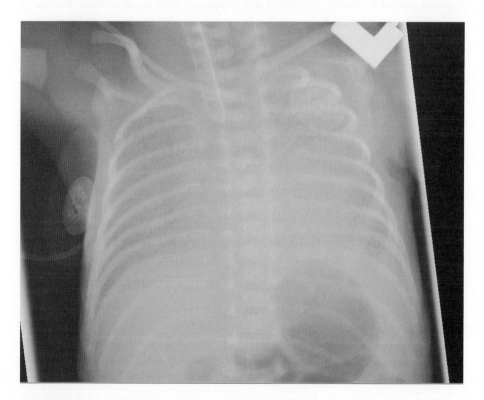

FIGURE 13.5. **Respiratory distress syndrome.** Frontal CXR in a neonate with respiratory distress syndrome, showing diffuse fine granular ("ground-glass") opacities and hypoaeration. (Reproduced, with permission, from USMLERx.com.)

- **Trisomy 18 (Edwards syndrome):**
  - Incidence: 1 in 6000–8000 live births, with females 3 times more likely to be affected than males.
  - Clinical features: Severe mental retardation, IUGR, hypertonicity, abnormal facies, overlapping fingers, and "rocker-bottom" feet.
  - Prognosis: Most affected infants die within the first year of life.
- **Trisomy 13 (Patau syndrome):**
  - Incidence: 1 in 6000 live births. Affects slightly more females than males.
  - Clinical features: Mental retardation, midline facial defects, polydactyly, syndactyly, blindness, deafness, and heart defects. Complications include seizures.
  - Prognosis: Most patients die within the first 6 months.
- **Klinefelter syndrome (XXY):**
  - Incidence: 1 in 1000 live births.
  - Clinical features: Affected individuals are phenotypically male until puberty, when they may be noted to have small testicles (microorchidism), gynecomastia, and ↓ facial hair. Mild mental retardation is common, but IQ may be normal.
  - Treatment: Testosterone replacement.
- **Turner syndrome (XO):**
  - Incidence: 1 in 10,000 live births. Most fetuses conceived with this disorder are spontaneously miscarried.
  - Clinical features: Presents with short stature, absence of 2° sexual characteristics, the characteristic **"shield chest,"** webbed neck, edema of the hands and feet, and coarctation of the aorta. Complications include amenorrhea and learning disabilities.
  - Treatment: Estrogen replacement is needed for sexual maturation, and growth hormone is used for the treatment of short stature.

AUTOSOMAL-DOMINANT DISORDERS

- **Neurofibromatosis type 1 (von Recklinghausen disease):** Neurofibromas are benign but have malignant potential and may compress nerves. Affected individuals are also at risk for other CNS tumors as well as for optic tumors and pheochromocytomas.
- **Neurofibromatosis type 2:** Acoustic neuromas and other CNS neoplasms. Cutaneous manifestations are much less prevalent.
- **Tuberous sclerosis:** Presents with cutaneous lesions (ash leaf spots and shagreen patches). Associated with mental retardation, seizures, CNS tumors, and tumors in the pancreas, kidney, liver, and spleen.
- **Marfan syndrome:** A triad of musculoskeletal changes (long limbs and ligamental laxity), lens dislocation, and aortic aneurysm. Penetrance is variable.

AUTOSOMAL-RECESSIVE DISORDERS

- **Cystic fibrosis (CF):** Occurs most frequently in whites in North America and northern Europe (incidence: 1 in 3000). May be caused by mutations in the CFTR protein (a chloride channel). In the past, the disease was generally fatal in childhood, but with improved therapy, median survival is now > 30 years.
- **Inborn errors of metabolism:** Absence of certain enzymes. The best-known type is phenylketonuria (PKU), in which affected individuals are unable to convert phenylalanine to tyrosine, which leads to CNS damage and mental retardation. Treatment involves avoidance of phenylalanine in the diet.

KEY FACT

Although women older than 35 years of age have an ↑ risk of having an infant with Down syndrome, most infants with Down syndrome are born to women with no risk factors.

MNEMONIC

Diagnostic criteria for neurofibromatosis type 1:

CAFÉ SPOT

Two or more of the following factors:

Café-au-lait spots (6 or more)
Axillary, inguinal freckling
Fibroma
Eye—Lisch nodules
Skeletal (eg, bowing leg)
Pedigree/**P**ositive family history
Optic **T**umor (glioma)

KEY FACT

Genetic screening can detect only the 20–30 most common gene mutations associated with CF. Sweat chloride testing remains the gold standard for diagnosis.

KEY FACT

Most families with hemophilia are aware that they carry the disease, but some remain unaware if the affected child has a new mutation or if the mutation has been passed from mother to daughter for several generations.

KEY FACT

Abnormal bleeding following circumcision or minor trauma in the early years may be the first clue to diagnosis.

X-LINKED DISORDERS

- **Duchenne muscular dystrophy:**
    - **Incidence:** 1 in 3500 live births.
    - **Clinical features:** Proximal muscle wasting and distal muscle hypertrophy developing in the second and third years of life. Progressive, with almost all affected individuals requiring the use of a wheelchair by age 12.
    - **Prognosis:** Life expectancy is in the 20s, with respiratory failure and cardiomyopathy the leading causes of death.
- **Hemophilia A and B:**
    - **Incidence:** 1 in 5000 live births. Hemophilia A (factor VIII deficiency) is much more common than hemophilia B (factor IX deficiency).
    - **Treatment:** Prevention of injury, factor replacement in the setting of active hemorrhage.
- **Fragile X syndrome:**
    - An example of genetic anticipation. Caused by a trinucleotide repeat on the long arm of the X chromosome that expands with each generation.
    - **Clinical features:** Female carriers may be mildly affected. Male offspring represent the full phenotype of mental retardation, macrocephaly, macro-orchidism, and behavioral problems.

OTHER CONGENITAL DISORDERS

- **Cleft lip/palate:** Isolated cleft palate is more likely than cleft lip plus palate to be part of a syndrome. Complications include feeding difficulties, speech delay, and recurrent otitis media.
- **Neural tube defects:** Encompass a broad range of defects, including myelomeningocele, spina bifida, encephalocele, and anencephaly. Causes include genetic abnormalities, folate deficiency, maternal diabetes, and exposures (alcohol, anticonvulsants). Often idiopathic.
- **Congenital hypothyroidism:** Most common cause of preventable mental retardation. Approximately 80% of cases are caused by thyroid agenesis or hypoplasia; less commonly related to inborn errors of metabolism or maternal antithyroid antibodies. Early diagnosis and treatment can prevent the severe mental retardation formerly known as cretinism.

EXPOSURE TO INTRAPARTUM DRUGS

- **Fetal alcohol syndrome:** Presents with short palpebral fissures, epicanthal folds, a flat midface, absent philtrum, a thin upper lip, mental retardation, behavioral problems, and poor coordination (Figure 13.6). Heart defects and epilepsy are sometimes seen.
- **Opiates:** Opiate withdrawal presents with diarrhea, irritability, shrill cry, tremulousness, hypertonicity, and seizures. Onset of symptoms depends on the half-life of the opiate used and time of the last dose. Treatment is with opiates, weaned gradually.

DEVELOPMENT AND BEHAVIOR

Common Issues in Child Development

COLIC

- **Sx/Exam:** Presents with the **rule of 3s:** crying for more than **3 hours** a day, **3 days** a week, for > **3 weeks.**
- **DDx:** If crying has developed suddenly, exogenous sources (eg, hair tourniquets, corneal abrasion, infection) should be ruled out.

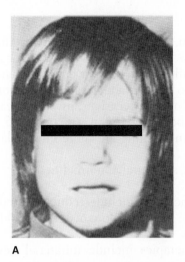
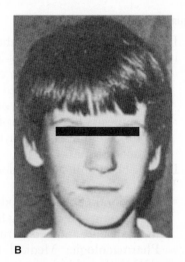
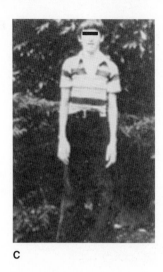

A   B   C

FIGURE 13.6. **Fetal alcohol syndrome.** (A) At 2½ years. (B, C) At 12 years. Note the persistence of short palpebral fissures, epicanthal folds, flat midface, hypoplastic philtrum, and thin upper vermilion border. This child also has the short, lean prepubertal stature characteristic of young males with fetal alcohol syndrome. (Reproduced, with permission, from Cunningham FG, et al. *Williams Obstetrics,* 23rd ed. New York: McGraw-Hill, 2010, Fig. 14-2.)

- **Tx:** Most cases are variations of normal behavior and resolve at about 4 months of age. Provide family support and close follow-up. Discuss methods to soothe colic (carrying, swinging, swaddling, changing formula or maternal diet in breast-feeding infants). Try ranitidine if GERD appears to be implicated.

ELIMINATION AND TOILET TRAINING

- Newborns typically have 6–8 wet diapers per day; older infants will usually have 4–6. Checking the number of diapers is a useful means of gauging hydration.
- Newborns often stool after every feed, but at 2–3 months stooling is much less frequent. Breast-fed infants can go as long as a week without stooling.
- Toilet training is generally initiated around 2–3 years of age but varies depending on the child's readiness and parental expectations.

ENCOPRESIS

- Defined as repeated stooling in inappropriate locations after 4 years of age or after successful toilet training. More common in males. Often related to constipation and other causes of painful defecation (eg, anal fissures), leading to overflow incontinence of stool.
- Behavioral causes include control issues and fear of using public toilets.
- Physiologic causes include dehydration, lack of stool bulk, anal fissure, GI disorders, and metabolic disorders such as hypothyroidism.
- **Tx:**
  - Treat underlying cause.
  - Treat constipation with stool softeners to make the passage of stool less painful.
  - May require disimpaction followed by regular use of a stool softener +/– a stimulant laxative to establish a regular routine of 1–2 soft bowel movements a day.
  - Behavioral modifications include sitting on the toilet after each meal. Referral to psychiatry may be necessary if significant behavioral problems persist.

KEY FACT

The colic rule of 3s:
  3 hours a day
  3 days a week
  3 weeks or more

ENURESIS

- Defined as involuntary urination. Nocturnal enuresis (bedwetting) is seen in 15% of 5-year-olds and 1%–2% of 15-year-olds. May be 1° or 2°.
  - **1° enuresis:** Enuresis in a child who has never had an extended period of dryness. May be related to small bladder capacity, abnormal ADH secretion, sleep disorders, or, on rare occasions, psychological issues.
  - **2° enuresis:** Recurrence of bedwetting after a period of 6 months or more. 2° enuresis and daytime wetting are more often related to psychosocial issues.
- **DDx:** UTI, neurologic disorders, structural abnormalities.
- **Tx:**
  - **Behavioral:** Behavior modifications include reducing fluid intake in the evening and emptying the bladder before bedtime; bladder training to ↑ capacity; and bed alarms.
  - **Pharmacologic:** Medical therapies include intranasal desmopressin (DDAVP) and imipramine.
  - Enuresis often recurs after medication is stopped, but medical treatment may be helpful for sleepovers or camp.

SLEEP

- Approximately 70% of infants sleep 8 hours at a time by 3 months of age, 80% by 6 months, and 90% by 12 months.
- Sleep disorders in children include the following:
  - **Night terrors:**
    - Occur during non-REM sleep in about 3% of children.
    - **Sx/Exam:** Children present with inconsolable screaming and thrashing. Episodes can last as long as 30 minutes and may be associated with sleepwalking. The next day, the child has no recollection of events.
    - **Tx:** Focused on reassurance of parents and prevention of injury to the child. Waking the child several minutes before the usual time of occurrence for several days may break the cycle.
  - **Nightmares:**
    - Occur during REM sleep in 25%–50% of children. Most common in children 3–5 years of age.
    - **Sx/Exam:** The child can be awakened and consoled.
    - **Tx:** Generally no intervention is required.

BEHAVIOR

- **Temper tantrums:**
  - Common in children 1–4 years of age, as children learn to express desires and frustrations. Most episodes ↓ with age.
  - **Tx:** Focused on protecting the child and others from harm and helping the child develop better forms of expression.
- **Breath holding:**
  - An involuntary response to minor injury or anger in which the child stops breathing after expiration. Loss of consciousness may occur.
  - **Dx:** Occasionally associated with pica or iron deficiency anemia. Most children grow out of this behavior by 6 years of age. If a child has frequent episodes, consider neurologic causes such as CNS tumor or seizure disorder.
  - **Tx:** Focused on preventing injury.

Developmental Milestones

Table 13.3 outlines major developmental milestones in pediatric patients 1 month to 5 years of age.

DEVELOPMENTAL SCREENING

- Primary care physicians must screen for delays and refer children with suspected delays for further evaluation.
- Parents' concern about developmental delays is very sensitive and specific.
- The Denver Developmental Screening Test II, the most commonly used screening tool, is not sensitive for identifying language delays. Other tools such as Ages and Stages or Parents' Evaluation of Development Status are more sensitive.

DEVELOPMENTAL DELAY

- Children who fail to meet developmental milestones must be evaluated early to initiate appropriate therapies.
- **DDx:** Environmental causes (abuse/neglect), sensory causes (vision/hearing loss), motor delay (coordination defect leading to speech delay), psychiatric conditions.

TABLE 13.3. Developmental Milestones

AGE	MOTOR	LANGUAGE/COGNITIVE	SOCIAL
1–2 months	Holds head up; rolls from side to back.	Vocalizes.	Spontaneous smile; recognizes parents.
3–5 months	Reaches for objects; sits with support; rolls from back to side.	Orients to voice.	Laughs; responds to facial expressions.
6–8 months	Sits alone briefly; rolls from back to stomach; passes objects between the hands.	Babbles.	Sleeps through the night; stranger anxiety begins.
9–11 months	Stands alone; pulls to stand; plays "pat-a-cake" and "peek-a-boo"; starts using pincer grasp.	Follows 1-word commands; uses "mama" and "dada" nonspecifically; develops the concept of object permanence.	Waves "bye-bye."
1 year	Walks independently; stacks 2 cubes.	Uses "mama" and "dada" appropriately.	Points to desired objects.
18 months	Stacks 3–4 blocks; throws ball; walks up/down stairs with help.	Uses 4–20 words; follows 2-step commands.	Feeds self with hands; stranger anxiety peaks.
2 years	Stacks 6–7 blocks; kicks ball; can stand on 1 foot.	Uses **2-word phrases;** uses pronouns; 50% of speech is comprehensible.	Helps dress self; mimics parents; stranger anxiety subsides.
3 years	Builds tower of 9–10 blocks; rides a tricycle.	Uses **3-word phrases;** copies a circle; knows own name.	Dresses self; feeds self with utensils.
5 years	Runs and turns without losing balance; can stand on 1 foot for 10 sec.	Counts to 4; answers questions appropriately.	Magical thinking; plays with peers.

- **Dx:** Workup includes a careful physical exam for features of genetic syndromes (Down, fetal alcohol, and Turner syndromes), possible chromosome analysis and fragile X testing, and testing of cognitive and adaptive skills. Loss of skills raises concern for a metabolic disorder or a neurodegenerative condition.
- **Tx:** Special education classes; appropriate occupational therapy.

SPEECH DELAY

- **DDx:** Hearing loss, isolated speech delay, autistic spectrum disorder.
- **Dx:** Any child with delay in speech milestones should receive a hearing evaluation.
- **Red flags:**
  - No babbling by 12 months.
  - No words by 15 months.
  - Speech not intelligible to a noncaretaker by 2 years.
- **Tx:** Speech therapy.

Developmental and Behavioral Disorders

AUTISM

- A pervasive developmental disorder characterized by deficits in interpersonal relationships as well as speech and language delay. It is an uncommon condition (incidence: 4 in 10,000) with a male-to-female ratio of 3:1. The cause is unknown; there is likely a genetic component. It is **not** linked to vaccinations.
- **Sx/Exam:** Presents at 1–3 years of age. Early signs are poor eye contact, lack of stranger anxiety, and poor attachment to parents. Later signs include peculiar interests, stereotypic behaviors, and low IQ (generally < 70).
- **DDx:** In Asperger syndrome, lack of awareness of others and poor social functioning are similar to that seen in autism, but mental retardation and language delay are generally absent.
- **Tx:** Early intervention with behavioral education focused on sensory clues and appropriate interactions.

ATTENTION-DEFICIT HYPERACTIVITY DISORDER (ADHD)

Characterized by a **triad of symptoms:** inattention, impulsivity, and hyperactivity. The disorder may be **classified as inattentive, impulsive, or combined.**

DIAGNOSIS

- Symptoms must be present in 2 areas of social interaction (home and school); must have been present before 7 years of age; must have persisted for longer than 6 months; and must be maladaptive or inappropriate for the child's developmental stage.
- Six of the symptoms in 1 or both of these categories must be present:
  - **Impulsivity/hyperactivity:**
    - Fidgetiness.
    - Difficulty remaining seated in class.
    - Excessive running or climbing.
    - Difficulty engaging in quiet activities.
    - Always "on the go."
    - Excessive talking.
    - Blurting out answers before questions have been completed.
    - Difficulty waiting for turn.
    - Interrupting and intruding on others.

KEY FACT

The MMR vaccine and its components do not cause autism.

MNEMONIC

Signs of AUTISM:

Aloneness
Understanding (lack of)
Touch (hypersensitivity to)
Irrelevant and metaphorical language
Sameness (desire for)
Memory (rote)

- **Inattentiveness:**
  - Failure to pay close attention to detail.
  - Difficulty sustaining attention in tasks.
  - Failure to listen when spoken to directly.
  - Failure to follow instructions.
  - Difficulty organizing tasks and activities.
  - Reluctance to engage in tasks that require sustained attention.
  - Losing utensils (eg, pencils, books) necessary for tasks or activities.
  - Easy distractibility.
  - Forgetfulness in daily activities.
  - Comorbid psychiatric problems are common and include mood and conduct disorders. All children should be evaluated for learning disabilities.

TREATMENT

- Components of treatment include medication, behavior modification (often with a token economy that rewards good behavior), and environmental interventions such as preferential seating and ↓ stimuli.
- The most commonly used medications are stimulants such as methylphenidate (Ritalin), which, however, can cause growth delay and loss of appetite.
- Intensive behavioral therapy may be helpful but is generally less effective than medication. Counseling is generally ineffective for ADHD itself but may be an important part of managing comorbid conditions such as depression and anxiety.

KEY FACT

Stimulants used for the treatment of ADHD are associated with anorexia and may inhibit growth. Some families opt not to use the medication on weekends or during holidays from school to let their children regain appetite and growth.

NUTRITION AND GROWTH

Normal Weight Gain/Feeding in Childhood

- **0–6 months of age:**
  - Weight loss in the first days is normal, but infants should be back to birth weight by the 10th day of life. Loss of > 10% of birth weight raises concern for dehydration.
  - "Breast is best." Breast-feeding ↓ the incidence of obesity and diabetes, improves immune defenses, ↓ allergies later in life, and facilitates mother–infant bonding.
  - Exclusive breast or formula feeding should continue until 6 months of age to meet the infant's nutritional needs and ↓ the risk of developing allergies.
  - Breast-fed infants 0–12 months of age should receive 200 IU of vitamin D daily. Formula is fortified with vitamin D.
  - Weight typically doubles by 6 months of age.
- **6–12 months of age:**
  - Begin to add enriched cereals, fruits, vegetables, and meats to the diet. Add only 1 new item per week to ↓ the incidence of food aversions and to allow allergic reactions to be readily correlated with a new food.
  - To prevent infant botulism, honey should not be introduced until after 1 year of age.
  - Continue breast-feeding. Formula should be continued until 1 year of age and should then be switched to cow's milk.
  - Iron-rich foods should be introduced by 6 months of age.
  - Birth weight triples by 1 year.

- **12 months and older:**
  - Whole milk is best from age 1–2 years, at which time low-fat milk should be introduced.
  - Growth decelerates dramatically. Use the growth curve to assess adequacy.

Failure to Thrive (FTT)

Defined as persistent weight loss, a weight curve that declines across 2 major percentile lines, or weight persistently below the 3rd percentile (Table 13.4).

DIAGNOSIS

- **Organic:** Consider GERD, problems with chewing/swallowing, malabsorption, protein-wasting nephropathy, genetic syndromes, and endocrine dysfunction.
- **Nonorganic:** Assess for inappropriate or inadequate feeding by caregivers. May be related to lack of knowledge about feeding, bonding issues, socioeconomic issues, or abuse. Can have a mixed picture, with frustration or anxiety over organic illness leading to inadequate feeding.
- Diagnostic testing should be guided by suspected etiology. Admission to observe weight gain with adequate calories may be helpful.

TREATMENT

Treatment depends on underlying etiology. Institute a high-calorie diet, with particular attention to protein intake. Outpatient treatment is often sufficient, but hospitalization may be necessary.

Obesity

- **Sx/Exam:** Defined as a body mass index (BMI) > 95th percentile for age and gender. At-risk children are between the 85th and 95th percentiles. Diagnosis is not made until 2 years of age, although at-risk children may be identified earlier.
- **Tx:** Lifestyle modification must involve the entire family. Limit sedentary activities like watching television. In most cases, the goal is to maintain current weight while linear growth catches up.
- **Cx:** Dyslipidemia, insulin resistance, type 2 DM, orthopedic problems, sleep apnea.

TABLE 13.4.   Causes of Failure to Thrive by Metabolic Process

INADEQUATE INTAKE	INADEQUATE ABSORPTION	EXCESSIVE LOSS	EXCESSIVE REQUIREMENT
Feeding mismanagement (eg, errors in formula feed, bizarre/restricted diet, neglect, poverty)	Pancreatic insufficiency (eg, cystic fibrosis, Schwachman-Diamond syndrome)	Vomiting (eg, CNS abnormality, intestinal obstruction, metabolic abnormality, gastroesophageal reflux)	Chronic illness (eg, cystic fibrosis, congenital heart disease, inflammatory bowel disease)
Inability to feed optimally (eg, developmental delay, cleft palate, bulbar palsy)	Small intestine disease (eg, dissacharidase deficiency, cow's milk protein intolerance, celiac)	Protein-losing enteropathy Chronic diarrhea	Thyrotoxicosis Chronic infection (eg, TB, HIV)
Anorexia (eg, chronic illness, anorexia nervosa)			Malignancy
Diencephalic syndrome			Burns

Reproduced, with permission, from Guandalini S. *Essential Pediatric Gastroenterolgy, Hepatology, and Nutrition.* New York: McGraw-Hill, 2005, 57.

Vitamin and Nutrient Deficiencies

- **Scurvy:** Vitamin C deficiency. Presents with bleeding gums, osteoid deficiency, and poor healing. Anorexia, FTT, irritability, and apathy may also be seen.
- **Rickets:** Vitamin D deficiency. Presents with craniotabes (thinning of the skull), rachitic rosary (thickening of the costochondral junctions), bowed legs, and tooth defects.
- **Kwashiorkor:** An isolated protein deficiency presenting with edema and FTT.
- **Marasmus:** A protein and calorie deficiency that presents with generalized wasting and FTT.
- **Calcium deficiency:**
  - Results in bone loss and failure to achieve maximal bone density. May contribute to later development of osteoporosis.
  - Premature infants and adolescents with poor dairy intake are at ↑ risk.
  - Absorption of calcium from breast milk is greater than that from cow's milk.

PREVENTIVE MEDICINE

Immunizations

Vaccine schedules are updated annually. Current recommendations may be found on the Center for Disease Control and Prevention Web site (www.cdc.gov/nip/ACIP). Contraindications to vaccines are outlined in Table 13.5.

Anticipatory Guidance

GROWTH

Plotting a child's growth on a standardized graph at all well-child checks is helpful in diagnosing FTT and growth abnormalities at a point when interventions may still be effective.

DENTAL CARE

- Teething typically begins at 3–12 months. Parents should start cleaning teeth as soon as they appear.
- Encourage use of a cup by 1 year of age. Do not allow a bottle in bed (can lead to "baby bottle tooth decay").

TABLE 13.5.   Contraindications to Vaccines

VACCINE	CONTRAINDICATIONS
All vaccines	A previous anaphylactic reaction to a specific vaccine or any part of that vaccine.
MMR and varicella	Pregnancy or known immunodeficiency. Anaphylactic reaction to neomycin or gelatin.
Influenza	Anaphylactic reaction to eggs.
HBV	Anaphylactic reaction to baker's yeast.
HAV	Anaphylactic reaction to aluminum or 2-phenoxyethanol.

- Fluoride supplementation should start at 6 months of age if the water supply is not fluoridated. Fluoride varnish may be applied at well-child checks.
- Dental caries is the most common chronic disease in childhood.
- Infants at higher risk for early dental caries should be referred to a dentist by 12 months of age. Risk factors include sleeping with a bottle, low socio-economic status, mother with multiple caries, visible plaques/staining on teeth.

INJURY PREVENTION

Injuries are the leading cause of death in children and adolescents after the first year of life. The well-child check is an opportunity to counsel parents on injury prevention strategies such as keeping poisons stored locked and out of reach, drowning prevention, and "baby-proofing" to prevent falls and aspirations. Specific strategies include the following:

- **Car seats/seatbelts:**
  - Car seats and booster seats should be in the back seat of the car.
  - Rear-facing infant seats should be used until a child is older than 1 year of age and weighs > 20 pounds.
  - Booster seats should be used for children who have outgrown car seats.
  - A combination lap/shoulder belt should be used when a child has grown enough to fit the seat belts (usually 4'9").
- **Bicycle helmets:**
  - Head trauma is the greatest cause of bicycle fatalities.
  - Although > 85% of brain injuries can be prevented by the use of bicycle helmets, < 25% of children wear a bike helmet when riding.
  - Community interventions can greatly influence the rate of helmet use.

KEY FACT

Injuries are the leading cause of death in children and adolescents after the first year of life.

SLEEP POSITION

Infants should sleep on their backs. This decreases the risk of sudden infant death syndrome (SIDS) by almost 50%.

TOBACCO EXPOSURE

- Exposure to second-hand smoke increases the risk of SIDS, asthma, pneumonia, bronchiolitis, otitis media, and hospitalizations in children.
- Children of smokers are also more likely to become smokers themselves.
- Primary care physicians should ask parents about smoking, advise them about the harmful effects, and encourage them to quit.

Laboratory Tests

IRON DEFICIENCY ANEMIA

- Risk factors include preterm or low-birth-weight births, iron deficiency in the mother, use of nonfortified formula or cow's milk before 12 months of age, and an infant diet that is low in iron-containing foods. Infants and toddlers consuming > 24 ounces of cow's milk per day are also at risk, as are children with chronic illness.
- Screen at-risk children at 9–12 months of age and again at 15–18 months. Screening may be done annually, if indicated, until 5 years of age. Premature and low-birth-weight infants may need testing before 6 months of age.
- Universal anemia screening at 9 and 15 months of age is appropriate for children in communities or populations in which anemia is found in ≥ 5% of those tested.

LEAD SCREENING

- The most common source of lead exposure is lead-based paint, which has been banned since 1977. Children may eat or inhale contaminated particles.
- High levels of lead are associated with seizures and coma. Moderate elevations are associated with behavioral problems and learning disabilities. Even low elevations are correlated with lower IQs.
- Screen all children in communities with a large number of old buildings or a high percentage of children with ↑ blood lead levels.

Child Abuse

PHYSICAL ABUSE

Physical indicators of abuse include the following:

- Injuries that do not correlate with the history.
- Specific pathognomonic injuries (eg, looped wire marks, cigarette burns, rib fractures, spiral fractures).
- Multiple injuries in varying stages of healing.
- Different types of injuries or disease (eg, burns and fractures).
- Overall evidence of poor care.
- Evidence of FTT.
- Infants who are severely shaken can present with sudden onset of seizure or coma with no signs of head trauma. They will typically have bilateral retinal hemorrhages and may have bilateral subdural hemorrhages on CT scan.
- When abuse is suspected, document all injuries, consider a skeletal survey, and report the case to Child Protective Services.

> **KEY FACT**
>
> Abuse may be physical, sexual, emotional, or by neglect. In early childhood, FTT may be the first indicator.

SEXUAL ABUSE

- Behavioral changes may be an indicator of sexual abuse.
- Preschool children may present with fear states (eg, fear of adult males), nightmares, precocious sexual behavior, enuresis, encopresis, or behavior regression.
- School-aged children may exhibit sexual behavior, sexual aggression toward other children, cross-dressing, school failure, truancy, running away, or depression.
- Adolescents may also develop problems with drugs, promiscuity, or prostitution.

COMMON ACUTE CONDITIONS

Respiratory Distress

In all cases of respiratory distress, look for nasal flaring, grunting, and retractions. Listen for wheezing, crackles, and ↓ air movement. Cyanosis around the mucous membranes and nail beds is a sign of significant hypoxia.

APNEA

Defined as cessation of breathing for > 20 seconds or for 10–20 seconds with signs of hypoxia. Subtypes are as follows:

- **Central:** Frequently identified early in infancy. May be related to infection, metabolic abnormalities, anemia, hypoxia, or CNS dysfunction.
- **Obstructive:** Occurs in later infancy and childhood. Obstruction causes cessation of airflow despite respiratory effort.
- **Mixed:** Both central and obstructive components are present.

DIAGNOSIS

- In infants, check for metabolic imbalance with a basic metabolic panel and BUN/creatinine test. Look for signs of infection (CBC, UA, and CXR; consider CT and LP); check for respiratory syncytial virus (RSV) and pertussis; consider an ECG.
- Consider an EEG if the patient has altered mental status or if a seizure focus is suspected. Admit for apnea monitoring.
- In older children, consider upper pharyngeal lesions such as tonsillitis and pharyngitis or laryngomalacia.

APPARENT LIFE-THREATENING EVENTS (ALTEs)

- Defined as an episode of apnea, change in muscle tone, and change in color (cyanosis or pallor).
- Differential includes infectious, cardiac, metabolic, and neurologic disorders. In 50% of cases, no diagnosis is found. GERD is often a diagnosis of exclusion.
- A single ALTE is not associated with ↑ risk of SIDS.

UPPER AIRWAY OBSTRUCTION

A panicked father presents to your office with his 2-year-old daughter, who is coughing and wheezing. The child was entirely well and playing "tea party" with her older sister when the father started doing laundry, but looked ill when he returned. She has no significant past medical history and no sick contacts. She is afebrile, slightly pale, and has an inspiratory wheeze. Her O_2 saturation is normal, and her CXR is significant only for mild hyperinflation of the right lung. What is your diagnosis?

This child almost certainly inhaled something radiolucent into her right bronchus while playing tea party. She needs urgent evaluation for removal of this object under direct visualization by ENT.

May be caused by a foreign body, epiglottitis, or croup; distinguished as follows (see also Figure 13.7):

- **Foreign body:**
    - **Sx/Exam:** Abrupt onset with no fever; not positional; presents with inspiratory **and** expiratory stridor.
    - **Dx:** Expiratory CXR shows possible object and hyperinflation. Bilateral decubitus views may be necessary to demonstrate hyperinflation in children who cannot cooperate with instructions for expiratory CXR (see Figure 13.8).
    - **Tx:** Removal via laryngoscopy or bronchoscopy.
- **Epiglottitis:**
    - Most common in children 2–5 years of age. Most often caused by *Streptococcus pyogenes*, *Streptococcus pneumoniae*, and *Staphylococcus aureus*; on rare occasions, *Haemophilus influenzae* may be implicated (a significant ↓ in incidence has been seen 2° to routine vaccination).
    - **Sx/Exam:** Rapid onset with high fever; presents with drooling and sore throat. Patients remain sitting or leaning forward. Primarily inspiratory stridor.
    - **Dx:** A lateral neck x-ray reveals the characteristic "thumbprint sign" (Figure 13.8).
    - **Tx:** Secure the airway, send blood cultures, and start broad-spectrum antibiotics.

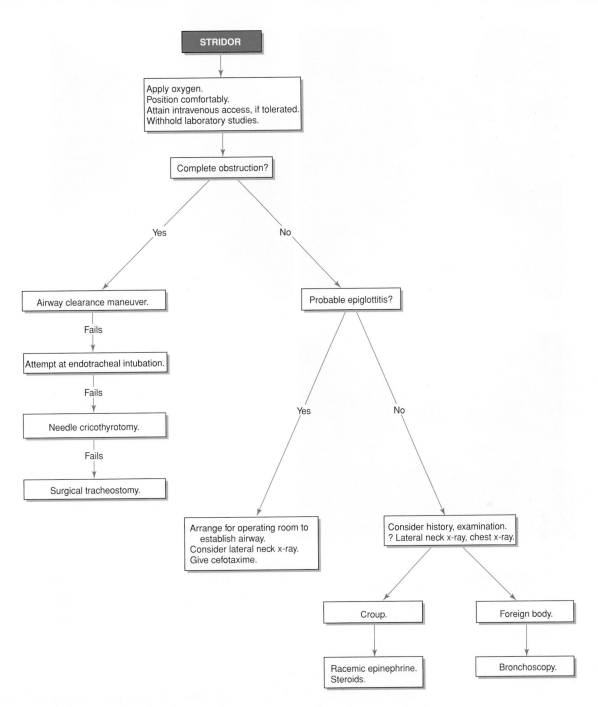

FIGURE 13.7. **Diagnosis and treatment of upper airway obstruction.** (Reproduced, with permission, from Stone CK, Humphries RL. *Current Emergency Diagnosis & Treatment,* 5th ed. New York: McGraw-Hill, 2004: 1054.)

- **Croup:**
  - Most common in children 6 months to 3 years of age, occurring during the fall and winter months. Caused by parainfluenza virus.
  - **Sx/Exam:** Barking (seal-like) cough, hoarseness, low-grade fever. Inspiratory and expiratory stridor may also be seen and may be provoked or worsened if the child is agitated or crying.
  - **Dx:** CXR shows subglottic narrowing, the "steeple sign" (see Figure 13.8).
  - **Tx:** Treat mild disease with humidified O_2. Moderate to severe disease should be treated with steroids and nebulized racemic epinephrine.

KEY FACT

The key feature of upper airway obstruction is inspiratory stridor.

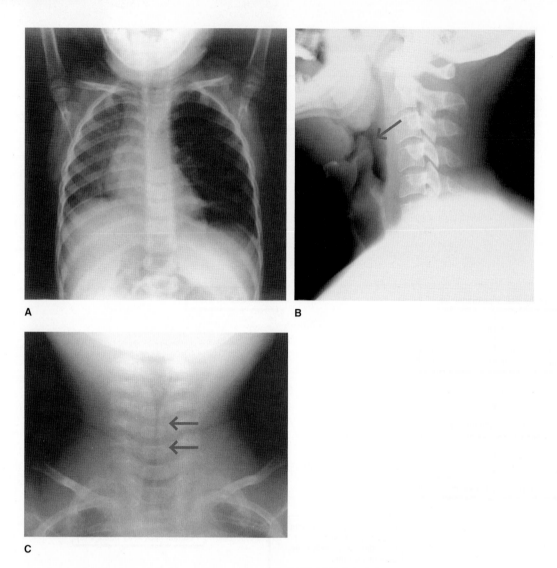

FIGURE 13.8.   **Airway obstruction.** (**A**) Aspirated peanut (not visible) in the left main stem bronchus, resulting in hyperinflated left lung with mediastinal shift. (**B**) Epiglottis, known as the "thumbprint" sign *(arrow)*. (**C**) Croup. Subglottic tracheal narrowing with an inverted "V" appearance below the larynx, the "steeple sign" *(arrowheads)*. (Image A reproduced, with permission, from Lalwani AK. *Current Diagnosis & Treatment in Otolaryngology,* 2nd ed. New York: McGraw-Hill, 2008, Fig. 38-2. Image B reproduced, with permission, from USMLERx.com. Image C reproduced, with permission, from Stone CK, Humphries RL. *Current Diagnosis & Treatment: Emergency Medicine,* 6th ed. New York: McGraw-Hill, 2008, Fig. 30-10.)

LOWER AIRWAY OBSTRUCTION

Causes in children include bronchiolitis, asthma, pneumonia, and foreign body obstruction. In infants, it can be associated with congenital anomalies of the airway (tracheal web, cysts, vascular rings, lobar emphysema).

- **Bronchiolitis:**
  - An acute lower airway respiratory disease that causes small airway obstruction, typically occurring in the winter. It primarily affects children < 12 months of age and is caused by RSV.
  - **Sx/Exam:** Cough, coryza, and upper respiratory symptoms, usually with fever, precede wheezing and dyspnea. May present as apnea in younger children.
  - **Dx:** CXR shows peribronchial cuffing, areas of hyperaeration, and atelectasis. Hypercapnia, hypoxemia, or both may be present. Obtain a nasal swab/wash for RSV.
  - **Tx:** Primarily supportive. Give O_2 for hypoxia. Nebulized albuterol can be helpful in patients with a history of wheezing. Corticosteroids may

provide added benefit in patients who respond to bronchodilators. Admit for low O_2 saturation, prematurity, age < 3 months, or toxic appearance. High-risk infants (premature infants and those with preexisting lung or heart disease) should receive palivizumab (Synagis), a monoclonal antibody, to ↓ the risk of contracting RSV.

- **Cx: Bacterial superinfection (pneumonia, otitis media).** There is a possible correlation between bronchiolitis in infancy and the subsequent development of reactive airway disease.

- **Asthma:**
  - **Sx/Exam:** Expiratory wheezing and shortness of breath. Inability to speak, cyanosis, accessory muscle use, pulsus paradoxus, or signs of infection may indicate more serious disease.
  - **Tx:** Exacerbations are treated with nebulized bronchodilators. Nebulized anticholinergics (ipratropium) ↓ hospitalizations. IV or PO steroids are required for moderate to severe exacerbations. For severe exacerbations, systemic bronchodilators (magnesium, terbutaline) may also help prevent intubation. Intubation is necessary in severe cases.

- **Pneumonia:**
  - Common causative organisms are as follows:
    - **Newborns:** GBS, gram-⊖ enteric bacteria, CMV, *Listeria monocytogenes.*
    - **Infants:** *Chlamydia trachomatis,* RSV, *S pneumoniae, S aureus.*
    - **Toddlers:** Viruses, *S pneumoniae,* nontypable *H influenzae.*
    - **Children (4–14 years):** *Mycoplasma pneumoniae, Pneumococcus, Chlamydia pneumoniae.*
  - **Sx/Exam:** Presents with fever and respiratory findings (crackles, egophony, dullness to percussion).
  - **Dx:** CXR shows evidence of parenchymal infiltrates.
  - **Tx:** Antibiotics; hospitalize if the patient is unable to maintain an O_2 saturation > 92% on room air. Some patients may respond to bronchodilators.

Fever

NEONATES (< 1 MONTH)

- Even well-appearing febrile children < 1 month of age are at high risk for occult serious bacterial illness (SBI).
- Rectal temperature > 38°C (100.4°F) is considered a fever in this age group.
- While viruses are the most likely source, consider late onset of congenitally acquired illnesses, such as rubella and CMV, or infections acquired at birth, such as GBS, *E coli,* and *Listeria.* Early infection may also be the first sign of a congenital abnormality (eg, in the GU system).
- **Dx:** CBC with differential, blood culture, UA, urine culture, LP. Also consider CXR, stool culture, and viral culture.
- **Tx:**
  - Admit and treat with broad-spectrum antibiotics while awaiting culture results.
  - Give ampicillin plus a third-generation cephalosporin or gentamicin.
  - Antibiotics may be discontinued at 48 hours if all cultures are ⊖ and the infant is clinically stable.

INFANTS (1–3 MONTHS)

- A positive viral test or a viral illness with a distinct phenotype may be considered the source of the fever.
- If no source is found, consider occult UTI, bacteremia, or meningitis.

- **Dx:**
  - UA and urine culture in all infants.
  - CBC with differential and blood culture if UA is ⊖ or if the child is ill-appearing. Also consider LP if child is ill-appearing or if antibiotics are being started empirically. As indicated: CXR, stool culture, and viral culture.
  - Start third-generation cephalosporin (eg, ceftriaxone) after collecting cultures if WBC > 15 or < 5, or if there are other concerns for infection.
  - Admit if the patient is ill-appearing or at risk for lack of follow-up.
  - Antibiotics may be discontinued at 48 hours if all cultures are ⊖ and the infant is clinically stable.

INFANTS AND TODDLERS (3–36 MONTHS)

- Rectal temperature > 39°C (102.2°F).
- Etiologies include viral infection, pneumonia, UTI, meningitis, and occult bacteremia. The source of the fever is more readily identifiable in this group than in younger children.
- **Dx:** In the absence of an obvious source of infection (eg, otitis media, infectious diarrhea), diagnose as follows:
  - **Females vaccinated against pneumococcus (2 or more doses):** Check UA and urine culture if the child is < 24 months of age.
  - **Males vaccinated against pneumococcus (2 or more doses):** Check UA and urine culture if the child is circumcised and < 6 months of age or uncircumcised and < 12 months.
  - If the child appears toxic or has not been adequately vaccinated against *Pneumococcus*, check CBC, blood cultures, UA, and urine culture. Also consider LP and CXR, based on clinical presentation.
- **Tx:** All toxic-appearing children should receive empiric IV or IM antibiotics while awaiting cultures. Unvaccinated children with WBC > 15,000 should also receive empiric antibiotics.

CHILDREN (> 36 MONTHS)

The risk of occult bacteremia is lower in this age group, and a source of fever is generally identifiable and treated as needed. In children < 5 years of age with persistent fever, consider Kawasaki disease.

Acute Otitis Media

- Commonly caused by *S pneumoniae*, *H influenzae*, and *Moraxella catarrhalis*.
- **Sx/Exam:** Presents with pain, fever, and hearing loss. May be preceded by a URI. Exam reveals a bulging tympanic membrane, with loss of visual landmarks. Loss of movement of the tympanic membrane, is both sensitive and specific.
- **Tx:** First-line treatment is high-dose amoxicillin (80–90 mg/kg/day). If children are high risk, have severe disease or bilateral disease (associated with *H influenzae*), or have been treated in the last 30 days, treat with amoxicillin-clavulanate. Recurrent infections may be an indication for referral to ENT for placement of tympanotomy tubes. In patients > 2 years of age without symptoms of systemic illness, acute otitis media may be treated supportively with pain control and close follow-up.
- **Cx:** Mastoiditis, hearing loss.

KEY FACT

Use of the pneumococcal conjugate vaccine and the Hib vaccine has dramatically ↓ the number of cases of invasive disease seen from *Pneumococcus* and *H influenzae* type B infections.

Diarrhea

- Rotavirus is the most common cause of acute diarrhea, particularly in the winter. Additional causes include other viruses, food poisoning, traveler's diarrhea, and diarrhea related to recent antibiotic use. Chronic diarrhea may be a sign of IBD, IBS, or celiac disease.
- **Dx:**
    - The history and physical are important to identify signs of dehydration. Ask about the number of wet diapers and the presence of tears when crying.
    - Fecal leukocytes and stool cultures are not always necessary, but may be helpful when a child has bloody diarrhea or appears significantly ill. The serum WBC count is generally higher in bacterial than in viral infection.
    - A Chem 7 can help identify electrolyte abnormalities in patients with severe disease.
    - The combination of bloody diarrhea and acute renal failure should raise suspicion of hemolytic-uremic syndrome (HUS) triggered by Shiga toxin–producing *E coli* O157:H7.
- **Tx:** The most important intervention is rehydration. This can usually be done with oral intake, but significant dehydration should be treated with IV fluids and occasionally with hospitalization. Most cases of infectious diarrhea will resolve without antibiotics. Even with bloody diarrhea, antibiotics should not be started empirically, as their role depends on the organism.

KEY FACT

Rotavirus accounts for as many as 50% of cases of acute diarrhea in winter. Enteric adenoviruses are the second most common viral pathogen in infants. In summer, most cases of diarrhea are caused by bacteria (including *E coli*, *Salmonella*, and *Shigella*).

Vomiting

- In infants and children, common causes of vomiting include gastroenteritis (may precede diarrhea by a few days), intussusception, appendicitis, UTI/pyelonephritis, Reye syndrome, and hepatitis.
- **Dx:** Consider CBC, electrolytes, UA, urine culture, and LFTs, as indicated clinically. Evaluate for dehydration, and consider imaging for underlying causes. "Currant jelly" stools are the classic late sign of intussusception. Ultrasound may be used in diagnosis. Barium enema is diagnostic and therapeutic.

Abdominal Pain

A mother brings her 8-month-old son to the emergency department. He has been having episodes of inconsolable crying during which he pulls his knees to his chest. Between episodes he is lethargic, and he has vomited twice. As you go in to examine him, the nurse tells you that he has just had an episode of bloody diarrhea. How do you proceed?

This presentation raises concern for intussusception. If the child does not appear toxic, a barium enema may be both diagnostic and therapeutic. If there is suspicion of necrotic bowel or perforation, air insufflation may be attempted or the child may need surgery.

- The most likely etiologies of abdominal pain vary by age group:
    - **Infants:** Colic, constipation, gastroenteritis, intussusception, viral syndrome, volvulus.
    - **Younger children:** Appendicitis, constipation, gastroenteritis, pneumonia, UTI, viral syndromes.
    - **School-aged children:** Appendicitis, pregnancy, gastroenteritis, pneumonia, peptic ulcer, PID.

- Rare causes include pancreatitis, Henoch-Schönlein purpura, and HUS.
- **Dx:** Check CBC and electrolytes if the child appears ill. Obtain imaging as indicated by the clinical presentation:
    - **AXR** (flat and upright or lateral): Helps identify free air (an indication of perforation) and air-fluid levels (an indication of obstruction).
    - **CXR:** To identify lower lobe pneumonia.
    - **Ultrasound or abdominal CT with IV contrast:** Ultrasound to identify appendicitis, intussusception, or pyloric stenosis. If ultrasound is not available, CT with IV contrast can be performed.
- **Testicular ultrasound:** To identify torsion.
- **Upper GI series:** To identify midgut malrotation +/− volvulus.
- **Barium enema:** To diagnose intussusception or reduce intussusception identified by ultrasound.

Head Trauma

Can be due to direct impact or acceleration/deceleration injuries. Direct injury to brain tissue and injury from pressure due to expanding hematomas or edema can be serious. The goals of evaluation and treatment are to promptly identify serious conditions and to monitor for and treat sequelae. Types of head trauma include the following:

- **Concussion:** A brief loss or alteration of consciousness due to head trauma, followed by a return to normal. Brain tissue is not damaged, and there are no focal findings. Amnesia, vomiting, confusion, dizziness, and sleep disturbances may be seen. A postconcussive syndrome may last for weeks to months. Children should avoid activity that would put them at risk for another event (eg, competitive sports) until they have remained asymptomatic for at least 1 week.
- **Contusion:** A bruise of the brain matter. The child's level of consciousness diminishes, and focal findings correspond to the area of the brain that is injured. Obtain a head CT and admit for observation.
- **Diffuse axonal injury:** Characterized by coma without focal signs on neurologic exam. There may be no external signs of trauma. The initial CT scan is normal or may demonstrate only small, scattered areas of cerebral contusion and areas of low density. Prolonged disability may follow diffuse axonal injury.
- **↑ ICP +/− herniation:** Etiologies include hemorrhage and generalized swelling in the setting of trauma. Symptoms include headache, vision changes, vomiting, gait difficulties, and a progressively decreasing level of consciousness. Cushing triad (bradycardia, hypertension, and irregular respirations) and papilledema are late findings.

DIAGNOSIS

- For children of all ages, obtain a CT scan in patients who are at high risk for intracranial injury. High-risk patients are those who have severe mechanism of injury, abnormal mental status (GCS < 14), or evidence of skull fracture.
- Children who are at moderate risk may be managed by observation for 4–6 hours or CT scan. Patients who are being observed may need a CT scan if symptoms persist or worsen.
- No further workup is needed in low-risk children.
    - **Age 0–2 years:** Neurologic exam may be normal. Children who are at moderate risk for intracranial injury include those with loss of consciousness for > 5 seconds, nonfrontal scalp hematoma, or abnormal activity per parents.
    - **Age 2–18 years:** Patients in this age group are considered moderate risk if they have loss of consciousness, vomiting, or severe headaches.

KEY FACT

Use CT scans judiciously in children. CT scans are associated with ↑ lifetime cancer risk in children. This risk is greater in younger children.

Seizures

STATUS EPILEPTICUS

- Continuous seizure activity or recurrent seizures without regaining consciousness for 30 minutes. There is some evidence that after 5 minutes, neurons begin to show signs of damage and seizures are unlikely to resolve without intervention.
- Children younger than 3 years of age are more likely to have an underlying cause such as CNS infection, vascular disorders, anoxia, trauma, intoxication, fever, or metabolic abnormalities. These conditions are often treatable.
- In older children, status epilepticus is more often the result of a chronic seizure disorder.
- **DDx:** Look for an underlying condition with a rapid blood glucose level, CBC, chemistry panel, LFTs, ammonia level, and toxicology screen.
- **Tx:** ABCs, anticonvulsants (benzodiazepines, phenytoin, barbiturates).

FEBRILE SEIZURES

- May be simple or complex.
    - **Simple febrile seizure:** Typically occurs as a generalized, self-limited tonic-clonic seizure of several minutes' duration.
    - **Complex febrile seizure:** Defined as a seizure that is focal, is associated with Todd paralysis, or lasts > 15 minutes. Also includes > 1 episode in 24 hours.
- Peak age is 8–20 months, although seizures may occur in children from approximately 6 months to 6 years of age.
- Often, underlying diseases are URIs or gastroenteritis. The seizure seems to be more the result of a rapid change in temperature than of absolute temperature and is independent of the underlying condition.
- **DDx:** Includes CNS infection and epileptic seizures.
- **Tx:** Simple febrile seizures are usually benign and require no therapy. Acetaminophen may be given PO or rectally as needed to address the fever. In rare cases, when children are prone to febrile seizure, diazepam can be used at the onset of a febrile illness and repeated as necessary until the fever resolves.
- **Cx:** Children with a history of complex febrile seizures have a higher risk of developing epilepsy.

Meningitis

Occurs when an organism invades the subarachnoid space. The most common route is hematogenous spread, but it may also occur by direct extension from a contiguous infection such as sinusitis or mastoiditis.

- **Sx/Exam:**
    - **Infants:** Clinical findings may be nonspecific and may include restlessness, irritability, poor feeding, emesis, lethargy, ↓ tone, respiratory distress, full fontanelle (late finding), and seizures. Obvious neck stiffness or other signs of meningeal irritation (eg, Kernig or Brudzinski sign) are not reliably present in infants < 18 months of age.
    - **Children > 18 months:** Neck stiffness, headache, nausea, vomiting, focal neurologic signs, fever, lethargy, and photophobia are common. Infants and children with *Neisseria meningitidis* infection often present with a petechial rash.
- **Dx:** LP with analysis of cell count, protein, and glucose as well as Gram stain and bacterial cultures.
- **Tx:** Table 13.6 outlines treatment options.

TABLE 13.6. Etiologies and Treatment of Childhood Meningitis

AGE	COMMON CAUSES	ANTIBIOTIC	OTHER CAUSES
Preterm to < 1 month	GBS, *E coli, Listeria*	Ampicillin + cefotaxime or gentamicin	Enterovirus, *Candida albicans*
1–3 months	GBS, *E coli, Listeria, S pneumoniae, N meningitidis, H influenzae* type B (rare)	Vancomycin + cefotaxime or ceftriaxone	Enterovirus
3 months–6 years	*S pneumoniae, N meningitidis, H influenzae* type B (rare)	Vancomycin + cefotaxime or ceftriaxone	Enterovirus, mumps, *Mycobacterium tuberculosis*
> 6 years	*S pneumoniae, N meningitides*	Vancomycin + cefotaxime or ceftriaxone	Enterovirus, mumps, *M tuberculosis*

Adapted, with permission, from Stone CK, Humphries RL. *Current Emergency Diagnosis & Treatment,* 5th ed. New York: McGraw-Hill, 2004: 1068.

CARDIOLOGY

Evaluation of a Murmur

You are seeing a 3-year-old girl for a routine well-child check. Her mother notes that she is now fully potty trained and about to start preschool. On exam, you note that her height and weight have been stable at the 50th percentile and that her developmental milestones are also appropriate for her age. On exam, you note that she has a quiet precordium, a regular rate, and normal S1 and S2, with a 2/6 systolic ejection murmur that is louder when she is supine. There is no radiation of the murmur to the neck, axillae, or back. What is your next step in management of this patient?

Reassure the parents that the murmur is innocent, and observe the patient.

Murmur is the most common cardiovascular finding that leads to a cardiology referral. Innocent heart murmurs (also known as functional murmurs) are extremely common. Between 40% and 45% of children have an innocent murmur at some time during childhood.

SYMPTOMS

Symptoms of **pathologic murmurs** include FTT, exercise intolerance, dyspnea with exertion/diaphoresis, syncope, dizziness, cyanosis, loss of consciousness, and tachypnea with feeds or activity.

EXAM

Assess the following factors: intensity, quality, timing in cycle, location, radiation, and variation with position (Table 13.7).

DIAGNOSIS

Indications of pathologic murmurs include the following (see also Table 13.7):

- Cyanotic, symptomatic (FTT, tachypnea).
- Grade III or more.

 MNEMONIC

Features of innocent murmurs:

The 8 Ss

Soft
Systolic
Short
Sounds (S1 and S2) normal
Symptomless
Special tests (x-ray, ECG) normal
Standing/**S**itting (vary with position)
Sternal depression (pectus excavatum)

TABLE 13.7. Types of Murmurs Based on Location of Loudest Intensity

Location/Diagnosis	Unique Features
Right upper sternal border	
Venous hum.	**Continuous;** disappears when the jugular vein is compressed, when the patient's head is turned, or when the patient is supine. Benign.
Aortic stenosis.	Systolic ejection quality (with audible S1 and S2); radiates to the neck; presents with thrill in the suprasternal notch. Often associated with a valve click.
Left upper sternal border	
Peripheral pulmonary stenosis.	Systolic ejection quality; usually seen in infants; often louder in the axillae than over the precordium. Benign.
Pulmonary stenosis.	Systolic ejection quality; radiates to the back and axillae; may be associated with a valve click.
PDA.	Continuous; **"machinery"** quality; bounding pulses.
ASD.	Systolic; fixed, split S2.
Coarctation of the aorta.	Systolic; radiation to the back; weak, delayed femoral pulses.
Left lower sternal border	
Still murmur.	**"Vibratory"** systolic ejection quality; no radiation; louder when the patient is supine. Benign.
VSD.	Holosystolic; harsh quality; often radiates all over the precordium; often louder as the defect gets smaller.
Hypertrophic obstructive cardiomyopathy.	Systolic ejection quality; louder when the patient is upright; often radiates to the apex; may be heard in patients who have chest pain with activity.
Apex	
Mitral regurgitation.	Holosystolic, decrescendo, **"cooing dove"** quality.

Reproduced, with permission, from Le T, et al. *First Aid for the Pediatric Boards,* 1st ed. New York: McGraw-Hill, 2006: 61.

- Diastolic murmur.
- Abnormal CXR or ECG.
- Comorbid syndrome with a high incidence of heart defects (eg, Down, Turner, Marfan, Williams, Noonan syndromes).

TREATMENT

Refer pathologic murmurs to a pediatric cardiologist; observe benign murmurs.

Ventricular Septal Defect (VSD)

The most common congenital heart malformation, accounting for approximately 30% of all cases of congenital heart disease. Defects in the ventricular septum occur both in the membranous portion of the septum (most common) and in the muscular portion, permitting blood in the high-pressure left ventricle to shunt into the low-pressure right ventricle. Eisenmenger syndrome and shunt reversal occurs in approximately 25% of cases.

SYMPTOMS

- **Small to moderate shunts:** Often asymptomatic and acyanotic.
- **Moderate shunts:** May cause pulmonary vascular disease and right-sided failure.
- **Large left-to-right shunts:**
  - Patients are ill early in infancy (with frequent upper and lower respiratory infections), growing and gaining weight slowly.
  - Dyspnea, exercise intolerance, and fatigue are common. CHF develops between 1 and 6 months of age.
  - With severe pulmonary hypertension and shunt reversal, cyanosis is present.

KEY FACT

Eisenmenger syndrome is a general term applied to pulmonary hypertension and shunt reversal in the presence of a congenital defect.

EXAM

- A systolic thrill is heard.
- **Small to moderate defects:** A loud, grade II–IV/VI holosystolic murmur is heard that is maximal along the lower left sternal border. Occasionally, a mid-diastolic flow murmur is heard.
- **Large defects:** Right ventricular volume and pressure overload may lead to pulmonary hypertension, CHF, and cyanosis. A grade II–IV/VI holosystolic murmur is maximal at the lower left sternal border. P2 is usually accentuated.

DIFFERENTIAL

Mitral regurgitation; mitral valve prolapse.

DIAGNOSIS

- **ECG:** LVH and/or RVH if the shunt is reversed.
- **CXR:** ↑ pulmonary vascularity.
- **Echocardiography:** Doppler is diagnostic and can assess the magnitude of the shunt as well as pulmonary arterial pressure.
- **Cardiac CT and MRI:** Can visualize the defect and other anatomic abnormalities.
- **Cardiac catheterization:** Reserved for those with at least moderate shunting; can measure pulmonary vascular resistance and the degree of pulmonary hypertension.

TREATMENT

- Small shunts do not require closure in asymptomatic patients.
- Symptomatic children should be managed with hypercaloric feeds, diuretics, and ACEIs.
- If symptoms persist despite maximal medical therapy or if there is ↑ pulmonary vascular resistance (affects approximately 50% of patients), the defect should be surgically or percutaneously repaired. The shunt should not be repaired if Eisenmenger syndrome has developed.
- Children who do not have surgery should be followed to assess for spontaneous closure of the defect or for the development of complications.
- Because infections can worsen heart failure, all children > 6 months of age should receive the influenza vaccine, and all children < 2 years of age should receive RSV prophylaxis.
- Endocarditis occurs more often with smaller shunts; antibiotic prophylaxis is mandatory for all patients.

COMPLICATIONS

Endocarditis; pulmonary hypertension/Eisenmenger syndrome. Surgical mortality is 2%–3%, but ↑ to ≥ 50% if pulmonary hypertension is present.

Atrial Septal Defect (ASD)

A communication between the right and left atria. The most common type is persistent ostium secundum, a defect of the midseptum. Initially results in a left-to-right shunt as oxygenated blood from the higher-pressure left atrium passes into the right atrium. Over time, a large defect may lead to pulmonary overcirculation, pulmonary hypertension, Eisenmenger syndrome, right-to-left shunting, and cyanosis.

SYMPTOMS

Small ASDs are typically not hemodynamically significant and do not cause symptoms. Large ASDs may present with exertional dyspnea, arrhythmias, syncope, and heart failure.

EXAM

- **A fixed, split S2** is heard.
- A systolic ejection murmur may be heard in the second and third interspaces. A right ventricular heave may also be present.

DIAGNOSIS

- **Echocardiography:** Usually diagnostic. Saline bubble contrast and Doppler flow can demonstrate shunting.
- **ECG:** Shows incomplete or complete right bundle branch block, right axis deviation, and RVH.
- **CXR:** Demonstrates large pulmonary arteries, $\uparrow$ pulmonary vascularity, and an enlarged right atrium and ventricle.
- **Cardiac catheterization:** Can show an $\uparrow$ in O_2 saturation between the vena cava and the right ventricle; can also quantify the shunt and measure pulmonary vascular resistance.

TREATMENT

- Although there is no evidence of benefit from closure of small shunts, large shunts generally require closure. Percutaneous closure devices are now available.
- There is no increased risk of infective endocarditis unless mitral regurgitation is present as well, so antibiotic prophylaxis is recommended only in these cases.

COMPLICATIONS

- Pulmonary hypertension, right-sided heart failure, **Eisenmenger syndrome,** and right-to-left shunting.
- Paradoxical emboli.
- $\uparrow$ risk of complications with scuba diving and at high altitudes.

Cyanotic Heart Disease

> A 2-year-old girl from Mexico is brought to the ER after a spell of intractable crying and irritability. Her mother mentions that she has a heart problem and that whenever doctors examine her, they hear a loud murmur. Pulse oximetry reveals an O_2 saturation of 62%. On auscultation, you hear a 1/6 murmur in systole at the left upper sternal border. What is your therapeutic strategy?
>
> You recognize that this girl is likely having a hypercyanotic spell associated with tetralogy of Fallot. You bring her knees up to her chest and administer a single dose of IV morphine, and her O_2 saturation rapidly improves to 92%.

Cyanosis is seen when > 5 g/dL of hemoglobin in the capillaries is deoxygenated. The most common causes of cyanotic heart disease in the newborn period are transposition of the great vessels, total anomalous pulmonary venous

Causes of cyanotic heart disease:

5 terrible Ts

Transposition of the great vessels
Total anomalous pulmonary venous return
Tetralogy of Fallot
Truncus arteriosus
Tricuspid atresia

return, truncus arteriosus (some types), tricuspid atresia, and pulmonary atresia or critical pulmonary stenosis. Infants with these disorders present with early cyanosis. The hallmark of many of these lesions is cyanosis in an infant without associated respiratory distress.

SYMPTOMS/EXAM

Table 13.8 outlines the common causes of cyanotic heart disease as well as its clinical presentation and treatment.

DIAGNOSIS

Differentiate between cardiac and noncardiac causes:

- **Hyperoxia test:** Obtain an ABG; then place the patient on 100% O_2 for 10 minutes and perform a repeat ABG. If the cause of cyanosis is pulmonary, the PaO_2 should ↑ by 30 mmHg. If the cause is cardiac, there should be minimal improvement in PaO_2.
- **CXR:** Vasculature on CXR provides information about pulmonary blood flow.

TABLE 13.8.   Causes, Presentation, and Treatment of Cyanotic Heart Disease

	DEFINITION	SYMPTOMS/EXAM	TREATMENT
Tetralogy of Fallot	Includes VSD, pulmonary stenosis, overriding aorta, and RVH.	Cyanosis, dyspnea, loud pulmonary stenosis murmur; a VSD (holosystolic) murmur may also be heard. Variable degree of cyanosis, depending on the amount of right-to-left shunting.	Surgical repair through placement of a transannular patch across the pulmonary valve.
Tricuspid atresia/ hypoplastic right heart	Complete or partial agenesis of the right ventricular cavity in which the left ventricle provides pulmonary blood flow through the ductus arteriosus.	Tachypnea, dyspnea, anoxic spells, and evidence of right heart failure; cyanosis; a grade II–VI harsh blowing murmur heard best at the lower left sternal border.	Anticongestive therapy. The Fontan procedure (connection of the systemic venous return to the pulmonary artery) is performed when increasing cyanosis occurs.
Transposition of the great vessels	Connection of the left ventricle to the pulmonary artery and the right ventricle to the aorta, causing the systemic and pulmonary circulations to operate in parallel.	Cyanosis; a single S2 and no murmur.	Early corrective surgery is recommended through an arterial switch operation of the great vessels.
Total anomalous pulmonary venous return	All pulmonary veins terminate in a systemic vein or the right atrium.	Tachypnea, feeding difficulties, and heart failure; widely fixed, split S2 and grade II–III/VI ejection-type systolic murmur.	Surgery is always required.
Truncus arteriosus	A single arterial trunk arises from the ventricles and divides into the aorta and pulmonary arteries.	Mild or no cyanosis, early CHF, systolic ejection click, wide pulse pressure.	Anticongestive treatment and surgical repair.

- **ECG:** Provides information about rhythm and, grossly, ventricular size. Examine both the axis and the magnitude of the deflections. Remember that right axis deviation is normal for a neonate.
- **Echocardiography:** The gold standard of diagnosis, as well as a noninvasive means of assessing the cardiac anatomy.

TREATMENT

For cyanotic heart disease in which circulation is ductus dependent (requiring a patent ductus arteriosus), immediate treatment with prostaglandins, which delay closing of the ductus, may be lifesaving while the child is transported to a facility for cardiac surgery.

Kawasaki Disease

A 5-year-old boy presents to your clinic with a 5- to 6-day history of persistent high fever and irritability. Three days ago, he was given antibiotics for presumed acute otitis media, but his fever did not resolve. On exam, he is found to have an erythematous rash, cracked lips, and a "strawberry tongue." He refuses to stand on both feet and cries every time he attempts to walk. Both ear canals appear red, which you attribute to the child's excessive crying. Do you continue the course of antibiotics?

Recognizing that this child has Kawasaki disease, you discontinue antibiotics and admit the boy to the hospital for appropriate therapy.

Previously called mucocutaneous lymph node syndrome, Kawasaki disease is an acute febrile vasculitis of childhood involving small and medium-size arteries, with characteristic involvement of the coronary arteries. The cause is unclear, and no specific diagnostic test is available. Approximately 80% of affected patients are younger than 5 years of age, and the male-to-female ratio is 1.5:1.

SYMPTOMS/EXAM

The condition is defined by the presence of fever for at least 5 days and at least 4 of the following features (see Figures 13.9 and 13.10):

- Bilateral, painless, nonexudative conjunctivitis.
- Lip or oral cavity changes (eg, lip cracking and fissuring, strawberry tongue, inflammation of the oral mucosa).
- Cervical lymphadenopathy ($\geq$ 1.5 cm in diameter and usually unilateral).
- Polymorphous exanthema.
- Extremity changes (redness and swelling of the hands and feet, with subsequent desquamation).

DIFFERENTIAL

Juvenile rheumatoid arthritis, infectious mononucleosis, scarlet fever, viral exanthems, leptospirosis, Rocky Mountain spotted fever, toxic shock syndrome, staphylococcal scalded-skin syndrome, erythema multiforme, serum sickness, SLE, Reiter syndrome.

KEY FACT

Right axis deviation is normal for a neonate.

MNEMONIC

Diagnosis of Kawasaki disease:

CRASH and Burn

Conjunctivitis—perilimbic sparing
Rash
Adenopathy—usually cervical
Strawberry tongue
Hand and foot changes
Burn—fever for > 5 days

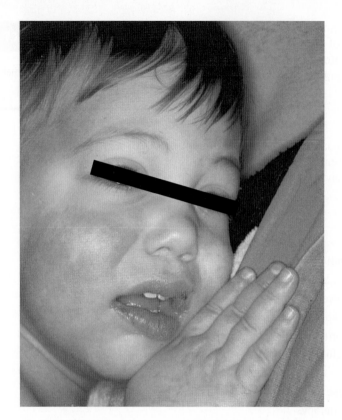

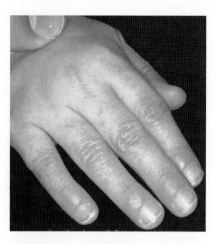

FIGURE 13.10.   Manifestation of Kawasaki disease in digits. Erythema and edema of the distal digits are an early manifestation of Kawasaki disease. Later the skin on the fingers may become cracked. (Reproduced, with permission, from Wolff K, et al. *Fitzpatrick's Dermatology in General Medicine,* 7th ed. New York: McGraw-Hill, 2008, Fig. 168-3.)

FIGURE 13.9.   Kawasaki disease. Cherry-red lips with hemorrhagic fissures in a boy with prolonged high fever. This child also had a generalized morbilliform eruption, infected conjunctivae, and strawberry tongue (not shown). Note erythema and edema of the fingertips. (Reproduced, with permission, from Wolff K, Johnson RA. *Fitzpatrick's Color Atlas & Synopsis of Clinical Dermatology,* 6th ed. New York: McGraw-Hill, 2009, Fig. 14-44.)

DIAGNOSIS

- Patients often have pyuria, transaminitis, normocytic anemia, and reactive thrombocytosis.
- Hyponatremia can be associated with an ↑ risk of cardiac complications.
- Screen with echocardiography or angiography for coronary artery aneurysms.

TREATMENT

- High-dose ASA and IVIG in the acute phase, followed by low-dose ASA for 6–8 weeks or until the coronary aneurysm resolves.
- Corticosteroids are not recommended, as they may be associated with an ↑ incidence of aneurysms.
- Serial echocardiograms at the time of diagnosis, at 2–4 weeks, and at 6–8 weeks. More frequent imaging may be required if abnormalities are present.

COMPLICATIONS

- **Coronary artery lesions:** Range from mild transient dilation of a coronary artery to large aneurysm formation. Untreated patients have a 25% risk of developing an aneurysm of the coronary arteries. Those at greatest risk for aneurysm formation are males, young children (< 6 months), and those not treated with IVIG.
- **Other:** Also associated with myocarditis, pericarditis, and valvular heart disease (usually mitral or aortic regurgitation).

PULMONARY DISEASE

Asthma

 An 8-year-old girl is brought to your office by her father. She has been to the ER twice in the last month for wheezing and has missed 3 or 4 days of school. She has a nebulizer at home, but lost her albuterol inhaler. Her father thinks she has a cold because she has woken up coughing during the night once or twice in the last week. On exam, she is comfortable and has some faint expiratory wheezes. What is your evaluation and management?

This child has persistent asthma. She needs to be placed on an inhaled steroid in addition to her rescue inhaler. Above all, she and her family need asthma education and an action plan.

Asthma is one of the most common diseases of childhood. Up to 25% of children will have 1 or more attacks, with 3%–5% continuing to have symptoms into adulthood. Asthma is a chronic inflammatory disorder of the airways characterized by reversible bronchoconstriction, ↑ mucus production, and basement membrane thickening (Figure 13.11). Risk factors include poverty and nonwhite ethnicity.

> **KEY FACT**
>
> Asthma causes up to 5000 deaths a year in the United States. African American teens are at highest risk.

SYMPTOMS/EXAM

- Acute attacks present with dyspnea, expiratory wheezing, nasal flaring, retractions, hypoxia, and a prolonged expiratory phase. Some patients present only with cough, and some are symptomatic only during or after exercise.

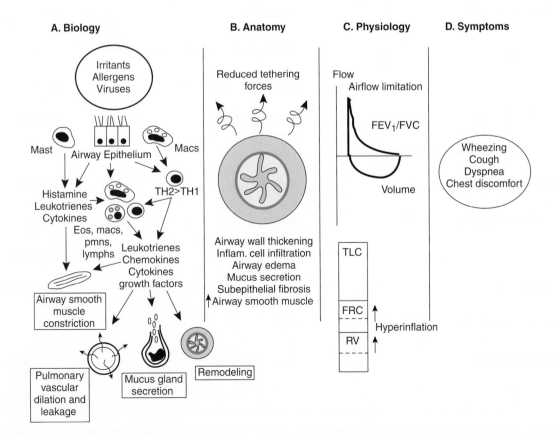

FIGURE 13.11. **Overview of asthma pathophysiology.** (Reproduced, with permission, from Hanley ME, Welsh CH. *Current Diagnosis & Treatment in Pulmonary Medicine,* 1st ed. New York: McGraw-Hill, 2003: 68.)

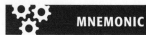

MNEMONIC

Precipitating factors for asthma:

ASTHMA

Allergies (dust mites, pollens, dander)
Sports
Temperature (cold, wet, windy weather)
Heredity
Microbes (eg, viruses, *Mycoplasma*)
Anxiety

- The disease is often associated with other forms of atopy (eg, allergies, atopic dermatitis).

DIFFERENTIAL

Croup, foreign body aspiration, reflux disease, CF, tracheomalacia.

DIAGNOSIS

- ↓ FEV_1/FVC ratio and > 10% improvement in FEV_1 following administration of a short-acting bronchodilator.
- In equivocal cases, a methacholine challenge may be diagnostic.

TREATMENT

Use of a stepwise approach and an action plan is most effective (Table 13.9).

COMPLICATIONS

In the long term, asthma results in airway remodeling and loss of lung function, as measured by FEV. Aggressive management may limit this progression.

TABLE 13.9. Preferred Stepwise Approach for Asthma Management

STEP	0–4 YEARS	5–11 YEARS	12+ YEARS
1	Short-acting β-agonist (SABA) PRN	SABA PRN	SABA PRN
2	Low-dose inhaled corticosteroids (ICS)	Low-dose ICS	Low-dose ICS
3	Medium-dose ICS	Low-dose ICS + LABA, leukotriene modifier, or theophylline OR Medium-dose ICS	Low-dose ICS + LABA OR Medium-dose ICS
4	Medium-dose ICS + Long-acting β-agonist (LABA) or montelukast	Medium-dose ICS + LABA	Medium-dose ICS + LABA
5	High-dose ICS + LABA or montelukast	High-dose ICS + LABA	High-dose ICS + LABA + ? Omalizumab
6	High-dose ICS + LABA or montelukast + Oral corticosteroids	High-dose ICS + LABA + Oral corticosteroids	High-dose ICS + LABA + Oral corticosteroids + ? Omalizumab

Adapted from the National Heart, Lung, and Blood Institute (NHLBI). *NAEPP Expert Panel Report 3: Guidelines for the Diagnosis and Management of Asthma,* 1st ed. Bethesda, MD: NIH, 2007.

Asthma-Associated Conditions

Asthma is an atopic condition. It is often associated with other atopic conditions, including allergies and atopic dermatitis.

ALLERGIES

- An array of disorders related to heightened immune response, including rhinoconjunctivitis, atopic dermatitis, urticaria, angioedema, and anaphylaxis. Exposure to an allergen causes the production of IgE and eosinophils and subsequent release of allergic mediators from mast cells and basophils. Common allergens include dust, pollens, animal dander, medications, foods, and insect bites.
- **Sx:** Sneezing, hives, wheezing, vomiting, anaphylaxis.
- **Tx:** Intranasal steroids or oral antihistamines. Immunotherapy is used when desensitization might be helpful. Anaphylaxis may be treated in the field using diphenhydramine (Benadryl) and an epinephrine pen, and referral to an emergency department is often required for the **ABCz: A**drenaline (epinephrine), **B**enadryl, **C**orticosteroids, **Z**antac.

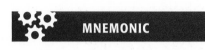

MNEMONIC

The ABCz of anaphylaxis treatment:

Adrenaline (epinephrine)
Benadryl
Corticosteroids
Zantac (an H_2 antagonist)

ATOPIC DERMATITIS (ECZEMA)

- Genetic susceptibility and environmental factors combine to produce skin with ↓ ability to hold water. The stratum corneum shrinks, leaving cracks in the epidermal barrier. Affected skin is at risk for 2° infection.
- **Sx/Exam:** Patients present with areas of dry, cracked skin (Figure 13.12), with distribution varying by age. In infants, the cheeks and trunk are most often affected; in children, the flexor surfaces are most frequently involved. In adolescents, the hands are the most common site.
- **Tx:** For flares, use topical steroids, moisturizers, and antibiotics as needed. For chronic treatment, prevent excessive drying with short, less frequent baths and showers, nonirritant soaps and lotions, and frequent moisturizing. Topical immunesuppressants (eg, tacrolimus) may be used for a limited time in children > 2 years of age.

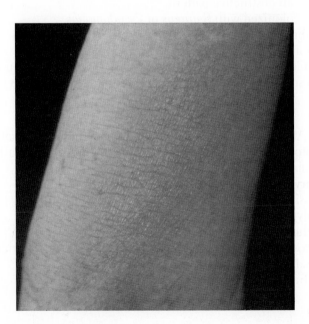

FIGURE 13.12. **Atopic dermatitis.** (Reproduced, with permission, from Wolff K, et al. *Fitzpatrick's Color Atlas & Synopsis of Clinical Dermatology,* 5th ed. New York: McGraw-Hill, 2005: 39.)

Cystic Fibrosis (CF)

The most common lethal genetic disease in the United States, with an incidence of 1 in 3000–4000 among whites. It is characterized by the triad of COPD, pancreatic exocrine insufficiency, and abnormal sweat chloride. The most common mutation is the **delta F508,** a deletion of 3 base pairs at position 508 in the gene. Life expectancy has ↑ from 4 years to 35 years owing to advances in therapy.

SYMPTOMS/EXAM

- GI:
    - Abdominal distention and discomfort, greasy or floating stools, ↑ flatulence 2° to exocrine pancreatic insufficiency and malabsorption.
    - Meconium ileus (15%) at birth.
    - Intestinal obstruction (meconium in the terminal ileum).
    - Hypoalbuminemia, anemia, edema, and hepatomegaly.
    - FTT (50%).
- Pulmonary:
    - **Frequent respiratory and sinus infections.** Cough, tachypnea, rales, wheezing, clubbing, difficulty breathing, ↑ sputum production, ↓ exercise tolerance.
    - RSV infections (associated with added morbidity in early infancy).
    - Hemoptysis due to bronchiectasis, cor pulmonale.

DIFFERENTIAL

Foreign body, carcinoma, pneumonia, sinusitis, COPD, asthma, α_1-antitrypsin deficiency, bronchiolitis, celiac sprue.

DIAGNOSIS

- **A positive sweat chloride test is the gold standard.** A result of "likely CF" is a sweat chloride level of > 60 mmol/L. **A positive test must be confirmed by a second sweat chloride test or a test for genetic mutation.**
- PFTs show an obstructive pattern.
- Lungs are colonized with *S aureus* or *Pseudomonas*.
- CXR findings are consistent with bronchiectasis, and CT shows bronchiectasis and mucous plugging (Figure 13.13).
- Mutated CFTR gene (most labs test for the 20–30 most common defects).
- Newborn screen for elevated blood levels of immunoreactive trypsin.

TREATMENT

- **General:** Attention to nutritional status and psychosocial situation.
- **GI symptoms:** Pancreatic enzyme supplementation; cathartics and enemas for obstructive symptoms.
- **Pulmonary symptoms:**
    - Aggressive antibiotic use.
    - Mucolytics and chest PT.
    - Bronchodilators and anti-inflammatory therapies.
    - Corticosteroids (adverse effects include glucose intolerance, frank diabetes, and ↓ linear growth).
    - Lung transplant for end-stage disease.

COMPLICATIONS

- Intussusception.
- Infertility in > 95% of males (due to lack of development of the vas deferens).
- Progressive pulmonary disease (the cause of death in 95% of cases).

MNEMONIC

Presentation of cystic fibrosis:

CF PANCREAS

Chronic cough and wheezing
Failure to thrive
Pancreatic insufficiency (symptoms of malabsorption such as steatorrhea)
Alkalosis and hypotonic dehydration
Neonatal intestinal obstruction (meconium ileus)/**N**asal polyps
Clubbing of fingers/**C**hest radiograph with characteristic changes
Rectal prolapse
Electrolyte elevation in sweat; salty skin
Absence or congenital atresia of the vas deferens
Sputum with *Staphylococcus* or *Pseudomonas* (mucoid)

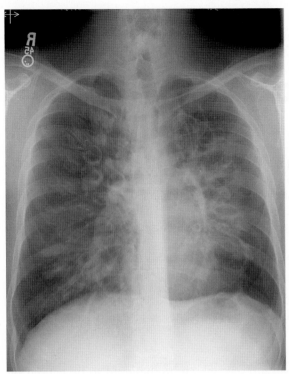
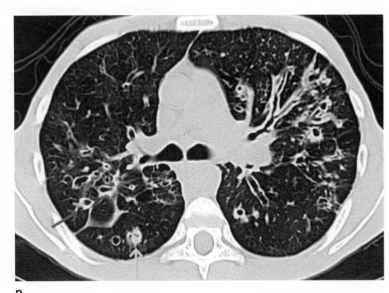

A   B

FIGURE 13.13.   **Cystic fibrosis.** (A) Frontal CXR showing central cystic bronchiectasis *(arrow)* in a patient with CF. (B) Transaxial CT image showing cystic bronchiectasis *(red arrow)* with some bronchi containing impacted mucus *(yellow arrow)*. (Reproduced, with permission, from USMLERx.com.)

Bronchopulmonary Dysplasia (BPD)

A chronic lung disorder that can develop in children who received prolonged mechanical ventilation to treat RDS. Risk factors include preterm delivery, low birth weight, and RDS, with an incidence of approximately 30% for infants with a birth weight of < 1000 g. Although neonates with BPD have an ↑ risk of mortality, lung function is normalized in early childhood in most survivors.

SYMPTOMS/EXAM

- Patients present with dyspnea, tachypnea, cyanosis, and hypoxia.
- Exam reveals hypoxia with ↑ O_2 requirement.

DIFFERENTIAL

Meconium aspiration syndrome, persistent pulmonary hypertension, congenital infection (eg, CMV), cystic adenomatoid malformation, recurrent aspiration, congenital heart disease, overhydration, idiopathic pulmonary fibrosis.

TREATMENT

- Inhaled corticosteroids with occasional use of β-adrenergic agonists.
- Chest physiotherapy is used for the thick secretions that may contribute to airway obstruction or recurrent atelectasis.
- RSV prophylaxis.
- Comprehensive interdisciplinary planning on discharge to ensure adequate follow-up.

COMPLICATIONS

Pulmonary hypertension, recurrent respiratory infections, cor pulmonale, exercise intolerance, ↑ risk of COPD, neurodevelopmental problems.

GASTROINTESTINAL DISEASE

Pyloric Stenosis

- Most common in firstborn sons.
- **Sx/Exam:** Usually presents at 2 weeks to 2 months of life with projectile, nonbilious vomiting. An olive-sized mass may be felt in the epigastrium.
- **Dx:** Ultrasound is diagnostic (Figure 13.14). Check electrolytes; hypochloremia and hypokalemia may be severe.
- **Tx:** Pylorotomy is curative. Correct electrolyte abnormalities before surgery.

Intestinal Obstruction

Forms of intestinal obstruction in infants can be distinguished according to clinical and radiographic findings, as discussed below (see also Table 13.10).

BOWEL ATRESIA

- Most obstructions are bowel atresias, which are believed to be caused by an ischemic event during development. Approximately 30% of cases of duodenal atresia are associated with Down syndrome.

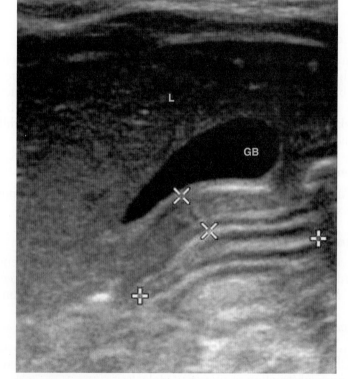
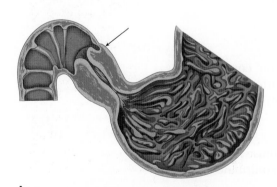

A

B

FIGURE 13.14. **Hypertrophic pyloric stenosis.** **(A)** Schematic representation of a hypertrophied pylorus. The arrow denotes protrusion of the pylorus into the duodenum. **(B)** Longitudinal ultrasound of the pylorus showing a thickened pyloric musculature (*X's*) over a long pyloric channel length (*plus signs*). GB = gallbladder; L = liver. (Image A reproduced, with permission, from Doherty GM. *Current Diagnosis & Treatment: Surgery,* 13th ed. New York: McGraw-Hill, 2010, Fig. 43-9. Image B reproduced, with permission, from USMLERx.com.)

TABLE 13.10.   Differential Diagnosis of Intestinal Obstruction in Infants

SITE OF OBSTRUCTION	CLINICAL FINDINGS	PLAIN RADIOGRAPHS	CONTRAST STUDY
Duodenal atresia	Down syndrome (30%); early vomiting that is sometimes bilious.	"Double bubble" sign (dilated stomach and proximal duodenum; no air distal).	Not needed.
Malrotation and volvulus	Bilious vomiting with onset at any time in the first few weeks.	Dilated stomach and proximal duodenum; paucity of air distally (may be a normal gas pattern).	UGI shows a displaced duodenojejunal junction with a "corkscrew" deformity of twisted bowel.
Jejunoileal atresia, meconium ileus	Bilious gastric contents of > 25 mL at birth; progressive distention and bilious vomiting.	Multiple dilated loops of bowel; intra-abdominal calcifications if in utero perforation occurred (meconium peritonitis).	Barium or osmotic contrast enema shows microcolon; contrast refluxed into the distal ileum may demonstrate and relieve meconium obstruction (successful in about 50% of cases).
Meconium plug syndrome, Hirschsprung disease	Distention; delayed stooling (> 24 hr).	Diffuse bowel distention.	Barium or osmotic contrast enema outlines and relieves plug; may show a transition zone in Hirschsprung disease. Delayed emptying (> 24 hr) suggests Hirschsprung disease.

Reproduced, with permission, from Hay WW, et al. *Current Diagnosis & Treatment in Pediatrics,* 18th ed. New York: McGraw-Hill, 2007: 47.

■ **Sx/Exam:** Proximal atresias have earlier bilious vomiting and less distention; distal atresias present later and have more distention.
■ **Dx:** AXR shows distended bowel loops and air-fluid levels (Figure 13.15).
■ **Tx:** Surgical resection of the affected area.

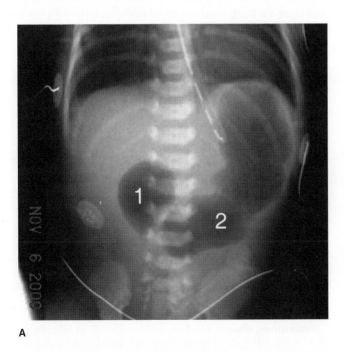
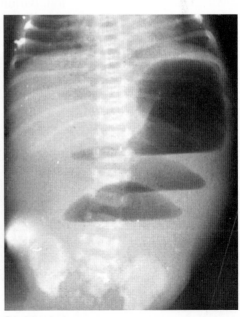

FIGURE 13.15.   Neonatal bowel obstruction. (A) Characteristic "double bubble" appearance (*1* and *2*) of duodenal atresia in an infant with bilious emesis. **(B)** Multiple dilated loops of small bowel with air-fluid levels in an infant with jejunal atresia. (Image A reproduced, with permission, from Brunicardi FC, et al. *Schwartz's Principles of Surgery,* 9th ed. New York: McGraw-Hill, 2010, Fig. 39-13. Image B reproduced, with permission, from Brunicardi FC, et al. *Schwartz's Principles of Surgery,* 9th ed. New York: McGraw-Hill, 2010, Fig. 19-14.)

HIRSCHSPRUNG DISEASE

> You are preparing to discharge a 2-day-old boy delivered by the normal spontaneous vaginal route when the nurse tells you that he has not yet passed any stool. The baby is breast-feeding, but seems to spit up most of what goes down, and his mother is becoming discouraged. You examine the infant and note that his belly is somewhat distended. You are not sure if you can feel a mass in the left side of the abdomen. What is the next step in evaluation?
>
> This scenario raises concern for Hirschsprung disease or an atresia. An AXR would be a good starting point, although a contrast enema may also be needed to make a definitive diagnosis.

A disease resulting from an absence of ganglion cells in the mucosal and muscular layers of the colon caused by the failure of neural crest cells to migrate appropriately. The aganglionic segment of bowel is usually narrowed, with dilation of the proximal normal colon. The disease is 4 times more common in boys than in girls, and 10%–15% of patients have Down syndrome.

SYMPTOMS/EXAM

- Early signs include delay or failure to pass meconium, vomiting, abdominal distention, and reluctance to feed.
- Later signs may include fever and explosive diarrhea. A dilated colon full of stool may be palpable through the abdomen, but no stool will be appreciated in the rectum on digital exam.

DIAGNOSIS

AXR may reveal a dilated proximal colon and absence of gas in the pelvic colon. Barium enema shows a narrowed segment distally, with a sharp transition to a dilated proximal colon (Figure 13.16).

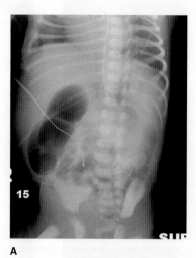 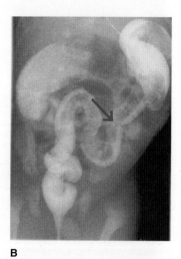

A   B

FIGURE 13.16. **Hirschsprung disease.** (A) AXR showing dilated, air-filled right colon in an infant with infrequent stools. (B) Barium enema showing relatively large transverse colon caliber, with transition to small-caliber colon at the splenic flexure. Note the stool *(arrow)* in the aganglionic sigmoid colon and rectum. (Reproduced, with permission, from USMLERx.com.)

TREATMENT

Surgery to resect the aganglionic section of bowel.

MALROTATION/VOLVULUS

Malrotation occurs early in development and may lead to volvulus. Volvulus occurs when a section of bowel rotates, occluding the superior mesenteric artery. Associated congenital anomalies (especially cardiac) occur in > 25% of symptomatic patients.

SYMPTOMS/EXAM

- Early signs include recurrent bile-stained vomiting or acute small bowel obstruction.
- Later signs include blood in stool, intermittent intestinal obstruction, malabsorption, protein-losing enteropathy, and diarrhea.

DIAGNOSIS

An upper GI series shows the duodenojejunal junction on the right side (Figure 13.17).

TREATMENT

Malrotation is treated surgically, even when volvulus is not immediately present, because of the risk of developing volvulus. Midgut volvulus is a surgical emergency, as it may result in bowel necrosis.

MECONIUM ILEUS

Obstruction of the terminal ileum with meconium. Approximately 90% of cases occur in patients with CF.

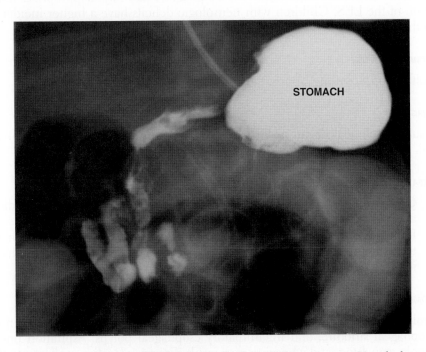

FIGURE 13.17.   Midgut malrotation. Frontal radiograph from an upper GI study shows a spiral pattern of duodenal and proximal jejunal loops in the right abdomen, consistent with midgut malrotation. The duodenojejunal junction should normally be to the left of the patient's spine. (Reproduced, with permission, from USMLERx.com.)

SYMPTOMS/EXAM

Absent or delayed passage of meconium, abdominal distention, vomiting.

DIAGNOSIS

- Barium enema is diagnostic and therapeutic.
- Sweat chloride testing for CF.

TREATMENT

Enema is first-line therapy. Surgical repair may be required.

Meckel Diverticulum

An ileal diverticulum that may contain ectopic gastric tissue. Males are affected more often than females.

SYMPTOMS/EXAM

- Painless rectal bleeding.
- Intussusception leading to intestinal obstruction.

DIAGNOSIS

A technetium scan can identify ectopic gastric tissue.

TREATMENT

Surgical resection of symptomatic lesions (asymptomatic diverticula do not need to be removed).

Gastroesophageal Reflux Disease (GERD)

Reflux of stomach contents into the esophagus caused by inappropriate relaxation of the LES. Children with neurologic deficits have a higher incidence of this condition.

SYMPTOMS/EXAM

Spitting up, vomiting, apnea, colic, FTT.

DIAGNOSIS

Usually a clinical diagnosis. pH testing may be useful if symptoms are atypical. EGD is helpful in identifying esophagitis.

TREATMENT

- Conservative treatment includes small feeds at shorter intervals. Medical options include H_2 receptor antagonists and PPIs.
- Indications for surgery include persistent vomiting with FTT, esophagitis, and apnea or pulmonary symptoms that persist after several months of medical treatment.

COMPLICATIONS

Prolonged symptoms may lead to esophagitis, occult blood loss, anemia, esophageal stricture, and inflammatory esophageal polyps. Aspiration pneumonia, coughing, and wheezing may result if gastric secretions reflux into the airways.

MNEMONIC

Meckel diverticulum rule of 2s:

2 inches long
2 feet from the ileocecal valve
2 types of tissue
Peak incidence at age **2**

KEY FACT

Reflux disease in children is usually self-limited. Approximately 85% of cases resolve by 6–12 months.

Cow's Milk Allergy

Most common food allergy in infancy. More likely in patients with a family history of atopy.

SYMPTOMS/EXAM

Usually presents by the first month after introduction of cow's milk, but may take several months to develop. Presents with colic, GERD, hematochezia, or rash.

DIAGNOSIS

Food challenge.

TREATMENT

Dietary changes that avoid cow's milk protein should lead to improvement within 3 weeks. Do not change to soy protein, as there is a 50% likelihood that patients who are allergic to cow's milk will also be allergic to soy.

ENDOCRINE DISORDERS

Growth Delay

Although height and weight percentiles may adjust during the first 2 years of life, a persistent ↑ or ↓ in height percentiles between 2 years of age and the onset of puberty warrants further evaluation (Figure 13.18).

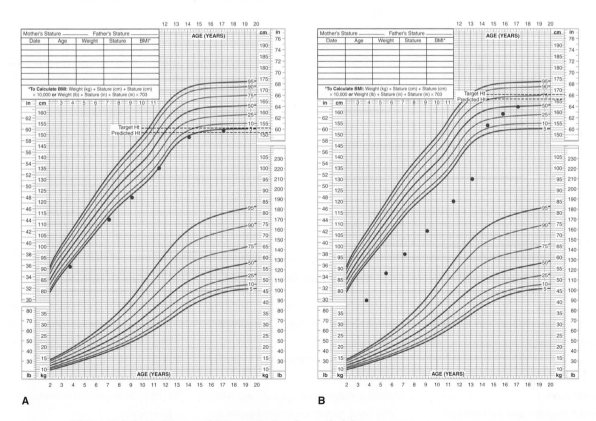

FIGURE 13.18. **(A) Familial short stature and (B) constitutional growth delay.** (Reproduced, with permission, from Hay Jr WW, et al. *Current Diagnosis & Treatment: Pediatrics*, 19th ed. New York: McGraw-Hill, 2009, Fig. 32-2 and 32-3.)

Workup includes hand x-rays for bone age, CBC and ESR to evaluate for infection, kidney function and UA to assess for occult renal disease, stool studies to examine for malabsorption, karyotype for girls to assess for Turner syndrome, TSH to evaluate for hypothyroidism, and IGF-1 to look for growth hormone deficiency. Table 13.11 compares 3 common causes of growth delay.

Ambiguous Genitalia

- The most common cause is congenital adrenal hyperplasia (CAH), which can lead to both XX virilization and XY feminization. Other causes include testicular regression syndrome, androgen insensitivity, testosterone biosynthesis disorders, and chromosomal abnormalities.
- CAH is a group of autosomal-recessive enzyme deficiencies that lead to problems with adrenal hormone synthesis. Most forms include cortisol deficiency. Depending on the type of CAH, there may be symptoms of either mineralocorticoid deficiency or excess and androgen deficiency or excess.

SYMPTOMS/EXAM

Initial evaluation should include a history, physical exam, and karyotype. Measure gonadotropins (LH, FSH), adrenal steroids (cortisol, 17-OHP, ACTH stimulation test), testosterone precursors (DHEA, androstenedione), testosterone, dihydrotestosterone, and hCG (hCG stimulation test).

TREATMENT

- Replace glucocorticoids, mineralocorticoids, and sodium as necessary in CAH.
- Provide hormone replacement as needed.
- Surgical reassignment is controversial. In the past, early surgery was recommended, but as children reached adolescence, some rejected their gender assignment. This has raised the issue of waiting and allowing the child to express a preference.
- A sensitive multidisciplinary team approach is crucial.

Diabetes Mellitus (DM)

- Type 1 DM is more common among children; it is immune mediated and associated with an interaction between genetic susceptibility and environmental factors, leading to the production of autoantibodies.

TABLE 13.11.   Common Causes of Growth Delay

FAMILIAL SHORT STATURE	CONSTITUTIONAL GROWTH DELAY	GROWTH HORMONE DEFICIENCY
Parents are short.	Parents are not necessarily short, but there may be a family history of late growth ("late bloomers").	Characterized by ↓ growth velocity and delay in skeletal maturation. Growth delay may begin in infancy or later in childhood.
Children are typically born with normal weight and length, but adjust to a lower percentile in the first 2 years of life. They will then have normal growth along that growth curve.	Growth pattern is similar to that of familial short stature.	May be isolated or occur with other pituitary hormone deficiencies.
Skeletal maturation and the timing of puberty are consistent with chronologic age.	Skeletal maturation and puberty are delayed, and linear growth continues beyond the typical age for reaching full height.	Treatment is recombinant human growth hormone.
No treatment is necessary.	No treatment is necessary.	

- Type 2 DM is seen more often in adults and teens; it is associated with insulin resistance and caused by genetic predisposition and obesity. Mature-onset diabetes of the young includes a number of inherited autosomal-dominant forms of type 2 DM that present early in life.
- **Sx/Exam:** Presents with polyuria, polydipsia, weight loss, hyperglycemia, and glycosuria +/− ketonuria and acidosis.
- **Dx:** Fasting glucose ≥ 126 mg/dL, HbgA1C > 6.5, glucose ≥ 200 after an oral glucose tolerance test, or random glucose ≥ 200 mg/dL in a patient with symptoms of hyperglycemia. When concerned for type 1 DM, test for autoantibodies.
- **Tx:** Education, monitoring, medications (insulin for type 1; oral medication is first-line treatment for type 2).
- **Cx:** Long-term complications include vision loss, kidney failure, cardiovascular disease, peripheral neuropathy, and gastroparesis. Acute complications include DKA, hyperosmolar nonketotic state, and hypoglycemia.

HEMATOLOGY/ONCOLOGY

Anemia in Children

Table 13.12 outlines the common types of anemias that can occur in children.

Sickle Cell Disease

An autosomal-recessive disorder characterized by production of abnormal hemoglobin HbS. Deoxygenated HbS polymerizes, leading to distorted RBC morphology and ↑ blood viscosity. Affects approximately 1 in 400 African American children.

SYMPTOMS/EXAM

The earliest symptom is often dactylitis (pain in the hands or feet). Pain crises, which are triggered by hemolysis and episodes of vaso-occlusion, may affect any part of the body.

TABLE 13.12. Anemia

↓ RBC PRODUCTION	↑ RBC LOSS (BLOOD LOSS, DESTRUCTION, SEQUESTRATION)
Nutritional deficiency	Hemoglobinopathies
Iron	Sickle cell disease
Vitamin B_{12}	Thalassemias
Folate	RBC membrane disorders
Bone marrow problems	Hereditary spherocytosis and elliptocytosis
Aplastic anemia	Enzyme defects
Diamond-Blackfan anemia	G6PD deficiency
Bone marrow infiltration (eg, leukemia)	Pyruvate kinase deficiency
Lead poisoning	Autoimmune hemolytic anemia
Anemia of chronic disease	Microangiopathic hemolytic anemia
Kidney disease	Blood loss (acute or chronic)
Other chronic inflammatory states	

Common complications of sickle cell anemia:

HbS PAIN CRISIS

Hemolysis, **H**and-foot syndrome

Bone marrow hyperplasia/infarction

Stroke (thrombotic or hemorrhagic)

Pain episodes, **P**riapism, **P**sychosocial problems

Anemia, **A**plastic crisis, **A**vascular necrosis

Infections—CNS, pulmonary, GU, bone, joints

Nocturia, urinary frequency from hyposthenuria

Cholelithiasis, **C**ardiomegaly, **C**ongestive heart failure, **C**hest syndrome

Retinopathy, **R**enal failure, **R**enal concentrating defects

Infarction—bone, spleen, CNS, muscle, bowel, renal

Sequestration crisis involving the spleen or liver

Increased fetal loss during pregnancy

Sepsis

KEY FACT

Acute chest syndrome is the leading cause of morbidity and mortality in patients with sickle cell anemia.

DIAGNOSIS

- Neonatal screening by hemoglobin electrophoresis detects the disease.
- Other lab abnormalities include mild to moderate anemia, hyperbilirubinemia, and ↑ reticulocyte count.

TREATMENT

- **Acute:** Acute vaso-occlusive crisis may require O_2, hydration, hydroxyurea, blood transfusion, and pain management. If there is evidence of acute chest syndrome or other underlying infection, treat with appropriate antibiotics.
- **Chronic:** Chronic management includes penicillin prophylaxis from 2 months to 5 years of age.
- The pneumococcal conjugate vaccine should be given in addition to other routine childhood vaccines.
- Health care maintenance also includes routine screening for eye, liver, and kidney disease beginning at 5 years of age as well as stroke risk assessment beginning at 2 years of age.

COMPLICATIONS

- Splenic infarction occurs in almost all patients, leading to functional asplenia, which ↑ susceptibility to infection from encapsulated organisms.
- Other complications include sepsis, stroke, avascular necrosis of the hip, MI, multiorgan failure, and acute chest syndrome (lung injury from vaso-occlusion, infarct, embolism, or infection).

Leukemia

Acute lymphoblastic leukemia (ALL) is the most common malignancy in children. Peak incidence in children is from 2–5 years of age.

SYMPTOMS/EXAM

Presents with bruising, purpura, pallor, bone pain, fever. Exam may show lymphadenopathy, petechial rash, and hepatosplenomegaly.

DIAGNOSIS

- Labs reveal abnormal WBC count (low or high), anemia, thrombocytopenia, and elevated LDH and uric acid.
- Bone marrow biopsy shows at least 25% blasts.

TREATMENT

Chemotherapy. Prognosis is good, with most ALL patients entering complete remission after induction chemotherapy.

Brain Tumor

The most common solid tumor in childhood. Children who have tuberous sclerosis or neurofibromatosis or have received brain radiation are at greatest risk.

SYMPTOMS/EXAM

- **Before 2 years of age: typically infratentorial.** Vomiting, unsteady gait, and cranial nerve palsies may be seen.
- **After 2 years of age: typically supratentorial.** Headache, vomiting, seizures, motor deficits, and changes in behavior. Headaches are classically daily, severe headaches that are worse with lying down and awakening from sleep.

DIAGNOSIS

- CT or MRI of the brain with contrast; MRI is more sensitive.
- Biopsy of the lesion is sometimes indicated.

TREATMENT

Depends on tumor type. Most require surgical resection and/or radiation. Chemotherapy is also helpful in certain tumors.

Osteosarcoma

The most common malignant bone tumor in children. Peak incidence is in adolescence.

SYMPTOMS/EXAM

- Presents with pain and swelling at the site of the tumor. Typically involves **ends** of the bone (distal femur, proximal humerus).
- **No systemic symptoms.**

DIAGNOSIS

- Aggressive lytic bone lesion with **"sunburst"** pattern of periosteal reaction on x-ray, typically in the metaphysis of a long bone (Figure 13.19).
- Bone biopsy.

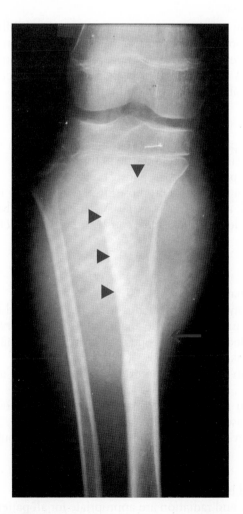

FIGURE 13.19.   Osteosarcoma. Lytic lesion of the proximal tibial metaphysis *(arrowheads)* with a Codman triangle of incomplete periosteal reaction *(arrow)*. (Reproduced, with permission, from Doherty GM. *Current Diagnosis & Treatment: Surgery,* 13th ed. New York: McGraw-Hill, 2010, Fig. 40-38.)

TREATMENT

Surgical resection and chemotherapy.

Ewing Sarcoma

The second most common malignant bone tumor in children. Peak incidence is at 10–20 years of age. Older age is a poor prognostic feature.

SYMPTOMS/EXAM

- Presents with pain and swelling at the site of the tumor. Typical locations are **midshaft** of long bones, pelvic bones, and ribs.
- **Systemic symptoms** often seen.

DIAGNOSIS

- X-ray demonstrates an aggressive lytic bone lesion, most commonly in the diaphysis of a long bone. Often associated with "**onion-skinning**" periosteal reaction.
- Bone biopsy reveals a small, round blue cell.

TREATMENT

Surgical resection, chemotherapy, and radiation.

Rhabdomyosarcoma

The most common soft tissue sarcoma occurring in childhood. It can occur anywhere in the body and accounts for 10% of solid tumors in childhood. The peak incidence is at 2–5 years of age; 70% of children are diagnosed before age 10 years. A second, smaller peak is seen in adolescents with extremity tumors. Males are affected more often than females.

SYMPTOMS/EXAM

- Presenting symptoms and signs of rhabdomyosarcoma result from disturbances of normal body function due to tumor growth.
- Presents with a painless, progressively enlarging mass.
- Orbital invasion may cause proptosis; mucosal invasion may cause chronic drainage (nasal, aural, sinus, vaginal). Cranial nerve palsies are also seen.
- Bowel or bladder invasion may cause urinary obstruction, constipation, and hematuria.

DIAGNOSIS

- Biopsy of the mass.
- When rhabdomyosarcoma imitates striated muscle and cross-striations are seen on light microscopy, the diagnosis is straightforward. Immunohistochemistry, electron microscopy, or chromosomal analysis is sometimes necessary to make the diagnosis.
- CT or MRI can determine the extent of the 1° tumor and assess regional lymph nodes.
- A lung CT can rule out pulmonary metastasis, the most common site of metastatic disease at diagnosis.
- A skeletal survey and a bone scan are obtained to rule out bony metastases.

TREATMENT

- Tumors should be excised if possible.
- Chemotherapy and radiation are appropriate for all patients and can shrink large tumors before surgery is attempted.

Neuroblastoma

The third most common pediatric malignancy. Accounts for approximately 10% of all childhood cancers. More than 80% of cases present before 4 years of age, and the peak incidence is at 2 years of age. Neuroblastomas arise from the neural crest cells of the adrenal medulla or sympathetic ganglia. The tumor most frequently originates in the adrenal glands, neck, chest, or pelvis. Prognosis is generally poor, with overall survival < 30%.

Symptoms/Exam

- Systemic symptoms.
- Can present with an asymptomatic or painful abdominal mass. The tumor/abdominal mass may cross the midline.
- Bone pain results from metastases.
- Tumor can invade the spinal cord, leading to muscle weakness or sensory changes.
- The majority of patients already show signs of metastatic disease at presentation.

Diagnosis

- ↑ levels of serum catecholamines or urinary catecholamine metabolites (VMA and HVA).
- Biopsy of the mass.
- CT or MRI can determine the local extent of disease, and nuclear medicine MIBG imaging can assess for distant metastases (Figure 13.20).

Treatment

Depends on staging. Often includes chemotherapy and surgical resection of tumor. If bone marrow is involved, may require autologous bone marrow transplantation.

KEY FACT

Neuroblastoma is an extremely malignant neoplasm. Most patients do not present with symptoms of the 1° lesion, but with complications of metastatic disease.

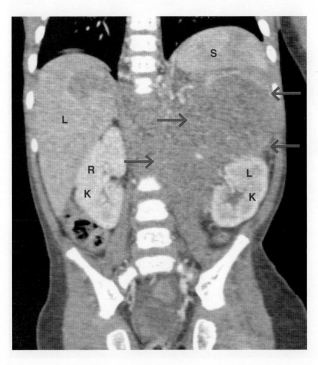

FIGURE 13.20.   Neuroblastoma. Coronal reformat from contrast-enhanced CT shows a massive left suprarenal mass displacing the left kidney inferiorly. L = liver; LK = left kidney; RK = right kidney; S = spleen. (Reproduced, with permission, from USMLERx.com.)

Wilms Tumor

Second most common abdominal malignancy after neuroblastoma. A tumor of the kidney consisting of a variety of embryonic tissues. Approximately 75% of children affected are < 5 years of age; the peak incidence is at 2–3 years of age. The constellation of Wilms tumor, aniridia, GU anomalies, and mental retardation (WAGR syndrome) is associated with deletion of chromosome 11p13.

SYMPTOMS/EXAM

- Presents with abdominal enlargement +/– pain, hematuria, malaise, weakness, anorexia, weight loss, and fever.
- Hypertension is noted in more than one-half of patients.
- An abdominal mass is felt that does not cross the midline.

DIFFERENTIAL

Abdominal masses, including hydronephrosis, multicystic or duplicated kidneys, neuroblastoma, teratoma, hepatoma, and rhabdomyosarcoma.

DIAGNOSIS

CT is required to determine the extent of the mass as well as to assess for bilateral disease, venous invasion, and metastases (Figure 13.21).

TREATMENT

- Surgical excision (nephrectomy) to completely remove the tumor and ureter.
- Very large tumors may be treated preoperatively with radiation therapy and chemotherapy to ↓ their size.

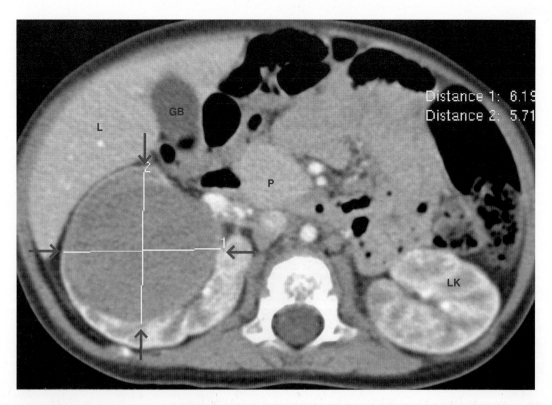

FIGURE 13.21. **Wilms tumor.** Wilms tumor centered in the right kidney (*arrows*) on transaxial image from contrast enhanced CT. GB = gallbladder; L = liver; LK = left kidney; P = pancreas. (Reproduced, with permission, from USMLERx.com.)

- Metastatic foci in the lung or liver may be resected or treated with radiation therapy.
- Overall survival is 85%.

MUSCULOSKELETAL DISORDERS AND RHEUMATOLOGY

Developmental Dysplasia of the Hip

- Inadequate pressure of the femoral head against the acetabulum that leads to a shallow socket, with risk of future dislocation and gait abnormalities.
- Risk factors include a ⊕ family history, breech presentation, and female gender.
- **Sx/Exam:** Look for an asymmetric skin fold in the thigh and gluteal region. Perform Barlow and Ortolani maneuvers to assess for a dislocatable hip. In older children, 1 knee may be lower than the other when patients are examined on their backs with the hips and knees flexed (Galeazzi test).
- **Dx:** Ultrasound is used for diagnosis until 4 months of age, since radiographs do not detect the uncalcified femoral head before this time (Figure 13.22).
- **Tx:** A Pavlik harness is used to hold the hips in abduction. Triple diapering is contraindicated because it may maintain the hip in a dislocated position.

Foot Problems

Most flexible deformities are 2° to intrauterine posture and usually resolve spontaneously.

METATARSUS ADDUCTUS (METATARSUS VARUS)

- A common congenital foot deformity characterized by inward deviation of the forefoot.

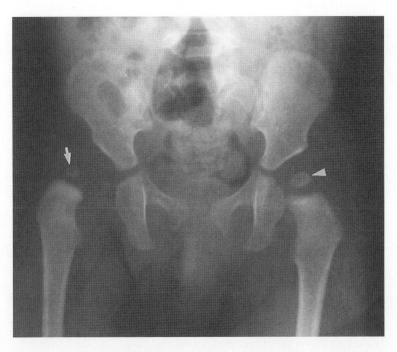

FIGURE 13.22. **Developmental dysplasia of the right hip, severe.** The right femoral epiphysis *(arrow)* is smaller than the left *(arrowhead)* and laterally displaced away from the acetabulum, and the right acetabular roof is shallow in comparison to the left. (Reproduced, with permission, from Chen MYM, et al. *Basic Radiology.* New York: McGraw-Hill, 2004, Fig. 7-11.)

- **Sx/Exam:** Convexity along the lateral border of the foot. In advanced cases, a vertical crease in the arch may be seen. The angulation is at the level of the base of the fifth metatarsal, and this bone will be prominent.
- **Tx:**
  - In most cases, the problem corrects itself as normal use of the foot develops.
  - Stretching exercises may be needed in cases that do not self-resolve, and the foot can be easily moved into a normal position.
  - Rarely, there is a rigid deformity that cannot be corrected with stretching exercises. In these cases, casting and even surgery may be needed, and a pediatric orthopedic surgeon should be involved.
- **Cx:** Approximately 10%–15% of affected children also have hip dysplasia.

TALIPES EQUINOVARUS (CLUBFOOT)

- May be idiopathic, neurogenic, or syndromic (eg, arthrogryposis, Larsen syndrome). Idiopathic clubfeet may be hereditary.
- **Dx:** Presents with a foot that turns inward and downward. Plantar flexion of the foot at the ankle joint (equinus), inversion deformity of the heel (varus), and adduction of the forefoot and hindfoot (varus) are seen (Figure 13.23). Infants should be carefully examined for associated anomalies, especially of the spine.
- **Tx:** Treat with manipulation of the foot to stretch the contracted tissues and with casting. Serial casting (the Ponseti technique) is generally effective, but if the deformity is rigid, surgical release may be necessary.

Rotational and Angular Disorders of the Lower Extremities

- **Genu varum and genu valgum:** Varum (bowlegs) is normal until age 2 years, after which many children develop genu valgum (knock knees), which may persist until about age 8. Persistence of either condition beyond these ages requires referral and possible surgical repair or splinting.

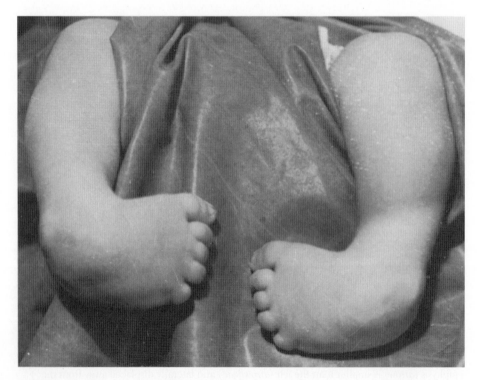

FIGURE 13.23.   **Talipes equinovarus (clubfoot).** (Reproduced, with permission, from Brunicardi FC, et al. *Schwartz's Principles of Surgery,* 8th ed. New York: McGraw-Hill, 2005: 1718.)

- **Tibial torsion:** Internal rotation of the leg between the knee and the ankle is normal in the newborn, but justifies referral for splinting if it persists beyond 18 months.
- **Femoral anteversion:** Internal rotation at the hip causes the appearance of intoeing. Treatment is generally not necessary unless passive external rotation is not possible.

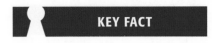

In genu valGUM, the knees are GUMmed together.

Limping

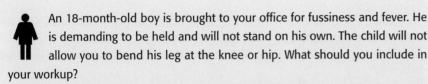 An 18-month-old boy is brought to your office for fussiness and fever. He is demanding to be held and will not stand on his own. The child will not allow you to bend his leg at the knee or hip. What should you include in your workup?

Workup should include CBC, radiographs, and ESR. In this child, suspicion must be high for osteomyelitis or septic joint. The infection may be in either joint (knee or hip), with pain in the other joint being an example of referred pain. Even if the x-ray is ⊖, it is often necessary to proceed with MRI (sensitive for osteomyelitis) and/or joint aspiration (for septic joint). Start broad-spectrum antibiotics while awaiting blood culture results. At this age, *S aureus* or *H influenzae* is the most likely culprit.

LEGG-CALVÉ-PERTHES DISEASE

- Avascular necrosis of the proximal femur. Most frequently occurs in boys ages 4–8 years.
- **Sx/Exam:** Presents with persistent pain, limp, and limited ROM. Can be painless.
- **Dx:** X-ray changes occur over several weeks. At several weeks, ↓ bone density, a necrotic center, and femoral head sclerosis are apparent (Figure 13.24).

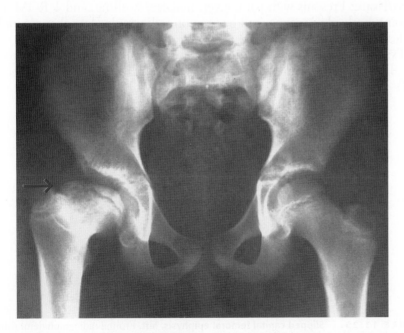

FIGURE 13.24. **Legg-Calvé-Perthes disease.** Note the sclerosis, fragmentation, and collapse of the right femoral epiphysis (*arrow*) in comparison with the left femur. (Reproduced, with permission, from Chen MYM, et al. *Basic Radiology.* New York: McGraw-Hill, 2004, Fig. 7-48.)

■ **Tx:** The goal is to keep the femoral head in the acetabulum and preserve ROM. In most cases, observation is adequate with ↓ weight bearing. In children older than 6 years of age, a brace is recommended. Some patients require surgery.

OSGOOD-SCHLATTER SYNDROME

■ Overuse injury that leads to inflammation at the tibial tuberosity at the insertion site of the patellar tendon. Seen in girls 11–13 and boys 12–15 years of age.
■ **Sx/Exam:** Presents with pain at the tibial tubercle, especially with activities that involve climbing and jumping.
■ **Dx:** X-rays are typically normal but may reveal fragmentation at the tibial tubercle.
■ **Tx:** Rest, ice, anti-inflammatories.

SLIPPED CAPITAL FEMORAL EPIPHYSIS (SCFE)

■ Disruption at the growth plate that leads to displacement of the proximal femoral head. Most common in overweight adolescent boys.
■ **Dx:** Generally presents with vague progressive pain and limp, but may occur suddenly with trauma. Check bilateral AP and frog-lateral x-rays. X-rays reveal the classic appearance of an ice-cream scoop slipping off its cone. Approximately 30% of patients with SCFE also have asymptomatic SCFE on the other side (Figure 13.25).
■ **Tx:** Surgical pinning.
■ **Cx:** Avascular necrosis may occur in up to one-third of cases.

SEPTIC ARTHRITIS

■ Causative organisms vary with age:
  ■ **Younger than 4 months:** *S aureus* and GBS.
  ■ **4 months to 4 years:** *H influenzae* and *S aureus*.
  ■ **4 years and older:** *S aureus* and *S pyogenes*.
  ■ **Adolescence:** Consider *Gonococcus*.
■ **Sx/Exam:** Presents with pain, fever, malaise, swelling, and ↓ ROM of the joint. Early changes may not be seen on radiographs; late changes include destruction of the joint space.
■ **Tx:** Drainage is key. The knee may be aspirated or washed arthroscopically, but the hip generally requires surgical drainage. Use broad-spectrum IV antibiotics while awaiting cultures.

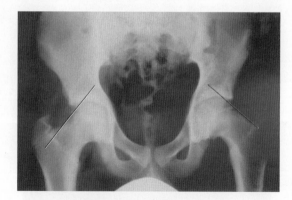

FIGURE 13.25. **Slipped capital femoral epiphysis, left.** Frontal radiograph demonstrates medial displacement of the left femoral epiphysis. The "Klein line" is drawn in red. Note that the abnormal left femoral epiphysis does not protrude lateral to this line, whereas the right epiphysis does intersect this line. (Reproduced, with permission, from Skinner HB. *Current Diagnosis & Treatment in Orthopedics*, 4th ed. New York: McGraw-Hill, 2006, Fig. 11-14.)

OSTEOMYELITIS

- Infection occurring in the bone resulting from either direct or hematogenous spread of bacteria. The metaphyses of long bones, especially the femur and tibia, are the most common locations in children.
- *Staphylococcus* infection is most common, but *Streptococcus* and *Haemophilus* are also seen. In patients with sickle cell, think *Salmonella*. In patients with a puncture wound, consider *Pseudomonas*.
- **Sx/Exam:** Infants may present with fussiness and pseudoparalysis of a limb. Older children will generally have fever and acute tenderness and will refuse to bear weight on the affected limb.
- **Dx:** ↑ WBC, CRP, and ESR. ⊕ blood culture in 40%–50%. X-ray findings lag behind clinical findings. MRI and bone scan are more sensitive. Aspiration of the bone for culture can help identify an organism and narrow the antibiotic spectrum.
- **Tx:** IV antibiotics with surgical debridement as indicated.

Scoliosis

- Defined as lateral curvature of the spine > 10 degrees. Idiopathic disease is most common and usually presents at 8–10 years of age.
- There is an association with Marfan syndrome, cerebral palsy, muscular dystrophy, and neurofibromatosis. The disease is seen 4 times more often in girls and frequently runs in families.
- **Dx:** First noted by the family or on exam. Forward bending test may show elevation of the rib cage on one side. To assess severity, check x-rays to calculate the angle of defect. There is no evidence to support universal screening.
- **Tx:** Treatment should be based on symptoms, obviousness of the deformity, and the likelihood of progression. Refer to orthopedics for a curve > 20 degrees. Mild disease may be followed with serial exams and bracing; more severe disease may require surgery to correct the deformity and preserve respiratory capacity.

Juvenile Idiopathic Arthritis (JIA)

The majority of cases of JIA improve with age, and many patients become asymptomatic after puberty. However, joint damage acquired during active disease may contribute to later disability, even in the absence of an ongoing disease process. JIA is defined by age < 16 years, arthritis, and symptoms persisting > 6 weeks. Subtypes are as follows:

- **Systemic JIA:**
    - Also known as Still disease.
    - **Sx/Exam:** Presents with fever, rash, arthritis, hepatosplenomegaly, and leukocytosis. Systemic symptoms generally regress within 1 year. Arthritis may regress, but may also continue and become extremely destructive.
    - **DDx:** Reactive or postinfectious arthritis; other connective tissue disease (eg, SLE); malignancy (eg, leukemia).
    - **Dx:** Daily symptoms for > 6 weeks. ANA and rheumatoid factor (RF) are usually ⊖.
    - **Tx:** NSAIDs, corticosteroids, methotrexate, other immune-modifying agents.
- **Polyarticular JIA:**
    - **Sx/Exam:** Involves ≥ 5 joints. Presents with **symmetric** chronic arthritis that may wax and wane. Systemic symptoms may be present but are generally mild. Iridocyclitis rarely occurs.
    - **Dx:** ↑ ESR; mildly ⊕ ANA.

KEY FACT

Unlike adults, children with RA generally have a ⊖ RF.

- **Tx:** NSAIDs; disease-modifying medications (eg, methotrexate, TNF-α blockers).
- **Pauciarticular JIA:**
    - **Sx/Exam: Asymmetric** chronic arthritis in **1–4 joints** (typically weight bearing). Iridocyclitis is a significant risk, and children require frequent ophthalmologic exams.
    - **Dx:** ESR and WBC are normal; RF is ⊖ but ANA is ⊕. Other causes of arthritis (eg, reactive) must be ruled out.
    - **Tx:** Treatment is the same as that for polyarticular JIA.

NEUROLOGY

Disorders of Head Growth

MICROCEPHALY

- Defined as a head circumference > 2 SDs below the mean or a declining rate of head growth over time. The fontanelle may close early, and sutures may be prominent.
- Etiologies include trisomies, fragile X syndrome, TORCHeS infections, fetal alcohol syndrome, metabolic disorders, perinatal infections (GBS meningitis, herpes encephalitis), anoxic brain injury, and neurodegenerative disorders (eg, Tay-Sachs disease). Treatable causes include hypopituitarism, hypothyroidism, and severe protein-calorie undernutrition.
- **Dx:** TORCHeS titers, metabolic workup, head CT, karyotype. Screen for maternal PKU.
- **Tx:** Correct endocrine or metabolic disorders if present. Otherwise, treatment is largely supportive. Follow for possible mental retardation.

MACROCEPHALY

- Defined as a head circumference > 2 SDs above the mean.
- Etiologies include progressive hydrocephalus, subdural effusion, arachnoid cyst, porencephalic cyst, brain tumor, external hydrocephalus, benign enlargement of the subarachnoid spaces, neurofibromatosis, and tuberous sclerosis.
- **Sx/Exam:** An excessive rate of growth suggests ↑ ICP (hydrocephalus, extra-axial fluid collections, neoplasms). Macrocephaly with normal head growth rate suggests familial macrocephaly.
- **Dx:** Imaging is not necessary if the infant is normal neurologically and head growth is consistent with catch-up or familial macrocephaly. Ultrasound may be used if the fontanelle is still open. Otherwise, CT or MRI is appropriate.
- **Tx:** Surgical resection or drainage of lesions as appropriate.

Hearing Loss

- Many states mandate universal hearing screening at birth. Routine clinical screening at well-child checks is essential. A child should turn toward a sound at 6 months and locate the source of a sound by 9 months. Speech delay can be a sign of hearing loss.
- **Sx/Exam:** Distinguish conductive from sensorineural hearing loss.
- **Conductive hearing loss:**
    - Most often 2° to otitis media and its sequelae (middle ear effusion). May also be caused by canal stenosis, impaction (cerumen or foreign body), and middle ear abnormalities (stapes fixation, ossicular malformation).

- Hearing loss 2° to middle ear effusion is typically mild and temporary, but may affect language acquisition if it occurs during critical developmental periods.
- **Sensorineural hearing loss:**
    - A result of damage to or abnormal development of the inner ear or the auditory nerve (CN VIII). May be congenital or acquired (more often congenital). Etiologies include congenital or neonatal infections, ototoxic drugs, trauma, genetic syndromes (eg, Alport syndrome), and inner ear dysplasia.
    - Most cases are autosomal recessive and nonsyndromic. Inner ear dysplasia is the most common defect.
- **Dx:** Hearing tests include otoacoustic emissions for screening. Auditory brain stem evoked response (ABER) is done if hearing loss is suspected.
- **Tx:** Language acquisition programs (verbal and sign). For conductive hearing loss, correct the underlying cause (eg, tympanostomy tubes for middle ear effusion). For sensorineural hearing loss, treatment is hearing aids and possible surgical implants.

Strabismus

- Misalignment of the visual axes of the eyes. **Esotropia** is a form of strabismus characterized by convergent axes; **exotropia** refers to strabismus with divergent axes.
- **Dx:** Intermittent esotropia may occur in normal infants up to 5–6 months of age. To confirm suspected strabismus, check the following:
    - **Light reflex:** The corneal light reflex from a penlight held along a toy that the child focuses on should appear symmetric.
    - **Cover test:** In an abnormal test, when the dominant eye is covered, the weaker eye will move to focus on an object.
- **Tx:** Esotropia is more serious and often requires surgery. Exotropia may initially be treated with patching and exercises but may also need surgical correction.
- **Cx:** Amblyopia (↓ visual acuity in the less dominant eye); diplopia (double vision); contracture of the extraocular muscles. Acquired strabismus (occurring after the first year of life) is of more concern and may be the result of a significant visual deficit or CNS disease.

Cerebral Palsy

- A spectrum of disorders that are nonprogressive and originate from some type of cerebral insult or injury. The injury may occur before birth, during delivery, or in the perinatal period.
- **Sx/Exam:** The most common form involves spasticity of the limbs. The second most frequent presentation is ataxia. Associated neurologic deficits can include seizure, mental retardation, speech delay, and sensory loss.
- **Tx:** Physical, occupational, and speech therapy; orthopedic interventions as necessary.

Adolescent Medicine

DEVELOPMENT

Normal Growth and Development

Stages of normal growth and development are as follows (see also Table 13.13):

TABLE 13.13. **Stages of Adolescence**

	EARLY ADOLESCENCE	**MIDADOLESCENCE**	**LATE ADOLESCENCE**
Characteristics	2° sexual characteristics have begun to appear.	2° sexual characteristics are well advanced.	Physically mature; statural and reproductive growth are virtually complete.
Growth	Growth rapidly accelerating; reaches peak velocity.	Growth decelerating; stature reaches 95% of adult height.	

- **Early adolescence:**
  - Occurs at 11–13 years of age and merges with midadolescence at 14–15 years.
  - Characterized by **concrete thinking** and **body image disruption.**
- **Midadolescence:**
  - Begins around 14–15 years of age and blends into late adolescence at about 17 years of age.
  - Issues involve **autonomy;** may lead to parental conflict.
- **Late adolescence:**
  - Begins at approximately 17–21 years of age. The upper end is particularly variable and depends on cultural, economic, and educational factors.
  - Adolescents begin to think about the future and form stable, intimate relationships.

Tanner Staging

Describes the development of pubic hair and breasts for girls (see Figures 13.26 and 13.27) and pubic hair and genitalia for boys. Progression through

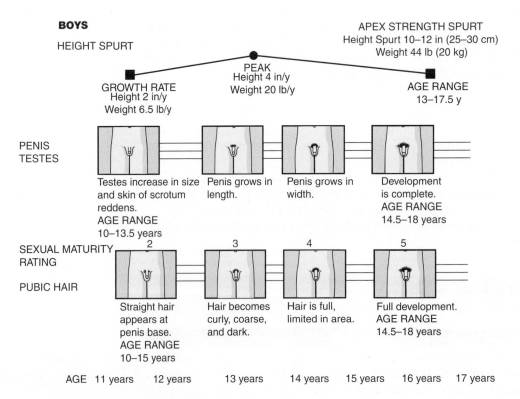

FIGURE 13.26. **Sexual maturation and growth in boys.** (Reproduced, with permission, from Hay Jr WW, et al. *Current Diagnosis & Treatment: Pediatrics,* 19th ed. New York: McGraw-Hill, 2009, Fig. 3-3.)

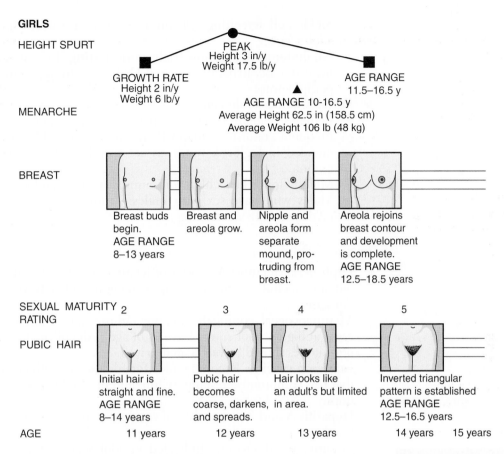

FIGURE 13.27.   Sexual maturation and growth in girls. (Reproduced, with permission, from Hay Jr WW, et al. *Current Diagnosis & Treatment: Pediatrics,* 19th ed. New York: McGraw-Hill, 2009, Fig. 3-4.)

the 5 stages is predictable. Lack of this predictable progression can indicate a pubertal disorder and may require further examination and possible referral to an endocrinologist.

PREVENTIVE MEDICINE

Routine Screening

Guidelines for routine screening of adolescents are as follows:

- **All adolescents:**
  - Measure BP.
  - Conduct subjective hearing tests at every well-child visit; conduct objective tests at 8, 10, 12, 15, and 18 years of age.
  - Conduct a Snellen test for visual acuity.
  - Calculate BMI.
- **High-risk or symptomatic adolescents:** TB, anemia, cholesterol.

Laboratory Tests

Often **not** necessary in the asymptomatic teenager, screening laboratory tests should be kept to a minimum.

- **General guidelines:**
  - **Hemoglobin or hematocrit:** Anemia screening is recommended at the first encounter or at the end of puberty.
  - **UA:** Obtain at the first encounter or at the end of puberty.

- **Sickle cell screening:** Obtain at the first visit with African American adolescents.
- **Cholesterol and fasting triglyceride testing:** Indicated in teens with heart disease, hypertension, and DM (or a strong family history of hyperlipidemia).
- **Sexually active adolescents:**
  - **Females:** Patients should receive a Pap smear starting at age 21 years. Frequent gonorrhea/chlamydia testing (every 6–12 months) is recommended in high-risk youth, as are syphilis testing and a vaginal wet mount.
  - **Males:** Gonorrhea, chlamydia, annual syphilis serology.
  - **Males who have sex with males:** Annual syphilis, gonorrhea, chlamydia, and HBV screening.

Immunizations

- **Diphtheria, tetanus:** A booster of tetanus toxoid, reduced diphtheria toxoid, and acellular pertussis (Tdap) is recommended 10 years after the initial series.
- **Meningococcal conjugate vaccine:** Administer to unvaccinated adolescents at high school entry (15 years of age). All college freshmen living in dormitories should be vaccinated as well.
- **Influenza vaccine:** Recommended for adolescents with certain risk factors that can compromise respiratory function or handling of respiratory secretions.
- **Hepatitis A and B:** Administer if vaccines were not received during childhood.
- **Pneumococcal vaccine:** Indicated in adolescents with chronic illnesses (sickle cell disease, HIV, asplenia, B-cell immune deficiency) and, in particular, in those with cardiovascular or pulmonary disease.
- **HPV vaccine:** Provisional recommendations are that all females 11–12 years of age should receive the 3-dose series.
- **Rubella:** Indicated for previously nonimmunized females.

HEADSS Assessment

Adolescence is generally a period of extremely good physiologic health and well-being. Underlying psychosocial issues may thus have more significance than physical ones during this period. The areas of sex, school performance, family, peer group, identity, and future should all be explored. The **HEADSS** assessment is a systematic approach to these issues.

Safety

Injuries are the most significant health problem of adolescents. A strong need for peer approval and lack of ability to appreciate consequences may lead youths to participate in a variety of risk-taking behaviors. Providing safety guidelines for teens is thus crucial in decreasing mortality from high-risk behavior. Guidelines are as follows (see also the mnemonic **SAFE TEENS**):

- **Motor vehicle safety:** Focus on the roles of driver, passenger, and pedestrian as well as on the influence of substance abuse and the importance of using seat belts.
- **Sexual activity:** Offer education regarding contraception, teen pregnancy, STI, unwanted intercourse, sexual readiness, sexual abuse, and sex with older partners.

MNEMONIC

Adolescent psychosocial screening:

HEADSS

Home
Education/employment
Activities
Drugs
Sexuality
Suicide/depression screen

- **Recreational athletic activities:** Counsel regarding the use of adequate equipment, protective gear and clothing, helmets, safe facilities, proper rules of safe play, and rational approaches toward activities requiring advanced skill levels.
- **Substance use:** Instruct patients in the potential dangers (including sudden death) that may occur not only with regular substance abuse but also with experimental use of drugs and alcohol. Include a discussion of nicotine and steroids.
- **Firearms:** Adolescents with firearms in the home need to learn proper use, safety, and legal issues associated with guns.

Anticipatory Guidance

Adolescents should receive health guidance annually, but information shared with them should be kept confidential. Recommendations for health guidance are designed to help adolescents approach development with greater knowledge and understanding, particularly as they develop cognitively and psychologically. The goals of anticipatory guidance are to:

- Promote a better understanding of physical growth, psychosocial and psychosexual development, and the importance of becoming actively involved in health care decisions.
- Reduce injuries by encouraging the use of helmets, seat belts, and sunscreen.
- Provide information regarding dietary habits, the benefits of a healthy diet, and ways to achieve a healthy diet and manage weight safely.
- Provide information about the benefits of fitness and physical activity.
- Educate adolescents about responsible sexual behaviors.
- Discourage use of illicit substances.

Consent and Confidentiality

Adolescents may fail to seek or delay seeking health care for a number of reasons. In addition to lack of access, finances, and awareness of clinical services, they may have concerns about confidentiality. Adolescents are more likely to seek care about sensitive issues if they feel that the health provider will not disclose that information to their parents. Laws about confidentiality vary from state to state.

- Minors have the right to consent for reproductive health care, treatment of STIs, treatment of rape or incest, and emergency health care. No parental consent is required in these cases.
- Minors who are considered "emancipated" do not require parental consent for medical decisions. Although this varies by state, emancipation may be based on whether a minor is a parent, is or has been married, is financially independent, or is in the armed forces.
- In most states, the age of maturity is considered to be 18 years, although in a few states, it is younger (14 in Alabama, 15 in Oregon, and 16 in South Carolina except for surgery). In Nebraska, the age of consent is 19 years.

Issues of confidentiality and consent are best managed in the context of a long-term physician–family relationship. Consent and confidentiality issues do not bind the physician to provide care that may violate the physician's own moral code. Teens should be aware of the physician's legal responsibility to report situations in which patients are at risk for suicide or homicide or are victims of sexual or physical abuse.

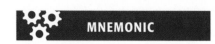

MNEMONIC

SAFE TEENS

Sexuality
Accident
Firearms/homicide
Emotions/suicide
Toxins
Environment (school, home, friends)
Eating (**N**utrition)
Shots/immunizations

SEXUALITY

Adolescence is a time of significant physical and emotional turmoil. At the same time, differing family values, cultural values, and personal experiences may give rise to varying sex education needs, which may include understanding body functions, exploring personal values, and setting sexual limits with partners. However, parents and clinicians may be unprepared to discuss sex-related health issues with adolescents. Additionally, teens may be uncomfortable discussing sexual issues with their peers and with adults. At the same time, a lack of comprehensive sex education programs as well as differences in cognitive and physical maturity put adolescents at ↑ risk for unwanted or unhealthy consequences of sexual activity.

Sexual Development

Table 13.14 outlines the stages of sexual development by time period.

TREATMENT

- Provide information to parents and adolescents, both together and separately. Emphasize the healthy expression of sexuality.
- Issues to discuss include timing of the initiation of sexual activity, abstinence resources (sex education, family planning clinics, professional education), contraception, education on STIs, and violence prevention.
- Discuss the use of latex condoms to prevent STIs, including HIV infection.

COMPLICATIONS

Teen pregnancy, STIs, unwanted sexual experiences such as sexual abuse or exploitation.

TABLE 13.14.   Stages of Sexual Development in Adolescence

STAGE	CHARACTERISTICS
Preadolescence	Low investment in sexuality.
	Information about sexuality comes from friends, school, and family.
	Physical appearance is prepubertal.
Early adolescence	Physical maturation begins.
	Curiosity about one's own body persists.
	Sexual fantasies are common.
	Masturbation begins.
	Sexual activities are often nonphysical (eg, phone calls, e-mail).
Late adolescence	Full physical maturation.
	Sexual behavior and thoughts are more expressive.
	Intimate physical and sharing relationships may develop.
	Sexual behavior can include masturbation, petting, oral sex, anal intercourse, and vaginal intercourse.

CHAPTER 14

Psychiatry and Behavioral Science

Pebble Kranz, MD

Mood Disorders

MAJOR DEPRESSIVE DISORDER (MDD)

Defined as **severe depression** that has a significant effect on a patient's ability to function. Variable age of onset. There is a 2- to 3-fold ↑ risk in 1st-degree family members. Full recovery from an episode is achieved within 6 months in one-half of all cases. Up to half of people with a major episode will relapse, and 15%–33% will not respond to multiple interventions.

SYMPTOMS

Defined as 1 or more episodes of **depressed mood** or **anhedonia** (loss of interest or pleasure) for **at least 2 weeks,** as well as by at least 5 of the **SIG E CAPS** symptoms of depression:

SIG E CAPS

Sleep—hypersomnia/insomnia.
Interest—loss of interest or pleasure in activities (anhedonia).
Guilt—a feeling of worthlessness or inappropriate guilt.
Energy—low energy.
Concentration—poor concentration.
Appetite—↑ or ↓ appetite.
Psychomotor agitation or retardation.
Suicidal ideation.

DIFFERENTIAL

- **Adjustment disorder with depressed mood:** A reaction to a specific incident or psychosocial stressor, leading to depressed mood. Symptoms begin within 3 months of the stressor and lessen within 6 months (after removal of stress or adaptation).
- **Bereavement:** After the loss of a loved one, depressive symptoms consistent with major depression may occur but should not last > 2 months or have suicidality or psychosis as features.
- **Mood disorder due to a medical condition:** May occur 2° to a variety of disorders (eg, anemia, hypothyroidism, pancreatic cancer, Parkinson disease).
- **Substance abuse mood disorder:** Major depressive symptoms due to use of or withdrawal from an abused substance.
- **Bipolar disorder:** Episodes of major depressive symptoms alternating with manic periods.
- **Schizoaffective disorder:** Predominantly a psychotic disorder with accompanying mood symptoms.

TREATMENT

- **Behavioral:** Many forms of individual, family, and group psychotherapy are appropriate and are as effective as medication in mild and moderate depression. Therapy in combination with medication has a significantly improved response rate over either modality separately.
- **Pharmacologic:** Antidepressants are associated with a response rate of 60%–80%. Select the medication with the most tolerable side effect profile while maximizing efficacy (see Table 14.1). The latest data indicate that sertraline is favored for efficacy and acceptability. Allow at least 4–6 weeks to assess the efficacy of a medication and continue antidepressants for at least 6 months after remission in moderate and severe depression. A

TABLE 14.1.   **Common Antidepressants and Side Effects**

CLASS	EXAMPLES	COMMON SIDE EFFECTS	MEDICALLY SERIOUS SIDE EFFECTS
SSRIs	Paroxetine (Paxil), fluoxetine (Prozac), sertraline (Zoloft), citalopram (Celexa), escitalopram (Lexapro), fluvoxamine (Luvox), others.	Headache, sedation or activation, weight gain, GI discomfort, orgasmic or ejaculatory delay.	Serotonin syndrome (tachycardia, hypertension, fever, hyperthermia, myoclonus, convulsions, coma).
SNRIs	Duloxetine (Cymbalta), venlafaxine (Effexor).	Same as SSRIs, and constipation, dizziness.	Lowered seizure threshold, hypertension.
TCAs[a]	Amitriptyline (Elavil), nortriptyline (Norpramin), clomipramine (Anafranil).	Dry mouth, constipation, bladder problems, sexual problems, blurry vision, drowsiness, orthostatic hypotension.	Tachycardia, arrhythmias, rhabdomyolysis. In overdose, cardiotoxicity.
MAOIs	Isocarboxazid (Marplan), phenelzine (Nardil), tranylcypromine (Parnate).	Orthostatic hypotension, edema, weight gain, GI distress, dizziness, headache, sedation.	Hypertensive crisis: Avoid tyramine-containing foods and medicines: cheese, wine, pickles, decongestants, OTC cold meds. Never combine with SSRI because of the risk of hyperserotonemia.
Other	Bupropion (Wellbutrin).	Insomnia, "jitteriness."	Lowered seizure threshold.
	Mirtazapine (Remeron).	↑ appetite, sedation, dry mouth, constipation.	Lowered seizure threshold.
	Trazodone (Desyrel).[a]	Sedation (often used for sleep), GI distress, headache.	Prolonged QT, dysrhythmias, priapism, serotonin syndrome.

[a]Consider a baseline ECG before prescribing a TCA or trazodone, particularly in the elderly, to evaluate for congenital prolonged QT. Consider interactions when prescribing another QT prolonging medication!

change in treatment should be considered if there has been no response in 4–12 weeks.

- **SSRIs** (eg, paroxetine, fluoxetine, sertraline): Generally 1st-line treatments owing to their **lower side effect profile. SNRIs, TCAs,** and **MAOIs** have all demonstrated a level of efficacy similar to that of SSRIs. Table 14.2 compares SSRIs and other pharmacologic treatments.
- **Adjunct therapies** for refractory depression: Atypical antipsychotics, mood stabilizers, and levothyroxine may be added, although this is usually done under the care of a psychiatrist.
- **Antidepressant discontinuation syndrome** can occur within days after abrupt medication cessation if a patient has been taking a medication for > 6 weeks. Supervised tapering over 6–8 weeks may be required to minimize symptoms of antidepressant discontinuation syndrome, which include symptoms from the mnemonic **FINISH:**
  - **F**lulike symptoms.
  - **I**nsomnia.
  - **N**ausea.
  - **I**mbalance.
  - **S**ensory disturbances (eg, paresthesias, "electric shocks").
  - **H**yperarousal (agitation).
- **Electroconvulsive therapy (ECT):** Primarily used for patients who show a lack of response to several antidepressants or have **severe depression** with

KEY FACT

Don't forget to ask about manic symptoms before prescribing an antidepressant. Initiating an antidepressant can launch a clinically important manic episode.

KEY FACT

ALERT! Many recent questions on the Family Medicine Boards have addressed choosing appropriate antidepressants, especially within a specific class (eg, "Which SSRI would be the most appropriate for . . . ?").

TABLE 14.2. **Medication Choices**

CONSIDERATION	CHOICE OF SSRI
Depression with low energy level.	An activating SSRI (like fluoxetine) or bupropion.
Depression with anxiety symptoms.	A calming SSRI like paroxetine or a TCA like imipramine; avoid bupropion.
OCD features.	Any SSRI or clomipramine.
Trouble sleeping.	Trazodone or mirtazapine.
Comorbid chronic pain.	Consider duloxetine (however, evidence that this is more effective than any other SSRI is slim).
Sexual side effects are problematic.	Bupropion.
Need to quit smoking or lose weight.	Bupropion (do not use for those with anorexia or bulimia!).
Seizure disorder.	Do NOT use bupropion, mirtazapine, or SNRIs.
Did it work for a close relative?	Give that medication a try.

psychosis, a high risk of suicide, or prior response to ECT. More effective than antidepressants (about 80%). ECT is not only effective but also very safe. Primary side effect is temporary retrograde amnesia as well as post-treatment confusion that lasts for minutes to hours. Permanent memory loss is rare.

- **Treatment phases of MDD:**
  - **Acute phase:** About 12 weeks.
  - **Continuation phase:** Full remission of symptoms, but at high risk for relapsing within the next 4–6 months. Continue antidepressant treatment at acute-phase doses and eventually taper down.
  - **Maintenance phase:** For patients with a high risk of relapse (eg, those with a history of 1 or more episodes of MDD), continue antidepressant treatment at acute-phase doses for prevention.

COMPLICATIONS

- **Psychosis:** Patients with severe MDD can develop psychotic symptoms such as auditory hallucinations, paranoia, and delusions. In such cases, the response rate is 40% with antidepressants alone, 20% with antipsychotics alone, and 70% with both taken together.
- **Suicidality:** Severe untreated MDD can lead to suicidality. Women tend to attempt more suicides, whereas men tend to succeed more often.
  - Risk factors for suicide include:
    - Prior attempts.
    - Family history of completed suicide.
    - Degree of premeditation or plan.
    - Access to a weapon or proposed plan.
    - Active substance abuse.
    - Impulsivity.
    - Recent psychiatric inpatient discharge.

- Protective factors include social support and family connectedness, parenthood, religiosity.
- If a high risk of suicidality is present, the clinician must hospitalize the patient to ensure his or her safety.
- Safety contracts are not effective in preventing suicide. Do a thorough suicide assessment including risks and protective factors.

KEY FACT

Always assess suicide risk! Ask directly about suicidal thoughts and plans!

DYSTHYMIA

A 24-year-old white female college student presents to your office complaining, "I never have any energy, even though I sleep all the time. And I seem to inhale all the food around me—I don't want to be this way! I don't know why I stay in school; I'll never finish. I'm not worth the money my parents are spending on this! I have friends, and I like my classes, but I'm such a downer. I can't remember more than a day here and there in the past 2 years that I haven't felt this way. Will it ever get any better than this?" How do you respond?

Supportive counseling and referral for psychotherapy. Consider pharmacologic treatment.

Defined as **depressed mood** occurring on most days and lasting **at least 2 years**. Although **less severe** than MDD, dysthymia significantly impairs work and social functioning because of its chronicity.

SYMPTOMS

Diagnostic criteria for dysthymia are as follows:

- **Two** of the following symptoms must be present, most of the day, more days than not, for at least **2** years:
  - Poor appetite or overeating.
  - Insomnia or hypersomnia.
  - Low energy, fatigue.
  - Poor concentration.
  - Low self-esteem.
  - Hopelessness.
- During a 2-year period, affected patients must **not have had a symptom-free period** for > 2 months.
- Symptoms must lead to significant impairment in daily functioning.

DIFFERENTIAL

- **Major depression:** A more severe form of depression.
- **Depression due to a medical condition:** Depressive symptoms may be similar to those of dysthymia, but are caused by a medical condition (eg, hypothyroidism, anemia).
- **Bipolar disorder:** Characterized by periods of mania or hypomania in addition to the depressive symptoms.
- **Substance abuse disorders:** Presentation is often similar to that of dysthymia, but symptoms are precipitated by the use of or withdrawal from alcohol or an illicit substance.

KEY FACT

Dysthymia is a "low-grade" depression commonly encountered in the 1° care setting that lasts years, with few symptom-free periods.

TREATMENT

- **Behavioral:** Various forms of individual and group psychotherapy may be of benefit.
- **Pharmacologic:** SSRIs; other classes of antidepressants.

Types of bipolar disorder:
Type I: At least 1 manic episode with or without major depression.
Type II: At least 1 hypomanic episode with a major depressive episode.

Hypomania consists of manic symptoms that do not lead to social or occupational dysfunction.

Even if patients experience only 1 manic episode, they are diagnosed with bipolar disorder. The diagnosis is made regardless of the number of manic episodes experienced.

BIPOLAR DISORDER

Characterized by **manic or hypomanic behaviors** that are sometimes accompanied by a depressive disorder. Lifetime prevalence is 1%, and the male-to-female ratio is 1:1. Individuals are at higher risk if family members are affected. The mean age of onset is around 19 years.

SYMPTOMS

- The symptoms of a manic episode of bipolar disorder are expressed in the mnemonic **DIG FAST**:
  - **D**istractibility.
  - **I**njudiciousness or **I**mpulsivity (poor judgment—eg, spending sprees, sudden travel, sexual indiscretion, reckless driving).
  - **G**randiosity (↑ self-esteem).
  - **F**light of ideas (racing thoughts).
  - **A**ctivities—psychomotor agitation; ↑ goal-directed activities (eg, socializing, hypersexuality, ↑ productivity).
  - **S**leep—↓ need for sleep.
  - **T**alkativeness—pressured speech.
- To qualify as mania, symptoms **must last 4–7 days** and must produce social or occupational dysfunction. If there is no social or occupational dysfunction, the symptoms qualify as **hypomania.**

DIFFERENTIAL

- **MDD:** Characterized by depressive symptoms without manic or hypomanic episodes.
- **Schizophrenia:** Although bipolar patients may exhibit signs of psychosis during a manic phase, schizophrenics do not experience mania.
- **Attention deficit/hyperactivity disorder (ADHD):** Distractibility and impulsivity are components of bipolar disorder, but ADHD patients do not exhibit other manic symptoms.
- **Cyclothymia:** Consists of mood swings between dysthymia and hypomania. However, depressive symptoms are not of sufficient severity to warrant a diagnosis of MDD, and manic symptoms do not reach the threshold sufficient for a manic episode.
- **Medical conditions leading to manic symptoms:** Include use of illicit substances (methamphetamines, cocaine), thyroid disorders, Cushing syndrome, HIV or HSV encephalitis, antidepressant treatment, steroid treatment, and neurologic disorders such as MS, frontal lobe syndromes, and temporal lobe epilepsy.

TREATMENT

- **Pharmacologic: Mood stabilizers** (lithium, valproic acid, carbamazepine, lamotrigine, atypical antipsychotics; see Table 14.3) **treat at least 1 phase**

TABLE 14.3. Mood-Stabilizing Medications and Side Effects

DRUG CLASS	DRUG	SIDE EFFECT	MEDICALLY SERIOUS SIDE EFFECTS
Mood stabilizer	Lithium	Cognitive dulling, tremor, sedation, nausea, diarrhea, T-wave flattening.	Lithium toxicity, **hypo**thyroidism (in long-term use), nephrogenic diabetes insipidus (DI).
Mood stabilizer/ anticonvulsant	Valproic acid (Depakote) Carbamazepine (Tegretol)	Weight gain, sedation, cognitive dulling.	Thrombocytopenia. SIADH, agranulocytosis, Stevens-Johnson rash.

of bipolar disorder (mania or depression) **without worsening the other phase.** Antidepressants are **not** mood stabilizers, as they are known to precipitate mania.

■ **Behavioral:** Individual therapy, CBT, and interpersonal therapy are useful in the treatment of bipolar patients. Establishing a therapeutic alliance is key.

COMPLICATIONS

■ Associated with a high rate of **completed suicides** (up to 15%).
■ Although bipolar disorder is not associated with a downward drift of socioeconomic status, patients have high divorce rates, multiple jobs, and a high incidence of achievement followed by decline.
■ Bipolar disorder is associated with several **comorbid conditions;** 60% have **substance abuse,** and 50% have **anxiety disorders.**

KEY FACT

Antidepressants lead to rapid cycling, in which patients have more manic-depressive episodes. It is therefore important to have a history that is ⊖ for manic episodes before starting a depressed patient on antidepressants.

PREMENSTRUAL DYSPHORIC DISORDER (PMDD)

A severe form of premenstrual syndrome (PMS) defined by nonspecific psychological, behavioral, and somatic symptoms occurring only during the luteal phase of the menstrual cycle. Affects 3%–5% of menstruating women. The condition tends to remain stable over time, with the majority of women seeking care in their 30s.

SYMPTOMS

■ Presents with depressed mood, feelings of hopelessness, self-deprecating thoughts, anxiety, tension, ↑ emotional lability, persistent and significant anger or irritability, anhedonia, lethargy, appetite changes, poor concentration, sleep disturbances, and a sense of being overwhelmed.
■ Physical symptoms include bloating, breast tenderness, hot flashes, headache, and joint pain.

DIFFERENTIAL

■ **PMS:** Characterized by mild luteal symptoms that do not interfere with performance or interpersonal relationships.
■ **Mood disorders:** Symptoms do not resolve with menses.
■ **Medical conditions:** Include dysmenorrhea, migraine, IBS, fibrocystic breast disease, and hypothyroidism.

DIAGNOSIS

■ Specified symptoms must be present and limited to the luteal phase.
■ Must lead to significant impairment in 1 or more areas of daily life.
■ Rule out medical etiologies or other psychiatric conditions.

TREATMENT

■ Recommend lifestyle changes such as aerobic exercise, ↓ caffeine, ↓ sodium intake, smaller and more frequent meals, and a diet rich in complex carbohydrates.
■ Stress reduction, anger management, and individual and group therapy may be of benefit.
■ Nutritional supplementation, with a daily multivitamin, vitamins D and E, calcium, and magnesium. Vitamin B_6 is also thought to be helpful, but recent data suggest that there may be harm from too much B_6—safe intake is 100 mg daily.

- Pharmacologic treatment with antidepressants or anxiolytics. NSAIDs can be used before or at onset to relieve physical symptoms. Spironolactone may be useful for significant bloating. OCPs or medroxyprogesterone acetate may stabilize hormonal swings.
- Ovulation suppression with GnRH agonists; danazol for severe symptoms refractory to other treatments.
- Bilateral oophorectomy should be used only in the most severe and refractory cases.

POSTPARTUM MAJOR DEPRESSION (PMD)

A major depressive episode with onset within 6 months of childbirth. Affects 1 in 10 childbearing women. Onset can begin 24 hours to several months after delivery, lasting several months to the 2nd year postpartum.

SYMPTOMS

Presents with depressed mood, anhedonia, sleep disturbance, ↓ energy, weight loss, a sense of hopelessness or guilt, ↓ concentration, thoughts of suicide or death, and thoughts of harming the infant.

DIFFERENTIAL

- Normal physiologic response to childbirth.
- **"Baby blues"**: Mild symptoms that usually peak after postpartum day 4 or 5 and resolve by postpartum day 10. Affects 30%–80% of childbearing women.
- Preexisting psychiatric disorders.
- Medical conditions such as thyroid dysfunction and anemia.
- **Puerperal psychosis:** Affects 0.2% of postpartum women. Constitutes a psychiatric emergency.

TREATMENT

- **Behavioral:** Individual or group therapy; couples therapy if indicated.
- **Pharmacologic:** Used in patients with moderate to severe PMD; treatment is the same as that for major depression (SSRIs, TCAs). There is no evidence of morbidity in breast-fed infants with SSRIs or TCAs, but the drugs and their metabolites have been found in breast milk. Weigh the risks and benefits, and discuss options with the patient.
- **Referral:** For any woman with suicidal/infanticidal ideation, no response to antidepressant therapy, or psychotic symptoms, immediate referral to psychiatry should be initiated and inpatient treatment considered.

PREVENTION

Identify at-risk women before delivery (eg, those with poor family support, stressful life events, a history of a mood disorder, or previous PMD).

COMPLICATIONS

Untreated PMD can have serious adverse effects on the mother and can also adversely affect the emotional and psychological development of the child.

PSYCHOTROPIC MEDICATIONS DURING PREGNANCY AND BREAST-FEEDING

Women and their physicians tend to **overestimate the teratogenic risk** of psychotropic medications during pregnancy and to **underestimate the risk of untreated maternal mental illness.**

- Antidepressants:
  - **TCAs: Not associated with major congenital malformations.** Some reports link TCA use to postpartum irritability, shakiness, and urinary and bowel obstruction.
  - **SSRIs:** Extensive research has shown **no association between major congenital malformations and fluoxetine,** but preliminary studies show a possible ↑ in persistent pulmonary hypertension (PPH) in the newborn when SSRIs are given **after 20 weeks' gestation. Paroxetine is contraindicated in pregnancy** in the wake of recent studies showing an association with cardiac malformations. Case reports link SSRIs with perinatal irritability, hypoglycemia, and shakiness.
  - Both SSRIs and TCAs have also been shown **not to have neurobehavioral toxicity,** and children exposed in utero have been found to develop normally. In contrast, studies have shown that untreated depression does have a negative effect on children's development.
- Mood stabilizers:
  - **Carbamazepine and valproic acid:** Both have a **well-established risk of neural tube defects** (1% and 5%, respectively). Carbamazepine may also ↑ the risk of neonatal hemorrhage.
  - **Lithium:** Use during the first trimester is associated with a **10%–20% higher risk of Ebstein anomaly** (tricuspid valve malformation). However, the **overall risk is still low (0.1%),** as the incidence of this anomaly is low to begin with.
    - Lithium remains the preferred medication for the treatment of pregnant patients with severe bipolar disease, as benefit outweighs the risks.
    - In other patients, it may be safer to discontinue the medication in the first trimester and resume it in the second or third trimester.
    - In the perinatal period, hypotonia, cyanosis, and diabetes insipidus have generally been reported to be rare and self-limited.
- Antipsychotics:
  - **High-potency neuroleptics** are considered **safe** in pregnancy. By contrast, study data are limited regarding the atypical antipsychotics (olanzapine, risperidone, quetiapine).
  - **Perinatal toxicities** (tremor, restlessness, dystonia) have been reported, but tend to resolve within weeks. Limited data exist regarding the neurobehavioral effects of these agents.
  - Again, the **benefits** (such as ↓ substance abuse and continuity with prenatal care) must be **weighed against the above risks.**
- ECT: Considered safe and effective during pregnancy.
- Medication use and breast-feeding:
  - All psychotropic medications are **secreted in breast milk.** Therefore, infants of mothers taking such medications must be **monitored for behavioral changes.** Check drug levels in infants with symptoms.
  - **Carbamazepine** and **valproic acid** are **not contraindicated** in breast-feeding but are associated with infant **thrombocytopenia** and **anemia.**

KEY FACT

Patients who do stay on lithium during their pregnancy should have a 2nd-trimester level II ultrasound to screen for congenital anomalies.

KEY FACT

Breast-feeding while taking lithium is considered a relative contraindication in light of the ↑ risk of lithium toxicity in dehydrated infants.

Anxiety Disorders

GENERALIZED ANXIETY DISORDER

 A 60-year-old woman presents to your office, saying, "Everyone knows I have a PhD in worry! If I know you're supposed to arrive at 3 PM, I start worrying at 1 PM that you've had a crash. You could have fallen asleep while driving. You could have forgotten to pick up the groceries; it could start snowing any minute! Sometimes I get so worried that I can't sleep. I can't even go to work! I don't know what is going to happen next with the world—it's all so out of control!" What counseling could you provide in the office?
Explore the worst-case scenarios and encourage accurate risk perception.

Defined as excessive worrying that is out of proportion to the situation and lasts **at least 6 months.** There is a 2:1 female predominance, usually beginning in childhood or adolescence. The condition is generally **chronic,** but has flares of worsening severity.

SYMPTOMS

Presents with **excessive worrying and anxiety** about a variety of subjects, more days than not, with difficulty controlling the worry. Three of the following symptoms—at a functionally impairing—level must be present:

- Restlessness
- Easy fatigability
- Poor concentration
- Muscle tension
- Insomnia
- Irritability

DIFFERENTIAL

- **Posttraumatic stress disorder (PTSD):** Must have a precipitating traumatic event.
- **Major depression:** Accompanied by depressive symptoms.
- **Panic disorder:** Consists of discrete, short-lived panic attacks.
- **OCD:** Anxiety that is due to obsessions and is relieved by compulsions.

DIAGNOSIS

Rule out medical causes (eg, hyperthyroidism, substance abuse).

TREATMENT

- **Behavioral:** CBT, mindfulness-based stress reduction (MBSR).
- **Pharmacologic:** Antidepressants, buspirone, and long-acting benzodiazepines (eg, clonazepam).

PANIC DISORDER

 A 25-year-old man discloses to you, "I don't know what it is. Nothing happened. I was just sitting there watching TV. But all of sudden, I had a terrible feeling, my heart was racing, and I couldn't breathe. Both hands started tingling and I was sweaty all over. I knew I was having a heart attack and was going to die." What is the best nonpharmacologic treatment for this patient? CBT.

Characterized by **recurrent unexpected** panic attacks, with fear of additional ones occurring. Onset is from late adolescence through the 3rd decade of life.

SYMPTOMS

- Characterized by episodes of **abrupt anxiety** that peak after 10 minutes and are associated with several features of **autonomic arousal.**
- Must include at least 4 of the following features of autonomic arousal: **palpitations**, tachycardia, chest discomfort, **shortness of breath**, nausea, a choking sensation, trembling, dizziness, **paresthesias**, sweating, chills, hot flashes, dissociation, and **fear of losing control or dying.**

DIFFERENTIAL

- Psychiatric:
  - **PTSD:** Must have a precipitating traumatic event.
  - **Generalized anxiety disorder:** Characterized by continuous anxiety, but no discrete attacks.
  - **Phobia:** A specific trigger for panic is present (eg, fear of flying, fear of heights, fear of bridges, fear of spiders).
- Medical:
  - **Endocrine:** Hypoglycemia, hyperthyroidism, pheochromocytoma.
  - **Cardiac:** Arrhythmia, MI.
  - **Pulmonary:** COPD, asthma, pulmonary embolus.
  - **Pharmacologic:** Side effects of medications (eg, SSRIs, albuterol); acute intoxication with a stimulant.

DIAGNOSIS

Rule out medical causes first (eg, ECG, CXR, metabolic panel).

TREATMENT

- **Behavioral:** CBT.
- **Pharmacologic:** SSRIs (fluoxetine, sertraline, paroxetine), benzodiazepines.

OBSESSIVE-COMPULSIVE DISORDER (OCD)

 A 32-year-old woman says, "I can't stop cleaning my house! I spent 4 hours yesterday cleaning the kitchen sink. This is crazy!" For which complications of this illness should you monitor?
Depression and substance abuse.

KEY FACT

Agoraphobia, which is sometimes a complication of panic disorder, is fear of being in a place from which escape would be difficult, or where it might be difficult to get help if a panic attack were to occur.

KEY FACT

Panic attacks come "out of the blue," whereas PTSD is caused by a precipitating traumatic event.

KEY FACT

SSRIs or long-acting benzodiazepines such as clonazepam are used to prevent panic attacks; short-acting benzodiazepines such as alprazolam are used to relieve attacks.

A chronic syndrome of intrusive, recurrent, undesired thoughts (**obsessions**) and/or uncontrollable repetitive behaviors or rituals (**compulsions**) that lead to significant distress in a patient's daily life. Prevalence is 2%–3%, with a mean onset in the second decade. Rarely presents after 35 years of age.

Symptoms

- **Obsessions: Recurrent** and persistent ideas, impulses, thoughts, or images that are perceived to be intrusive and meaningless and cause anxiety or grief. Not anxieties about real-life problems.
- **Compulsions: Uncontrollable** repetitive behaviors or rituals. May temporarily relieve anxiety.

Differential

- **Obsessive-compulsive personality disorder:** Generally lacks the obsessions and compulsive behaviors and rituals common to OCD. Patients are perfectionists, with inflexibility and obsessive attention paid to detail. Patients typically are not disturbed by their symptoms, whereas in OCD, they often are.
- **Generalized anxiety disorder:** Anxiety tends to be generalized to all areas of the patient's life, and the patient does not present with ritual behaviors to relieve anxiety.
- **Schizophrenia:** The patient is typically unaware that the obsessions are a product of his or her own mind and will have other symptoms characteristic of schizophrenia, such as psychotic and ⊖ symptoms.

Diagnosis

KEY FACT

Patients with OCD recognize that their obsessions are the product of their own minds.

The following criteria must be met to characterize a disorder as OCD:

- The presence of obsessions or compulsions.
- The patient is able to recognize that the obsessions or compulsions are to the **point of excess or unreason.**
- The obsessions or compulsions **interfere with daily living,** cause anguish, or are significantly time consuming (> 1 hour in 1 day).

Treatment

- **Behavioral:** Begin with CBT, with the goal of stopping intrusive thoughts and behaviors.
- **Pharmacologic:** Generally, medications should be started once the patient has failed behavioral treatment. SSRIs are indicated and may need to be titrated to higher doses than those used to treat depression or other anxiety disorders. Clomipramine (a TCA) is also indicated in the treatment of OCD.

Complications

Can cause depression if untreated. Can also lead to significant impairment in one's life, such as loss of income, family stressors, and substance abuse.

POSTTRAUMATIC STRESS DISORDER (PTSD)

Avoidance, hyperarousal, and **reexperiencing** of a traumatic, life-threatening event that overwhelms the person's coping mechanisms. Risk factors include young age, a history of prior trauma, a history of mental illness, low IQ, and minimal social support. Experiences as a refugee and domestic and street violence are important to consider.

SYMPTOMS

- **Reexperiencing:** Frequent intrusive memories and sensations of the experience of the event (flashbacks, hallucinations, and nightmares).
- **Avoidance/numbing:** The patient avoids any reminder of the event, such as conversations, people, and places. For example, a patient who has experienced combat may avoid all films about war. He or she may also feel detached from others or emotionally restricted and have little hope for the future.
- **Hypervigilance:** The patient may be easily startled and has a persistently ↑ autonomic response, characterized by difficulty sleeping, irritability, anger, and difficulty concentrating.

DIFFERENTIAL

- **Acute stress disorder:** Similar to PTSD, but lasts < 1 month.
- **Adjustment disorder:** May have symptoms similar to those of PTSD, but they are not caused by a life-threatening, severely traumatic event.
- **OCD:** The patient experiences recurrent intrusive thoughts, but they are not the result of a severe trauma.

DIAGNOSIS

- Patients must have witnessed or **experienced a life-threatening or severe injury-threatening event** that elicited a response of intense horror, hopelessness, and fear.
- Avoidance symptoms must be present.
- Reexperiencing symptoms must be present.
- ↑ arousal symptoms must be present.
- Symptoms must last > 1 month.
- Symptoms must lead to severe impairment and significant distress in the patient's life.

TREATMENT

- **Behavioral:**
  - **CBT:** Effective, as is psychotherapy geared toward reducing survivor guilt, hopelessness, and anger.
  - **Family therapy:** May be helpful in reducing the negative effects of PTSD on family members who may not understand or be aware of the trauma inflicted on the patient.
  - **Eye movement and desensitization reprocessing (EMDR):** A technique used to ↓ negative responses to trauma with rapid eye movements. The method of action is not well understood, and opinions vary as to its efficacy.
- **Pharmacologic:**
- SSRIs (fluoxetine) or TCAs (desipramine, amitriptyline) can be used to treat depression.
- For mood swings, mood stabilizers such as carbamazepine or valproic acid are effective. β-blockers such as propranolol can help ↓ hypervigilance, and benzodiazepines (alprazolam, clonazepam) can be used for anxiety.

COMPLICATIONS

Comorbid conditions associated with PTSD include alcohol and substance abuse, MDD, somatoform disorders, dissociative disorders, other anxiety disorders, and ongoing trauma.

KEY FACT

Acute stress disorder is diagnosed when symptoms occur within 1 month of the event, but do not last > 1 month. In PTSD, symptoms last > 1 month.

SPECIFIC PHOBIAS

Persistent and notable **fear of a specific object or situation** that leads to marked anxiety and avoidance that impair the patient's life. Fear of animals or natural environments (eg, snakes, heights, water) and fear of blood and injections usually start in childhood, whereas fear of situations (eg, flying, small spaces) may start in the 2nd decade of life.

SYMPTOMS

- Presents with persistent, marked fear that is **excessive** and unreasonable in relation to the object and situation.
- Exposure to the feared object or situation causes **extreme** anxiety and panic.
- The patient recognizes that the fear is unreasonable.
- The object or situation is avoided or dreaded.

DIFFERENTIAL

- **Panic disorder:** Panic attacks are not related to fear of a specific object or situation.
- **PTSD:** Panic symptoms are triggered by severe trauma.
- **Generalized anxiety disorder:** Anxiety is generalized and is not related to a specific situation or object.

TREATMENT

- **Behavioral:** CBT is geared toward extinguishing the anxiety response to the specific situation. This is done through **desensitization** or repeated exposures to the inciting agent.
- **Pharmacologic:** Antianxiety medications such as benzodiazepines can help ↓ anxiety and ↑ exposure to the offending object or situation. These medications are best used in the short term before or during triggering situations.

Psychotic Disorders

DELUSIONAL DISORDER

A chronic disorder of delusions (**fixed false beliefs**) that form a coherent system characterized by a certain level of plausibility. An uncommon disorder, with a prevalence of 0.01%–0.05%.

SYMPTOMS

- Presents with highly specific delusions that form a coherent belief system that seems somewhat plausible.
- Patients are otherwise normal and maintain a high level of functioning.

DIFFERENTIAL

- **Schizophrenia:** Associated with more functional impairment, auditory hallucinations, and thought disorders.
- **Substance-induced delusions:** Seen primarily with CNS stimulants such as cannabis and amphetamines.
- **Medical conditions:** Include thyroid disorders, Huntington disease, Parkinson disease, Alzheimer disease, CVAs, metabolic causes (uremia, hepatic encephalopathy, hypercalcemia), alcohol withdrawal, and other causes of delirium.

TREATMENT

- Patients are often resistant to treatment or medications.
- The first goal is to create a strong physician–patient alliance. Avoid directly challenging the patient's beliefs, but do not pretend to be in full acceptance of the delusions.
- Low-dose **antipsychotics** are indicated (atypicals such as olanzapine or risperidone are preferred). **Antidepressants,** especially clomipramine, may be helpful.
- The goal of medications is to help the patient avoid acting on the delusion.

SCHIZOPHRENIA

A **chronic** disorder characterized by **delusions, hallucinations, behavioral disturbances,** and **impaired social function** (without any mental status changes). Prevalence is 1%, manifesting earlier (18–25 years of age) and more severely in males and later (26–45 years of age) in females, with an equal male-to-female ratio (1:1). **Prevalence is higher** in the presence of a ⊕ **family history** (10% if there is a sibling or parent with schizophrenia).

SYMPTOMS

- Patients must have at least a **6-month period** of continuous symptoms.
- Symptoms include the following:
    - **Hallucinations:** Mostly auditory.
    - **Delusions:** Fixed false beliefs that are not shared by others in the same culture and that persist despite evidence to the contrary.
    - **Disorganized speech:** "Word salad."
    - **Catatonic** or bizarre behavior.
    - **Negative symptoms:** Flat affect, alogia (poverty of speech), avolition, lack of purposeful action.

DIFFERENTIAL

- **Mood disorders:**
    - **Bipolar disorder:** Psychotic symptoms can occur during manic or depressive episodes.
    - **Schizoaffective disorder:** Predominantly a mood disorder (mania or depression), with psychotic symptoms (lasting at least 2 weeks) during normal mood.
    - **Depression with psychotic features:** Depression predominates, with superimposed psychotic features. Patients are not psychotic when depression improves or resolves.
- **Delusional disorder:** Delusions tend not to be bizarre, and there are no associated symptoms such as hallucinations, thought disorders, or negative symptoms.
- **Drug-induced psychosis:** Amphetamines or cocaine can lead to paranoia and hallucinations. LSD, PCP, ketamine, and MDMA (ecstasy) can all lead to psychosis. Typically accompanied by other signs of substance abuse.
- **Organic causes:** Include medical conditions such as neurosyphilis, dementia, delirium, complex partial seizures, Huntington disease, heavy metal exposure, neoplasms, and medications (eg, prednisone).
- **Negative symptoms:** If the patient has negative symptoms only, other disorders should be ruled out, including Parkinson disease, depression, hypothyroidism, frontal lobe injury, PTSD, and substance abuse.

MNEMONIC

The 4 A's of schizophrenia:

Affective flattening
Asociality
Auditory hallucinations
Alogia (poverty of speech)

KEY FACT

Schizophrenia often starts with negative symptoms without the delusions or hallucinations (positive symptoms). This is called the **prodromal** or **residual** phase.

DIAGNOSIS

- Diagnosis is made by the history. Patients must have either bizarre delusions or hallucinations or 2 or more of the above symptoms (thought disorder, disorganized speech, catatonia, negative symptoms).
- Initially, **medical causes must be ruled out.** Consider BMP, calcium, CBC, TFTs, LFTs, VDRL, vitamin B_{12}, folate, HIV, a toxicology screen, brain imaging (CT or MRI), and EEG (if clinically indicated).

TREATMENT

- Antipsychotics are the treatment of choice. **Atypical neuroleptics,** or 2nd-generation antipsychotics, are **often 1st-line agents** (eg, olanzapine, quetiapine, risperidone), but typical or 1st-generation antipsychotics (eg, haloperidol, fluphenazine, chlorpromazine) are often just as effective, though with some intolerable side effects.
- Acutely, the goal of therapy is to **minimize symptoms and side effects** and, once the patient is stable, to titrate to the lowest effective dose that will maintain maximal functioning and prevent recurrence.
- Since 25%–50% of schizophrenics continue to have residual symptoms and impaired functioning, psychosocial treatment is a component of therapy and includes **CBT, individual therapy, group therapy, family therapy,** and **social skills training.** In more severe cases, a **multidisciplinary team** (case manager, nurse, and physician) is often needed to prevent hospitalization.
- "Potency" in typical antipsychotics refers to their potency, in binding to the D_2 dopamine receptor—the higher the potency, the greater the likelihood of extrapyramidal symptoms. Atypical antipsychotics (also called 2nd-generation antipsychotics [SGAs] have fewer extrapyramidal symptoms.

TABLE 14.4. Typical and Atypical Antipsychotics and Side Effects

CLASS/POTENCY	DRUG	SIDE EFFECT	MEDICALLY SERIOUS SIDE EFFECTS
Typical, high-potency antipsychotics	Haloperidol (Haldol), fluphenazine (Prolixin).	Sedation, akathisia.	Acute dystonic reactions, neuroleptic malignant syndrome, tardive dyskinesia (in long-term use).
Typical, midpotency antipsychotics	Thioridazine (Mellaril), chlorpromazine (Thorazine).	Sedation, anticholinergic side effects (dry mouth, constipation, urinary retention, tachycardia).	Acute dystonic reactions, neuroleptic malignant syndrome, tardive dyskinesia (in long-term use), prolonged QT interval.
Typical, low-potency antipsychotics	Thiothixene (Navane), perphenazine (Trilafon), trifluoperazine (Stelazine).	Orthostatic hypotension and other anticholinergic effects, sedation, hyperlipidemia.	Acute dystonic reactions, neuroleptic malignant syndrome, tardive dyskinesia (in long-term use).
Atypical antipsychotics (SGA)	Olanzapine (Zyprexa). Risperidone (Risperdal). Quetiapine (Seroquel). Clozapine (Clozaril). Aripiprazole (Abilify) Ziprasidone (Geodon).	Weight gain, sedation, anticholinergic at high doses, hyperlipidemia. Weight gain, hyperprolactinemia. Weight gain, sedation, anticholinergic at high doses, hyperlipidemia. Drooling, sedation, anticholinergic effects, hyperlipidemia. Fewest side effects, though has the typical ones. Hyperprolactinemia.	Diabetes mellitus. Side effects of typical antipsychotics (when used in high doses). Cataracts. Agranulocytosis. Prolonged QT interval.

There is no fundamental difference in efficacy. Table 14.4 compares typical and atypical antipsychotics by side effects and toxicity.

- All antipsychotic medications have risk of sedation, sexual dysfunction, postural hypotension, cardiac arrhythmias, and sudden cardiac death. Avoid combining with other medications that prolong the QT interval.
- Aripiprazole and ziprasidone have the least effect on weight gain of all the atypical antipsychotics. Weight gain is the worst with clozapine and olanzapine.
- Clozapine is most effective for treatment-resistant psychosis.

KEY FACT

Atypical (SGA) antipsychotics treat negative symptoms more effectively than typical or 1st-generation antipsychotics.

COMPLICATIONS

- Without treatment, patients with schizophrenia may experience "**downward drift**" in socioeconomic class.
- **Tardive dyskinesia** (involuntary movements of the tongue, lips, face, trunk, and extremities) can be caused by long-term treatment with typical antipsychotics such as haloperidol. This complication can be minimized through use of atypical antipsychotics or by adding benztropine concurrently with typical antipsychotic medication.
- Individuals with schizophrenia have ↑ **rate of violence** that is seen more often with uncontrolled paranoia and disorganized symptoms.

Substance Abuse Disorders

> A 55-year-old man was admitted to your service for cellulitis 2 days ago and now complains of nausea, vomiting, and diarrhea. He appears feverish and diaphoretic and is yawning repeatedly. Exam reveals no abdominal tenderness, rebound, or guarding. You note that his eyes and nose are watering, and his pupils are unusually dilated. On further questioning, you find that the patient takes oxycodone, which he buys from a friend. What treatment do you give him to relieve his symptoms?
> Daily methadone.

- **Substance abuse** is the compulsion to use substances despite adverse consequences. **Substance dependence** is physiologic and/or emotional reliance on the substance.
- **Abuse can be present without dependence:** For example, a person who expends significant energy acquiring and using cocaine, with adverse legal, financial, work, and interpersonal consequences, but only uses cocaine sporadically, has substance abuse, but not dependence. Commonly abused substances include the following:
  - **Alcohol:**
    - The prevalence of alcoholism is 6% in women and 12% in men. Alcohol-related deaths are the **3rd leading cause of preventable deaths** in the United States. While there is no direct genetic link, it is clear that alcoholism tends to run in families and is likely the product of a complex and poorly understood gene–environment interaction.
    - In men, "safe" levels of alcohol consumption equal **2 drinks per day**; in women, "safe" levels of alcohol consumption equal **1 drink per day**.

KEY FACT

Substance abuse can be characterized either by brief episodes or by more chronic patterns.

KEY FACT

CAGE questionnaire for alcohol abuse:

C: Have you ever felt the need to **C**ut down on your drinking?

A: Do you get **A**nnoyed when people talk to you about your drinking?

G: Do you feel **G**uilty or bad about your drinking?

E: Do you ever have an **E**ye opener (a drink first thing in the morning)?

■ **Opiates:** The prevalence of opiate abuse is 6%, with a male-to-female ratio of 3:1. The age of onset is generally in the teens, with the death rate among opioid abusers 20 times greater than that in the nonusing population.

■ **Stimulants:** Twelve percent of people have used cocaine at least once in their lifetimes, 3% in the last year, and 1% in the last month.

SYMPTOMS/EXAM

Table 14.5 outlines the presentation and treatment of common substance abuse disorders.

DIAGNOSIS

■ All patients should be screened for substance abuse disorders. Questions should be asked in a **nonjudgmental** manner and in a **confidential** environment to ensure the most open responses. The **CAGE questionnaire** is an example of a tool used to screen for alcohol abuse disorders.

■ **Substance abuse** requires at least 1 of the following criteria:
  ■ Continued use in **physically dangerous** situations (eg, drinking and driving).
  ■ **Legal problems** due to use.
  ■ Continual **failure to complete important obligations.**
  ■ Persistent use despite detrimental social or interpersonal impact.

TABLE 14.5. Presentation and Treatment of Substance Abuse Disorders

DRUG	MEDICAL COMPLICATIONS	WITHDRAWAL SYMPTOMS	TREATMENT
Alcohol	**General:** Cirrhosis, pancreatitis, ataxia, delirium, GI bleed, hepatitis, hypertension, cardiomyopathy, anemia, sexual dysfunction, depression, peripheral neuropathy, memory loss, depression, ↑ risk of cancer (esophageal, stomach, lung, colon). **In pregnancy:** Fetal alcohol syndrome.	**Early** (8 hours after last drink): Sweating, flushing, sleep disturbances, hallucinations, seizures, mild mental status changes. **Late** (48 hours after last drink): DTs (tremor, hallucinations, delirium, ↑ autonomic tone).	**Withdrawal:** Benzodiazepines (long-acting, eg, chlordiazepoxide). **Long-term treatment:** **Naltrexone:** ↓ cravings and relapse. **Disulfiram:** Causes flushing, nausea, and vomiting when mixed with alcohol. **SSRIs:** ↓ cravings.
Cocaine	**General:** Hypertension, tachycardia, arrhythmias, vasospasm of coronary arteries (MI) and cerebral arteries (CVA), hemoptysis, chest pain, nasal septum necrosis, dehydration, malnutrition, weight loss. **In pregnancy:** Fetal hypoxia and placental abruption.	Depressed mood, fatigue, disturbing dreams, ↑ appetite, insomnia or hypersomnia, agitation, or retardation.	No specific treatment for withdrawal; no pharmacologic treatments for dependence.
Opiates	**IV use:** Endocarditis, HIV, HBV/HCV, cellulitis, abscesses, septic arthritis, osteomyelitis, pneumonia, meningitis, pulmonary emboli, nephrotic syndrome. **In pregnancy:** Infant withdrawal.	Depressed mood, nausea, vomiting, diarrhea, yawning, insomnia, myalgias, runny nose, watering eyes, dilated pupils, sweating, fever.	**Withdrawal:** Methadone, clonidine, buprenorphine, clonidine-naltrexone. **Long-term treatment:** Methadone maintenance, buprenorphine, naltrexone.

- **Substance dependence** requires **3 or more** of the following criteria:
  - Physiologic **tolerance** or **withdrawal.**
  - Persistent desire or unsuccessful **attempts to cut down** or stop using.
  - Use for a **longer amount of time** or in larger amounts than was originally intended.
  - Main activities are **centered on the substance** (eg, intoxication or obtaining drugs).
  - **Giving up important activities** for drugs (eg, work).
  - **Persistent use,** regardless of the knowledge that continued use can lead to physical or psychological problems.

TREATMENT

Before formulating an approach toward substance abuse, it is important for the clinician to understand what **phase of behavioral change** the patient is in. It is also crucial to recognize that substance abuse has a **relapsing and remitting pattern.**

- **Psychotherapy:** Methods include the following:
  - **Therapeutic communities:** Residential treatment centers. Treatment duration is generally 6–18 months; communities tend to have strict limits and are highly structured. Associated with high dropout rates, but successful for highly motivated individuals.
  - **Group therapy.**
  - **Individual therapy:** Includes CBT, harm reduction (minimizing negative effects of behaviors), and psychoeducation.
  - **Family support/education:** Essential in the treatment of abusers, as family members are strongly affected by negative behaviors. Education (eg, Al-Anon) helps families recognize what to expect and how best to be supportive.
  - **Peer support groups:** Self-help organizations such as Alcoholics Anonymous. Such groups tend to focus on relapse prevention and maintenance of sobriety. Users are supported by peer mentors who have maintained abstinence. They may then graduate to peer lead the groups.

Child and Adolescent Psychiatry

DEPRESSION IN CHILDREN AND ADOLESCENTS

The intensity of feelings and emotions during childhood and adolescence makes it difficult to differentiate severe depression from normal sadness. In less severe depression, unhappiness associated with problems of everyday life is generally short lived, with symptoms usually resulting in only minor impairment in school performance, social activities, and relationships with others. These symptoms, even if they seem minor, must be evaluated and may respond to support and reassurance. Depression can be the precursor to suicide attempts. With more severe forms of depression, psychological referral may be useful.

SYMPTOMS/EXAM

- Serious depressive symptoms in youth may be similar to those in adults, with vegetative signs such as depressed mood.
- May also present with the following:
  - A sense of emptiness and meaninglessness.
  - Negative expectations of oneself and the environment.
  - Isolation.

- Persistent psychosomatic complaints (abdominal pain, chest pain, headache, lethargy, weight loss, dizziness, syncope).
- Other behavioral manifestations (depressive equivalents) of masked depression include truancy, running away from home, defiance of authority, self-destructive behavior, vandalism, drug and alcohol abuse, sexual acting out, and delinquency.

DIFFERENTIAL

- Eating disorders.
- **Organic CNS disorders:** Tumors, vascular lesions, closed head trauma, subdural hematomas.
- **Metabolic and endocrinologic disorders:** SLE, hypothyroidism, hyperthyroidism, Wilson disease, hyperparathyroidism, Cushing syndrome, Addison disease, PMS.
- **Infections:** Infectious mononucleosis, syphilis.
- **Other:** Drug use or withdrawal; other mental health disorders such as schizophrenia; a family history of depression, suicide, or bipolar affective disorder.

DIAGNOSIS

Lab workup is the same as in adults.

TREATMENT

- Counsel adolescents and parents if depression is mild or results from an acute personal loss or frustration.
- For MDD, suicidal thoughts, or psychotic thinking, psychological referral is necessary.
- SSRIs may be prescribed for patients who will be closely followed. Fluoxetine was the first antidepressant approved by the FDA for use in children (over 8 years old) and adolescents. Escitalopram is also now FDA approved for use in patients 12–17 years old. However, many others have been used safely. Clinical response varies from 2 to 6 weeks. The FDA recommends that paroxetine **not** be used for treatment of MDD in children and adolescents.
- In 2004, the FDA issued a black-box warning regarding the risk of ↑ suicidality in children and adolescents prescribed antidepressant medications. However, this warning must be balanced with the risk of suicidality related to the depression.

BIPOLAR DISORDER IN CHILDREN AND ADOLESCENTS

- **Sx:** Hyperactivity, irritability, or temper tantrums (the most common behavioral manifestation of mania in children is hyperactivity). Mixed manic-depressive states are more common in children.
- **DDx:** ADHD, conduct disorder, and schizophrenia.
- Manic symptoms in adolescents are similar to those in adults. It may be challenging to differentiate substance abuse and schizophrenia from bipolar disorder. Also, the normal risk-taking behavior of adolescents may appear similar to the recklessness of mania.
- **Dx, lab evaluation, and Tx** of bipolar disorder is the same as in adults.

SUICIDALITY

With the normal mood swings of adolescence, short periods of depression are common, and a teenager may have thoughts of suicide. **Suicide is the 3rd leading cause of mortality among adolescents.** The suicide rate of teen males is 5 times higher than that of females, and white males have the highest rate. The incidence of unsuccessful suicide attempts is 3 times higher in females than in males. Firearms account for the majority of suicide deaths in both males and females.

Teens with same-sex orientation are at significant risk for suicidal thoughts and suicide attempts. Those who have not "come out" (have not claimed a nonheterosexual identity) are at the highest risk. GLBT teens are at higher risk for victimization and bullying, which is also thought to contribute to an ↑ risk of suicidality. Accompanied by an ↑ risk of depression and substance abuse.

SYMPTOMS/EXAM

Inability to keep up with schoolwork; social withdrawal; symptoms of depression; anger; a history of a previous suicide attempt.

DIAGNOSIS

Determine the extent of the patient's depression and assess the risk of inflicting self-harm. The history should include medical, social, emotional, and academic background. Inquire about the following:

- Common signs of depression.
- Recent stressful events.
- Evidence of long-standing problems in the home, at school, or with peers.
- Drug or substance use and abuse.
- Signs of psychotic thinking, such as delusions or hallucinations.
- Evidence of marked depression, such as rebellious behavior, running away from home, reckless driving, or other acting-out behavior.

TREATMENT

- Medical therapy should be aimed at treating medical complications of the suicide attempt.
- Physical protection is needed to avoid harm to self if a plan is in place.
- Provide emergency psychological consultation for any teenager who is severely depressed, psychotic, or acutely suicidal.
- Safety contracts are not effective in preventing suicide. Do a thorough suicide assessment for risks and protective factors, as with adults.

SELF-INJURIOUS BEHAVIOR

- Only 1%–4% of adults participate in self-injurious behavior; however, approximately 15% of adolescents report some form of self-injury. Behavior includes cutting, skin carving, burning, severe abrading/scratching, or punching/hitting as well as more severe forms of self-injury. Typical age of onset is between 14 and 24 years.
- **Comorbid conditions:** Borderline personality disorder, dissociative disorders, eating disorder, MDD, alcohol dependence.
- **The relationship with suicidality is complex.** Many who self-injure are not suicidal, but as the severity of self-injury ↑, the risk of suicide ↑. Therefore, it is critical to evaluate self-injury severity.

MNEMONIC

STOPS FIRE for evaluating risk in self-injury:

Suicidal ideation during or before self-injury
Types of self-injury in which the patient engages
Onset of self-injury
Place on the body of injury
Severity of damage caused by self-injury
Functions of the self-injury for the patient
Intensity or frequency of urges to self-harm
Repetition of behavior
Episodic frequency of injury

TREATMENT

- Therapeutic alliance is key. Work to develop an understanding of the behavior, including recognition that the self-injurious behavior is serving a function for the patient.
- Motivational interviewing techniques may be helpful. Reflectively listen and validate emotions with a nonjudgmental attitude. It is also important not to be overly concerned, as this may be a reinforcing behavior.
- Pharmacological treatments: Topiramate, clozapine, naltrexone.
- Psychotherapeutic treatments: DBT (most evidence available, though with mixed results), CBT, other therapy techniques with a focus on addressing underlying psychological dysfunction and skill building.

PSYCHOSIS IN CHILDREN

Prepubertal onset of schizophrenia is extremely rare. Psychosis can occur among children with major depression or mania.

DIFFERENTIAL

Substance intoxication, medical conditions such as SLE, thyrotoxicosis, and temporal lobe epilepsy, as well as auditory and visual hallucinations can occur in nonpsychotic children under extreme stress.

TREATMENT

Should be under the care of a psychiatrist, as antipsychotics are indicated. Children seem to have a weaker response to antipsychotics than adolescents and adults. Family support and education, as well as the proper educational setting for a child, is crucial to treatment success.

EATING DISORDERS

A 17-year-old high school senior is brought to your clinic because her mother is concerned about her daughter's abnormal eating habits. The girl denies that she has a problem, stating that she is just picky with her food and is attempting to become a vegetarian. She has lost 18 pounds over the past 6 months, and her periods have stopped. What is your advice for her anxious mother?

Interview the girl alone, and look for signs and symptoms of an eating disorder.

Teenagers and younger children continue to develop eating disorders at an alarming rate. The spectrum of eating disorders includes **anorexia nervosa, bulimia nervosa, eating disorders not otherwise specified, and binge-eating disorder.** The relationship between biology and environment in the development of eating disorders is complex. Contributing factors appear to include the influence of the media (television, magazines, movies, videos), in which thin young women are often depicted as the norm. Anorexia and bulimia are distinguished as follows:

- **Anorexia nervosa:** Diagnosis requires the following 4 diagnostic criteria, as defined in the DSM-IV:
  - Refusal to maintain weight within a normal range for height and age (> 15% below ideal body weight).
  - Fear of weight gain.

- Severe body image disturbance (body image is the predominant measure of self-worth, along with denial of the seriousness of the illness).
- In postmenarchal females, absence of the menstrual cycle, or amenorrhea (> 3 cycles).
- **Bulimia:** Defined as episodic and uncontrolled ingestion of large quantities of food, followed by recurrent inappropriate compensatory behavior to prevent weight gain, such as self-induced vomiting, diuretic or cathartic use, strict dieting, or vigorous exercise.

SYMPTOMS

- **Anorexia:** Amenorrhea, depression, fatigue, weakness, hair loss, bone pain, constipation, abdominal pain.
- **Bulimia:** Normal or near-normal body weight, mouth sores, dental caries, heartburn, muscle cramps and fainting, hair loss, easy bruising, intolerance to cold, menstrual irregularity, abuse of diuretics and laxatives, misuse of diet pills (leading to palpitations and anxiety), frequent vomiting (resulting in throat irritation and pharyngeal trauma).

EXAM

- Assess vitals to evaluate for bradycardia, hypotension, or orthostatic hypotension.
- Perform a detailed physical and dental exam, including height, weight, and BMI.
- **Anorexia:** Signs include brittle hair and nails; dry, scaly skin; loss of subcutaneous fat; fine facial and body hair (lanugo hair); and breast and vaginal atrophy.
- **Bulimia:** Signs include a callused finger (Russell sign; results when the finger is used to induce vomiting); dry skin; periodontal disease; and sialadenosis (swelling of the parotid glands).
- Obtain a psychiatric history to assess for substance abuse and mood/anxiety/personality disorders.
- Ask about suicidal ideation.

DIAGNOSIS

- Explore body image, exercise regimen, eating habits, sexual history, current and past medication use, diuretic and laxative use, binging and purging behavior, and substance use.
- Obtain electrolytes, CBC, LFTs, and ECG to evaluate for arrhythmias and electrolyte disturbance.

TREATMENT

- The goal of treatment is restoration of normal body weight and eating habits, along with resolution of psychological difficulties.
- **Behavioral therapy:** Intensive psychotherapy and family therapy.
- **Pharmacotherapy:** TCAs, SSRIs, lithium carbonate.
- Enteral or parenteral feeding in patients with severe malnutrition.
- Hospitalization as indicated in cases of severe malnutrition or failed outpatient therapy.

COMPLICATIONS

Severe malnutrition, cardiac arrhythmias, suicide attempt, osteopenia, heart failure, dental disease.

FEMALE ATHLETE TRIAD

A 16-year-old girl comes to your clinic for 2° amenorrhea. She tells you that she feels better than ever after joining her neighborhood gym. The girl is sexually active and uses condoms for contraception. You obtain a urine pregnancy test, which is ⊖. How do you work up her amenorrhea?

Obtain a better history about the type and amount of exercise to determine the cause of amenorrhea in a young female.

Many young women engage in exercise to control body weight and improve exercise capacity. The consequences of excessive exercise can include amenorrhea, infertility, and delay of puberty and menarche. The likelihood of amenorrhea varies with the type and amount of exercise as well as with the rapidity of ↑ in exercise. Activities that are associated with low body weight and amenorrhea include running, ballet dancing, and figure skating. Gradual ↑ in exercise is less likely to lead to amenorrhea than acute ↑. Amenorrhea occurs only when there is relative caloric deficiency due to inadequate nutritional intake for the amount of energy expended.

TREATMENT

- Educate patients on the need for adequate caloric intake to match energy expenditure.
- Take an interdisciplinary approach with sports coaches, family, school, and school counselors.
- Estrogen replacement for women with amenorrhea (OCPs).
- Patients should be encouraged to take 1200–1500 mg of calcium daily, along with supplemental vitamin D (400 IU daily).

COMPLICATIONS

Exercise-induced amenorrhea; loss of bone density.

> **KEY FACT**
>
> The "female athlete triad" consists of an eating disorder, amenorrhea, and osteoporosis.

SUBSTANCE USE AND ABUSE IN ADOLESCENTS

Use of substances during adolescence may compromise physical, cognitive, and psychosocial aspects of adolescent development and can be a risk factor for substance abuse later in life. Commonly used substances include alcohol,

TABLE 14.6. Presentation of Substance Use and Abuse

VARIABLE	PRESENTATION
Physical	Fatigue, insomnia or hypersomnia, runny nose, shortness of breath, injected eyes, pinpoint pupils.
Emotional	Personality change, sudden mood changes, irritability, irresponsible behavior, low self-esteem, poor judgment, depression, withdrawal, general lack of interest.
Family	Breaking rules or withdrawing from the family, high family conflict, lack of bonding.
School	Truancy, academic failure, lack of commitment to school and education, early persistent behavioral problems.
Social/behavioral	Peer group involvement with drugs and alcohol, problems with the law.

marijuana, opioids, cocaine, amphetamines, sedative-hypnotics, hallucinogens, inhalants, nicotine, anabolic steroids, γ-hydroxybutyrate (GHB), and 3,4-methylenedioxymethamphetamine (ecstasy). When discussing substance use with adolescents, physicians must be aware of state confidentiality laws.

DIAGNOSIS

Clinical history, specific physical examination findings (see Tables 14.6 and 14.7), and a drug screen if drug abuse is suspected.

TABLE 14.7. Physiologic Effects of Common Illicit Substances

SYMPTOM	SUBSTANCE
Eyes/pupils	
Mydriasis	Amphetamines, MDMA or other stimulants, cocaine, jimsonweed, LSD; withdrawal from alcohol or opioids.
Miosis	Alcohol, barbiturates, benzodiazepines, opioids, PCP.
Nystagmus	Alcohol, barbiturates, benzodiazepines, inhalants, PCP.
Conjunctival injection	LSD, marijuana.
Lacrimation	Inhalants, LSD; withdrawal from opioids.
Cardiovascular	
Tachycardia/hypertension	Amphetamines, MDMA, cocaine, LSD, marijuana, PCP; withdrawal from alcohol, barbiturates, or benzodiazepines.
Hypotension	Barbiturates, opioids; withdrawal from depressants. Orthostatic hypotension—marijuana.
Arrhythmia	Amphetamines, MDMA, cocaine, inhalants, opioids, PCP.
Respiratory	
Depression	Opioids, depressants, GHB.
Pulmonary edema	Opioids, stimulants.
Core body temperature	
↑	Amphetamines, MDMA, cocaine, PCP; withdrawal from alcohol, barbiturates, benzodiazepines, or opioids.
↓	Alcohol, barbiturates, benzodiazepines, opioids, GHB.
PNS response	
Hyperreflexia	Amphetamines, MDMA, cocaine, LSD, marijuana, PCP; withdrawal from alcohol or benzodiazepines.
Hyporeflexia	Alcohol, benzodiazepines, inhalants, opioids.
Tremor	Amphetamines, cocaine, LSD; withdrawal from alcohol, benzodiazepines, or cocaine.
Ataxia	Alcohol, amphetamines, MDMA, benzodiazepines, inhalants, LSD, PCP, GHB.
CNS response	
Hyperalertness	Amphetamines, MDMA, cocaine.
Sedation/somnolence	Alcohol, benzodiazepines, inhalants, marijuana, opioids, GHB.
Seizures	Alcohol, amphetamines, MDMA, cocaine, inhalants, opioids; withdrawal from alcohol or benzodiazepines.
Hallucinations	Amphetamines, MDMA, cocaine, inhalants, LSD, marijuana, PCP; withdrawal from alcohol or benzodiazepines.
Gastrointestinal	
Nausea/vomiting	Alcohol, amphetamines or other stimulants, cocaine, inhalants, LSD, opioids, peyote, GHB; withdrawal from alcohol, benzodiazepines, cocaine, or opioids.

TREATMENT

- Counsel about the dangers of substance use and abuse.
- Family therapy.
- **Smoking:** Nicotine patches, gum.
- **Alcohol:** Recommend participation in Alcoholics Anonymous or Alateen.
- **Illicit drug use:** Recommend drug rehabilitation programs.

COMPLICATIONS

Death and injury (from motor vehicle accidents, other unintentional injuries, homicide, and suicide); physical and sexual abuse; ↑ sexual activity (teen pregnancy, STIs); alterations in mood, sleep, and appetite; frank psychosis indistinguishable from schizophrenia; irreversible cardiomyopathy; noncardiogenic pulmonary edema; pulmonary hypertension; drug overdose with multiorgan system failure.

PSYCHOTROPIC MEDICATIONS IN CHILDREN AND ADOLESCENTS

Pharmacokinetics in children and adolescents are different from pharmacokinetics in adults. Children have greater hepatic capacity, ↑ glomerular filtration rate, and less fatty tissue. Half-lives may be shorter.

- **Mood disorders:** SSRIs have overall been found to be safe in children and adolescents, even given black-box warnings regarding ↑ risk of suicide. Fluoxetine has been shown to have the most favorable risk-to-benefit ratio in children and adolescents. The risks and benefits of both treating and not treating psychiatric disorders must be fully explained to children/teens and their caretakers. Manic episodes are treated as they are among adults.
- **OCD and anxiety disorders:** SSRIs are 1st-line treatments; buspirone and long-acting benzodiazepines can also be used.
- **Psychosis and schizophrenia:** The best-studied medications are chlorpromazine and haloperidol; however, overall, atypical antipsychotics are preferred in children. Risperidone is used for psychosis as well as behavior disorders. Be sure to check BMI, lipids, and fasting blood glucose, and monitor for weight gain.

Behavioral Disorders

PERSONALITY DISORDERS

A 35-year-old woman comes to your office for an initial visit. Her chart is lengthy and shows multiple 1° care providers, numerous ER visits for self-mutilation, and a history of alcohol abuse. The woman states that she was referred to you by a friend, and throughout the visit she continually praises you, saying that you are not like the other doctors, who were just interested in prescribing pills and making a cut from the drug companies. On further questioning, the patient tells you that she hasn't had any stable partners because they all turned out to be shallow, empty users who didn't care about her. As she tells you more about herself, you begin to remember complaints about this patient and her inappropriate behavior in the waiting room. What is the most likely diagnosis? Borderline personality disorder.

Distinguished by **persistently inadequate adaptive capacities** and patterns of behavior, leading to significant impairment in areas such as social relationships and occupational performance. Disorders start in **early childhood** and persist through adulthood. They are **coded on Axis II.**

SYMPTOMS

Personality disorders are classified into 3 clusters that share characteristics:

1. **Cluster A** (odd and eccentric):
   - Paranoid
   - Schizoid
   - Schizotypal
2. **Cluster B** (dramatic, emotional, and erratic):
   - Antisocial
   - Borderline
   - Histrionic
   - Narcissistic
3. **Cluster C** (anxious and fearful):
   - Avoidant
   - Dependent
   - Obsessive-compulsive

DIFFERENTIAL

- Distinguish from personality changes caused by a medical condition, mental retardation, and Axis I disorders.
- Personality disorders have an early-childhood onset and possess characteristics not found in Axis I disorders, such as intact reality testing, normal abstracting ability, and the absence of formal thought disorders.

DIAGNOSIS

The diagnosis is made after several visits, when the persistent patterns of behavior become apparent.

TREATMENT

- Because personality disorders are developed across an individual's life span, patients are often **resistant to treatment** and require a multidisciplinary approach for effective management.
- **Dialectical behavior therapy,** in group and individual treatment, has the best evidence of efficacy among psychotherapeutic treatments and focuses on learning to manage emotions and reactions. **Psychoanalysis** and psychodynamic psychotherapy may help the patient recognize and change maladaptive behavior patterns.
- Although of limited utility, **pharmacologic treatments** are used in some cases. In **antisocial** and **borderline** personality disorder, mood stabilizers such as lithium and carbamazepine are sometimes used; in **paranoid** and **schizotypal personality disorder,** low-dose **antipsychotics** have been given.

KEY FACT

Personality disorders are classified into 3 clusters: cluster A ("weird"—odd and eccentric); cluster B ("wild"—dramatic, emotional, and erratic); and cluster C ("wimpy"—anxious and fearful).

Somatoform Disorders

A 22-year-old woman is brought to the office by her mother. She complains of sudden onset of bilateral blindness. She denies any trauma. Her mother states, "I can't believe this is happening. First, her father is dying of cancer, and now this." As the patient moves toward the exam table, you are struck by how easily she avoids all obstacles that lie between her and the table. On exam, you note normal bilateral pupillary responses, and you are surprised that she has none of the expected bruises or scrapes. You order a visual evoked potential, and it comes back normal. What is the most likely explanation for your patient's symptoms?

Conversion disorder.

A group of psychiatric disorders that share the common feature of **overimportance of physical symptoms (with no clear medical etiology)** in a patient's life. This often leads to a feeling of being misunderstood by health providers. Somatization can lead to inappropriate workups, hospitalizations, and procedures (up to $30 billion per year) and may cause the patient harm.

SYMPTOMS

Generally categorized as follows:

- **Somatization disorder:** A **chronic** disorder characterized by **multiple clinically significant symptoms** (a completely ⊕ ROS: especially GI, sexual, musculoskeletal, and neurological symptoms) that vary over time and are **not explained by medical findings.** Patients usually have an extensive treatment history, with age of onset < 30 years of age. Higher prevalence in women.
- **Conversion disorder:** Usually characterized by self-limited symptoms that affect voluntary motor or sensory systems and **suggest a neurologic disorder,** but are **not consistent with anatomic structures.** Age of onset is 10–40 years of age. **Preceded by stress or trauma.**
- **Hypochondriasis:** A chronic preoccupation with or **fear of having a serious medical disease** that is not relieved by appropriate evaluation or reassurance. Usually begins in early adulthood.
- **Body dysmorphic disorder:** Chronic preoccupation with **an imagined defect in physical appearance;** usually begins in adolescence. Is **not** the same as an eating disorder.
- **Chronic pain syndrome:** Long-standing **pain without an identified organic cause** is the central feature.

KEY FACT

Somatoform disorders are motivated by inner psychic gain; symptoms are unintentional or involuntary and are precipitated by stress.

DIFFERENTIAL

- **Malingering:** Motivated by external gain (eg, drug seeking, insurance fraud); symptoms are intentional, with poor cooperation in evaluation.
- **Factitious disorder (Munchausen syndrome):** Motivated by assumption of the sick role, in which symptoms are fabricated or self-inflicted. Histories are often vague, and patients go from hospital to hospital seeking care.

DIAGNOSIS

A careful assessment and evaluation should be performed using standard medical workups, with an emphasis on avoiding exhaustive and unnecessary testing.

TREATMENT

- Stress empathy, along with the importance of establishing and maintaining a strong 1° care relationship. Schedule routine, frequent visits to ↓ "emergency" visits and calls.
- Avoid stratifying the diagnosis as mental or physical; address in "stress" terms or emphasize the mind–body connection.

- Comorbid psychiatric disorders should be addressed and treated.
- Consider a psychiatry referral to provide a framework for treatment (not to take the place of the 1° care provider).
- Individual or group therapy may be of benefit, as may stress identification and reduction.
- Prevent iatrogenesis by limiting workup and treatments to objective findings (not complaints).

Mind–Body Syndromes

CHRONIC FATIGUE SYNDROME

Etiology is unknown, although an infectious source is suspected. Many report sudden onset of symptoms after a severe flulike illness. All potential endocrine, neurological, infectious, and psychiatric disorders must be ruled out.

DIAGNOSIS

Diagnosis is made by observation of severe unexplained fatigue for at least 6 months that is not resolved by rest and is functionally impairing, plus 4 or more of the following criteria:

- Impaired memory or concentration.
- Sore throat.
- Tender or enlarged lymph nodes.
- Muscle pain and arthralgias.
- Headache.
- Sleep disturbance.
- Postexertional malaise.
- Causes at least a 50% reduction in activities.

TREATMENT

Similar to somatoform disorders as well as other supportive treatments. Do not continue treatment indefinitely without evidence of clinical response.

FIBROMYALGIA

Fibromyalgia is a noninflammatory soft tissue pain disorder of > 3 months' duration, widespread musculoskeletal pain, and tenderness in at least 11 of 18 anatomic sites. There is a female predominance. Typically occurs between 30 and 60 years of age. Risks include gender, low socioeconomic status, poor functional status, and stressful life events. In 50%, it starts after a negative event of a flulike illness.

DIAGNOSIS

Diagnosis is based on tenderness in at least 11 of 18 trigger points with 4 kg pressure (whitens examiner's nail bed) in the setting of a normal lab evaluation (CBC, ESR or CRP, CK, TSH, normal renal and liver function). Sleep study may be indicated to rule out OSA or narcolepsy as the cause of fatigue.

May be accompanied by any of the following:

- **Nonrestorative sleep,** with early morning awakening.
- **Generalized fatigue.**
- Pain is ↑ with anxiety/stress and improved with mild physical activity or relaxation (eg, on vacations).

KEY FACT

While mind–body syndromes like chronic fatigue and fibromyalgia don't have a clearly agreed-upon etiology or pathology, they require a multidisciplinary approach and are clearly exacerbated by stress and emotional pain.

- Chronic headache.
- Symptoms of IBS.
- Subjective complaints of swelling, numbness.
- Dizziness.
- Depression/anxiety.
- Reduced physical endurance.
- ↓ social interaction.
- May have general hyperalgesia.

DIFFERENTIAL

- **Chronic fatigue:** Pain is less prominent.
- **Myofascial pain:** Pain is more localized.
- **Common comorbid conditions:** Connective tissue diseases, mental illness, sleep disorders, Lyme disease, TMJ, IBS.

TREATMENT

- **Treatment with antidepressants:** Duloxetine, milnacipran, any other SSRI.
- **Pharmacologic treatment of pain:** Pregabalin, amitriptyline or desipramine, cyclobenzaprine, tramadol. NSAIDs unlikely to be helpful. Avoid narcotics!
- **Behavioral treatments:** Psychoeducation about illness, low-impact aerobic exercise, CBT, stress management, sleep hygiene, psychosocial support, may require job/workplace modifications.
- **Complementary therapies:** Evidence exists for acupuncture, hypnotherapy, biofeedback, balneotherapy, and massage.

KEY FACT

Serotonin syndrome is a rare but sometimes fatal syndrome that presents as nausea, hyperthermia, hyperreflexia, agitation, autonomic dysfunction, muscle rigidity, delirium, and coma.

Therapeutic Drugs in Psychiatry

DRUG–DRUG INTERACTIONS

Table 14.8 shows psychotropic drugs that can potentially interact with other medications.

TABLE 14.8. Drug Interactions

DRUG	LEVEL RAISED BY	LEVEL LOWERED BY	OTHER INTERACTIONS
Lithium	Thiazides, ACEI, NSAIDs, metronidazole.	Theophylline, anything causing urinary alkalinization ($NaHCO_3$).	Can cause neurotoxicity (rare): Antipsychotics, carbamazepine, methyldopa, calcium channel blockers; can cause serotonin syndrome (rare): SSRIs, TCAs.
Valproic acid	ASA, erythromycin, ibuprofen.	Phenobarbital, phenytoin, carbamazepine.	↓ efficacy of AZT, warfarin, benzodiazepines.
Carbamazepine	Valproic acid, antifungals, calcium channel blockers, INH, protease inhibitors, grapefruit juice.	Phenytoin, phenobarbital.	↓ efficacy of warfarin, benzodiazepines, many AEDs, antidepressants, OCPs.
SSRIs	↑ risk of serotonin syndrome with MAOIs, lithium, other serotonergic agents.		

Abuse and Violence

It is essential that physicians understand the role they play in recognizing and reporting abuse of any kind. Guidelines are as follows:

- **Child abuse:** Mandatory reporting laws exist for all suspected cases of child abuse or neglect, and physicians are required to report all such cases.
- **Domestic violence:** Reporting laws regarding domestic violence vary from state to state, with few states requiring reporting. Nonetheless, domestic violence should by no means be considered a "private matter," and physicians must screen for it in 1° care visits. In this context, physicians should not judge their success on the basis of whether a patient leaves his or her partner, but they should let victims know that the abuse is not their fault; that they do not merit such treatment; and that the violence they are confronting is unacceptable.
- Pregnancy is a known period of heightened risk for domestic violence.
- **Who and when to screen:** As part of a routine health history; with every new intimate relationship; all females > 14 years of age; with each pregnancy. Some questions to ask on the topic of abuse, suggested by the Family Violence Prevention Fund: Do you feel controlled or isolated by your partner? Do you ever feel afraid of your partner?
- **Elder abuse:** Approximately 1–2 million older Americans are victims of abuse or neglect by their 1° caretakers. Physicians are **mandatory reporters** of elder abuse and neglect.
- Don't forget to ask your adolescent patients about gang violence and their sense of safety in school and in their neighborhoods.

The Patient–Physician Relationship

COMMUNICATION

Good communication is key to strong patient–physician relationships. A good relationship with your patients leads to **higher adherence** and **greater patient satisfaction** (not to mention ↓ **likelihood of litigation!**). Components of effective communication:

- **Make eye contact** and a brief personal connection at the beginning.
- **Avoid interrupting the patient** while keeping patients on track.
- Do not appear rushed. Sit down with the patient.
- **Manage expectations** by asking patients about their expectations.
- **Empower patients** to ask questions and make decisions about their own medical care.
- **Respect confidentiality:** Do not disclose information to family members who may also be under your care (especially important to remember with adolescent patients).
- **Provide information:** Summarize the plan, review medication dosages, use patient handouts. **Assess literacy level** before providing written materials.
- Don't talk excessively (or at all) about yourself—the encounter is about the patient!
- Be attentive to nonverbal forms of communication.

KEY FACT

When victims of domestic violence leave their abusers, they have a 75% ↑ risk of being murdered.

KEY FACT

One in 7 women is a victim of domestic violence.

MNEMONIC

Guidelines for domestic violence surveillance:

RADAR

Remember to ask about partner violence.
Ask directly about violence.
Document information in the patient's chart.
Assess the patient's safety.
Refer the patient to outside resources (eg, legal services, support groups, shelters).

KEY FACT

An exception to the requirement for confidentiality occurs when physicians feel that patients may be at risk of hurting themselves or others.

CULTURAL COMPETENCE

It may not be realistic for physicians to be familiar with all of their patients' cultural backgrounds; however, it is important for clinicians to understand how culture affects the patient–physician relationship and hence treatment outcomes. Above all, you must take care **not to apply stereotypes** or prejudices to patients whose gender, race, ethnicity, sexual orientation, or culture may differ from your own. It is important to be knowledgeable about cultural issues prevalent in populations in your community. Be aware of your own feelings, biases, and prejudices as you interact with patients.

Techniques to **minimize cultural misunderstandings** include the following:

- Be respectful (address all patients as Ms. or Mr.).
- Where feasible, use competent interpreters who are not only bilingual but also bicultural.
- Spend more time with the patient if needed.
- Ask patients to explain what the symptom or illness means to them and how it might be treated in their culture.
- Anticipate that patients may have had negative interactions with the medical system in the past.
- Review treatment plans carefully and have patients demonstrate an understanding of these plans.
- Be nonjudgmental and accepting of patients' cultural differences.
- Work to create a culture of safety for transgender patients by respecting the pronoun and name they choose to use. When possible, use patient forms that have options for "partnered" as well as married or single. Do not make assumptions about the gender of a patient's sexual partner(s).

KEY FACT

Harm reduction is a method by which physicians seek a middle ground between what they feel is best and what the patient wants. This method helps the patients modify behaviors to ↓ self-harm (eg, ↓ smoking vs. smoking cessation; using clean needles vs. quitting heroin). The physician must **understand and respect** the patient's wishes, as such understanding will foster a stronger relationship and ↑ the likelihood of adherence.

CHAPTER 15

Geriatric Medicine

Kristen Thornton, MD

Sensory Disorders

CATARACTS

Opacity of the lens that ↓ visual acuity. Caused by oxidative damage to the lens, leading to ↑ deposition of insoluble proteins in otherwise transparent tissue. Risk factors include smoking, diabetes, and corticosteroid therapy.

- **Sx/Exam:** Presents with painless blurred vision. Symptoms are progressive, developing over months or years. Lens opacities can be grossly visible or seen as a diminished red reflex.
- **Dx:** Diagnosed with slit-lamp biomicroscopy during ophthalmologic exam.
- **Tx:** Decision to treat is based on the degree of functional impairment imposed by the cataracts. Surgery consists of removal of the cataract and placement of an intraocular lens; improves visual acuity in 95% of cases.

AGE-RELATED MACULAR DEGENERATION (MD)

A 79-year-old white male ex-smoker presents to your office with several months of deteriorating eyesight. On further questioning, he describes his bilateral vision as blurred and notes ↓ ability to read fine print. He also finds it difficult to discriminate features when he looks at objects straight on, but reports intact peripheral vision. His visual impairment has not affected his driving. On exam, you find opaque deposits on both retinas. What is the most likely diagnosis?

Age-related macular degeneration, which is the leading cause of permanent visual loss in the elderly. Its exact cause is unknown, but risk factors include age > 50 years, white race, female gender, ⊕ family history of macular degeneration, and a history of cigarette smoking.

Deterioration of the macula, leading to **bilateral central vision loss.** The leading cause of permanent legal blindness in the elderly. May be **atrophic** (dry) or **exudative** (wet); atrophic MD is the **more common** type.

SYMPTOMS

- Blurred vision is the earliest symptom of atrophic MD, whereas the classic early symptom of exudative MD is the perception of straight lines as bent or crooked.
- Reading vision is lost, but peripheral vision is often maintained (eg, patients have difficulty reading but less difficulty driving).

EXAM

Small, yellow-white deposits called **drusen** appear underneath the retina (see Figure 15.1).

TREATMENT

- Limited treatment exists for **atrophic** MD.
- Antioxidant multivitamins may slow progression in **exudative** MD.
- Early laser photocoagulation surgery may delay or reverse visual loss in **exudative** MD.

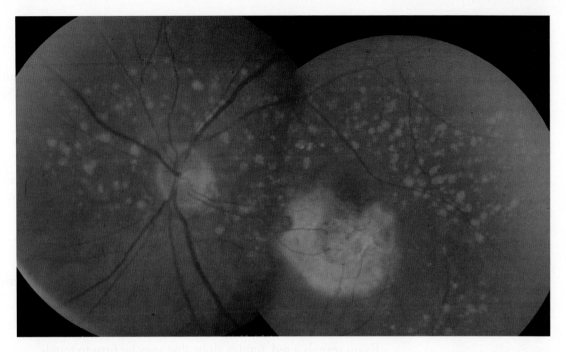

FIGURE 15.1.   Macular degeneration. Composite fundoscopic photogram showing drusen associated with atrophy and fibrosis of the macula. (Reproduced, with permission, from USMLERx.com.)

GLAUCOMA

A group of disorders characterized by ↑ intraocular pressure, leading to irreversible damage to the optic nerve. The 2 forms most relevant to geriatrics are **open-angle** and **angle-closure glaucoma.**

Open-Angle Glaucoma

↑ intraocular pressure due to abnormal aqueous drainage through the trabecular meshwork of the eye. The **most common form of glaucoma,** accounting for > 90% of cases. Prevalence is ↑ in 1st-degree relatives of affected individuals and in persons with diabetes. May also develop after uveitis or trauma. Risk factors: Age > 65 years, ⊕ family history of glaucoma, black ancestry, and diabetes.

SYMPTOMS

- Insidious onset; patients are often asymptomatic until vision is seriously compromised.
- Characterized by bilateral peripheral vision loss, leading to ↑ tunnel vision.
- Patients may also complain of "halos around lights."

DIAGNOSIS

- Diagnosis is made through visualization of an anatomically normal or "open" anterior chamber angle and through excavation or "cupping" of the optic nerve in the setting of ↑ intraocular pressure.
- Periodic ophthalmologic exams are the best way to diagnose the disease, especially in **high-risk** individuals.

TREATMENT

- **Avoid** anticholinergics that can worsen glaucoma.
- **Medications** (see Table 15.1).
- **Surgical treatments:** Surgical intervention improves aqueous outflow; recommended in patients whose intraocular pressure remains ↑ despite medical therapy.

Angle-Closure Glaucoma

An ophthalmologic emergency due to a closed anterior chamber angle. The only type of glaucoma that is curable. Accounts for approximately 10% of glaucoma cases in the United States. More prevalent among Asians.

SYMPTOMS

- Rapid onset; usually unilateral.
- Presents with severe pain and profound vision loss.
- As intraocular pressure ↑, patients may experience nausea, vomiting, and abdominal pain that may be mistaken for an acute abdomen.

EXAM

- Exam reveals a red, tender globe that may be firm to touch.
- A steamy or hazy cornea and a nonreactive, dilated pupil may be seen.
- Tonometry or palpation of the globe reveals ↑ intraocular pressure.

DIFFERENTIAL

Angle-closure glaucoma must be differentiated from acute conjunctivitis, uveitis, and corneal disorders.

TREATMENT

- Constitutes a **medical emergency,** requiring immediate referral to an ophthalmologist. Delay of treatment can cause irreversible vision loss.
- Therapy for 1° acute angle-closure glaucoma consists of immediate reduction of intraocular pressure via IV acetazolamide in conjunction with a topical agent, followed by laser peripheral iridotomy. Usually leads to permanent cure.

TABLE 15.1. Antiglaucoma Agents

MEDICATION CLASS	EXAMPLE	NOTES
β-blockers	Timolol (topical drops).	↓ aqueous production and intraocular pressure. May have side effects similar to those of systemic β-blockers.
Carbonic anhydrase inhibitors	Acetazolamide (oral) and dorzolamide (topical drops).	↓ aqueous production. Topical preparations have largely replaced oral systemic ones. Systemic therapy may induce kidney stones or acidosis.
Prostaglandin analogs	Bimatoprost (topical drops).	↑ aqueous outflow.
Cholinergic agonists	Pilocarpine (topical drops).	↑ aqueous outflow. Fewer systemic effects, but less effective than topical β-blockers; may cause myopia and ↓ visual acuity.
α-adrenergic agonists	Brimonidine (topical drops).	↓ aqueous production and ↑ outflow. Use with caution in patients with coronary or cerebrovascular insufficiency.

RETINAL DETACHMENT

Results from separation of the sensory portion of the retina from its pigment epithelium. Most often occurs in people > 50 years of age. Risk factors include aging, myopia, cataract surgery, trauma, and a ⊕ family history of retinal detachment.

SYMPTOMS

- Presents with unilateral blurred vision described by patients as a "curtain coming down" over the eye.
- Marked by flashes of light and a shower of floaters.

EXAM/DIAGNOSIS

- Exam reveals the retina hanging in the vitreous like a gray cloud.
- Diagnosis is based on an ophthalmoscopic exam in addition to the **clinical triad** of **eye flashes, floaters,** and a **visual field defect.**

TREATMENT

Retinal detachments require immediate referral to an ophthalmologist. Treatment is surgical and is directed at closing retinal tears via cryotherapy or laser photocoagulation. Approximately 80% of uncomplicated cases can be cured with a single surgery.

KEY FACT

Classic signs and symptoms in retinal detachment are eye flashes, floaters, and a visual field defect.

HEARING LOSS

Sensorineural Hearing Loss

> A new patient arrives at your practice in tears. She is 76 years of age, and her companion states that except for some minor arthritis pain, she is in excellent health and usually very lively. However, over the past year she has stopped participating in social activities at their independent living facility because of her embarrassment at being unable to understand her peers. She often perceives that others are mumbling, and she dreads the idea of needing a hearing aid, stating that it will make her feel old. Her last complete physical was 3 years ago. What is the most likely diagnosis?
>
> Sensorineural hearing loss. A thorough exam to rule out easily treated causes of conductive hearing loss (eg, cerumen impaction) and referral for audiometry are warranted. Timely screening may have prevented this patient's isolation.

Caused by disease of the cochlea or the 8th cranial nerve (CN VIII). Affects almost one-half of individuals > 75 years of age, making it the most common disability among the elderly. Timely treatment can help prevent social isolation, depression, and functional dependence on caregivers. Risk factors include:

- Older age.
- Noise exposure.
- Ototoxic medications.

KEY FACT

Sensorineural hearing loss is the most common type of hearing loss in the elderly.

SYMPTOMS

- Presents with bilateral, gradual, and usually symmetric hearing loss.
- Loss of speech discrimination is experienced in noisy environments.
- Patients have ↓ ability to hear high-frequency (> 4000-Hz) sounds.

EXAM

- Otoscopic exam may reveal findings that suggest conductive hearing loss (eg, cerumen occlusion) or anomalies of the ear canal or tympanic membrane (eg, otitis media, tumors, tympanosclerosis, perforation).
- Tuning fork tests such as the Rinne and Weber tests can be performed, but should not be solely relied upon when making a diagnosis.

DIFFERENTIAL

Metabolic derangements (eg, diabetes, hypothyroidism, dyslipidemia, renal failure), infections (eg, measles, mumps, syphilis), and radiation therapy are less common but potentially reversible causes of sensory hearing loss.

DIAGNOSIS

- Although not sufficient for diagnosis, tuning fork tests can be useful in differentiating conductive from sensorineural hearing losses:
  - **Weber test:** A tuning fork is placed on the forehead. In conductive losses, the sound appears louder in the poorer-hearing ear, whereas in sensorineural losses, sound radiates to the better-hearing ear.
  - **Rinne test:** A tuning fork is placed alternately on the mastoid bone and in front of the ear canal. In conductive losses, bone conduction exceeds air conduction (ie, BC > AC); in sensorineural losses, the opposite is true (ie, AC > BC).
- Audiometry is a standardized tool for recording hearing thresholds at different frequencies (see Table 15.2 and Figure 15.2). Frequencies **most important** for human speech are in the 250- to 6000-Hz range.
- Hearing loss accompanied by pulsatile tinnitus may signify a serious vascular abnormality such as carotid vaso-occlusive disease, aneurysm, AVM, or glomus tumor, warranting workup via MRA to establish the diagnosis.

TABLE 15.2. General Guidelines for the Interpretation of Audiometric Findings

DECIBEL MEASURE	AUDIOMETRIC FINDING
0–25 dB	Hearing within normal limits.
26–50 dB	Mild hearing loss. Patients will have trouble with soft sounds, with background noise, and when at a distance from the source of the sound.
51–70 dB	Moderate hearing loss. Patients will have significant difficulties with normal conversational-level speech and will rely on visual cues.
71–90 dB	Severe hearing loss. Patients cannot hear conversational speech and miss all speech sounds; however, they can hear environmental sounds, such as dogs barking and loud music.
91+ dB	Profound hearing loss. Patients can hear only loud environmental sounds, such as jackhammers, airplane engines, and firecrackers.

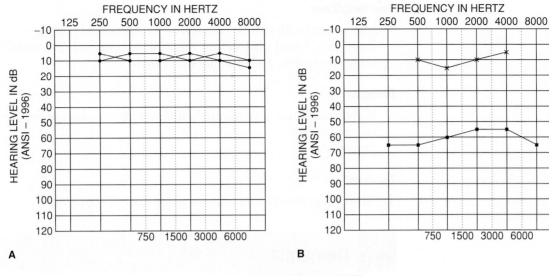

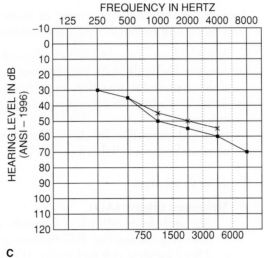

FIGURE 15.2. **Common audiograms.** Examples of audiograms: **A.** Normal audiogram. **B.** Conductive hearing loss. **C.** Sensorineural hearing loss. ✻ = bone conduction. ■ = air conduction. (Reproduced, with permission, from Lalwani A, et al. *Current Otolaryngology—Head and Neck Surgery,* 1st ed. New York: McGraw-Hill, 2004: Figure 44-2.)

TREATMENT

■ **Hearing aids:** The 1° treatment for presbycusis; however, < 50% of elderly patients who might benefit from hearing aids actually wear them.
 ■ **Behind-the-ear aids:** The most powerful ear-level units; easier to see and manipulate.
 ■ **In-the-canal aids:** Smaller and more expensive; the best choice for patients with mild to moderate hearing loss.
■ **Aural rehabilitation:** Most patients benefit from this treatment, which includes practical advice on how to optimize communication.

Conductive Hearing Loss

Hearing loss that occurs when sound is not conducted efficiently through the ear canal, tympanic membrane, or ossicles of the middle ear. This type of hearing loss can often be medically or surgically corrected.

SYMPTOMS/EXAM

- May present with painless sudden or gradual loss of hearing.
- Exam may reveal **obstruction** (eg, cerumen impaction), middle ear effusion, otosclerosis, and ossicular disruption.

DIAGNOSIS

- Weber and Rinne tests may help differentiate conductive from sensorineural hearing loss.
- Audiometry.

TREATMENT

Treatment is geared toward correcting the underlying cause.

Dementia

Acquired progressive impairment of memory that interferes with activities of daily living and causes at least 1 the following:

- Aphasia: Loss of the ability to understand and/or produce language.
- Apraxia: Difficulty with carrying out learned actions or movements in the absence of motor or sensory impairment.
- Agnosia: Failure to recognize or identify objects despite intact sensory function.
- Impaired executive function: Includes the abilities to initiate, monitor, plan, and organize behaviors.

Types of dementias:

- **Alzheimer disease (AD):**
  - Accounts for two-thirds of dementia cases; affects 6%–8% of individuals ≥ 65 years of age and 30% of those ≥ 85 years of age.
  - The 2 greatest risk factors for AD are advanced age and ⊕ family history of AD.
- **Vascular dementia:**
  - Accounts for 15%–25% of dementia cases.
  - Common risk factors for vascular dementia include hypertension, hyperlipidemia, diabetes mellitus, smoking, advanced age, and male sex.
- **Other (less common) dementias:**
  - Lewy body dementia (cognitive fluctuations, visual hallucinations, parkinsonism, neuroleptic sensitivity).
  - Frontotemporal dementia (personality and social behavior changes, nonfluent speech).
  - Neurodegenerative conditions, such as Huntington disease, and metabolic abnormalities.

SYMPTOMS/EXAM

Presents with **gradual, progressive memory loss** (may be stepwise, with periods of plateaus in vascular dementia). Other common features include:

- Word-finding and concentration problems.
- Emotional lability, personality changes, social withdrawal.
- Difficulties with dressing, cooking, balancing checkbook, maintaining hygiene.
- Visuospatial disturbances.

KEY FACT

Dementia is not an inherent aspect of aging.

DIAGNOSIS

- Complete history and physical; assess for mood disorders.
- Brief quantitative screening tests of cognitive function, such as the Mini Mental Status Exam (**MMSE**), may be useful and provide a baseline for future comparison. Accuracy depends on age and educational background.
- **Labs:** CBC, glucose, metabolic panel, albumin, LFTs, vitamin B_{12}, UA. Consider VDRL if patient is at risk for 3° syphilis.
- **Imaging:** Routine brain imaging is controversial. If obtained, noncontrast CT is usually adequate and can help identify subdural hematomas, hydrocephalus, and masses.

TREATMENT

- Discontinue nonessential medications, especially sedatives, hypnotics, and anticholinergics.
- Identify and treat coexisting depression, malnutrition, thyroid dysfunction, occult infections.
- Evaluate for home safety and minimize social isolation; consider screening for caregiver stress.
- **Medications:**
    - Cholinesterase inhibitors may slow decline in function and improve cognition in patients with mild to moderate AD and may also be useful in other types of dementia.
    - NMDA (**N-methyl-D-aspartic acid**) antagonists (eg, memantine, amantadine) may provide modest benefit to patients with moderate to severe AD.
    - Behavioral symptoms of dementia, such as paranoia, agitation, and irritability, are best managed by nonpharmacological strategies such as reducing overstimulation.

Delirium

Acute changes in mental status, marked by inattention, poor concentration, and fluctuating levels of consciousness. Commonly occurs in hospitalized elderly patients; one-third of patients > 70 years of age admitted to a general medical facility experience delirium.

SYMPTOMS/EXAM

- ↓ ability to focus, sustain, or shift attention.
- Rapid onset, fluctuating course.
- Rambling, irrelevant, or incoherent speech.
- Confusion.
- May have ↑ or ↓ level of arousal.
- **Hyperactive delirium:** Agitation prominent, may be mistaken for anxiety.
- **Hypoactive delirium:** Psychomotor activity is slowed.

DIAGNOSIS

- **Obtain a thorough history** from individuals close to the patient to determine the frequency and duration of mental status changes. Ask about alcohol and prescription and illicit drug use, as withdrawal can precipitate delirium.
- **Review medications.** Steroids, benzodiazepines, hypnotics, anticholinergics, and TCAs are common causes of delirium.
- Review complete physical exam, with assessment of vital signs and O_2 saturation.

- **Labs:** CBC, serum glucose and electrolytes, UA. Consider blood cultures and arterial blood gas levels.
- **Additional tests:** ECG and CXR may reveal cardiac or pulmonary causes of delirium. LP may also be considered.
- **Imaging:** Head CT may be indicated for high-risk patients (eg, those with head trauma or focal neurologic findings) or when etiology cannot be established.

TREATMENT

- Identify and treat underlying causes.
- Minimize physical and chemical restraints as much as possible.
- Encourage consistent presence of family or caregivers familiar to the patient, as well as clocks and calendars to help with orientation.
- Encourage patients to wear eyeglasses and hearing aids, if indicated.
- Target medications for delirium to specific behaviors (eg, physical aggression, distressing hallucinations).
- Low-dose antipsychotics such as haloperidol are preferred in hyperactive delirium. Use the minimal dose necessary.
- Benzodiazepines are last-line therapy, as they may worsen delirium.

COMPLICATIONS

- Patients with delirium during hospitalization have longer stays, higher mortality rates, and an ↑ risk for deconditioning, pressure ulcers, atelectasis, and malnutrition.
- Delirium may take weeks or months to fully resolve.

Parkinsonism

A syndrome characterized by **resting tremor, bradykinesia, muscular rigidity,** and **loss of postural reflexes.** A common disorder in patients > 60 years of age; affects both sexes and all racial groups. Results from the depletion of dopamine in the **substantia nigra,** leading to unopposed cholinergic activity.

Parkinsonism may be due to Parkinson disease or other neurodegenerative disorders (see Table 15.3) or 2° to drugs, small vessel disease of the brain, trauma, or metabolic disturbances.

SYMPTOMS/EXAM

- Presents with resting tremor or "pill rolling" that is less severe during voluntary movement.
- Bradykinesia commonly manifests as ↓ arm swing while walking.
- Rigidity is evident during passive movement of limbs (eg, "cogwheeling").
- Shuffling gait and impaired postural reflexes are seen.
- Masklike facial expressions are seen, with ↓ frequency of eye blinking.
- Seborrhea of the scalp and face is common.

DIAGNOSIS/TREATMENT

- Clinical diagnosis is made on the basis of symptoms and neurologic exam.
- Discontinue drugs that can worsen parkinsonism (eg, antipsychotics, metoclopramide).
- Regular exercise and physical therapy may aid with balance; occupational therapy may help patients use adaptive strategies and equipment to carry out activities of daily living.

MNEMONIC

Causes of delirium:

PS DELIRIUM

Pain
Sleep deprivation
Drugs—especially when a drug is introduced or changed
Electrolyte and physiologic abnormality—hyponatremia, hypoxemia, acidosis
Lack of medication—withdrawal
Infection—UTI, respiratory infection, sepsis
Reduced sensory input—blindness, deafness, isolation, change of surroundings
Intracranial problems—hemorrhage, meningitis, stroke, seizures
Urinary retention and fecal impaction
Myocardial problems—MI, arrhythmia, CHF

TABLE 15.3.   Clinical Features of Parkinson-Plus Syndromes

SYNDROME	KEY FEATURES
Dementia with Lewy bodies	Cognitive decline, **visual hallucinations,** misidentification of family/friends, marked **daily fluctuations** in mental status.
Progressive supranuclear palsy	Cognitive decline. Extraocular abnormalities, especially **vertical gaze.** Prominent **rigidity** of the entire body, leading to frequent **falls** and a characteristic **facial appearance** ("wide-eyed" scared expression).
Corticobasal degeneration	Cognitive decline, **"alien limb"** phenomenon; **limb apraxia;** inability to perform learned motor tasks (eg, brush teeth, salute).
Multiple-system atrophy Shy-Drager syndrome Olivopontocerebellar atrophy Striatonigral degeneration	Encompasses a group of Parkinson-plus syndromes. **Autonomic dysfunction**, especially orthostatic hypotension. **Ataxia;** incoordination with mild parkinsonism. **Isolated parkinsonism;** no tremor; **no response to levodopa.**

- Medications:
    - **Levodopa/carbidopa:** 1st-line treatment that has been shown to improve all major features of parkinsonism. Levodopa, a precursor of dopamine, is administered with carbidopa, a decarboxylase inhibitor that inhibits peripheral conversion of dopamine, thereby reducing the amount of levodopa required for treatment while lowering the risk of side effects.
    - **MAOIs:** Selegiline may be used as an adjunct to levodopa by inhibiting the degradation of levodopa; sometimes used to improve declining response to levodopa.
    - **Dopamine agonists:** Pramipexole and ropinirole may be considered for initial monotherapy in mild disease to delay the use of levodopa and appearance of levodopa-related dyskinesias and motor fluctuations.
    - **Amantadine:** An antiviral medication that may be used to treat dyskinesias in patients with advanced disease.
    - **Anitcholinergics:** Useful for tremor in younger patients; avoid in elderly patients due to potential adverse effects on cognition.
- **Surgical measures:** Patients who become unresponsive to medical treatment or have intolerable side effects may be helped by brain stimulators or thalamotomy or pallidotomy.

Incontinence

A disorder characterized by the unintentional loss of urine. Causes are multifactorial:

- **Transient factors** include inadequate mobility, motivation, or dexterity; confusion; and medications.
- **Chronic factors** include detrusor overactivity/underactivity, insufficient sphincter tone, or outlet obstruction. Urinary incontinence ↑ risk of decubitus ulcers. Social implications include loss of self-esteem and social isolation.

URGE INCONTINENCE

The most common type of incontinence in geriatric patients. Due to detrusor overactivity.

SYMPTOMS/EXAM

- Patients feel an abrupt urge to urinate, but cannot get to the toilet in time.
- May have nocturia.
- Pelvic and rectal exam should be performed.

DIFFERENTIAL

Mixed, overflow, or stress incontinence; diuretic effect of caffeine or medications.

DIAGNOSIS

- Bladder diary to establish severity of problem, exacerbating factors, etc.
- UA to rule out UTI.
- PSA testing in men.
- Postvoid residual > 200 mL indicates urinary retention.
- Cystoscopy indicated in patients with hematuria or pelvic pain to rule out irritative processes such as stones or cancer.

TREATMENT

- **Nonpharmacologic** methods should be attempted first:
  - Frequently scheduled voids.
  - Bladder retraining, such as urge suppression exercises.
  - Behavior modifications, such as reducing or eliminating caffeine and alcohol and late-night fluid intake.
- **Pharmacologic:**
  - **Anticholinergics** such as **oxybutynin** and **tolterodine** antagonize acetylcholine at muscarinic receptors, leading to bladder smooth muscle relaxation.
  - Tolterodine may cause less dry mouth than oxybutynin.
  - Neuromodulation of the sacral nerve may be helpful in severe, otherwise refractory cases.

STRESS INCONTINENCE

Involuntary loss of urine during a stress maneuver (eg, sneezing, coughing, laughing) due to weak pelvic floor muscles or insufficient internal urethral sphincter strength. More common in women, although it may develop in men following prostate surgery.

SYMPTOMS/EXAM

- Nocturnal symptoms are uncommon.
- Pelvic exam may reveal weak pelvic floor muscle strength or cystocele.

DIAGNOSIS

Look for evidence of pelvic prolapse and causes of intrinsic sphincter deficiency such as use of α-adrenergic antagonists (eg, terazosin), radiation, or surgical trauma.

TREATMENT

- Treat chronic cough if it is a precipitant.
- Kegel exercise to strengthen pelvic floor muscles. Reinforce these exercises, as patients often give up too early.
- Pessaries may benefit women with stress incontinence exacerbated by bladder or uterine prolapse.
- Surgery offers highest cure rates. Options include bladder neck suspension, suburethral slings, and tension-free vaginal tape.
- Periurethral injection of collagen-like substance is a short-term alternative that focally expands pressure to the proximal and mid-urethra.

OVERFLOW INCONTINENCE

Unpredictable dribbling of urine or weak urine stream due to underactive bladder and/or outlet obstruction. The 2nd most common cause of incontinence in older men. Underactive bladder may be due to medications (eg, calcium channel blockers, anticholinergics) or detrusor denervation or injury. Outlet obstruction may be due to enlarged prostate gland, tumors, urethral stricture, or chronic constipation.

SYMPTOMS/EXAM

Thorough history and exam, including digital rectal exam to assess for fecal impaction and abnormalities of the prostate.

DIAGNOSIS

- UA and cytology.
- Postvoid residual. If PVR > 200 mL, renal ultrasound should be obtained to rule out hydronephrosis.
- PSA in males, particularly if > 50 years of age.
- Cystoscopy may help identify masses.
- Urodynamic testing may reveal detrusor underactivity.

TREATMENT

- If possible, discontinue anticholinergics and narcotics that promote urinary retention.
- Prazosin and terazosin are α-blockers that induce internal sphincter relaxation and may relieve retention associated with benign prostatic hyperplasia.
- 5α-reductase inhibitors such as finasteride may partially relieve symptoms associated with BPH, but require months for onset of effect.
- Acute urinary retention and acontractile bladders require indwelling or intermittent catheterization.
- Address constipation, if present.
- Surgical decompression may be required for obstruction.

Osteoporosis

> An 83-year-old woman with a history of hypertension presents with sudden onset of severe left-sided back pain that radiates to her left buttock. Her symptoms occurred when she bent over to pick up a laundry basket. She denies a loss of urine, but reports numbness in her left leg. On exam you note a short, overweight woman in obvious pain, especially when sitting. You are unable to perform a straight-leg test because of her discomfort. What is the diagnosis?
>
> This patient has a vertebral fracture secondary to osteoporosis. Her age and sudden onset of back pain are core features of symptomatic disease. Although osteoporosis affects > 10 million individuals in the United States, only a small proportion are properly diagnosed and treated.

Age-related decline in bone mass, leading to bone fragility and ↑ fracture risk. **Risk factors** include smoking, excessive alcohol consumption, sedentary lifestyle, estrogen deficiency, female gender, white or Asian race, and prolonged corticosteroid use.

SYMPTOMS

- Typically asymptomatic until fractures occur.
- Patients may complain of "getting shorter"; hip, neck, and back pain.
- Sudden acute back pain while performing routine activities such as lifting or bending may indicate a vertebral compression fracture.

EXAM

Classic findings include thoracic kyphosis and loss of height in thin older women; however, men may be affected as well.

DIFFERENTIAL

Osteomalacia, osteopenia, multiple myeloma. 2° osteoporosis may be caused by medications, hyperthyroidism, hyperparathyroidism, and hypogonadism.

DIAGNOSIS

- CBC, chem 7, TSH, and PTH.
- **Dual-energy x-ray absorptiometry (DEXA) scan:** Measures loss of bone mineral density (BMD); the **most accurate and precise method** to diagnose osteoporosis. Routine screening is recommended for women > 65 years of age and women > 60 years of age with significant risk factors.
- **T-scores:** Compare patient's values with normal and healthy bones of young adults.
- Osteoporosis represents a T-score ≤ 2.5 (ie, a BMD that is 2.5 SDs below normal).
- **Z-scores:** Compare patient's BMD values with those of age- and sex-matched controls. Used to track accelerated osteoporosis and treatment response.

TREATMENT

- **Nonpharmacologic therapy:**
  - **Diet:** Should include adequate protein, calcium (1500 mg/day), and vitamin D (800 IU/day).
  - **Exercise:** Weight-bearing exercise such as walking can help strengthen bones.
  - **Smoking cessation.**
- **Pharmacologic therapies:**
  - **Bisphosphonates:** Alendronate and risedronate are 1st-line treatments that $\uparrow$ bone mass and $\downarrow$ the incidence of vertebral and nonvertebral fractures. Effective in women with established osteoporotic fractures.
  - **Selective estrogen receptor modulators (SERMs):** Raloxifene $\uparrow$ BMD and $\downarrow$ total LDL cholesterol concentrations while $\downarrow$ the incidence of vertebral fractures. Less effective than bisphosphonates.
  - **PTH:** Teriparatide is a recombinant human PTH that stimulates bone formation. It is a good choice for high-risk patients who have failed previous treatment. Drawbacks include high cost, daily injection, and $\uparrow$ risk of osteosarcoma. Contraindicated in patients with Paget disease.
  - **Calcitonin:** 2nd-line therapy for the treatment of osteoporosis, but can be used for its analgesic effect in patients who have substantial pain from an acute osteoporotic fracture.

Constipation

Attributable partly to normal physiologic changes such as $\uparrow$ rectal compliance and weakening of pelvic floor and abdominal muscles. Often exacerbated by underlying medical and surgical conditions.

SYMPTOMS

- Characterized by $\downarrow$ stool frequency, difficult passage of feces, and/or a feeling of incomplete evacuation.
- Severe fecal impaction can cause symptoms of intestinal obstruction, colonic ulceration, overflow fecal incontinence, and paradoxical diarrhea.

EXAM

- Thorough physical exam, including rectal exam.
- Hemorrhoids, anal fissures, and rectal prolapse may result from excessive straining.

DIAGNOSIS

- Identify misperceptions about normal bowel movement frequency.
- Chem 8 and TSH tests to exclude metabolic factors.
- Abdominal x-ray to identify the distribution of stool and findings that warrant surgical consultation.
- Colonoscopy to evaluate for structural lesions.

Treatment

Dietary and **behavioral changes** are the **1st-line** approach to correcting constipation:

- ↑ hydration and foods high in fiber; fiber supplementation if needed.
- ↑ physical activity.
- Stop constipating medications, if possible.
- Daily osmotic laxatives such as lactulose and sorbitol are useful for chronic slow-transit constipation.
- Stool softeners (eg, docusate) are helpful for patients who are on opiates or who are bedridden.
- Stimulant laxatives (eg, senna, bisacodyl) are best reserved for short-term use.
- Enemas are best employed when fecal impaction is present.

Falls

Falls are a major cause of morbidity and mortality among elderly patients, especially women. More than 50% of community-dwelling seniors > 80 years of age fall each year, and falls are the 6th leading cause of death in the elderly. Table 15.4 lists common causes of falls and their appropriate interventions.

Complications

Falls commonly lead to fractures of the wrist, vertebrae, and hip. Older persons have a 20% ↑ in mortality rate in the 1st year following a hip fracture.

TABLE 15.4. Causes and Treatment of Falls

Risk Factors	Medical Interventions	Rehabilitative/Environmental Interventions
↓ visual acuity	Corrective lenses; cataract extraction.	Home safety assessment.
↓ hearing	Cerumen removal; audiologic evaluation.	Hearing aid.
Vestibular dysfunction	Avoid drugs affecting the vestibular system; ENT evaluation.	Physical therapy for habituation.
Proprioceptive dysfunction	Screen for cervical spondylosis and vitamin B_{12} deficiency.	Gait and balance exercises.
Dementia	Avoid sedative drugs.	Gait and balance exercises.
Postural hypotension and syncope	Assess medications and consider carotid and cardiac ultrasounds to assess for carotid artery and aortic valve stenosis; rehydration.	
Medication assessment	↓ polypharmacy; select the least centrally acting drugs; prescribe the lowest effective dose. Frequent reassessment of risks and benefits.	

Adapted, with permission, from Tierney LM, et al. *Current Medical Diagnosis & Treatment,* 40th ed. New York: McGraw-Hill, 2000: 60.

Pressure Ulcers

Skin breakdown often attributable to ↓ subcutaneous fat, poor nutrition, and poor circulation in the setting of prolonged pressure and friction over bony prominences such as the ischial tuberosities and sacrum. Immobilization and incontinence are major risk factors for the development of pressure ulcers.

SYMPTOMS/EXAM

Staging is as follows:

- **Stage 1:** Nonblanchable erythema of intact skin.
- **Stage 2:** Partial-thickness superficial skin loss up to subcutaneous tissue.
- **Stage 3:** Full-thickness skin loss through subcutaneous tissue.
- **Stage 4:** Tissue loss down to the level of muscle, tendon, or bone.

DIFFERENTIAL

Infectious ulcers, thermal burns, malignant ulcers (cutaneous lymphoma, basal cell carcinoma, or squamous cell carcinoma), rectocutaneous fistula, ulcers 2° to vascular disease.

TREATMENT

- ↓ pressure, friction, and shearing forces via frequent repositioning and use of protective devices such as pillows, foam or sheepskin, and special mattresses.
- ↓ moisture by treating bladder and bowel incontinence.
- Ensure adequate nursing care to keep affected areas clean.
- Optimize nutrition.
- Mobilize the patient as soon as possible.
- When ulcers are not healing or have persistent exudates after 2 weeks of optimal cleansing and dressing changes, consider antimicrobials (topical for superficial infection, systemic for deep tissue infections).

Insomnia

Impaired ability to fall and stay asleep. Up to 50% of elderly people report sleep problems. Factors that contribute to sleep disorders include the following:

- **Psychiatric:** Bereavement, social isolation, anxiety, depression.
- **Neurologic:** Dementia, leading to nocturnal agitation.
- **Medication:** Including sedative-hypnotics, bronchodilators, diuretics, decongestants.
- **Pain syndromes:** Neuropathic pain, arthritic pain, malignancy syndromes.
- **Respiratory:** Dyspnea from cardiac and pulmonary conditions.
- **Alcohol.**
- **Caffeine.**

Sleep consists of alternating types: non–rapid eye movement (NREM) and rapid eye movement (REM) sleep.

- Majority of time is spent in NREM sleep.
- NREM sleep has 4 stages: stages 1 and 2, defined as light sleep, and stages 3 and 4, consisting of deep restorative sleep.
- Age-related changes in normal sleep include an unchanging percentage of REM sleep and a marked ↓ in stage 3 and 4 NREM sleep.

SYMPTOMS/EXAM

Presents with difficulty falling asleep, intermittent wakefulness during the night, early-morning awakening, and daytime sleepiness.

DIAGNOSIS/TREATMENT

- Evaluate for stress, depressed mood, level of physical activity, and dietary habits.
- Consider sleep apnea and/or restless leg syndrome in the patient and/or patient's partner.
- Identify sleep hygiene patterns that may worsen insomnia and recommend the following:
  - Adherence to regular sleep time and morning rise time.
  - Limitation of daytime napping.
  - Avoidance of caffeine, alcohol, and nicotine in the evening.
  - Limitation of nighttime fluid intake.
  - Limitation of noise, uncomfortable beds, and inappropriate temperature settings.
  - Avoidance of benzodiazepines and antihistamines that ↑ the likelihood of falls and hip fractures.

Postherpetic Neuralgia (PHN)

Exquisite pain that persists after the initial rash of herpes zoster has healed. Can occur at any age, but has a peak incidence in patients 50–70 years of age. The duration and severity of PHN ↑ sharply with age.

- **Sx/Exam:** Symptoms vary but can include constant pain; deep, aching, burning pain; spontaneous intermittent lancing pain; or hyperesthesia. Pain is unilateral. There are no specific exam findings.
- **Dx:** History of a vesicular rash that resolves and is followed by the pain syndrome.
- **Tx:** Once established, PHN is difficult to treat. The most effective treatment is prevention with early and aggressive antiviral therapy. Capsaicin ointment, lidocaine patches, gabapentin, pregabalin, and TCAs are helpful. Narcotics and regional anesthetic blocks +/− steroids can also be considered for resistant cases.
- **Prevention:** Live attenuated varicella virus vaccine (Zostavax) is recommended for patients > 60 years of age to ↓ risk of herpes zoster and subsequent PHN.

Polypharmacy

Defined as problems that occur when patients are taking more medications than needed, rendering them prone to dosage errors and adverse drug reactions and interactions. Changes in physiologic function and pharmacokinetics ↑ sensitivity to medications, thereby ↑ the possibility of iatrogenic illness. Such factors include the following:

- **Distribution:**
  - ↓ in total body water, leading to ↑ concentration of water-soluble drugs.
  - ↑ in body fat, leading to longer half-lives of fat-soluble drugs.
  - ↓ albumin levels limits protein binding of some drugs (eg, warfarin, phenytoin), leaving more free drug available.
- **Metabolism:**
  - **Phase I:** Hepatic enzyme activity (eg, cytochrome P-450) is ↓ and thus affects the metabolism of drugs with high 1st-pass metabolism (eg, propranolol).
  - **Phase II:** Conjugation by acetylation, glucuronidation, or sulfation is not affected by aging.
  - **Excretion:** ↓ GFR leads to ↓ excretion of drugs.

SYMPTOMS/EXAM

May present with delirium, nausea, anorexia, weight loss, hypotension, fatigue, and acute renal failure.

DIAGNOSIS

- Adverse drug reactions must be considered as a potential cause of ill presentations in the elderly.
- Obtain a thorough history of both prescribed and OTC medications, including antihistamines that can have anticholinergic effects.

TREATMENT

- Ensure that the symptom requiring treatment is not due to another drug.
- Use drug therapy only after nonpharmacologic methods have been tried.
- Slowly titrate doses.
- Simplify dosage schedule and number of pills and avoid frequent medication changes.

Palliative and End-of-Life Care

Palliative care focuses on relief of pain and other distressing symptoms of serious illnesses. Palliative care may be used during, but is not limited to, the end of life.

ETHICAL AND LEGAL ISSUES

End-of-life care is guided by the same ethical principles that inform other types of medical care. In addition, there are 3 unique ethical considerations that are relevant to end-of-life care:

- **Medical futility:** A unilateral decision by the physician to forgo futile interventions. This decision may create conflict between the physician and the patient or family, but such conflict can usually be resolved through timely, frequent, and consistent communication.
- **Withdrawal of care:** The principle that the patient has the right to stop unwanted treatments once begun as well as to refuse those treatments before they are started.
- **Doctrine of double effect:** The argument that the potential to hasten imminent death is acceptable if it comes as an unintended consequence of a 1° intention to provide comfort and relieve suffering.

Decision-Making Capacity

Considered intact when a patient can communicate a choice that takes into account the risks, benefits, and consequences of that choice. Must be consistent with the patient's values and goals.

Informed Consent

A process by which a patient is given information about the nature of the intervention, the expected risks and benefits, the likely consequences, and the alternatives to the interventions.

Advance Directives

Documents that allow patients to express their preferences and values to guide care in the event they can no longer make informed decisions. Types of advance directives include the following:

- **Living will:** Allows patients to direct their physicians to withhold or withdraw life-sustaining treatment in the event they develop a terminal condition or enter a persistent vegetative state.
- **Durable power of attorney for health care:** Allows patients to designate a surrogate to make proxy decisions in the event they themselves are unable to communicate their wishes **or** lose decision-making capacity. Applies to all health situations, not just terminal illness.
- **Do not resuscitate (DNR) orders:** Allows patients to request to not receive CPR if their heart stops beating or they stop breathing. DNR orders are accepted by doctors and hospitals in all states. Only 15% of all patients who undergo CPR in the hospital survive to hospital discharge. Patients should be informed of mortality outcomes as well as the potential consequences of surviving CPR (eg, neurologic disability, damage to internal organs, and the likelihood of requiring other aggressive interventions).

HOSPICE CARE

- Patient and family centered; emphasizes the provision of comfort and pain relief rather than an attempt to cure illness and prolong life.
- Requires physicians to estimate the patient's probability of survival as < 6 months.

SYMPTOM MANAGEMENT

Common end-of-life symptoms that should be addressed to maximize quality of life and comfort include the following:

- **Pain:**
  - Assess for pain frequently. Consider use of numeric and visual facial pain scales.
  - Allow the patient to set goals of pain management.
  - Regularly assess and treat side effects of opioids such as nausea and constipation.
  - There is no maximum allowable dosage for opioids such as morphine sulfate; doses should be titrated to achieve adequate pain relief.
- **Dyspnea:**
  - A sensation of dyspnea is common among dying patients.
  - Identify treatable causes (eg, pneumonia, pleural effusion).
  - Buccal morphine sulfate is highly effective; benzodiazepines may help anxiety.
  - Consider supplemental O_2 or open windows for fresh air.

- **Nausea and vomiting:**
    - If opioid related, consider substituting an equianalgesic dose of another opioid or a sustained-release formulation or add a dopamine antagonist antiemetic (eg, haloperidol) to block the chemoreceptor trigger zone.
    - If due to an intra-abdominal process such as constipation, gastroparesis, or gastric outlet obstruction, consider NG suction, laxatives, prokinetic agents, high-dose corticosteroids, and ondansetron.
    - Around-the-clock dosing of antiemetics and as-needed benzodiazepines are also highly effective.
- **Constipation:**
    - Opioids, poor dietary intake, and physical inactivity make constipation common among the dying.
    - Anticipate and prevent constipation via prophylactic bowel regimens of stool softeners and stimulant laxatives when opioid treatment is begun.
    - Consider simple considerations such as privacy, undisturbed toilet time, and a bedside commode in appropriate patients.
- **Delirium and agitation:**
    - Many terminally ill patients experience delirium before death.
    - Nonpharmacologic strategies to help orient patients may be sufficient to ↓ delirium when no other reversible causes are identified.
    - Haloperidol or risperidone can be highly effective.
    - It may be acceptable to do nothing if the delirium does not negatively affect the family or patient.

NUTRITION AND HYDRATION

- Individuals at the end of life have the right to refuse nutrition and hydration.
- Eating without hunger and artificial nutrition can cause potential complications such as nausea, vomiting, choking, and aspiration.
- Starvation is associated with ketonemia, which can cause a sense of well-being, analgesia, and mild euphoria.
- Allow the family to express concerns, and remind them that withholding nutrition at the end of life engenders little hunger or distress.

WITHDRAWAL OF SUPPORT

- Requests for withdrawal of care from informed and competent patients or their surrogates must be respected.
- Physicians may determine medical futility and cease further medical intervention.
- Educate the patient and family on the expected course of events following withdrawal of support.

PSYCHOLOGICAL, SOCIAL, AND SPIRITUAL ISSUES

- Family meetings may help family members and patients during end-of-life transitions.
- Remain attentive to patients' spiritual need to understand the underlying meaning of their lives and their experience in the world.
- Attempt to understand how cultural beliefs and ethnic traditions can affect the experience of dying.

Elder Abuse

An intentional or unintentional act that causes harm to an elderly person. It is estimated that between 1 and 2 million elderly Americans are abused each year; however, it is often unreported. Abuse may be verbal, physical, or sexual; it may also be in the form of neglect and financial exploitation. Domestic and institutional **risk factors** for abuse include isolation, poverty, physical or emotional dependence of the victim on the caregiver, lack of community resources, a low staff-to-patient ratio, and caregiver or staff burnout. Table 15.5 lists the types of elder abuse and their clinical presentations.

SYMPTOMS/EXAM

- Symptoms are wide ranging and may include unexplained withdrawal from normal activities, depressed mood, or a strained or tense relationship with the caregiver or spouse.
- Exam may reveal poor hygiene, unusual weight loss, bedsores, bruises, pressure marks, broken bones, and abrasions.

DIAGNOSIS

Ask screening questions **while the patient is alone.** Inquire about perceived safety and violence in the family. Ask about the patient's dependency on caregivers, friends, and family.

T A B L E 1 5 . 5 . **Types and Characteristics of Elder Abuse**

TYPE	DESCRIPTION
Domestic	Maltreatment of an older adult living at home or in a caregiver's home.
Institutional	Maltreatment of an older adult living in a residential facility.
Self-neglect	Behavior of an older adult who lives alone that threatens his or her own health or safety.
Physical abuse	Intentional infliction of physical pain or injury.
Financial abuse	Improper or illegal use of the resources of an older person without his/her consent, benefiting a person other than the older adult.
Psychological abuse	Infliction of mental anguish (eg, humiliating, intimidating, threatening).
Neglect	Failure to fulfill a caretaking obligation to provide goods or services (eg, abandonment, denial of food or health-related services).
Abandonment	Desertion of an elderly person by someone who has assumed responsibility for providing care to that person.
Sexual abuse	Nonconsensual sexual contact of any kind.

TREATMENT

- Document the type, frequency, and severity of abuse. Assess the decision-making capacity of the victim.
- Health care providers are mandated by law to report suspected elder mistreatment. Reports should be given to the state or county division of Adult Protective Services. In the absence of such services, the reporter should contact the county or state extension office of Child and Family Services.
- **If the patient has the capacity** to make decisions and refuses intervention:
  - Educate the patient about the incidence of mistreatment of the elderly and the tendency for mistreatment to ↑ in frequency and severity over time.
  - Provide written information about emergency assistance numbers.
  - Develop and review a safety plan.
  - Refer the patient to agencies that provide respite care, support for personal care, and transportation.
- **If the patient does not have the capacity** to make decisions, the physician should initiate the process of separating the victim from the perpetrator while arranging supportive services for the whole family, including the abuser.

CHAPTER 16

Reproductive Health

Leticia Cantu, MD
Diana Coffa, MD

Obstetrics

PRECONCEPTION ISSUES

Given that nearly 50% of pregnancies are unplanned, any medical visit with a female patient of childbearing age is an opportunity to offer basic counseling on preconception health.

Preconception Risk Assessment

A thorough preconception risk assessment includes:

- **Past medical history:** Ask about metabolic and autoimmune diseases, cardiac disease.
- **Dietary habits:** Determine body mass index (BMI), food restrictions, and diabetic risk; ascertain if caffeine intake is > 250 mg daily.
- **Medication history:** Ask about prescription drugs, OTC medications, and herbal supplements.
- **Substance abuse:** Inquire about EtOH and illicit drug use.
- **Environmental exposures:** Evaluate exposure to toxins (eg, organic solvents or lead), radiation, or infectious agents (eg, toxoplasmosis, rubella, parvovirus).
- **Age and reproductive history:** Ask about past gynecologic or pregnancy complications and DES exposure.
- **Family history:** Ask about CF, thalassemia, sickle cell anemia, birth defects, endocrine disorders, thromboembolic disease, and multiple gestation.
- **Psychosocial history:** Inquire about domestic violence, financial stability, emotional support, and barriers to care.

Preconception Lab Workup

- **Routine preconception/prenatal labs:** CBC, ABO/Rh, rubella titer, hepatitis B antigen, RPR, Pap smear, chlamydia screening in women < 25 years of age or at risk, gonorrhea in women at risk, and HIV testing.
- The following labs are appropriate in certain situations:
  - **Varicella titer:** If patients have no known history of varicella vaccination or disease.
  - **Hepatitis C antibody:** If patients are at high risk for HCV (eg, if they have a history of IV drug use, have tattoos, or received blood products before 1992).
  - **Fasting blood glucose:** If patients are at high risk for diabetes (eg, if they are obese; have a strong family history of diabetes; or have a prior history of gestational diabetes, macrosomic infant, or fetal demise/ structural anomalies).
  - **PPD +/– CXR:** For patients who are at high risk for TB (eg, immigrants and those with known exposure).
  - **Toxoplasmosis titer:** For patients who are exposed to cat feces or undercooked meat.
  - **CMV/parvovirus titer:** For patients at risk (eg, those who work at day care centers).
  - **Genetic carrier testing:** For familial heritable diseases if indicated (eg, Tay-Sachs disease, sickle cell anemia).

Preconception Interventions

The goal of preconception medical care is to minimize risk, thereby ensuring a healthy outcome for both mother and baby. Recommended interventions include the following:

- Discontinue teratogenic medications.
- Control medical conditions (obtain specialty consultation if indicated).
- Provide dietary and/or substance abuse counseling where applicable.
- Vaccinate against teratogenic illnesses. (Patients should wait 1 month to attempt conception after receiving live attenuated rubella or varicella vaccines.)
- Refer for genetic counseling if indicated (eg, advanced maternal age; family or individual history of congenital problems or heritable diseases).

FIRST-TRIMESTER ISSUES

Diagnosis of Pregnancy

Common symptoms of pregnancy include breast tenderness, fatigue, and nausea or vomiting. Signs on physical exam in the early first trimester include Chadwick sign (blue cervix) or Goodell sign (cervical softening), and uterine enlargement.

Diagnose with urine qualitative hCG assay (98% sensitivity 7 days after implantation), serum quantitative β-hCG assay (sensitivity 4–5 days after implantation), or pelvic ultrasound (a gestational sac is usually visible 5–6 weeks after the last menstrual period [LMP]).

The estimated date of delivery can be established by several methods:

- LMP + 40 weeks, adjusting for cycle length if ≠ 28 days.
- Pelvic ultrasound (the most reliable method):
    - Gestational sac diameter (in millimeters) + 30 = gestational age (in days) **or**
    - Crown-rump length (in millimeters) + 42 = gestational age (in days) (most accurate at 9–12 weeks) **or**
    - Biparietal diameter or femur length (most accurate at 12–15 weeks) **or**
    - Abdominal circumference (most accurate at > 15 weeks).
- Uterine size.
- The presence of fetal heart tones on Doppler ultrasound (audible after 9–12 weeks).
- The presence of fetal movement (felt by the mother by 16–20 weeks).

First-Trimester Routine Prenatal Care

The goals of the initial prenatal visit are 4-fold: to identify patients with undesired pregnancies and refer for adoption counseling/abortion if applicable; to identify any medical or psychosocial problems that merit immediate attention; to establish the gestational age of the pregnancy; and to begin patient education.

- **Physical exam:** A full exam, including a thyroid, breast, and pelvic exam, along with BP screening, should be performed within 1–2 weeks of the diagnosis. After 9–12 weeks of gestation, fetal heart tones should be auscultated at each visit with a Doppler ultrasound.

KEY FACT

Accuracy of ultrasound measurement:
- **First-trimester ultrasound:** Accurate to within approximately **1** week.
- **Second-trimester ultrasound:** Accurate to within approximately **2** weeks.
- **Third-trimester ultrasound:** Accurate to within approximately **3** weeks.
- The most accurate ultrasound measurement is a crown-rump length performed between 9 and 12 weeks, which is accurate to within 3–5 days.

- **Initial labs/studies** should include the following:
  - Preconception labs as above, if not already done.
  - A maternal serum antibody test (if Rh ⊖, give RhoGAM at 28 weeks, with any bleeding during pregnancy, and postpartum to prevent Rh isoimmunization).
  - A complete UA with culture.
  - A 1-hour 50-g glucose challenge for diabetic screening in high-risk patients.
  - Pelvic ultrasound for dating if the LMP is unknown.
  - A urine dipstick at each visit to screen for proteinuria and glucosuria.
- **Prenatal counseling:**
  - **Overview of prenatal care:** Patients should be counseled regarding the frequency of prenatal visits, routine pregnancy monitoring, how to reach after-hours care, and other resources that may be available (eg, childbirth classes).
  - **Nutrition:** Patients should follow a healthy, balanced diet, aiming for a 25- to 35-pound total weight gain for a singleton pregnancy (10–15 pounds for a BMI > 26; 35–45 pounds for a BMI < 19.8). They should also be counseled to avoid uncooked food, unpasteurized dairy products, mercury-containing fish, and excess vitamin A. A daily prenatal vitamin with at least 400 µg of folic acid can help prevent neural tube defects.
  - **Drug/alcohol cessation:** Alcohol use is associated with growth retardation, small-for-gestational-age (SGA) babies, fetal alcohol syndrome, and fetal alcohol effects. Illicit drug use is also associated with ↑ neonatal morbidity and mortality and is primarily related to preterm birth, respiratory problems, mental retardation, and poor growth. Promptly refer patients to appropriate substance abuse treatment where applicable.
  - **Tobacco cessation:** Smoking during pregnancy is associated with low birth weight, prematurity, and an ↑ risk of miscarriage and thromboembolic events. Nicotine patches or gum may be used to aid in tobacco cessation; the use of bupropion is not well studied in pregnancy.
  - **Safety:** Screen all patients for domestic violence. Patients should avoid trauma (no contact sports; use seat belts), environmental toxins (organic solvents, lead, radiation), extremes of temperature (no hot tubs), and prolonged immobility. Toxoplasmosis and *Listeria* precautions should also be discussed (eg, avoid raw meat/fish, unpasteurized dairy products, and cat litter), as should safe sex practices.
  - **Genetic counseling:** All women should be offered nuchal translucency testing for Down syndrome and quadruple screening with serum AFP, hCG, estriol, and inhibin A. If these tests suggest a high risk of genetic disorders, additional testing and services should be offered, including genetic counseling, amniocentesis, chorionic villus sampling, and a detailed anatomic survey by ultrasound.

First-Trimester Fetal Development

Milestones of first-trimester fetal development are outlined in Table 16.1.

Common Problems of the First Trimester

Hyperemesis Gravidarum

Defined as persistent vomiting with weight loss and ketonuria, usually starting at < 10 weeks of gestation. Affects 1 in 200 pregnancies and is especially associated with molar pregnancies and multiple gestations. Advanced maternal age and nicotine use may be protective.

KEY FACT

Assessing gestational age by uterine bimanual exam during the first trimester:
- At 6 weeks, the uterus is the size of a large lemon.
- At 8 weeks, it is the size of an orange.
- At 10 weeks, it is the size of a grapefruit.

KEY FACT

Elevated β-hCG levels probably account for the ↑ incidence of hyperemesis gravidarum in molar and multiple-gestation pregnancies.

TABLE 16.1.   Fetal Development Milestones

Weeks	Milestones
1–2	Implantation with the beginning of placental development.
3–4	Gestational sac with distinct ectoderm, mesoderm, and endoderm layers.
4–5	Primitive brain.
5–6	Fetal pole with cardiac activity.
4–8	Primitive eyes, ears, abdominal organs, and limb buds.
7	Fetal movement is visible.
8–9	Spine/limb formation and organogenesis are complete.
10	The palate is formed.
12	Breathing, swallowing, sucking motions; the fetus is able to move the head, arms, hands, legs, and feet. Formation of fingernails and toenails.
14	Blinking, meconium accumulation, cardiac/digestive systems fully functional.

SYMPTOMS/EXAM

- Presents with persistent vomiting accompanied by weight loss > 5% of prepregnancy weight.
- Determine orthostatic BPs and fluid status.

DIFFERENTIAL

Normal nausea of early pregnancy; GI disorders (gastroenteritis, hepatitis, appendicitis, biliary disease); metabolic disorders (DM, porphyria); pyelonephritis or other infections; neurologic or psychiatric disease; medication side effects; preeclampsia or HELLP syndrome if diagnosed after 20 weeks; fatty liver of pregnancy.

DIAGNOSIS

- **Labs:** Obtain urine ketones, TSH/T_4, and serum electrolytes.
- **Imaging:** Ultrasound to rule out molar pregnancy or multiple gestation.

TREATMENT

- Initial treatment consists of avoiding triggers; eating small, salty meals with clear fluids; consuming ginger; and using Sea-Bands and acupressure.
- Antiemetics (eg, vitamin B_6, doxylamine, H_2 blockers, promethazine, ondansetron) may be of benefit.
- Patients with severe dehydration and/or > 5% weight loss should be hospitalized with IV/enteral fluids and nutrition.
- Corticosteroids are the last resort for treatment.

COMPLICATIONS

Hypokalemia, metabolic alkalosis, Wernicke encephalopathy, Mallory-Weiss esophageal tears. Mild hyperthyroidism and hyperparathyroidism may also be associated with the condition.

MNEMONIC

Causes of recurrent miscarriage:

RIBCAGE

Radiation
Immune reaction
Bugs (infection)
Cervical incompetence/**C**lotting disorder
Anatomic anomalies (eg, uterine septum)
Genetic (eg, aneuploidy, balanced translocation)
Endocrine

KEY FACT

Any patient who has had > 2–3 spontaneous abortions should be worked up for thromboembolic disorders and chromosomal anomalies.

KEY FACT

Most ectopic pregnancies present between 6 and 8 weeks of gestation.

MNEMONIC

Risk factors for ectopic pregnancy:

PID

Prior ectopic pregnancy/**P**rior abdominal or gynecologic surgery
IUD/**I**nfection
DES exposure in utero/**D**amaged tubes

FIRST-TRIMESTER VAGINAL BLEEDING

- Any vaginal bleeding that occurs prior to 15 weeks of gestation, which can range from spotting to life-threatening hemorrhage. See Table 16.2 for the causes of first-trimester bleeding.
- The immediate goals of management are to maintain maternal hemodynamic stability and to rule out ectopic pregnancy or trophoblastic disease. In the case of spontaneous, incomplete, or missed abortion, uterine evacuation may be performed if the patient desires or if bleeding does not resolve spontaneously or with the administration of misoprostol.

ECTOPIC PREGNANCY

A 20-year-old woman with a recent history of chlamydial cervicitis presents to your clinic with several days of increasing right lower abdominal pain. Her last menstrual period was > 6 weeks ago, and her urine pregnancy test is ⊕. Pelvic ultrasound reveals an empty uterus and an ectopic tubal pregnancy with a visible fetal pole, a tubal mass size of 2.0 cm, and no cardiac activity. How should she be treated?

Appropriate management of this patient would include treatment of her chlamydial infection and a dose of methotrexate with serial serum β-hCG levels (to ensure resolution of the tubal pregnancy) or surgical intervention to remove the tubal pregnancy. If methotrexate administration is unsuccessful or if there are signs of hemodynamic instability, immediate surgical intervention is indicated.

A condition in which an otherwise normal embryo implants outside of the uterus, most frequently in one of the fallopian tubes, but sometimes in the peritoneal cavity. Tubal pregnancies never survive to term and if left untreated will lead to rupture of the fallopian tube, which is considered an **obstetric emergency.** Risk factors for ectopic pregnancy include:

- Previous ectopic pregnancy.
- Current use of an IUD. IUDs do not increase the risk of ectopic pregnancies, but if a woman becomes pregnant with an IUD inserted (an extremely rare occurrence), she is more likely to have an ectopic pregnancy than a pregnant woman without an IUD.
- Prior abdominal/gynecologic surgery or invasive procedures.
- A prior history of PID.
- In utero DES exposure.
- Tubal/uterine pathology or unusual anatomy.

SYMPTOMS/EXAM

Presents with pelvic pain, vaginal bleeding (variable), and nausea/vomiting.

DIAGNOSIS

- **Imaging:** Ultrasound shows an empty uterus and may reveal an enlarged adnexal mass.
- **Labs:** ⊕ qualitative or ↑ quantitative β-hCG (+/– abnormal doubling time for β-hCG in early pregnancy).

TREATMENT

- Give IM methotrexate if the ectopic pregnancy is small (< 3 cm) and unruptured, with no fetal cardiac activity, and if the patient is stable and likely to be compliant. Follow with serial β-hCG measurements to ensure resolution.

KEY FACT

The absence of an adnexal mass on ultrasound does not necessarily rule out an ectopic pregnancy.

TABLE 16.2. **Common Causes of First-Trimester Bleeding in an Intrauterine Pregnancy**

CAUSE	DEFINITION/PRESENTATION	TREATMENT
Physiologic bleeding	Vaginal spotting in the early first trimester without any other cause; no cramping or other symptoms. Closed cervix on pelvic exam.	Pelvic exam; ultrasound for prolonged spotting; expectant management. The differential includes threatened SAB, ectopic pregnancy, and gynecologic pathology.
Spontaneous abortion (SAB)	The most common complication of early pregnancy (occurs in roughly 20% of recognized pregnancies). Defined as expulsion of an embryo/fetus < 500 g (usually at < 20–22 weeks). Generally presents with moderate bleeding, cramping, and passage of tissue. An open cervix is seen on pelvic exam.	Pelvic exam; ultrasound with serial serum β-hCG if the history of tissue passage is uncertain; D&C for prolonged or heavy bleeding. Risk factors include advanced maternal age, prior SAB, multiparity, toxin/teratogen exposure, and invasive intrauterine procedures.
Threatened abortion	Vaginal bleeding with a closed cervix but no passage of tissue. Cramping is variable. Fetal cardiac activity is present, and uterine size is appropriate for gestational age.	Pelvic exam; ultrasound and/or β-hCG; expectant management. The differential includes SAB, physiologic bleeding, gynecologic pathology, and ectopic pregnancy. Most threatened abortions do **not** result in loss of pregnancy.
Inevitable abortion	Usually painful uterine cramps, increasing bleeding, and a dilated cervix with gestational tissue often visible at the cervical os.	Pelvic exam; removal of tissue at the os may stop bleeding. D&C is indicated for significant cramping or blood loss; otherwise, treat with expectant management or misoprostol.
Incomplete abortion	Embryonic demise with partial passage of tissue. Cramping/bleeding is variable; uterine size is less than dates; retained placental tissue may be visible. Usually occurs at > 12 weeks.	Expectant or medical management can be offered. D&C indicated for significant cramping or blood loss or for retention of gestational products for a prolonged period.
Septic abortion	Uterine infection. Presents with fever, chills, pelvic pain, bleeding, purulent vaginal discharge, a boggy and tender uterus with a dilated cervix, and signs of sepsis.	Stabilize with IV fluids; broad-spectrum antibiotics; D&C. Usually a complication of nonsterile elective abortion or other invasive procedures.
Missed abortion ("blighted ovum")	Embryonic/fetal demise prior to 20 weeks or anembryonic pregnancy with retention of pregnancy. Presents with inadequate growth and absent fetal heart tones or empty gestational sac on routine monitoring. Closed cervix on exam.	Ultrasound to confirm diagnosis; may choose between expectant management, medical management with misoprostol, or D&C/D&E for prolonged retention/ unsuccessful medical management/patient preference.

Methotrexate treatment may be repeated in 1 week in cases of incomplete resolution.

- Laparoscopic injection of methotrexate is appropriate if the patient is unstable and/or unlikely to be compliant.
- Surgical removal is necessary if the ectopic is ruptured or if medical treatment is not indicated or is unsuccessful.

HYDATIDIFORM MOLAR PREGNANCY

A nonmalignant subtype of gestational trophoblastic disease in which an abnormal fertilization event leads to a tumor of fetal origin. Gestational trophoblastic disease must be ruled out in any patient with a ⊕ pregnancy test and significant vaginal bleeding. Molar pregnancies can be complete (no normal

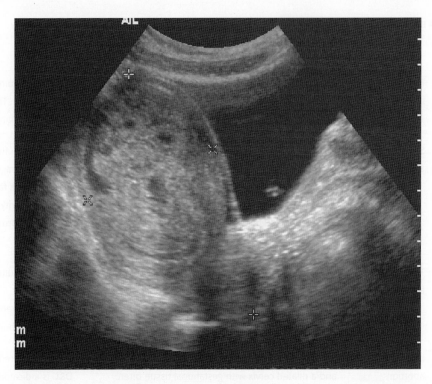

FIGURE 16.1. Molar pregnancy on sagittal ultrasound. Notice the uterus distended by a heterogeneous mass with hypoechoic foci.

fetal tissue is present) or partial (some fetal tissue is present). Risk factors include nulliparity, a history of prior gestational trophoblastic disease, and extremes of maternal age (< 20 or > 35 years).

SYMPTOMS/EXAM

Presents with vaginal bleeding +/– anemia; pelvic pressure or pain; hyperemesis gravidarum; hyperthyroidism; and early-onset preeclampsia.

DIAGNOSIS

- **Imaging:** Ultrasound reveals enlarged ovaries with theca-lutein cysts and an enlarged uterus containing a heterogeneous mass with anechoic areas (Figure 16.1).
- **Labs:** CBC reveals anemia; β-hCG is ↑. Tissue pathology confirms the diagnosis.

TREATMENT

Hemodynamic stabilization; expeditious uterine evacuation; serial β-hCG measurements to ensure resolution; CXR. Consider a repeat pelvic ultrasound.

SECOND- AND THIRD-TRIMESTER ISSUES

Second- and Third-Trimester Routine Prenatal Care

Because the second trimester is the time of most rapid fetal growth, continued self-care and good nutrition are key to ensuring a healthy pregnancy.

Physical Exam During the Second and Third Trimesters

The second- and third-trimester physical exam includes the following elements:

- **Fundal height measurement:** By 20 weeks, the uterine fundus should be palpable at the umbilicus. After 20 weeks, fundal height (in centimeters) should correspond to gestational age (in weeks) +/– 2 cm until the fetus descends into the pelvis at 34–36 weeks.
- **Other:**
  - BP screening; fetal heart rate auscultation (normal is 120–160 bpm); examination for the presence of edema.
  - Additional measures include Leopold maneuvers to determine fetal position after 36 weeks and/or a digital cervical exam to determine the extent of cervical ripening if an induction is planned.

Second- and Third-Trimester Labs/Studies

- Urine dipstick for glucosuria and proteinuria at each visit.
- Offer a "quadruple screen" at 15–18 weeks to measure maternal serum α-fetoprotein, hCG, unconjugated estriol, and inhibin A levels; findings help predict the risk of Down syndrome, neural tube defects, and trisomy 18.
- One-hour 50-g glucose challenge test at 26–28 weeks.
- Check hematocrit; treat with iron if anemic.
- Where applicable, obtain a test of cure for UTIs or genital tract infections; repeat gonorrhea/chlamydia screen in high-risk patients.
- Periodic urine toxicology screens are necessary for high-risk patients.
- Ultrasound for routine anatomic survey is recommended by many providers, although there is no evidence that this measure has any effect on morbidity or mortality.
- Obtain a vaginal/rectal swab for group B streptococcus (GBS) at 36 weeks.

Second- and Third-Trimester Counseling

- **Second trimester:**
  - Continue to discuss nutrition, weight gain, and exercise recommendations.
  - Conduct ongoing screening for domestic violence.
  - Offer education on maternal physiologic changes.
  - Administer influenza vaccine when seasonally available.
- **Third trimester:** As above, plus the following:
  - **Fetal kick counts:** To monitor fetal well-being.
  - **Travel:** Caution patients to avoid airline travel after 35–36 weeks.
  - **Sex:** Sexual activity may stimulate uterine contractions, but is safe in uncomplicated pregnancies with intact membranes.
  - **Work:** Most women are eligible for disability or family leave for the last 3–4 weeks of pregnancy. Patients should also be cautioned to avoid excessive exertion.
  - **Labor plans:** Discuss emotional support (including plans for a doula if available), anesthesia options, fetal monitoring during labor, the labor process, and orientation to the hospital or birth center.
  - **Postpartum birth control:** Discuss options; obtain signed consent for tubal ligation if desired.
  - **Breast-feeding:** Encourage all patients to try breast-feeding; provide patients with information on the advantages of breast-feeding both for the infant and for the mother.
  - **Other postpartum measures:** Discuss routine postpartum and newborn care as well as postpartum follow-up.

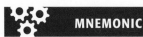

MNEMONIC

The ABCs of second- and third-trimester prenatal visits:

Amniotic fluid leakage?
Bleeding vaginally?
Contractions?
Dysuria?
Edema?
Fetal movement?

Second- and Third-Trimester Fetal Development

Table 16.3 lists significant milestones associated with second- and third-trimester fetal development.

ANTENATAL TESTING

Methods and indications for antenatal testing are as follows:

- **Biophysical profile (BPP):** The BPP is a series of biophysical variables measured by ultrasound that, taken together, can help predict fetal well-being. The scoring includes the following criteria:
  - Fetal tone: Two points for movement extension and flexion of a joint, including opening and closing a hand, in 30 minutes.
  - Fetal movements: Two points for 2 episodes of gross limb or body movements in 30 minutes.
  - Fetal breathing motions: Two points for 1 or more episodes of > 20 seconds in 30 minutes.
  - Nonstress test (NST) assessment of fetal heart rate: Two points in a term pregnancy for a "reactive" NST (2 accelerations of 15 bpm lasting 15 seconds during a 20-minute period).
  - Measurement of amniotic fluid index (AFI): Two points for 1 or more fluid pockets > 2 cm vertically.
- **Modified BPP:** Consists of NST and AFI; currently indicated on a biweekly basis after 36–37 weeks of gestation for pregnancies complicated by gestational diabetes, a hypertensive disorder, multiple gestation, cholesta-

TABLE 16.3. Second- and Third-Trimester Milestones

WEEK	MILESTONES
18	Sleep/wake cycles, hair growth, egg development in females, fully formed placenta.
20	Rapid brain and bone growth; testicular descent in males; thumb sucking.
22	Continuing growth; ability to hear maternal sounds.
24	Tooth buds; beginning of lung maturation.
26	Brain growth; eyes open.
28	Rhythmic breathing motions; disappearance of lanugo; fat accumulation.
30	Head hair develops; lack of space → "fetal position"; brain development.
32	Continued brain growth; immune system development.
34	Vertex position; lungs fully mature.
36	Descent into the maternal pelvis begins.
38	Vernix (sebaceous secretion protecting the skin from the amniotic fluid) is gone.
40	Term gestation.

sis of pregnancy, poly- or oligohydramnios, preeclampsia, or other serious medical or obstetrical conditions.

- An abnormal NST/AFI should be followed by a full BPP.
- If the BPP is normal (10/10), the NST/AFI should be repeated in 2–3 days. If the BPP is 8/10 due to inadequate fluid, rule out ruptured membranes, hydrate, and repeat the NST/AFI in 2–3 days.
- A BPP < 8/10 with adequate amniotic fluid indicates a pregnancy at risk for fetal asphyxia. The patient should be admitted for observation, a BPP should be repeated, and a contraction stress test (CST) should be conducted (see below).
- **CST:** A CST is performed to evaluate fetal ability to tolerate labor. External fetal heart monitors are placed, and either nipple stimulation or IV Pitocin is used to stimulate uterine contractions until either 3 strong uterine contractions occur in 10 minutes with no decelerations in fetal heart rate **or** ≥ 2 fetal heart rate decelerations occur.
  - One fetal heart rate deceleration associated with uterine contraction is considered an equivocal test and should be repeated.
  - A ⊕ CST is a contraindication to labor, and operative delivery should be considered.

Common Problems of the Second and Third Trimesters

THIRD-TRIMESTER BLEEDING

A 35-year-old G8P6 with no history of prenatal care in this pregnancy presents to labor and delivery complaining of heavy vaginal bleeding. Her BP is 90/60, pulse 115, and temperature 37°C (98.6°F); a fetal strip is nonreactive with ↓ variability and tachycardia. The patient has a scar from a prior C-section and has a steady flow of bright red blood from her vagina. How should she be treated?

Initial management of this patient, who has a presumed diagnosis of placenta previa, includes placement of 2 large-bore IVs, typing and crossing of 2–4 units of blood, a call to anesthesia for a stat C-section, and expeditious ultrasound determination of placental position where possible.

Third-trimester bleeding most commonly results from placenta previa, placental abruption, and vasa previa. Table 16.4 outlines the etiologies, presentation, and treatment of these conditions as well as the risk factors associated with each. Low-lying placentas (ie, those in the lower uterine segment, but not covering or immediately adjacent to the os) are also at ↑ risk for bleeding (Figure 16.2).

INTRAUTERINE GROWTH RETARDATION (IUGR)

Defined as fetal weight below the 10th percentile for gestational age. Occurs in about 7% of pregnancies. Etiologies for true growth restriction are classified as fetal, maternal, or placental. Fetal factors include congenital anomalies, genetic syndromes, and multiple gestations; maternal factors include substance abuse, smoking, poor nutrition, hypoxemia, thrombotic and hypertensive disorders, and infections. Placental causes include abruption, hematoma, structural anomalies, and a 2-vessel cord.

TABLE 16.4. **Presentation and Management of Third-Trimester Bleeding**

Cause	Definition	Presentation	Risk Factors	Management
Placenta previa	Placental tissue completely or partially covering the internal cervical os. Diagnosed by ultrasound.	Asymptomatic, or presents with generally painless vaginal bleeding late in the second or third trimester. Incidence is 1 in 4000 pregnancies.	Advanced maternal age, multiparity, multiple gestation, uterine anomalies, prior gynecologic surgery. May be complicated by placenta accreta (placenta ingrown into the uterine wall).	**If no bleeding:** Complete pelvic rest (no intercourse, tampons, or douching) until resolution of the previa is confirmed on serial ultrasounds or until cesarean delivery. **If actively bleeding:** Admit and stabilize the mother; immediate C-section delivery if fetal/maternal status is nonreassuring. **If bleeding resolves:** Conservative inpatient management with bed rest, corticosteroids, and serial ultrasounds; C-section once fetal lung maturity is confirmed at approximately 34 weeks.
Placental abruption	Separation of the placenta prior to delivery of the infant. An **obstetric emergency;** second-trimester abruption is associated with an extremely poor fetal prognosis.	Constant severe uterine contractions +/– vaginal bleeding (80%); CBC and coags may suggest occult bleeding or consumptive coagulopathy; nonreassuring fetal heart tracing. Partial abruption may be difficult to distinguish from early labor. Diagnosis is clinical; ultrasound is insufficiently sensitive to rule out abruption.	Abdominal trauma, maternal hypertension, smoking, advanced maternal age, thrombophilic disease, increasing parity, cocaine or methamphetamine use, polyhydramnios with sudden rupture of membranes (ROM), preterm premature rupture of membranes (PPROM), multiple gestation, previous abruption.	Stabilize the mother (IVs, type and cross, transfuse PRN); continuous fetal monitoring. **If nonreassuring maternal/fetal status:** Immediate C-section. **If term and stable:** May deliver vaginally in the OR. **If preterm and stable:** Inpatient conservative management.
Vasa previa	Amniotic blood vessels presenting in front of the fetal head.	Painless vaginal bleeding with ROM, often with fetal heart rate anomalies (a sinusoidal pattern is classic).	Low-lying or multilobed placentas; multiple gestations; in vitro fertilization.	**If term and/or unstable:** Immediate C-section. **If preterm and stable:** Inpatient conservative management; C-section when fetal lungs are mature. Transvaginal ultrasound with color Doppler and/or Apt/Kleihauer-Betke tests to determine the origin of bleeding if the diagnosis is unclear. Rule out DIC.

Symptoms/Exam

Uterine fundal measurements > 2 cm less than expected for gestational age; confirm with ultrasound. If dates are unknown, serial ultrasounds may be needed every 2 weeks for evaluation.

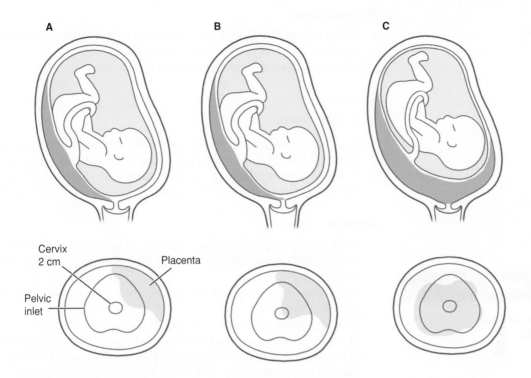

FIGURE 16.2. **Placenta previa.** (A) Marginal placenta previa. (B) Partial placenta previa. (C) Complete placenta previa. (Reproduced, with permission, from DeCherney AH, Nathan L. *Current Diagnosis & Treatment: Obstetrics & Gynecology,* 10th ed. New York: McGraw-Hill, 2007.)

DIAGNOSIS

▪ A detailed fetal anatomic survey by ultrasound can confirm the diagnosis, distinguish symmetric from asymmetric growth restriction, and evaluate the patient for placental causes of IUGR.

▪ Determine fetal karyotype, especially in severe cases and/or those associated with polyhydramnios.

▪ Obtain maternal serum infection titers if rubella, CMV, or syphilis is suspected.

▪ Doppler flow velocimetry of the umbilical artery can determine the systolic-to-diastolic ratio to rule out placental insufficiency.

TREATMENT

▪ Give corticosteroids for lung maturity if the fetus is preterm; follow with antenatal testing.

▪ Deliver by 40 weeks or sooner if there is evidence of placental insufficiency or nonreassuring antenatal testing.

GESTATIONAL DIABETES MELLITUS (GDM)

Defined as glucose intolerance beginning or first recognized during pregnancy. Women with a family history of diabetes and a personal history of glucose intolerance, polycystic ovarian syndrome (PCOS), obesity, glucocorticoid use, or prior macrosomic infants are at high risk. Hispanics, Native Americans, and African Americans are also at ↑ risk. Universal preliminary screening with a 1-hour 50-g glucose challenge should be performed at 24–28 weeks of gestation, but should be done earlier in high-risk patients. If a 1-hour glucose challenge test is ↑ (> 140 mg/dL after 1 hour), a 3-hour glucose tolerance test should be performed within 1 week to confirm the diagnosis.

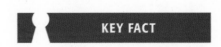

KEY FACT

Any one of the diagnostic criteria for GDM is sufficient to make the diagnosis.

SYMPTOMS/EXAM

- Often asymptomatic. May present with polydipsia/polyuria or frequent infections, especially UTIs or yeast infections.
- Obesity and acanthosis nigricans may be seen.

DIAGNOSIS

Diagnostic criteria:

- Random blood glucose > 200 mg/dL on 2 separate occasions **or**
- Fasting blood glucose > 126 mg/dL on 2 separate occasions **or**
- A 100-g glucose challenge with ≥ abnormal values: > 95 mg/dL fasting, > 180 mg/dL at 1 hour, > 155 mg/dL at 2 hours, or > 140 mg/dL at 3 hours.

TREATMENT

- Offer nutritional counseling. Aim for 30 kcal/kg/day in women of normal weight, with carbohydrates making up no more than 40% of total caloric intake.
- Encourage regular blood sugar monitoring and exercise regimens; offer diabetic education.
- If fasting blood glucose is > 95 mg/dL **or** postprandial glucose is > 130 mg/dL on > 2 occasions, start insulin (bedtime NPH for high fasting glucose at a starting dose of 0.2 U/kg; mealtime regular/lispro for high postprandial glucose at a starting dose of 1.0–1.5 U/10 g of carbohydrates).
- **Peripartum management:** IV saline, NPO, and hourly blood glucose monitoring should be initiated with a goal of 70–110 mg/dL. Most laboring diabetic patients do not require insulin.
- **Postpartum management:** Continue diet and exercise counseling, weight control, and diabetic education, as women with GDM have a significantly ↑ risk of developing subsequent type 2 DM. Check a 2-hour 75-g glucose tolerance test 6 weeks postpartum, and check fasting blood glucose yearly thereafter.

COMPLICATIONS

Preeclampsia, polyhydramnios, fetal macrosomia with ↑ risk of birth trauma/operative delivery, neonatal metabolic complications and ↑ perinatal morbidity, subsequent maternal development of type 2 DM.

MACROSOMIA

Defined as a fetal weight at term exceeding 4.5 kg. Incidence is roughly 9% in the United States. May be associated with maternal DM and congenital anomalies, although many cases of macrosomia are simply constitutionally large.

SYMPTOMS/EXAM

Maternal impression of ↑ fetal weight; uterine fundal height > 2 cm greater than the number of weeks of gestation.

DIAGNOSIS

Clinical assessment by Leopold maneuvers; ultrasound (fetal abdominal circumference is the most accurate parameter).

MNEMONIC

Cornerstones of GDM management:

DIABETIC

Diet
Information
Antenatal testing
Baby growth monitoring
Exercise
Test home blood glucose
Insulin
Check postpartum blood glucose

KEY FACT

Maternal assessment is a more accurate measure of fetal weight than Leopold maneuvers or ultrasound.

TREATMENT

- Maintain tight control of maternal diabetes if applicable.
- Induction or elective C-section at term should be considered only in severe cases.
- In the case of vaginal births, prepare for shoulder dystocia.

COMPLICATIONS

Shoulder dystocia; maternal traumatic injury. ↑ morbidity is associated with a fetal weight > 4 kg.

POLYHYDRAMNIOS

Defined as an accumulation of excess amniotic fluid. Affects 0.2%–1.6% of pregnancies, with potential causes including fetal malformations (especially those that cause problems with fetal breathing or swallowing), fetal anemia, maternal DM, and multiple gestations.

KEY FACT

Most idiopathic cases of polyhydramnios resolve spontaneously.

SYMPTOMS/EXAM

Presents with a uterine size measuring large for dates; may be accompanied by ↓ fetal movement.

DIAGNOSIS

- Ultrasound to evaluate AFI, as well as fetal surveillance to look for fetal GI obstruction (eg, esophageal or duodenal atresia or gastroschisis) or neurologic abnormalities.
- Glucose challenge test if one has not already been done.
- Kleihauer-Betke test to look for fetomaternal hemorrhage.
- Maternal serology for infectious agents and hereditary metabolic abnormalities; amniocentesis for karyotype analysis if severe.

TREATMENT

- Monitor AFI every 1–3 weeks.
- Amnioreduction is appropriate for cases that are symptomatic and severe.
- Give indomethacin, especially if severe and/or preterm.

COMPLICATIONS

Maternal respiratory compromise, preterm labor, PPROM, fetal malposition, umbilical cord accidents, postpartum hemorrhage.

OLIGOHYDRAMNIOS

Defined as inadequate amniotic fluid. Incidence of approximately 1 in 200 pregnancies. Oligohydramnios is usually idiopathic, but can be associated with uteroplacental insufficiency (maternal hypertension, medications, placental abruption or infarction) or fetal factors such as intrauterine fetal demise, chromosomal/congenital anomalies, and twin-twin transfusion. Postdate pregnancy and unrecognized rupture of amniotic membranes should also be considered.

SYMPTOMS/EXAM

Presents with a uterine size measuring small for dates and ↓ fetal movement.

DIAGNOSIS

Inadequate AFI measured on ultrasound; consider amniocentesis for karyotype analysis.

TREATMENT

- Maternal hydration; amnioinfusion if necessary for adequate ultrasound assessment of the fetus. Antepartum surveillance with biweekly AFI measurements.
- Labor induction is indicated at term or earlier if there is evidence of non-reassuring fetal status.

COMPLICATIONS

Meconium aspiration, cord accidents, fetal growth restriction.

PRETERM LABOR

Defined as uterine contractions leading to cervical change prior to 37 weeks of gestation. Approximately 10% of births in the United States are preterm. Preterm labor is the second leading cause of perinatal mortality (after congenital anomalies) and is the leading cause of perinatal morbidity. See Table 16.5 for risk factors.

DIAGNOSIS

- UA and culture to rule out pyelonephritis; sterile speculum exam to rule out PPROM (pooling/ferning/nitrazine).
- Obtain cervical swabs for gonorrhea, chlamydia, and bacterial vaginosis.
- Obtain a fetal fibronectin (fFN) specimen between 24 and 35 weeks.
- Ultrasound to measure cervical length.
- Serial sterile vaginal exams if membranes are unruptured to evaluate cervical change.

TREATMENT

- **Initial management of preterm contractions:** See Figure 16.3.
- **Active management of preterm labor:**
  - Give antibiotics to treat any UTI or genital infections as indicated; GBS prophylaxis.

MNEMONIC

Risk factors for preterm labor:

PIMS

Placental abruption/**P**olyhydramnios
Infection/**I**nadequate cervix
Multiple gestation/**M**ultiple years
   (advanced maternal age)
Single, **S**ad, or **S**tressed/**S**ubstance abuse

TABLE 16.5. Risk Factors for Preterm Labor

RISK CATEGORY	RISK FACTORS
Socioeconomic	Single, anxiety/depression, emotional stress, poor nutrition, maternal age > 40 or < 18, substance abuse, tobacco, African American, extreme physical exertion.
Uterine/placental	Multiple gestation, polyhydramnios, uterine anomalies (especially those → uterine overdistention), cervical incompetence, placental abruption, or placenta previa.
Infectious	Bacteriuria/pyelonephritis, STIs, bacterial vaginosis, periodontal disease.
Fetal	Congenital anomalies, growth restriction.

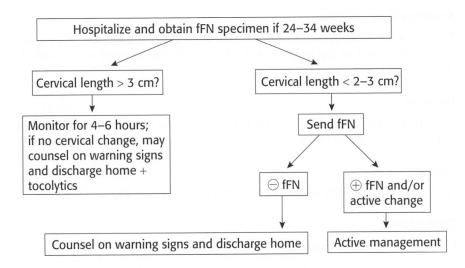

FIGURE 16.3.   Algorithm for the treatment of preterm contractions.

- Administer corticosteroids (betamethasone 12 mg QD × 2; maximum benefit is derived 48 hours after the first dose) if prior to 34 weeks' gestation.
- Bed rest (unproven benefit); tocolytics prolong labor 48 hours to 7 days, but have not been shown to improve outcomes (Table 16.6). They are standard of care and should be used to give time for the administration of steroids, transfer to an appropriate facility, or resolution of a known cause of preterm labor (ie, trauma, abdominal surgery).

PREMATURE RUPTURE OF MEMBRANES (PROM)

Defined as rupture of amniotic membranes before the onset of uterine contractions. PPROM refers to PROM that occurs prior to 37 weeks of gestation. The incidence of PROM is 1 in 10 pregnancies; most patients will enter labor spontaneously within 24 hours. Risk factors are similar to those for preterm labor and include genital tract infection, a prior history of PPROM, smoking, cervical incompetence, polyhydramnios, multiple gestation, and antepartum hemorrhage.

KEY FACT

fFN is a protein that acts as a trophoblastic "glue" between the uterine lining and the chorionic membranes; its presence in the vagina between 24 and 34 weeks may indicate chorionic-decidual separation. If the test is performed correctly, it has a 98% negative predictive value.

TABLE 16.6.   Guidelines for Treatment with Tocolytics

MEDICATION	CLASS	LOADING DOSE	MAINTENANCE DOSE	SIDE EFFECTS/COMPLICATIONS
Terbutaline	β-adrenergic agonist.	2.5–5.0 µg IV.	Up to 25 µ/min or until contractions abate.	Contraindicated in women with cardiac disease.
Magnesium sulfate		4–6 g IV.	IV infusion 2–4 g/hr; monitor serum magnesium levels and DTRs.	Magnesium toxicity (loss of DTRs, respiratory paralysis, cardiac arrest).
Nifedipine	Calcium channel blocker.	30 mg PO.	20 mg q 4–8 hr.	Fewest side effects.
Atosiban	Oxytocin receptor antagonist.	Not available in the United States.	Not available in the United States.	Considered first-line treatment outside the United States owing to favorable side effects; efficacy is similar to that of terbutaline.

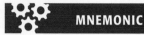

MNEMONIC

Contraindications to tocolysis:

OH SH**

Pregnancy **O**ver (intrauterine fetal demise or lethal anomaly)
Hypertension (severe preeclampsia or eclampsia)
Small baby (IUGR)
Hemorrhage (especially with maternal hemodynamic instability)
Infection (chorioamnionitis)
Troubled baby (nonreassuring fetal heart tracing)

SYMPTOMS/EXAM

Presents with leaking or gushing of clear fluid from the vagina and pooling of amniotic fluid in the vaginal vault. Avoid a digital cervical exam until the patient is in labor!

DIAGNOSIS

⊕ **nitrazine testing** (blood or semen may also turn nitrazine paper ⊕); **ferning** of amniotic fluid; pooling of fluid in the vaginal vault.

TREATMENT

An algorithm for the treatment of PPROM is outlined in Figure 16.4.

COMPLICATIONS

Chorioamnionitis, endometritis, preterm delivery.

HYPERTENSIVE DISORDERS OF PREGNANCY

A spectrum of complex multisystem diseases of uncertain etiology that complicate up to 1 in 5 pregnancies and are associated with greatly ↑ fetal and maternal morbidity and mortality. Milder forms (eg, transient gestational hypertension) are often a precursor to more severe forms (eg, preeclampsia).

TRANSIENT GESTATIONAL HYPERTENSION

Defined as a BP ≥ 140/90 on 2 occasions 6 hours apart, with onset after 20 weeks of pregnancy, in the absence of other causative factors. Severe gestational hypertension is defined as BPs > 160/105. Risk factors include a prior or family history of hypertension.

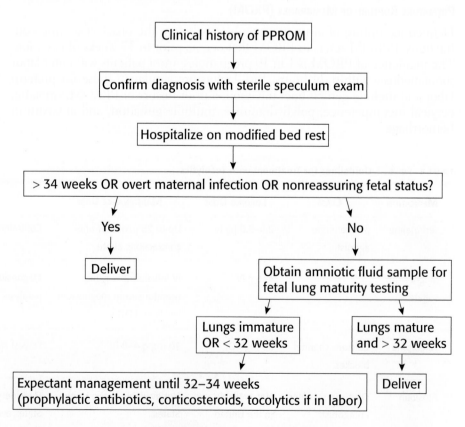

FIGURE 16.4.   Treatment of premature rupture of membranes.

DIAGNOSIS

- Elevated BP, as above.
- Obtain CMP, CBC, and urine dipsticks to test for proteinuria. Consider 24-hour urine collection for baseline protein level in case preecclampsia is suspected later in pregnancy.

TREATMENT

- Diet and exercise counseling.
- Labetalol or methyldopa if systolic BP persistently elevated above 160 mmHg.
- Antepartum surveillance.
- In severe cases, consider delivery by 38–39 weeks.

PREECLAMPSIA

A 36-year-old G3P1 with a history of gestational hypertension presents to labor and delivery at 36 weeks of gestation with a complaint of intense frontal headaches, progressive pedal edema, and nausea over the past week. On initial evaluation, her BP is 176/92, her cervix is favorable, and her urine dip reveals 2+ proteinuria. External fetal monitoring shows a reactive strip. How should she be managed?

Appropriate management of severe preeclampsia at term includes hospital admission, obstetrical consultation, initiation of 24-hour urine collection and GBS swab if this has not previously been done, induction of labor , and IV magnesium for seizure prophylaxis.

Defined as a BP ≥ 140/90 accompanied by proteinuria > 300 mg/24 hours with onset after 20 weeks of pregnancy. Severe preeclampsia is diagnosed in the presence of any of the following: BP > 160/110, CNS or pulmonary symptoms, thrombocytopenia, IUGR, hepatic involvement, oliguria, or proteinuria > 5 g/24 hours.

Risk factors include primigravidity, a past history of preeclampsia, obesity, pre-existing hypertension or renal disease, multiple gestations, diabetes, advanced maternal age, antiphospholipid antibody syndrome, chronic autoimmune disease, and a partner with a prior history of fathering a preeclamptic pregnancy.

SYMPTOMS/EXAM

Patients may present with edema, blurry vision, epigastric pain, nausea, headache, and hyperactive deep tendon reflexes (DTRs).

DIAGNOSIS

- Screen with a urine dipstick for proteinuria on each visit; obtain 24-hour urine protein if dipstick is elevated.
- LFTs, CBC with smear, creatinine, uric acid.

TREATMENT

- **Mild preeclampsia:** Give labetalol, hydralazine, or nifedipine to control BP; supplement with antepartum surveillance and frequent weight checks. Deliver at term; consider $MgSO_4$ for seizure prophylaxis.

- **Severe preeclampsia:**
  - Immediate delivery with continuous fetal monitoring; consider a 48-hour delay only to give steroids for fetal lung maturity.
  - Restrict fluids and monitor urine output; control BP with hydralazine or labetalol; give $MgSO_4$ for seizure prophylaxis; monitor magnesium q 4–6 h; repeat LFTs and creatinine. Aggressive furosemide treatment is appropriate in the presence of pulmonary edema.

COMPLICATIONS

Pulmonary edema, neurologic deterioration, coma, seizure, stroke.

ECLAMPSIA

- Onset of grand mal seizures in a preeclamptic patient in the absence of any other cause. Approximately 1 in 50 severely preeclamptic patients will progress to seizures.
- **Tx:** Check ABCs; stabilize the mother; administer $MgSO_4$ (6 g IV) for seizure control accompanied by fetal monitoring. If $MgSO_4$ is not effective, consider benzodiazepines.

HELLP SYNDROME

A hypertensive disorder characterized by **H**emolysis, **E**levated **L**iver enzymes, and **L**ow **P**latelets. Its incidence is approximately 1 in 1000 pregnancies, and it develops in up to 10%–20% of women with preeclampsia. HELLP syndrome is usually diagnosed during the third trimester, but may present earlier or even postpartum.

SYMPTOMS/EXAM

Patients may present with nausea/vomiting, edema, headache and blurry vision, and ↓ urine output.

DIFFERENTIAL

Acute fatty liver of pregnancy; gastroenteritis or appendicitis; cholecystic or hepatic disease; HUS/TTP.

DIAGNOSIS

- Look for the presence of preeclampsia.
- **Labs:** Hemolytic anemia, platelet count < 100,000, and either LDH > 600 and total bilirubin > 1.2 or AST > 70.
- **Imaging:** Obtain CT/MRI if hepatic infarction, rupture, or hematoma is suspected.

TREATMENT

- Hospitalize and stabilize the mother; assess the fetus.
- Consider corticosteroids for fetal lung maturity if < 34 weeks.
- Hypertensive medications to control maternal BP; platelet transfusion if platelet count is < 20,000 or there is maternal bleeding.
- Expeditious delivery is indicated at > 34 weeks of gestation or in the setting of nonreassuring fetal status or severe maternal disease.

COMPLICATIONS

Associated with a maternal morbidity rate of 1%. See also the **4 H's** mnemonic.

CHOLESTASIS OF PREGNANCY

A syndrome of pruritus and ↑ serum bile acids that typically develops after 30 weeks of gestation. Cholestasis of pregnancy is associated with fetal prematurity and sudden intrauterine demise; its pathogenesis is unknown.

SYMPTOMS/EXAM

- Presents with intolerable itching, especially on the palms and soles, that usually worsens at night.
- May present with jaundice.

DIAGNOSIS

↑ bile acids. Total bilirubin, alkaline phosphatase, and AST/ALT may also be high.

TREATMENT

- Synthetic bile acids; cholestyramine; hydroxyzine for symptomatic relief.
- Deliver by 38 weeks or sooner if severe and fetal lung maturity is established.

PRURITIC URTICARIAL PAPULES AND PLAQUES OF PREGNANCY (PUPPP)

The most common dermatosis of pregnancy, with an incidence of 1 in 160. The cause is unknown. Usual onset is in the late third trimester. There is no associated risk of ↑ fetal/maternal morbidity.

SYMPTOMS/EXAM

- Presents with extreme pruritus, with erythematous papules coalescing to plaques within striae (Figure 16.5).
- The rash usually starts on the abdomen and spreads to the extremities.

DIFFERENTIAL

Pemphigoid gestationis, viral syndromes, allergic reactions, cholestasis.

TREATMENT

Topical steroids; antihistamines for symptomatic relief.

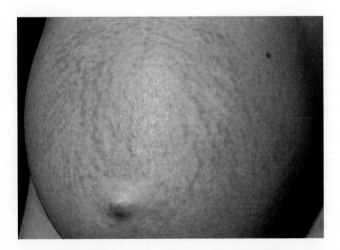

FIGURE 16.5.   Pruritic urticarial papules and plaques of pregnancy. (Reproduced, with permission, from Wolff K, et al. *Fitzpatrick's Dermatology in General Medicine,* 7th ed. New York: McGraw-Hill, 2008.)

BREECH PRESENTATION

Nonvertex presentation of the fetus occurs in 3%–4% pregnancies at term, with the frequency decreasing as the pregnancy approaches term. Risk factors include placental or uterine anomalies, fetal anatomic anomalies, multiple gestation, poly- or oligohydramnios, and a short umbilical cord. Frank, complete, and footling breech presentations are illustrated in Figure 16.6.

SYMPTOMS/EXAM

- The fetal head is not palpable on cervical exam.
- Breech position is found by Leopold maneuvers.

DIAGNOSIS

Confirm the position with ultrasound.

TREATMENT

- **If diagnosed prior to onset of labor,** external cephalic version at 36–39 weeks.
- **If cephalic version is unsuccessful,** schedule a C-section at 39–40 weeks.
- **If presentation is in active labor,** proceed to C-section.

COMPLICATIONS

Labor dystocia; maternal and/or fetal birth trauma. External cephalic version is associated with a risk of placental abruption, cord accident, or fetal distress.

MULTIPLE-GESTATION PREGNANCIES

Although the incidence of monozygotic (identical) twins has remained constant at roughly 1 in 250, dizygotic (fraternal) twinning varies from 1 in 30 to 1 in 100, depending on the population. Risk factors include high parity, family history of twins, assisted reproductive technology, advanced maternal age.

SYMPTOMS/EXAM

- Presents with ↑ uterine size for dates and > 1 fetal heart tone heard on Doppler.
- Also associated with prolonged or more severe nausea than is typical with a singleton pregnancy.

DIAGNOSIS

- Early ultrasound to establish amnionicity/chorionicity; level 2 ultrasound to detect congenital anomalies.
- Serial ultrasound should be obtained through the second and third trimesters every 4–6 weeks (for uncomplicated twin pregnancies) to look for discordant growth or twin-twin transfusion problems.

TREATMENT

- Recommend an extra 300 kcal daily over singleton pregnancies and a 35- to 45-pound weight gain by term for uncomplicated twin pregnancies.
- Antepartum testing with biweekly **NST/AFI** after 36 weeks has not been shown to be effective, but is nevertheless recommended by the American College of Obstetricians and Gynecologists (ACOG).

MNEMONIC

Complications of multiple-gestation pregnancies:

PAPA PIG

Preterm labor
Antepartum hemorrhage
Preeclampsia
Abortion (intrauterine fetal demise)
Polyhydramnios
IUGR
Gestational diabetes

KEY FACT

If division of the embryo occurs:

- **Up to 3 days after fertilization:** Diamniotic/dichorionic
- **Between 4 and 8 days:** Diamniotic/monochorionic
- **Between 8 and 12 days:** Monoamniotic/monochorionic (high risk for morbidity/mortality)
- **After 13 days:** Conjoined twins (extremely high risk; refer to a perinatologist)

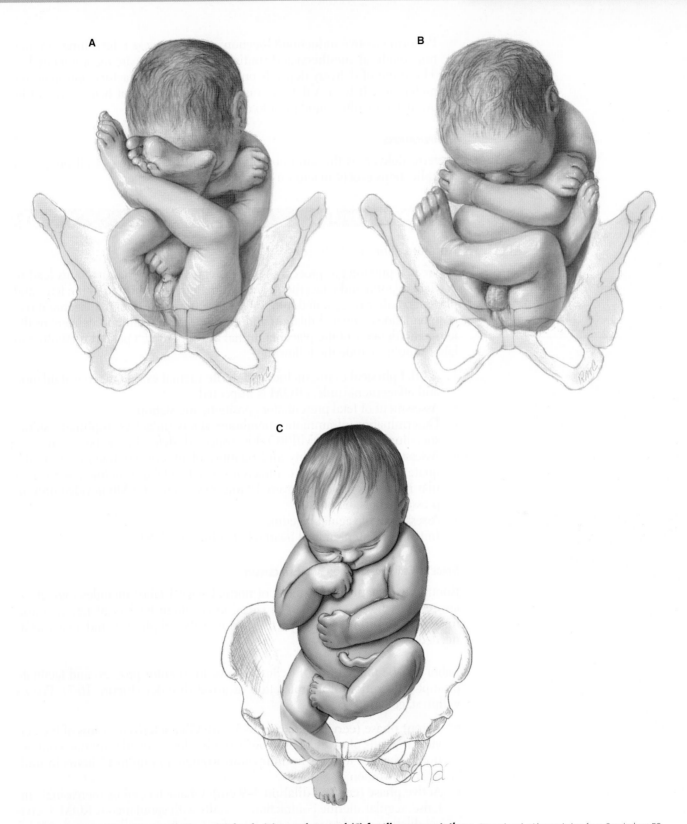

FIGURE 16.6. **Breech presentations: (A) frank, (B) complete, and (C) footling presentations.** (Reproduced, with permission, from Cunningham FG, et al. *Williams Obstetrics*, 23rd ed. New York: McGraw-Hill.)

- Perform elective induction/C-section at 37–38 weeks if fetal lungs are mature; epidural anesthesia and continuous monitoring are recommended.
- The route of delivery depends on presentation, risk factors, and maternal preference. If twin A delivers vaginally, the position of twin B should be evaluated by ultrasound prior to delivery.

COMPLICATIONS

Preterm delivery is the most common complication. ↑ risk of all pregnancy complications except macrosomia and postterm pregnancy.

PERIPARTUM ISSUES

Normal Labor and Delivery

Labor is a physiologic process in which regular uterine contractions lead to cervical dilation and effacement, and, ultimately, to expulsion of the fetus and placenta. Labor is separated into 3 stages, each with distinct management recommendations: cervical dilation and effacement, descent and delivery of the fetus, and delivery of the placenta. Initial assessment of a patient presenting in labor should include the following:

- A brief physical exam, including a sterile vaginal exam for cervical dilation and effacement (unless ROM is suspected).
- Assessment of fetal presentation, position, and station.
- Determination of amniotic membrane status (intact vs. ruptured); sterile speculum exam if ROM/PROM is suspected (defer the vaginal exam).
- Assessment of the quality and quantity of uterine contractions (an adequate number of uterine contractions in active labor is defined as 3–5 regular intense contractions every 10 minutes, each > 60 Montevideo units of pressure above baseline).
- Assessment of vaginal bleeding.
- Initial assessment of fetal heart rate tracing with NST.

STAGE I: CERVICAL DILATION AND EFFACEMENT

Routine expectant management of normal stage I labor includes vaginal exams every 4 hours to monitor progress, intermittent fetal heart rate monitoring (every 15 minutes during active and transitional phases), and analgesia as needed.

Labor can be plotted on a Friedman curve to monitor progress and facilitate prompt recognition of a protraction or arrest disorder (Figure 16.7). Phases within stage I are:

- **Latent phase (cervical dilation 0–3 cm):** Characterized by loss of the cervical mucous plug ("bloody show") and by slow, irregular uterine contractions. May last for days in nulliparous women and up to 14 hours in multiparous women.
- **Active phase (cervical dilation 3–9 cm):** Characterized by increasingly intense, regular uterine contractions, usually with spontaneous ROM. Cervical dilation should progress at a rate of ≥ 1 cm/hr in nulliparas and at ≥ 1.2 cm/hr in multiparas.
- **Transition (cervical dilation 9–10 cm):** Characterized by continued intense uterine contractions; cervical dilation may slow during this phase.

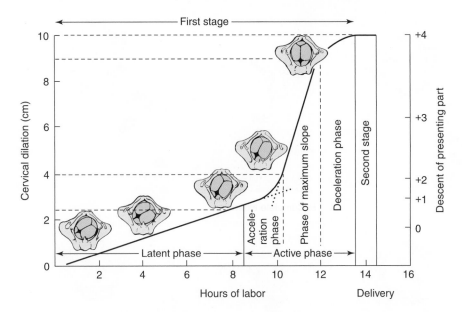

FIGURE 16.7. **Friedman curve showing normal progression of stage I labor in nulliparous women.** (Reproduced, with permission, from Morgan Jr GE, Mikhail MS, Murray MJ. *Clinical Anesthesiology,* 4th ed. New York: McGraw-Hill, 2006.)

STAGE II: DESCENT AND DELIVERY OF THE FETUS

Routine expectant management of a normal second stage of labor includes serial vaginal exams to monitor progress, more frequent fetal heart rate monitoring (every 5 minutes), analgesia as needed, and preparation for delivery of the fetus.

The second stage is characterized by an ↑ in bloody show, continuing intense uterine contractions, intrapelvic pressure, and a maternal urge to push. Accurate assessment of fetal position and station is important for anticipation of potential problems during stage II. Additional considerations are as follows:

- **Duration:** Stage II should last no longer than 1 hour in multiparas and 2 hours in nulliparas, although the presence of epidural/spinal anesthesia may prolong the second stage.
- **Assessment of fetal position:** The fetus undergoes a series of position changes during the end of stage I and stage II in order to pass through the birth canal (Figure 16.8). Most babies are born either right or left occiput anterior (ROA or LOA). Occiput posterior (OP) babies are associated with protracted labors and with an ↑ likelihood of maternal birth trauma. The key to determining position lies in palpation of the sutures of the fetal head.
- **Assessment of fetal station** (3+, 3, 2, 1, 0, –1, –2, –3): Refers to the relative position of the fetal head and maternal ischial spines in centimeters (0 = fetal head level with ischial spines).

STAGE III: DELIVERY OF THE PLACENTA

The third stage of labor should last no longer than 30 minutes. Active management is associated with ↓ rates of postpartum hemorrhage and includes oxytocin administration prior to placental delivery, early cord clamping, and controlled traction. Signs of imminent placental delivery include cord lengthening, a gush of blood indicating placental separation, and a ↓ in uterine fundal height. Collecting cord blood prior to placental delivery provides a sample of fetal blood if needed for testing.

 KEY FACT

The cardinal movements of labor— how to get engaged:

Descend to the floor.

Flex your knee.

Look down (internal rotation) at the ring you are about to give your beloved.

Extend your hand to give your beloved the ring.

Look up (external rotation) to see what the answer will be.

Straighten up (restitute) when the answer is yes!

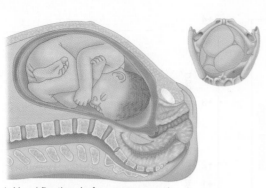

1. Head floating, before engagement

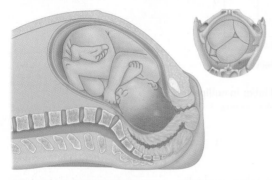

2. Engagement, descent, flexion

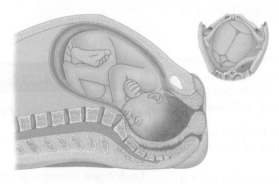

3. Further descent, internal rotation

4. Complete rotation, beginning extension

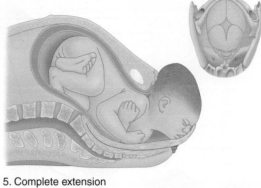

5. Complete extension

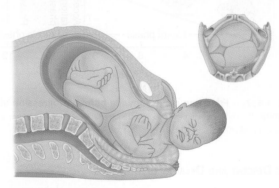

6. Restitution (external rotation)

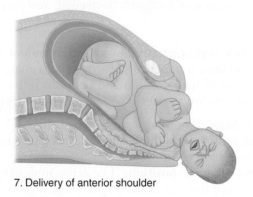

7. Delivery of anterior shoulder

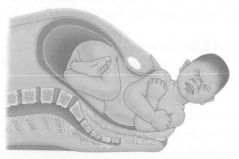

8. Delivery of posterior shoulder

FIGURE 16.8. **Cardinal movements of labor.** Cardinal movements consist of engagement, descent, flexion, internal rotation, extension, external rotation, restitution, and expulsion. (Reproduced, with permission, from Cunningham FG, et al. *Williams Obstetrics,* 22nd ed. New York: McGraw-Hill, 2005: 418.)

Fetal Monitoring

FETAL HEART RATE ASSESSMENT

Assessment of fetal heart rate during labor is a controversial practice, but has become accepted as the standard of care. Initially developed in an attempt to ↓ the rate of cerebral palsy and hypoxic birth injury, continuous electronic fetal monitoring has not been shown to be of benefit, and in uncomplicated labor it is associated with ↑ risk of operative delivery. Intermittent fetal auscultation has begun to replace continuous FHR assessment in some institutions that have sufficient nursing staffing and training.

- **Monitoring techniques:** Performed with an external ultrasound monitor or internal placement of fetal scalp electrodes (more accurate, but more invasive and requires ROM).
- **Monitoring recommendations:**
  - **Intermittent auscultation or external fetal monitoring:** Appropriate for uncomplicated labors; performed every 15 minutes in the active phase of stage I and every 5 minutes in stage II.
  - **Continuous external fetal monitoring:** Indicated if the mother is receiving IV Pitocin for labor induction or augmentation or with conditions known to be associated with ↑ fetal morbidity/mortality.
  - **Continuous internal fetal monitoring:** Use if fetal heart rate tracing cannot be consistently followed with external monitoring or if fetal heart rate tracing is not reassuring.
- **Categories of fetal heart tracing:**
  - **Category 1—normal:** Baseline pulse of 110–160, moderate variability, early decelerations may be present, but no other decelerations. FHR accelerations may or may not be present.
  - **Category 2—indeterminate:** Any of the following: Absent or minimal variability, marked variability, tachycardia, bradycardia without absent variability, absence of accelerations with stimulation, recurrent variable decelerations with minimal or moderate variability, recurrent late decelerations (Figure 16.9) with moderate variability, prolonged decel-

Fetal Heart Rate

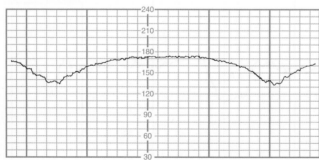

Tocometer

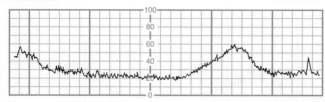

FIGURE 16.9.   Late decelerations on fetal heart rate tracing indicate uteroplacental insufficiency and fetal acidemia. Upper image shows a fetal heart rate with minimal variability and late decelerations reaching their nadir after maximal uterine contraction and slowly resolving. The bottom image displays a tocometer measuring the timing of uterine contractions. In this case, abruption was the cause and immediate C-section was performed. The umbilical artery pH was 7.05. (Reproduced, with permission, from Cunningham FG, Leveno KJ, Bloom SL, et al. *Williams Obstetrics,* 23rd ed. New York: McGraw-Hill, 2008.)

eration > 2 minutes but < 10 minutes, recurrent variable decelerations (Figure 16.10) with slow return to baseline or overshoot.

- ■ **Category 3—abnormal:** Either of the following: Sinusoidal pattern **or** absent variability with recurrent late decelerations or bradycardia.

Management of category 2 fetal heart rate tracing consists of IV fluid, moving the mother onto her left side, oxygen administration, discontinuation of exogenous Pitocin, and treatment of underlying conditions. An internal fetal scalp electrode should be placed for continuous accurate monitoring. Consider terbutaline administration to stop contractions. Consider warm saline amnioinfusion for variable decelerations on fetal heart tracing.

Category 3 fetal heart tracing is an indication for immediate delivery.

Labor Arrest and Protraction Disorders

A protraction disorder is defined as slower-than-normal labor; complete cessation of progress is termed arrest of labor.

MANAGEMENT OF STAGE I PROTRACTION/ARREST

- ■ Assess maternal/fetal well-being.
- ■ Perform a digital cervical exam every 1–2 hours.
- ■ Perform amniotomy if membranes are still intact.
- ■ Oxytocin administration is indicated if uterine contractions are inadequate; titrate the dose to effect.
- ■ An intrauterine pressure catheter (IUPC) is recommended for greater accuracy of oxytocin titration.
- ■ Adequate uterine contractions are typically defined as at least 3 contractions every 10 minutes, each ≥ 60 Montevideo units above baseline and lasting ≥ 10 seconds (200 Montevideo units in a 10-minute period).

Fetal Heart Rate

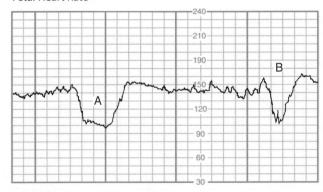

Tocometer

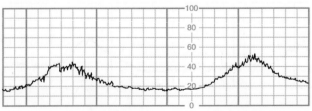

FIGURE 16.10. Variable decelerations on fetal heart tracing suggest cord compression and are not an indication of fetal distress. Top image shows FHR with steep decelerations that resolve rapidly. Bottom image shows tocometer indicating timing of uterine contractions. (Reproduced, with permission, from Cunningham FG, Leveno KJ, Bloom SL, et al. *Williams Obstetrics,* 23rd ed. New York: McGraw-Hill, 2008.)

- A C-section should be considered in the setting of complete arrest despite 4 hours of adequate uterine contractions, especially in the setting of fetal intolerance of labor.

MANAGEMENT OF STAGE II PROTRACTION/ARREST

- Observation is adequate as long as maternal/fetal status is reassuring and some progress has been made.
- Oxytocin administration with IUPC, as above, is appropriate in the presence of inadequate uterine forces.
- Attempt operative vaginal delivery (see below).
- A C-section should be performed if complete arrest is diagnosed, operative vaginal delivery is unsuccessful, or fetal intolerance of labor is diagnosed.

Pain Control During Labor and Delivery

Labor pain is caused primarily by distention of mechanoreceptors in the uterus and cervix during stage I and by stretching and/or tearing of the birth canal and pelvic ligaments during stage II. Fetal malpresentation and nulliparity are physiologic risk factors for ↑ pain, but fear or emotional distress can exacerbate pain as well. A feeling of control over the labor process can greatly improve patients' experience of labor; thus, early education about the labor process and pain control options, along with encouragement of maternal involvement in the decision-making process, is key. Treatment options are as follows:

- **Nonpharmacologic options:** Presence of a doula/labor support person, acupuncture, hypnosis, visualization, breathing exercises, family support, movement, bathing in warm water.
- **Pharmacologic options:** Vary according to stage.
  - **Stage I:**
    - Nalbuphine IV 10–20 mg q 3–4 hr.
    - Fentanyl 25–100 µg IV/IM q 1–2 hr.
    - Epidural anesthesia (continuous drip of local anesthetic and opiate, eg, bupivacaine and fentanyl). Requires bed rest, urinary catheter placement, and continuous fetal monitoring.
    - Spinal anesthesia (opioid injection alone during early labor, or combination opioid/local anesthetic later in labor and/or for C-section). Requires bed rest, urinary catheter placement, and continuous fetal monitoring.
  - **Stage II:**
    - Pudendal block (10 mL 1% lidocaine injected posterior to both ischial spines).
    - Local anesthetic into the perineum, especially if an episiotomy is to be performed.
    - Epidural/spinal anesthesia may be initiated during the second stage (see above), but is less desirable given the prolonged latency of medications and the potential for fetal respiratory depression.

Induction of Labor

Indicated when prolonging the pregnancy puts the mother, the fetus, or both at risk. The most common indication is for postterm pregnancy (≥ 40–42 weeks), but induction may be necessary at any gestational age. If possible, fetal lung maturity should be established either by accurate pregnancy dating or by amniocentesis, and, if necessary, corticosteroids should be administered for fetal lung maturity.

To choose a method for induction, check the Bishop score (Table 16.7).

- **Bishop score > 6:** Associated with a higher chance of success. Start IV Pitocin; cervical ripening agents are not needed.

MNEMONIC

Causes of protraction and arrest disorders:

The 3 P's

Power: Hypocontractile uterine activity, epidural anesthesia, chorioamnionitis
Passenger: Fetal macrosomia, malposition (especially occiput posterior fetus), postdate pregnancy
Pelvis: Pelvic contraction, cephalopelvic disproportion, short maternal stature, obesity

MNEMONIC

Contraindications to spinal/epidural:

BK PAIN

Blood pressure too low (uncorrected hypovolemia)
"Koagulopathy" (bleeding disorder)
Pressure (↑ ICP)
Anatomic back problems
Infection of the soft tissue overlying the epidural injection site
No (the patient refuses)

TABLE 16.7. The Bishop Scoring System

CERVIX	SCORE			
	0	**1**	**2**	**3**
Position	Posterior	Midposition	Anterior	–
Consistency	Firm	Medium	Soft	–
Effacement	0–30	40–50	60–70	≥ 80
Dilation	Closed	1–2	3–4	≥ 5
Station	–3	–2	–1, 0	+1, +2

- Bishop score < 6:
    - Consider a cervical ripening agent such as misoprostol.
    - Consider placement of a Foley bulb into the cervical os.
    - Failure rate is 10%–50%.
    - Continuous fetal monitoring is necessary throughout induction.

Peripartum Complications

GROUP B STREPTOCOCCUS (GBS) INFECTION

- GBS is normal vaginal flora, but used to be the most common cause of neonatal sepsis. It is transmitted during passage through the birth canal.
- Risk factors for neonatal sepsis with GBS are preterm delivery, prolonged ROM, and maternal colonization with GBS.

DIAGNOSIS

- Universal screening should be performed at 35–37 weeks.
- If GBS bacteruria is found on urine culture during this pregnancy, there is no need for vaginal swab, as the mother is considered positive.
- In threatened preterm labor, collect cultures and start treatment during tocolysis. If negative, discontinue treatment and rescreen at 35–37 weeks.

TREATMENT

See Figure 16.11 and Table 16.8.

SHOULDER DYSTOCIA

Defined as failure of the fetal shoulders to deliver spontaneously 1 minute after the delivery of the baby's head, usually because the baby's anterior shoulder is stuck behind the maternal pubic bone. **Considered an obstetrical emergency,** shoulder dystocia occurs in 0.5%–2.9% of deliveries, with most cases affecting babies weighing > 4 kg. Other risk factors include maternal obesity, maternal diabetes, and vacuum or forceps delivery.

Anticipate shoulder dystocia if there is prolonged fetal descent and/or "turtling" of the fetal head.

TREATMENT

See HELPER mnemonic.

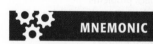

MNEMONIC

Management of shoulder dystocia:

HELPER

Help (ask for help)
Episiotomy
Legs up (perform McRoberts maneuver)
Pressure (suprapubic)
Enter the vagina to rotate with Wood's screw maneuver or to deliver the fetal arm
Return the fetal head to the pelvis for C-section (Zavanelli maneuver)

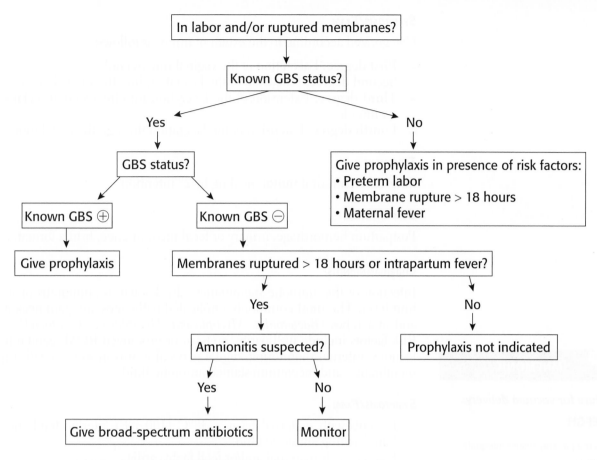

FIGURE 16.11.   Antibiotic prophylaxis for GBS infection.

COMPLICATIONS

Fetal hypoxia, fetal clavicular fracture, Erb palsy, and maternal perineal laceration.

GENITAL TRACT LACERATIONS

Injury to the birth canal during vaginal delivery is the one of the most common obstetrical complications. Perineal midline tears are most common, but periurethral, labial, and cervical lacerations also occur frequently. Risk factors include primiparity, precipitous delivery, fetal macrosomia or malpresentation, operative vaginal delivery, and maternal connective tissue disorders.

TABLE 16.8.   GBS Prophylaxis Regimens

	MEDICATION	INITIAL DOSE	MAINTENANCE DOSE
Preferred regimen	Penicillin G	5 MU IV	2.5 MU IV q 4 hr until delivery
Alternative regimen	Ampicillin	2 g IV	1 g IV q 4 hr until delivery
Penicillin-allergic patients with low risk of anaphylaxis	Cefazolin	2 g IV	1 g q 8 hr until delivery
Penicillin-allergic patients with high risk of anaphylaxis	Clindamycin	900 mg IV	900 mg IV q 8 hr until delivery

SYMPTOMS/EXAM

Categorized according to the extent of injury as follows:

- **First degree:** Laceration of the vaginal mucosa only.
- **Second degree:** Extension of the laceration into the vaginal deep tissue.
- **Third degree:** Extension of the laceration into the external rectal sphincter muscle.
- **Fourth degree:** Extension of the laceration through the rectal mucosa.

TREATMENT

Surgical repair, or if minor, healing by 2° intention.

COMPLICATIONS

Postpartum hemorrhage, urinary or fecal incontinence, fistula formation.

CHORIOAMNIONITIS

Infection of the amniotic membranes; also known as amnionitis or intrapartum fever. The most commonly implicated pathogens are gram-negative rods and anaerobes (*Bacteroides*, *Mycoplasma*, *Ureaplasma*, *Gardnerella*, GBS). Risk factors include nulliparity, preterm or prolonged ROM, genital tract infections, internal monitoring, digital cervical exams in women with ruptured membranes, and meconium-stained amniotic fluid.

SYMPTOMS/EXAM

- Presents with maternal fever > 38°C (100.4°F), uterine tenderness, and foul-smelling amniotic fluid.
- Exam reveals maternal and/or fetal tachycardia.

DIAGNOSIS

CBC; culture of amniotic fluid.

TREATMENT

Treat with broad-spectrum antibiotics (ampicillin and gentamicin) along with continuous fetal monitoring.

COMPLICATIONS

Fetal sepsis, fetal neurologic damage, ↑ C-section rate, wound infection, endomyometritis, postpartum hemorrhage.

OPERATIVE VAGINAL DELIVERY

Refers to application of a vacuum or forceps to assist in vaginal delivery. Criteria for operative delivery include a completely dilated cervix and a term fetus in vertex position and **at least 0 station,** with no shoulder dystocia anticipated. Complications include maternal birth trauma, fetal cephalohematoma, subgaleal hematoma, fetal retinal hemorrhage, and fetal intracranial hemorrhage.

CESAREAN SECTION

Defined as operative removal of the fetus through an abdominal incision. C-sections are indicated for a variety of reasons, classified as either fetal indications (malpresentation, intolerance of labor, fetal congenital anomalies; consider for estimated fetal weight > 4.5 kg) or maternal indications (failure to

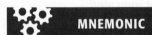

MNEMONIC

Procedure for vacuum delivery:

ABCDEFGH

Address the patient/ensure adequate **A**nalgesia
Bladder must be emptied
Cervix completely dilated, 0 station or more
Determine position of fetal head
Equipment check
Find **F**lexion point, apply vacuum, and engage
Gentle traction downward
Halt if 3 pulls without movement, 3 pop-offs, or 20 minutes

KEY FACT

Operative vaginal delivery should **not** be undertaken unless the provider is willing to abandon the attempt should it prove unsuccessful.

progress, placenta or vasa previa, 1° HSV infection, medical contraindications to labor, uterine/cervical abnormalities). Approximately 20%–25% of babies in the United States are delivered via C-section. Preoperative preparation includes the following:

- Informed consent (with consent for tubal ligation if desired by patient).
- Placement of a Foley catheter.
- Spinal/epidural anesthesia (general anesthesia if emergent).
- Removal of fetal monitors.
- Sterile prep/drape.

Complications of C-section include bleeding; infection; damage to the abdominal organs, especially the uterus, ureters, and bladder; prolonged maternal recovery time; anesthesia risks; and neonatal injury or respiratory depression.

Vaginal Birth After C-Section (VBAC)

Due to the risk of uterine rupture, VBAC should be performed only in hospitals with 24-hour on-site anesthesia and obstetric services and with patients with a history of no more than 1 low transverse or low vertical uterine incision.

Symptoms/Exam

Symptoms and signs of uterine rupture include fetal bradycardia, constant severe abdominal pain, vaginal bleeding, loss of uterine tone, a change in uterine shape, and hypovolemia.

Treatment

The management of VBACs includes continuous monitoring, avoidance of prostaglandin cervical ripening agents, and very close monitoring if oxytocin augmentation is used.

Meconium-Stained Amniotic Fluid

Occurring in roughly 14% of deliveries, meconium-stained amniotic fluid is associated with neonatal meconium aspiration syndrome. Risk factors include postdate gestation and nonreassuring fetal status.

Diagnosis

Diagnosed clinically by the characteristic thick, "pea soup" appearance of amniotic fluid.

Treatment

If there is no spontaneous cry at delivery, attempt intubation with a meconium suction device × 2 before initiating the Neonatal Advanced Life Support (NALS) protocol (Figure 16.12).

Placental Pathology

The placenta is the site of maternal and fetal nutrient exchange and, as such, contains many clues to intrauterine pathology. The basic placental exam includes an assessment of the weight/appearance of placental parenchyma and membranes, cord length, and number of vessels. Indications for a full pathology exam include abnormal placental appearance; preterm or postterm birth; stillbirth; fetal infection, hydrops, or congenital anomalies; oligo- or polyhy-

KEY FACT

Maternal indications for operative vaginal delivery:
- Mother **can't** push (eg, inability to push effectively due to epidural anesthesia)
- Mother **won't** push (eg, maternal exhaustion)
- Mother **shouldn't** push (eg, cardiac disease, ↑ ICP)

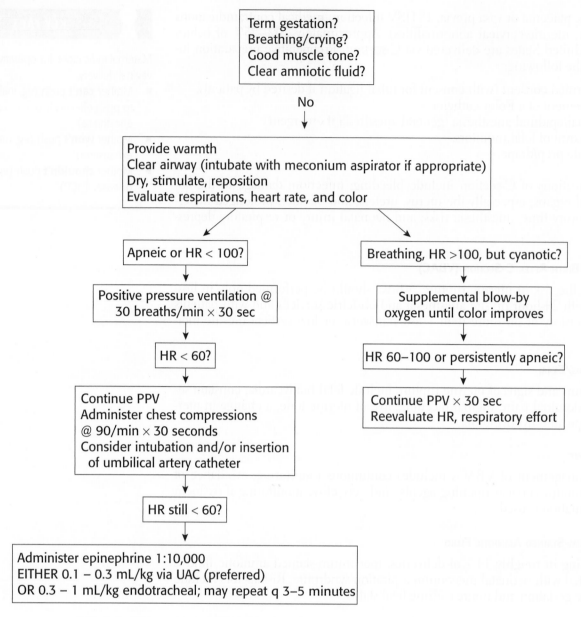

FIGURE 16.12. Neonatal Advanced Life Support protocol.

dramnios; antepartum hemorrhage; or severe hypertensive disorders. Abnormalities include the following:

- Cord abnormalities:
  - **Hypo- or hypercoiled cord/short cord:** Associated with poor fetal growth.
  - **Long cord:** Presents with a knotted or compressed cord.
  - **Abnormal cord insertion** (eg, marginal or velamentous): Associated with cord trauma or thrombi.
  - **Abnormal number of vessels:** Associated with congenital anomalies and IUGR.
- Membrane abnormalities:
  - **Abnormal color:** Associated with infection, meconium, or hemorrhage.
  - **Abnormal membrane insertion:** May be circummarginate (in which membranes originate from the inside margin of the placental disk) or

circumvallate (in which membranes are grooved from abnormally deep implantation in the disk).
- **Parenchymal abnormalities:**
  - **Small placenta:** Associated with inadequate placental perfusion.
  - **Missing lobe:** Presents with retained placental tissue in the uterus.
  - **Calcified placenta:** Associated with postterm pregnancy.
  - **Placenta succenturiata:** An additional lobe; associated with a retained placental lobe or with placenta or vasa previa.
  - **Duplex placenta:** Complete separation into 2 lobes; associated with velamentous cord insertion.
  - **Circumvallate placenta:** A small chorionic plate with growth of extra-chorial placental tissue; associated with premature separation and second-trimester bleeding.

POSTPARTUM ISSUES

Routine Postpartum Care

The postpartum period lasts 6 weeks after delivery. The main focus of routine care consists of mother-baby bonding, establishing breast-feeding, and delivering education regarding routine newborn and self-care. While most obstetrical problems resolve after delivery, you must keep in mind the possibility of persistent gestational diabetes, eclampsia, venous thromboembolism, infection, or hemorrhage.

POSTPARTUM PHYSICAL EXAM

Immediate postpartum examination of the mother should include an evaluation of the extent of bleeding, palpation of the uterine fundus for size and firmness, and assessment of the cervix and perineum for the presence of trauma (see the discussion on repair of vaginal lacerations). Prior to discharge, an exam should be conducted to assess and document the quantity and quality of continuing lochia, lower extremity edema, and any uterine tenderness or breast/nipple abnormalities. A complete physical, including a pelvic exam, should be conducted at approximately 6 weeks postpartum.

POSTPARTUM LABS

- Recheck hematocrit if there was postpartum hemorrhage.
- For women with GDM, a fasting blood glucose should be obtained the day after delivery, and a 2-hour 75-g glucose challenge obtained 6 weeks after delivery to ensure resolution of GDM.

POSTPARTUM COUNSELING

- Ask about common discomforts (eg, urinary retention, constipation, perineal care).
- Determine the frequency of breast-feeding and commonly encountered problems.
- Counsel patients with regard to routine newborn care, including how to take the baby's temperature, anticipate URIs, use car safety seats, and perform jaundice checks.
- Offer information about postpartum depression, family support, and emotional self-care.
- Counsel patients with regard to birth control methods. Estrogen-containing combined hormonal contraceptives are listed as Category 3 on the CDC medical eligibility criteria for contraception during the first 21 days after

MNEMONIC

Postpartum physical exam assessment:

BUBBBLES

Breast
Uterus
Bowel
Blues
Bladder
Lochia
Episiotomy
Surgical site (for cesarean section)

pregnancy because of the risk of clot and decreased breast milk supply. Progesterone-only contraceptives, such as Implanon, Mirena, and progesterone-only pills, do not have these same risks and are listed as Category 2.

- Discuss the duration of normal bleeding and recommend pelvic rest for 6 weeks.

Postpartum Complications

POSTPARTUM ENDOMETRITIS

Defined as uterine infection after delivery, usually caused by *Bacteroides*, *Enterobacter*, group A or B streptococcus, or *Chlamydia trachomatis* (late endometritis). Its incidence after a vaginal birth is < 3%, but is higher after a C-section; risk factors include operative delivery, prolonged ROM, and amnionitis.

SYMPTOMS/EXAM

Presents with fever, abdominal pain, and uterine tenderness without any other identifiable cause.

DIFFERENTIAL

UTI, retained placental products, wound/episiotomy infection, pelvic abscess, septic pelvic thrombophlebitis, drug fever, pulmonary embolism.

DIAGNOSIS

- CBC; UA and urine culture.
- Consider CXR and ultrasound.

TREATMENT

- Ampicillin, gentamicin, and clindamycin **or** ticarcillin/clavulanate.
- Continue antibiotics until the patient is afebrile for 24–48 hours.

POSTPARTUM HEMORRHAGE

Defined as ≥ 500 mL of blood loss 0–24 hours after delivery or blood loss sufficient to make the patient symptomatic (eg, lightheadedness, dizziness, tachycardia). Risk factors include prolonged or very rapid labor, large baby, multiple gestations, nulliparity or grand multiparity, use of endogenous oxytocin, uterine infection, retained placenta, or lacerations of the cervix and vagina. The most common causes are uterine atony and retained tissue or blood clot.

SYMPTOMS

Patients present with continued vaginal bleeding.

EXAM

- Perform a cervical and perineal exam for lacerations; do a bimanual exam to assess uterine tone.
- A placental exam, uterine sweep, and ultrasound can assess for clots/retained tissue.

DIAGNOSIS

Diagnosed through accurate assessment of blood loss postpartum (providers consistently **underestimate** blood loss for vaginal and cesarean deliveries).

MNEMONIC

Causes of postpartum hemorrhage:

The 4 T's

Tissue (retained placenta)
Tone (uterine atony)
Trauma (traumatic delivery, episiotomy)
Thrombin (coagulation disorders, DIC)

MNEMONIC

Treatment of uterine atony:

Arm Pits Help Me Pack Blood In

Arm (bimanual pressure)
Pits (Pitocin; may be given IV or IM)
Help (call for help) and **He**mabate (250 μg IM q 1.5–3.5 hr unless asthmatic)
Methergine (200 μg IM unless hypertensive) and misoprostol 800–1000 μg
Pack (the uterus)
Blood (type and cross; transfusion PRN)
Into the OR for emergent uterine ligation/hysterectomy; **in**terventional radiology for embolization.

TREATMENT

- **Retained placental tissue:** Evacuation or curettage.
- **Genital tract laceration:** Expeditious repair!
- **Uterine inversion** (Figure 16.13): Give terbutaline to relax the uterus; then replace the uterus in the pelvis. Do **not** remove the placenta while the uterus is inverted!
- **Uterine atony:** See the mnemonic **"Arm Pits Help Me Pack Blood In."**

RETAINED PLACENTA

Diagnosed when the third stage of labor lasts > 30 minutes or when the placental exam confirms retention of placental tissue. Occurs in 1%–2% of deliveries and is associated with uterine abnormalities and placenta accreta.

DIAGNOSIS

Ultrasound to determine whether the placenta is detached from the uterine wall.

TREATMENT

- **If the placenta is completely detached:** Manual traction on the umbilical cord.
- **If the placenta is partially or completely adherent:** Attempt manual removal.
- May require general anesthesia in the OR.

COMPLICATIONS

Postpartum hemorrhage, intrauterine infection.

BREAST-FEEDING ISSUES

Breast-feeding imparts passive immunity and complete nutrition to the newborn and promotes mother-baby bonding. Exclusive breast-feeding is recommended for the first 6 months of life and partial breast-feeding thereafter for

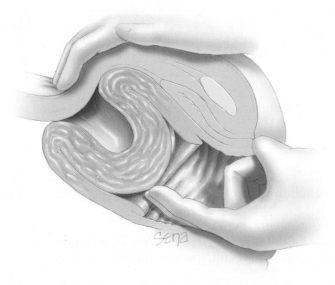

FIGURE 16.13. **Partial uterine inversion.** Partial uterine inversion is diagnosed by a crater-like depression on abdominal palpation and vaginal palpation of the fundal wall in the lower segment and the cervix. (Reproduced, with permission, from Cunningham FG, Leveno KJ, Bloom SL, et al. *Williams Obstetrics*, 23rd ed. New York: McGraw-Hill, 2008.)

the first year. Breast-feeding should be continued as long as mutually desired. Common problems encountered include the following:

- **Engorgement:** Treat with frequent and complete feeds along with cool compresses.
- **Plugged ducts:** Presents with a palpable tender lump. Treat with frequent feeds; aspiration may be required.
- **Mastitis:** Presents with a hard, red, tender area associated with fevers, chills, and malaise. Treat with frequent feeds along with dicloxacillin × 10–14 days.
- **Poor latch:** Improper seal of the infant's lips around the nipple. Address with a lactation consult.
- **Nipple soreness/trauma:** Keep nipples clean with water and saline; air dry; use lanolin cream and/or mupirocin (Bactroban) ointment for refractory cracking or soreness. Consider treating for a yeast infection with topical antifungals if the patient has pink skin surrounding the nipple or complains of stabbing pain during breast-feeding.

INFECTIONS IN PREGNANCY

A 27-year-old G3P2 with poorly controlled gestational diabetes presents to the ER at 30 weeks of gestation with a complaint of 12 hours of lower abdominal pain radiating to the back, accompanied by fever, chills, nausea, and vomiting. Her urine is cloudy, with 25–50 WBCs/hpf. How should she be treated?

Appropriate management of pyelonephritis includes hospital admission, IV fluid administration, fetal monitoring, and IV antibiotics until the patient has been afebrile for 24 hours. Urine should be sent for culture, and antibiotic treatment should be adjusted according to culture and sensitivity results.

Urinary Tract Infections and Asymptomatic Bacteriuria

Caused by the same pathogens as those that affect nonpregnant patients, UTIs complicate roughly 5% of pregnancies. Risk factors include bladder/kidney anomalies, gestational diabetes, and multiparity. Rapid progression to pyelonephritis is the main risk of UTIs in pregnancy.

DIAGNOSIS

Obtain a clean-catch urine culture; perform routine screening at the first prenatal visit.

TREATMENT

- Treat with 7 days of antibiotics (nitrofurantoin, amoxicillin, cephalosporins, or sulfisoxazole); adjust treatment in accordance with culture and sensitivity.
- Obtain follow-up urine cultures.
- Hospitalize for IV antibiotics if pyelonephritis is suspected.
- GBS bacteriuria requires intrapartum antibiotic prophylaxis.

COMPLICATIONS

Pyelonephritis, which is associated with increased risk of preterm delivery and hypoxic fetal events, in addition to severe sepsis and perinephric abscesses in

KEY FACT

Avoid TMP (a folic acid antagonist) in the first trimester, sulfonamides in the third trimester (may cause jaundice), and fluoroquinolones and tetracyclines throughout the pregnancy (potential teratogens).

the mother Bacteriuria is also associated with an ↑ risk of preterm birth and perinatal mortality.

Bacterial Vaginosis

Overgrowth of normal vaginal bacterial flora. Occurs in 10%–25% of pregnant women.

SYMPTOMS/EXAM

Generally asymptomatic; exam reveals a vaginal discharge with a fishy odor.

DIAGNOSIS

- ⊕ KOH "whiff test"; clue cells on wet mount.
- Vaginal discharge with pH > 4.5.

TREATMENT

- Oral metronidazole.
- Generally, treatment is indicated only in symptomatic women. If bacterial vaginosis is found incidentally on Pap, you should only treat women who are at high risk for preterm labor.

COMPLICATIONS

Higher incidence of PPROM; spontaneous abortion; preterm birth.

HIV Infection in Pregnancy

DIAGNOSIS

- Perform routine screening of all pregnant women at the first prenatal visit.
- If the patient has had no prenatal care, obtain a rapid HIV test at the time the patient presents to the hospital in labor.

TREATMENT

- Consultation with an HIV specialist.
- Offer mental health and drug abuse resources as well as behavioral interventions, as applicable.
- Assess current disease status with a CD4 cell count and viral load.
- Initiate antiretroviral treatment during pregnancy, as this dramatically reduces the risk of vertical transmission from 25%–30% to less than 5%.
- Give antibiotic prophylaxis as indicated for opportunistic infections (as with nonpregnant patients).
- Consider elective C-section in the presence of a high viral load.
- Adminster intrapartum antiretroviral prophylaxis.
- Avoid fetal scalp electrodes, episiotomy, or artificial ROM.
- Wash the baby **immediately** after birth.
- Breast-feeding is not recommended for HIV-positive mothers in the United States because of the risk of viral transmission. In developing countries, breast-feeding is still recommended because it is protective against gastroenteritis and other infections that are more common and morbid in these countries.

Genital Herpes Simplex Infection

See the STI discussion for signs, symptoms, and diagnosis.

TREATMENT

- During pregnancy, treat genital HSV outbreaks with acyclovir (400 mg PO BID–TID) or valacyclovir (500 mg PO QD) × 7–14 days for the first outbreak.
- Begin suppressive therapy at 36 weeks.
- A C-section should be performed if a 1° genital HSV outbreak occurs during labor.
- Consider C-section for any patient with active genital lesions.

COMPLICATIONS

Systemic neonatal herpetic infection from passage through the birth canal. Neonatal herpes has a 50% mortality rate.

Varicella-Zoster Infection (VZV)

Infection with varicella zoster, or "chickenpox," affects 1–5 in 10,000 pregnancies and is caused by respiratory transmission of VZV.

SYMPTOMS/EXAM

Normal symptoms of fever, malaise, myalgias, and vesicular rash may be more severe in pregnant women.

DIAGNOSIS

Diagnosed by viral titer.

TREATMENT

- Administer VZIG to neonates at risk and to nonimmune pregnant women who have been exposed to VZV.
- Avoid varicella vaccination during pregnancy.

COMPLICATIONS

Maternal varicella pneumonia (40% mortality), congenital varicella syndrome, neonatal varicella infection.

Syphilis

Given that perinatal transmission in mothers with 1° or 2° syphilis is 50%, universal screening for serology (RPR or VDRL) is recommended at the first prenatal visit.

TREATMENT

Penicillin. Desensitization to penicillin is recommended in penicillin-allergic patients.

COMPLICATIONS

Perinatal death, preterm birth (especially in the setting of a Jarisch-Herxheimer reaction), congenital anomalies, IUGR.

Gonorrhea and Chlamydia

Cervical infection with either *Neisseria gonorrhoeae* or *Chlamydia trachomatis* is associated with an ↑ risk of PROM and preterm labor, chorioamnionitis, endometritis, and neonatal ophthalmologic infection.

DIAGNOSIS

- Perform routine screening of all pregnant women at the first prenatal visit.
- Consider retesting later in pregnancy for patients at high risk.

TREATMENT

- Treat with ceftriaxone 250 mg IM × 1 and azithromycin 1 g PO × 1.
- Public health reporting is mandatory in most states for confirmed diagnosis of either pathogen.

OTHER MEDICAL ISSUES IN PREGNANCY

Depression in Pregnancy/Postpartum Depression

Three percent to 5% of pregnant women and 1%–5% of postpartum women experience major depression. Risk factors include a prior or family history of depression, social and psychological stressors, and intrapartum or neonatal complications.

DIFFERENTIAL

Bipolar disorder, hypothyroidism, generalized anxiety disorder, recreational substance use.

DIAGNOSIS

CBC, TSH, CMP; urine toxicology screen.

TREATMENT

- Counseling; family support; SSRIs (fluoxetine and sertraline are the best studied).
- Hospitalization may be necessary if the depression is severe and/or associated with psychosis.

COMPLICATIONS

- Noncompliance with medical care; impaired maternal-infant bonding; poor nutrition; suicidal/homicidal ideation and attempts; postpartum psychosis.
- Use of SSRIs is associated with persistent pulmonary hypertension of the newborn and may be associated with "neonatal behavioral syndrome," which consists of self-limited tremors, mild tachypnea, and, rarely, seizures.
- Paroxetine is contraindicated because of its association with fetal cardiac abnormalities.

Thromboembolic Disease

Pregnancy is considered a hypercoagulable state, and DVT or pulmonary embolism occurs in 0.2% of pregnancies. Risk factors include inherited thrombophilia, C-section, preterm delivery, and multiple births.

SYMPTOMS/EXAM

- **DVT:** Presents with lower extremity swelling or pain.
- **Pulmonary embolism:** Presents with dyspnea or cough.

DIAGNOSIS

- D-dimer has excellent negative predictive value.
- Lower extremity Doppler ultrasound for suspected DVT; V/Q scan for pulmonary embolism.

TREATMENT

- Anticoagulation with low-molecular-weight or unfractionated heparin up to 4–6 weeks postpartum.
- May switch to warfarin postpartum; titrate to an INR of 1.5–2.5.
- IVC filter for patients in whom anticoagulation is contraindicated.

Medications in Pregnancy

Medications are categorized according to their safety in pregnancy as well as in lactation. Accepted categories are as follows:

- **Pharmaceutical pregnancy categories:**
  - **A:** Safety established using human studies.
  - **B:** Presumed safety based on animal studies.
  - **C:** Uncertain safety; no human/animal studies to date show an adverse effect.
  - **D:** Unsafe; risk may be justifiable in certain clinical circumstances.
  - **X:** Highly unsafe; the risk of use outweighs all possible benefits.
- **Pharmaceutical lactation categories:**
  - ⊕: Generally accepted as safe.
  - ?: Safety is unknown or controversial.
  - ⊖: Generally regarded as unsafe.
- Medications generally accepted as safe for use in pregnancy are outlined in Table 16.9.

TABLE 16.9. **Medications Not Contraindicated in Pregnancy**

CATEGORY	EXAMPLES
Analgesics	Acetaminophen, narcotics (except if used on a long-term basis or in high doses at term).
Antimicrobials	Penicillin, cephalosporin, erythromycin, azithromycin, nystatin, clotrimazole, metronidazole, nitrofurantoin.
Cardiovascular	Labetalol, methyldopa, hydralazine, heparin.
Dermatologic	Erythromycin, clindamycin, benzoyl peroxide.
Endocrinologic	Insulin, levothyroxine, glyburide.
ENT	Chlorpheniramine, diphenhydramine, dextromethorphan, guaifenesin, intranasal steroids.
GI	Antacids, simethicone, H_2 blockers, metoclopramide, docusate, doxylamine.
Psychiatric	Fluoxetine, desipramine, doxepin.
Pulmonary	Albuterol, cromolyn, inhaled steroids, short-term prednisone.

Gynecology

FAMILY PLANNING

A 31-year-old woman presents to your office 5 weeks after the birth of her first baby. Breast-feeding is going well, and she occasionally supplements with formula. She and her partner had planned to remain abstinent until her 6-week postpartum checkup, but last night they had sex on the "spur of the moment" without a condom or any birth control. She feels strongly that they are not yet ready to have another baby. How would you counsel her?

Since she is not breast-feeding exclusively, she should not rely on lactational amenorrhea to prevent pregnancy. You can offer her several options for emergency contraception that are safe during breast-feeding and are available in the office. After that, she may choose from any number of maintenance birth control methods that will be safe both for her and for the baby. She should take a urine pregnancy test in 2–3 weeks.

Contraception

Planning when and if to have children is an important part of overall health maintenance for men, women, and adolescents. Whether through abstinence, natural family planning, or one of the many contraceptive options available, the goal of birth control is to prevent unintended pregnancy so that people may have children when they are ready to be parents.

EMERGENCY CONTRACEPTION

- Defined as postcoital contraception that ↓ the chance of pregnancy if used after unprotected sex or method failure (eg, a condom slips off or doses of oral contraceptives are missed).
- All methods of emergency contraception are more effective the sooner after intercourse they are used.
- Emergency contraception is effective **only** before implantation is established and does not interrupt or terminate an established pregnancy. Like other hormonal birth control methods, its 1° mechanism of action lies in preventing ovulation. It may also prevent fertilization or implantation.
- Emergency contraception may be most needed at night or on weekends, when clinics are closed. To prevent delay in obtaining such contraception, consider providing advance prescriptions (and refills) at routine office visits. Advance provision has been found to be safe and effective and does not ↑ high-risk sexual behavior.
- No clinical examination or pregnancy testing is necessary before an emergency contraception prescription is given. No scheduled follow-up is required after use of emergency contraception. Clinical evaluation is indicated if menses is delayed by a week or more or if lower abdominal pain or persistent irregular bleeding develops; rule out pregnancy, spontaneous abortion, or ectopic pregnancy.

■ Plan B and Ella are two products approved specifically as emergency contraception and can be obtained over the counter by patients 18 and over. Younger patients need prescriptions.

■ If these products are not available, high doses of combined or progestin-only OCPs can be prescribed.

■ Plan B has proven efficacy up to 5 days after intercourse.

■ There are no evidence-based contraindications to Plan B.

■ Common side effects: nausea, vomiting, and irregular bleeding.

■ Table 16.10 outlines options for emergency contraception along with their indications and effectiveness.

COMBINED HORMONAL METHODS

■ OCPs, the weekly patch (Ortho Evra), and the monthly ring (NuvaRing) all work by releasing estrogen and progestin into the bloodstream.

■ With > 99% effectiveness for perfect use and 92% for typical use, these contraceptives are among the most effective available and have also demonstrated good safety and tolerability.

■ **Mechanism of combined hormonal contraceptives:** Estrogen component inhibits ovulation by suppressing FSH and LH; progesterone component inhibits ovulation by suppressing LH, thickening cervical mucus, and inhibiting endometrial proliferation.

■ Conditions that contraindicate the use of combined hormonal methods include:

■ DVT, pulmonary embolism, thrombophlebitis, or a thromboembolic disorder.

■ Uncontrolled hypertension, especially if > 160/100 mmHg, or with vascular disease.

■ A history of MI, CVA, CAD, or valvular heart disease with thrombogenic complications.

■ Diabetes of > 20 years' duration or with vascular involvement (nephropathy, neuropathy, or retinopathy).

■ Heavy tobacco use (≥ 15 cigarettes per day) in patients > 35 years of age. Use caution in all smokers > 35 years of age.

■ History of estrogen-dependent cancer, including breast cancer.

■ Migraines with aura, or any migraines in patients > 35 years of age.

■ Hepatic adenoma, hepatic carcinoma, or acute or chronic hepatocellular disease with abnormal liver function.

■ Planned surgery with prolonged immobilization.

■ Pregnancy.

■ Undiagnosed abnormal vaginal bleeding.

TABLE 16.10. **Emergency Contraception Options**

	PROGESTIN ONLY (EMERGENCY CONTRACEPTION)	COMBINED HORMONAL ("YUZPE METHOD")	COPPER IUD (PARAGARD)
How supplied	Two pills of Plan B (0.75 mg of levonorgestrel) or 40 pills of Ovrette (norgestrel).	Multiple pills from OCP pack (each dose is equivalent to 100–120 µg of ethinyl estradiol and 0.50-0.75 mg of levonorgestrel).	Inserted by provider.
Effective if used	Within 5 days.	Within 5 days.	Within 5–8 days.
Pregnancy rate following use	1%–4%.	1%–4%.	< 1%.

- Use caution with breast-feeding mothers in the first 6 weeks postpartum and in all women in the first 3 weeks postpartum (in view of ↑ DVT risk).
- Noncontraceptive benefits include reduction in ovarian and endometrial cancer risk, regulation and reduction of menstrual bleeding, treatment of dysmenorrhea, reduced PMS/premenstrual dysphoric disorder (PMDD), treatment of pelvic pain due to endometriosis, prevention of menstrual migraines, reduced ovarian cysts (not used to treat existing functional ovarian cysts), and treatment of acne or hirsutism.
- Combined hormonal contraceptives may be safely used continuously—skipping the withdrawal bleed—to treat menses-related conditions or for convenience. This may ↑ the rate of breakthrough bleeding.
- Combined hormonal contraceptives can be started on any day of the menstrual cycle. For convenience, some people start on the first day of menses or the first Sunday after the beginning of menses. The Quick Start method, in which the patient takes her first dose during the visit with the provider, has been proven to ↑ adherence.
- If starting on the first day of a regular menstrual cycle, no backup method is needed. All others should use a barrier method or abstain for 7–14 days.
- Counseling to patient if she misses pill(s):
  - Missed single pill: Take the missed dose immediately and the next dose at the usual time.
  - Missed 2 pills: Take 2 pills immediately and 2 pills the next day.
  - Missed 3 or more pills: Discard pack of pills, allow withdrawal bleed then start new pack.
- Serious complications—including MI, CVA, and DVT—are exceedingly rare.

PROGESTIN-ONLY METHODS

- Available as medroxyprogesterone injected every 3 months (Depo-Provera IM or Depo-SubQ Provera 104) or as progestin-only pills ("minipills") taken daily.
- Associated with an effectiveness of > 99% with perfect use vs. 92% (for pills) and 97% (for injections) with typical use.
- Safe for breast-feeding mothers and their babies.
- Irregular spotting and amenorrhea are common.
- Depo-Provera users may have more weight gain than with other methods.
- When Depo-Provera is stopped, it usually takes 7–12 months for fertility to return.
- Current breast cancer is the only absolute contraindication. Use **caution** if patients have a history of the following conditions:
  - Multiple risk factors for cardiovascular disease.
  - Uncontrolled severe hypertension (≥ 160/110).
  - Current DVT or pulmonary embolism.
  - Ischemic heart disease or CVA.
  - Migraine with focal neurologic symptoms.
  - Unexplained vaginal bleeding prior to evaluation.
  - Past breast cancer.
  - Hepatic adenoma, hepatic carcinoma, active hepatitis, or severe cirrhosis.
  - Postpartum < 6 weeks and breast-feeding.
- Long-term use of Depo-Provera (> 2 years), especially in teens, may lead to ↓ bone mineral density (BMD) in a manner similar to that seen during pregnancy and lactation. Though there is good evidence that BMD returns to baseline after cessation of Depo-Provera, long-term risk is unknown. An FDA warning advises long-term use only if other birth control

methods are unacceptable. Encourage all users to take adequate calcium and vitamin D and to engage in weight-bearing exercise.

■ Progestin-only pills must be taken at the same time every day to be effective.

INTRAUTERINE CONTRACEPTION (IUC)

■ Copper-T (ParaGard) and levonorgestrel-releasing (Mirena) IUCs are the 2 available IUDs. Effectiveness is > 99% with perfect and typical use.

■ Mirena is approved for use up to 5 years, with newer evidence suggesting that its effectiveness lasts 7 years. ParaGard is approved for use up to 10 years, with evidence of effectiveness extending to 12 years. If a device is removed or spontaneously expelled at any time, fertility returns to baseline.

■ Counsel patients to use condoms if they are at risk for STIs. IUCs do not ↑ the risk of acquiring STIs or PID. With monofilament strings, modern IUCs do not cause the ascending infection that older devices are known for. Mirena decreases risk of PID through its effect on cervical mucus. PID complicating IUC insertion is uncommon, and the risk of PID increases only for the first 20 days after insertion.

■ *Actinomyces israelii*, a gram-positive anaerobe found in the GI tract, is more common in the genital tract of IUD users than in nonusers. It is considered a colonizing type of bacteria and does not need to be treated unless the patient has symptoms of infection.

■ Candidates for IUC use:
  ■ Multiparous and nulliparous women.
  ■ Women who desire long-term contraception.
  ■ Women who are not candidates for combined hormonal contraception for medical reasons.

■ Contraindications include the following:
  ■ Pregnancy.
  ■ Active infection (endometritis, PID, cervicitis).
  ■ Anatomic abnormalities or fibroids that distort the uterine cavity enough to make insertion difficult (most fibroids **are** compatible with IUC insertion).
  ■ Current gynecologic cancer.
  ■ Breast cancer (Mirena only).
  ■ Unexplained vaginal bleeding prior to evaluation.
  ■ Allergy to any component of IUC or Wilson disease (for copper-containing IUC).
  ■ For Mirena, all cautions of progestin-only methods apply.

■ IUCs ↓ the overall risk of ectopic pregnancy and are not contraindicated in women with a history of ectopic pregnancy or PID. If a pregnancy occurs, there is an ↑ likelihood that it will be ectopic if an IUC is in place.

■ Light or absent menses are common with Mirena, making it a good treatment for menorrhagia and dysmenorrhea. Irregular spotting, especially in the first 6 months, is common.

■ Heavier menses and cramps are expected with the ParaGard.

■ Routine prophylactic antibiotics during insertion are not indicated.

■ Risks associated with IUC use include uterine perforation, lack of visible strings, creating difficult removal of IUC, and expulsion of IUC.

MALE CONDOMS

■ When used alone, latex condoms are 98% effective with perfect use and 85% with typical use. All condom types have similar contraceptive effectiveness, but animal skin condoms do not protect against STIs (Table 16.11).

KEY FACT

Past use of an IUC does not ↑ the risk of an ectopic pregnancy. Current use of an IUC reduces the risk of pregnancy in general, including an ectopic pregnancy. However, if a pregnancy does occur in a woman with an IUC, it is more likely to be an ectopic pregnancy.

TABLE 16.11.   Condom Choices

	LATEX	**SYNTHETIC**	**ANIMAL SKIN**
Acceptable for latex-allergic users	No	Yes	Yes
Effective pregnancy prevention	Yes	Yes	Yes
Effective STI prevention	Yes	Yes	No
Acceptable lubricant	Water-based	Any	Any

- Educate patients about proper condom use and emergency (postcoital) contraception as a backup method. Avoid use with oil-based lubricants, which may weaken condom.
- Advantages include instant reversibility and protection against STIs.
- Disadvantages include lack of control by the female partner, possible diminishing of sexual pleasure for 1 or both partners, and relatively low effectiveness with typical use.

VAGINAL BARRIERS

- Women have a variety of choices if they wish to use a barrier method that is inserted prior to sexual contact (Table 16.12).
- All vaginal barrier methods confer some degree of protection against STIs, but only the female condom provides protection equivalent to or better than the male condom.
- Educate patients about proper use, cleaning, and storage, as well as the use of emergency (postcoital) contraception as a backup method.

TABLE 16.12.   Vaginal Barrier Choices

	DIAPHRAGM	**FEMALE CONDOM**	**SPONGE**	**CERVICAL BARRIERS**
Acceptable for latex-allergic users	No	Yes	Yes	Yes
Acceptable lubricant	Water-based	Any	Any	Any
Effectiveness (perfect use)	94%[a]	95%	91% nulliparous; 80% parous	Estimated 91%–98%
Effectiveness (typical use)	80%[a]	79%	84% nulliparous; 68% parous	Data not available
STI prevention	+/–	+	+/–	+/–
How to obtain	Fitted and prescribed by provider	OTC	OTC	Fitted and prescribed by provider

[a]When used as recommended with spermicidal jelly.

VAGINAL SPERMICIDES

- Sold as foams, creams, jellies, films, or suppositories.
- When used alone, they are 82% effective with perfect use and 71% effective with typical use.

IMPLANTS

- Implanon is a matchstick-sized single-rod implant that releases progestin slowly, providing up to 3 years of contraception. It is now available from providers trained in insertion and removal techniques.
- > 99% effective with perfect and typical use.
- Norplant, a progestin-releasing method that involved 6 implanted rods, is no longer distributed.

STERILIZATION

- Female sterilization can be accomplished by bilateral tubal surgery. Effectiveness is > 99%.
- Methods of occlusion include electrocoagulation, mechanical occlusion devices (rubber bands or clips), and ligation methods.
- Methods of surgical sterilization include laparoscopy, mini-laparotomy, transcervical fallopian tube coil insertion (Essure), and transvaginal approach.
- Tubal sterilization failure rates are comparable with IUCs.
- Male sterilization is by vasectomy and is also > 99% effective. Vasectomy is considered safer than tubal sterilization, as it is a less invasive procedure performed using local anesthesia.
- Sterilization is considered permanent. Patients should be sure they do not want to have children in the future, as reversal procedures are not reliable.

ABSTINENCE

- The only way to absolutely guarantee against pregnancy is the complete avoidance of penile-vaginal contact.
- Most currently abstinent patients will become sexually active in the future and may still wish information about other family planning methods.
- Those choosing abstinence can still be at risk for nonconsensual intercourse and should be aware of the availability of emergency (postcoital) contraception.

FERTILITY AWARENESS

- Defined as methods that chart fertility based on menstrual cycle timing or physical signs (cervical mucus, basal body temperature, breast and other body changes). The information thus derived can be used to plan a pregnancy, or to prevent pregnancy through use of barrier methods or abstinence during fertile periods.
- With perfect use, fertility awareness methods are 91%–99% effective at preventing pregnancy. With typical use, they are 75% effective.

LACTATION

- Exclusive breast-feeding with associated amenorrhea is > 98% effective at preventing pregnancy for the first 6 months of breast-feeding or until menses return.
- Pumping and supplementing both ↓ the contraceptive effectiveness of breast-feeding.

- Nonhormonal and progestin-only methods are safe for breast-feeding mothers and their infants.
- The estrogen in combined hormonal contraceptives (pills, ring, patch) may ↓ milk production. For nursing mothers who choose an estrogen-containing method, it may be best to delay initiation until 6 weeks postpartum in order to establish optimal breast-feeding.

WITHDRAWAL

- Coitus interruptus, in which the male partner withdraws his penis from his partner's vagina prior to ejaculating, ↓ the risk of pregnancy but does not prevent STIs.
- Provides approximately 96% effectiveness with perfect use and 73% with typical use.
- Disadvantages include lack of control by the female partner, possible diminishing of sexual pleasure for 1 or both partners, and possible transmission of sperm to female prior to ejaculation.
- Educate patients about emergency (postcoital) contraception as a backup method.

ABORTION

When the diagnosis of pregnancy is made, a woman should be offered all options—continuing the pregnancy and parenting, continuing the pregnancy and placing the baby for adoption, or terminating the pregnancy. Half of all pregnancies in the United States are unintended, and half of these are electively terminated. It is estimated that up to 40% of women have an abortion in their lifetimes. Up to the point of viability, abortion is legally protected; when performed by a trained provider, it is extremely safe, with overall complication rates < 1%.

FIRST-TRIMESTER ABORTION WITH ASPIRATION

- Dilation followed by aspiration, with or without sharp curettage, is the most common abortion procedure up to approximately 12 weeks' gestation and can be performed by electric suction or with a handheld manual vacuum aspirator (MVA).
- Analgesia includes local paracervical block plus the option of systemic agents such as NSAIDs, benzodiazepines, and/or narcotics.
- Perioperative antibiotics ↓ the risk of infection.
- The most common complications are incomplete abortion (continued pregnancy or retained tissue) and infection (combined < 1%). Perforation and the need for hospitalization are extremely rare (< 0.1%). Mortality is < 1 in 100,000.

FIRST-TRIMESTER ABORTION WITH MEDICATION

KEY FACT

Contrary to popular myth, abortion does not ↑ a woman's risk of breast cancer or future pregnancy complications.

KEY FACT

Approximately 88% of abortions in the United States are obtained in the first trimester.

A 40-year-old mother comes to your rural family medicine practice concerned because her period is late. Since the birth of their third child 6 years ago, she and her husband have been practicing natural family planning. Her period, which she reports comes every 28 days "like clockwork," is 5 days late. She has mild breast tenderness and nausea, but otherwise feels well, with no cramping or bleeding. A sensitive urine pregnancy test is ⊕. A pelvic exam is normal, with a small uterus consistent with a 5-week pregnancy. Upon learning she is pregnant, the patient is distraught. You provide supportive counseling and discuss her options, and several days later she returns with her husband. They have decided to terminate the pregnancy medically. What medical regimen do you offer her, and what, if any, further testing is needed?

Since her history and exam provide reliable pregnancy dating and there are no signs or symptoms of ectopic pregnancy, you can offer this patient medical termination with mifepristone followed by misoprostol. You can follow with history, exam as needed, and serial quantitative β-hCG levels to confirm completion of the abortion.

- A regimen of mifepristone (formerly RU-486) followed by misoprostol is FDA approved for pregnancy termination up to 7 weeks' (post-LMP) gestation. It is commonly used up to 9 weeks' gestation, based on abundant evidence of effectiveness and safety.
- Mifepristone acts as a progesterone receptor antagonist, and misoprostol acts as a prostaglandin analogue, which increases uterine contractility and softens and dilates the cervix.
- In commonly used evidence-based regimens, the patient takes mifepristone either vaginally or bucally in the provider's office and is then given misoprostol to take at home. Heavy cramping and bleeding follow the misoprostol, and the patient typically passes the pregnancy within several hours.
- Oral NSAIDs and acetaminophen-narcotic combinations are offered as analgesia.
- Prophylactic antibiotics are often used, but their benefit is uncertain.
- Potential side effects of the medications include pain, nausea, vomiting, diarrhea, dizziness, fatigue, headache, and warmth or chills. Complications include continuing pregnancy (1%–4%), infection, and heavy bleeding. Fatal toxic shock syndrome following mifepristone abortion has occurred, but is extremely rare. Medication abortion remains a very safe option for women.
- In the United States, mifepristone can be dispensed by or under the supervision of any physician who certifies that he or she can accurately assess gestational age, diagnose ectopic pregnancy, and offer access to a surgical provider if needed. Ultrasound capability is not required.
- If gestational cardiac activity is detected on vaginal ultrasound 2 weeks after treatment initiation, medical abortion is considered failed and surgical abortion is needed.
- Good patient follow-through is important for medical abortions, so selecting patients who can understand instructions and will be able to follow them is important. Patients must have access to emergency medical treatment if necessary, and surgical curettage should be available.

SECOND-TRIMESTER ABORTION

- Dilation and evacuation (D&E), which combines vacuum aspiration with forceps extraction, is the most commonly used procedure in the United States, with induction terminations also being utilized.
- Analgesia is usually with IV sedation or general anesthesia, but oral analgesics (plus local cervical block) may be adequate for early second-trimester procedures.
- After the first trimester, maternal morbidity and mortality associated with abortion ↑ with gestational age. Second-trimester abortion nonetheless remains very safe, with mortality (approximately 3 per 100,000) lower than that associated with childbirth.

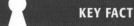

KEY FACT

With an early abortion, keep in mind the possibility of an ectopic or heterotopic pregnancy. Neither uterine aspiration nor mifepristone treats an ectopic pregnancy!

KEY FACT

All abortion patients with Rh-⊖ blood type should receive Rh(D) immune globulin (RhoGAM). Use 50 µg for women who are < 12 weeks' pregnant and 300 µg for those ≥ 12 weeks.

KEY FACT

Hormonal contraceptive methods can be started at the time of or immediately following an abortion procedure. IUDs can be placed at the conclusion of an aspiration procedure.

POSTABORTION CARE

- Pelvic rest is recommended for 2 weeks following an abortion, although there are no data indicating that this is necessary.
- Postabortion bleeding usually abates with time and may continue for up to 2–4 weeks. Patients with excessive bleeding should be assessed for retained products of conception. Monitor for anemia.
- Menses usually return to normal within 4–6 weeks of the abortion.
- Routine follow-up 2 weeks after an uncomplicated abortion is encouraged. At this visit, the provider should address contraceptive needs, offer testing and treatment for STIs, and discuss general social support issues, including patients' remaining questions or sentiments about the abortion.

KEY FACT

In patients diagnosed with gonorrhea, treat presumptively for chlamydia unless you can definitively rule it out.

SEXUALLY TRANSMITTED INFECTIONS (STIs)

A 23-year-old woman presents for a routine checkup and Pap smear. She is sexually active only with her boyfriend of 1 year and uses OCPs. She expresses concern about several small, painless growths on her labia. Her external genital exam reveals multiple nontender, cauliflower-like, skin-colored papules. Speculum and bimanual exams are unremarkable. What is the most likely diagnosis?

HPV-associated genital warts (Figure 16.14). You offer the patient treatment options of topical medications or cryotherapy as well as testing for other STIs.

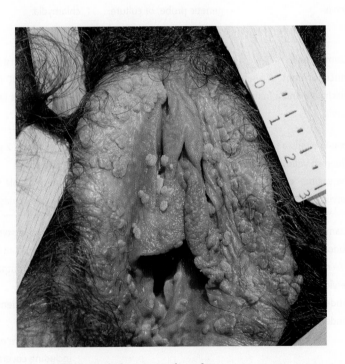

FIGURE 16.14. **Multiple genital warts on the vulva.** (Reproduced, with permission, from Wolff K, et al. *Fitzpatrick's Color Atlas & Synopsis of Clinical Dermatology*, 5th ed. New York: McGraw Hill, 2005: 888.)

The most common STIs are usually asymptomatic in women, so it is important to offer testing to high-risk patients. Routine screening for STIs is recommended for pregnant women and for women or men who are at high risk on the basis of the following risk factors:

- A history of a prior STI or a current diagnosis of another STI.
- New or multiple sex partners, or a partner with multiple partners.
- Age < 25 years.

SYMPTOMS/EXAM

- Evaluation of all patients of reproductive age should include a sexual history.
- The specific symptoms, signs, and diagnostic tests for each STI are listed in Table 16.13.

TREATMENT

Patients diagnosed with any STI should make sure their sexual partners are also treated to prevent reinfection.

TABLE 16.13. **Presentation, Diagnosis, and Treatment of Common STIs**

STI	SYMPTOMS	EXAM	DIAGNOSIS	TREATMENT
Gonorrhea (GC) (*Neisseria gonorrhoeae*); gram–negative intracellular diplococci	Usually asymptomatic in women, or may present with purulent discharge.	Exam reveals **mucopurulent discharge** and a friable cervix.	Test sample from urine or cervical swab using nucleic acid amplification tests, genetic probe, or culture.	Ceftriaxone, cefixime. Consider treating presumptively for chlamydia.
Chlamydia (*Chlamydia trachomatis*); obligate intracellular bacterium	Usually asymptomatic in women, or may present with purulent discharge.	Exam reveals **mucopurulent discharge** and a friable cervix.	Test sample from urine or cervical swab using nucleic acid amplification tests, genetic probe, or culture.	Azithromycin 1 g PO × 1. Doxycycline 100 mg PO BID × 7 days (avoid in pregnancy).
Trichomoniasis (*Trichomonas vaginalis)*; flagellated protozoan	Presents with a copious greenish-yellow vaginal discharge.	Exam reveals a frothy greenish-yellow fluid in the vagina, "strawberry cervix."	Wet mount reveals motile trichomonads and white blood cells.	Metronidazole 2 g PO × 1. Alternatively, metronidazole 500 mg PO BID × 7 days.
Pelvic inflammatory disease (PID); polymicrobial, including *C trachomatis* and *N gonorrhoeae*	Presents with lower abdominal pain +/– fever +/– nausea and anorexia.	Exam reveals diffuse abdominal tenderness +/– rebound with cervical motion tenderness +/– adnexal tenderness.	Diagnosis is clinical. GC and chlamydia cultures may or may not be ⊕.	Ceftriaxone, doxycycline, +/– flagyl. Can be treated as outpatient in stable cases. Consider inpatient IV treatment. Broad-spectrum antibiotics, including coverage for GC, chlamydia, and anaerobes.

TABLE 16.13.   Presentation, Diagnosis, and Treatment of Common STIs *(continued)*

STI	SYMPTOMS	EXAM	DIAGNOSIS	TREATMENT
Genital herpes (HSV-1 or -2)	Presents with painful vesicles (pain may precede eruption) +/− systemic symptoms (fever, myalgia) +/− vaginal discharge. May also be asymptomatic or present with nonspecific symptoms.	Exam reveals tender grouped vesicles on an erythematous base. Ruptured vesicles appear as shallow ulcers or abrasions. Inguinal lymphadenopathy is also seen.	Diagnosis is mainly clinical. Consider viral culture or Tzanck smear from vesicular fluid.	Oral acyclovir, valacyclovir, or famciclovir. Treatment resolves lesions but does not cure HSV; recurrence is common. Suppressive therapy for frequent outbreaks or during pregnancy. Topical therapy not effective.
Genital warts (HPV)	Presents with painless growths on the genitals, anus, or perineum (see Figure 16.14).	Exam reveals fleshy, skin-colored "cauliflower" papules or plaques on the vulva, vagina, or cervix.	Diagnosis is clinical. Rarely may need biopsy.	Treatment resolves lesions; recurrence is common. Treatment options include topical imiquimod or podofilox applied by the patient; podophyllin; cryotherapy; trichloroacetic acid; electrocautery; or excision.
Syphilis *(Treponema pallidum)*	**1°: Painless** genital ulcer. **2°:** Fever, malaise, diffuse rash. **Latent:** Asymptomatic. **3°:** Aortic aneurysm rupture, CNS symptoms.	**1°:** Nontender **chancre.** **2°:** Nonspecific maculopapular rash involving palms and soles of feet; **condylomata lata.** **Early latent (< 1 year):** Fourfold ↑ in titer. **Late latent (> 1 year or unknown):** Serology remains ⊕. **3°:** Aortitis, gummas, meningitis, encephalitis, tabes dorsalis, Argyll Robertson pupil.	Start with nonspecific RPR or VRDL (may be false ⊕). FTA-ABS or darkfield microscopy to confirm; LP if neurosyphilis is suspected.	Penicillin 2.4 MU IM × 1 for new infections; × 3 for infections of > 1 year duration. In penicillin-allergic patients, consider desensitization. For neurosyphilis, IV penicillin G (3–4 MU IV q 4 hr × 10–14 days).

(continues)

TABLE 16.13. **Presentation, Diagnosis, and Treatment of Common STIs** *(continued)*

STI	SYMPTOMS	EXAM	DIAGNOSIS	TREATMENT
Chancroid (*Haemophilus ducreyi*)	Presents as a **painful** genital ulcer.	Exam reveals a tender papule, pustule, or ulcer with an erythematous edge. Tender inguinal lymphadenopathy is also seen.	Diagnosis is largely clinical. Gram stain may help (streptobacillary chains). Rule out HSV and syphilis.	Azithromycin, ceftriaxone, ciprofloxacin (avoid in pregnancy).
Granuloma inguinale (*Calymmatobacterium granulomatis*); gram-negative intracellular bacterium	Presents as painless; progressive to ulcerative lesions.	Exam reveals painless nodule that progresses to beefy red ulcer.	Diagnosis requires visualization of dark-staining Donovan bodies on tissue biopsy.	Bactrim, doxycycline, tetracycline.
HIV/AIDS	Acute retroviral syndrome 3–6 weeks after infection; opportunistic infections.	Exam findings vary, depending on the cause of presentation.	Serology: ELISA and Western blot. Rapid test is available.	HAART; appropriate prophylaxis (see the Infectious Diseases chapter).
Hepatitis B (HBV)	Presents as acute hepatitis with flulike symptoms and jaundice.	Exam reveals acute hepatitis with jaundice and hepatomegaly.	HBsAg (may be used alone for screening).	See the Infectious Diseases chapter.
Pubic lice or "crabs" (*Phthirus pubis*)	Presents with an itch in the pubic hair. May also affect the axillae and other hair-covered areas.	Tiny white nits are attached to hair. Adult lice may be seen.	Diagnosis is clinical. Lice may be viewed under the microscope.	Topical permethrin, malathion, or lindane; decontaminate bedding and clothing.
Molluscum contagiosum (caused by *Poxvirus*)	Presents with multiple small bumps that are painless and nonpruritic.	Dome-shaped pearly papules with **central umbilication** are seen.	Diagnosis is clinical. Giemsa stain of material expressed from the lesion contains inclusion bodies.	Most resolve spontaneously and do not require treatment. Treatment options include imiquimod, cryotherapy, curettage, and electrodesiccation.

PREVENTION

- Complete sexual abstinence is the only way to ensure prevention of STIs.
- For patients who are sexually active, consistent use of latex condoms is the best protection against STIs.
- All children, as well as adults with risk factors, should be vaccinated against HBV.

- Vaccination against HPV is recommended for all girls by age 12, and for young women up to age 26. The 3-dose vaccine Gardasil protects against virus strains that cause most cervical cancer (types 16 and 18) and genital warts (types 6 and 11). It is more effective if given before the patient initiates sexual activity.

COMPLICATIONS

- Even without frank PID, gonorrhea and chlamydia infections ↑ the risk of tubal scarring, which can lead to infertility and ectopic pregnancy.
- PID can lead to multiorgan systemic illness and even death.
- Untreated syphilis and HIV are fatal.
- Untreated STIs in pregnant women can be transmitted to newborns.

MNEMONIC

Complications of PID:

I FACE PID

Infertility
Fitz-Hugh–Curtis syndrome
Abscesses
Chronic pelvic pain
Ectopic pregnancy
Peritonitis
Intestinal obstruction
Disseminated—sepsis, endocarditis, arthritis, meningitis

VULVOVAGINITIS

A 19-year-old woman complains of 1 week of yellow-gray vaginal discharge with a fishy odor. She has no urinary symptoms or vaginal itching or burning. She has tried douching with a vinegar preparation but finds that the symptoms return. She is not currently sexually active and denies a history of STIs. Speculum exam reveals copious discharge but an otherwise normal vulva, vagina, and cervix. Bimanual exam is unremarkable. Litmus paper applied to the discharge shows a pH of 5. Saline wet mount reveals epithelial cells with peripheral stippling. KOH applied to the slide releases a strong amine "fishy" odor. KOH prep is ⊖ for hyphae. What is the mostly likely diagnosis?

Bacterial vaginosis based on the presentation, the presence of "clue cells" on microscopy (Figure 16.15), and a ⊕ "whiff test." You offer the patient treatment with metronidazole and advise against douching.

With the exception of trichomoniasis, the causes of vulvovaginitis are normal flora that have overgrown rather than STIs. Therefore, patients' partners generally do not require treatment.

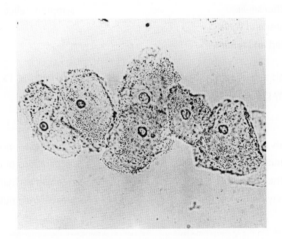

FIGURE 16.15. Clue cells of bacterial vaginosis. Note the stippled appearance. (Reproduced, with permission, from DeCherney A. *Current Obstetrics and Gynecology Diagnosis and Treatment,* 8th ed. Stamford, CT: Appleton & Lange, 1994: 692.)

SYMPTOMS/EXAM

The specific presentation of each cause of vulvovaginitis is given in Table 16.14. In general, the diagnosis should be considered for any of the following:

- Unusual vaginal discharge.
- Unusual vaginal/vulvar odor.
- Vaginal/vulvar itch or irritation.

PREVENTION

- Douching is associated with an ↑ risk of bacterial vaginosis and should be discouraged.
- Patients with bacterial vaginosis and candidiasis are generally advised to take measures to ↓ vulvar warmth and minimize moisture (eg, losing weight, wearing cotton underpants and loose-fitting clothing).

COMPLICATIONS

Bacterial vaginosis and trichomoniasis have been associated with an ↑ risk of preterm labor.

TABLE 16.14.   Presentation and Treatment of Vulvovaginitides

CAUSE	SYMPTOMS	EXAM	BEDSIDE TESTS	TREATMENT
Bacterial vaginosis (*Gardnerella* and other spp)	Presents with a malodorous discharge.	Discharge is thin and yellowish-gray. A fishy odor may be noticeable without KOH.	pH > 4.5. Wet mount shows **clue cells** (see Figure 16.15). KOH whiff test is ⊕ for a fishy amine odor.	Metronidazole 500 mg PO BID × 7 days is most effective. Metronidazole gel 5 g PV QD × 5 days. Clindamycin 5 g PV QHS × 7 days.
Yeast infection (*Candida albicans*)	Presents with vaginal itching and burning accompanied by a cheesy white discharge.	Exam reveals a white discharge adherent to the introitus. The discharge is thick and cottage cheese–like. The perineum and vulva may be red and tender.	pH 3.5–4.5. KOH prep shows "budding" hyphae.	Intravaginal azole antifungals; oral fluconazole (avoid in pregnancy). Antifungal cream may be applied externally for symptom relief.
Trichomoniasis (*Trichomonas vaginalis*)	Presents with a copious green discharge.	Exam reveals a discharge that is frothy green.	See Table 16.13.	See Table 16.13.
Atrophic vaginitis	Vaginal irritation and pain with intercourse in postmenopausal women.	Exam reveals a clear, thin discharge and a pale vaginal epithelium with patches of erythema.	pH > 7.	Water-based moisturizing preparations or estrogen vaginal cream. If vaginal bleeding is present, rule out malignant causes.

CHRONIC PELVIC PAIN

Defined as episodic or continuous pain for **6 months or longer** that is severe enough to affect daily functioning. Up to 20% of women of reproductive age are affected by pelvic pain. Although endometriosis is the most common associated condition, many women with pelvic pain have a history of abuse or depression. Etiologies are varied but include the following categories.

- Gynecologic:
  - **Uterine:** Adenomyosis, chronic endometritis, fibroids, IUD use, pelvic congestion, pelvic support defects, endometrial polyps.
  - **Extrauterine:** Adhesions, chronic pelvic infection, endometriosis, ovarian neoplasm, imperforate hymen, cervical stenosis, chronic functional cyst.
- **Urologic:** Interstitial cystitis, urethral syndrome, chronic UTI, stones, ureteral diverticuli or polyps, bladder carcinoma, detrusor overactivity.
- **GI:** Chronic appendicitis, constipation, diverticular disease, IBS, IBD (Crohn disease, ulcerative colitis), neoplasia.
- **Musculoskeletal:** Myofascial pain (trigger points, spasms), fibromyalgia, coccydynia, degenerative joint disease, low back pain, levator ani syndrome (spasm of the pelvic floor), nerve entrapment syndromes, osteoporosis (compression fractures), strains/sprains.
- **Other:** Abuse (physical or sexual, past or present), psychiatric disorders (depression, bipolar disorder), psychosocial stress (work stress, marital problems), herpes zoster, heavy metal poisoning (lead, mercury), lymphoma, sickle cell crisis, somatoform disorders, substance use (cocaine).

SYMPTOMS

- In all patients, evaluate exacerbating or ameliorating factors; the relationship of the pain to the menstrual cycle; worsening or improvement of pain with work, exercise, stress, intercourse, or orgasm; and associated symptoms such as bleeding, discharge, constipation, or diarrhea.
- A thorough pregnancy, surgical, psychiatric, and substance abuse history is needed, including a depression screening test. Pain in other parts of the body should be explored as well, as 90% of women with chronic pelvic pain have backaches, and up to 60% also have headaches.
- Specific symptoms to evaluate include the following:
  - Pain due to cervical, uterine, or vaginal pathology, often referred to the buttock or low back.
  - Pain from the ovaries or fallopian tubes, which is usually localized to one side and referred to the medial thigh.

EXAM

Conduct a complete physical exam, focusing on abdominal, back, vulvar, perineal, vaginal, bimanual, and rectovaginal exams.

DIAGNOSIS

- **Labs:** CBC, ESR, UA and culture, stool guaiac, gonorrhea and chlamydia cultures, vaginal wet mount, pregnancy test.
- **Imaging:** Ultrasound, CT, MRI, hysterosonogram.
- **Surgical:** D&C, diagnostic laparoscopy, cystoscopy, colonoscopy.

KEY FACT

Patients with chronic pelvic pain should be screened for depression.

TREATMENT

- Treat the underlying cause.
- **Pharmacologic:** Pain medications and antidepressants.
- **Surgical:** Pelvic denervation procedures; hysterectomy +/− salpingo-oophorectomy; pelvic floor reconstruction.
- **Other:** Psychotherapy, marriage and sex counseling, biofeedback, physical therapy.

PELVIC ORGAN PROLAPSE

Also known as genital prolapse, condition occurs with the descent of the bladder, uterus, or vagina from the anatomic location toward or through the vaginal opening. Prolapse is the most common indication for hysterectomy in the United States for women over the age of 55. Risk factors include multiparity, genetic predisposition, advancing age, prior pelvic surgery, menopause, obesity, chronic constipation with straining, repeated heavy lifting, pregnancy, and connective tissue disorders.

SYMPTOMS

Usually asymptomatic. May complain of feeling a bulge of tissue that protrudes to or past the vagina. May also experience pelvic pressure with straining, urinary incontinence, and/or difficulty with bowel movements.

EXAM/DIAGNOSIS

Speculum exam, bimanual exam, and rectovaginal exam identify pelvic abnormalities. May stage the pelvic organ prolapsed by the Baden-Walker System and Pelvic Organ Prolapse-Quantification System (Table 16.15).

TREATMENT

Asymptomatic or mildly symptomatic women may be observed. May recommend weight management, avoidance of heavy lifting and straining with bowel movements, and pelvic floor muscle training (Kegel exercises) to reduce symptoms. Pessaries may be used for all stages in women awaiting surgery, poor surgical candidates, or women who decline surgery. Obliterative or reconstructive surgery may be offered to symptomatic women.

TABLE 16.15. Pelvic Organ Prolapse Staging Systems

BADEN-WALKER SYSTEM		PELVIC ORGAN PROLAPSE-QUANTIFICATION SYSTEM	
GRADE	**DESCRIPTION**	**STAGE**	**DESCRIPTION**
0	No prolapse	0	No prolapse
1	Descent halfway to hymen	I	> 1 cm above hymen
2	Descent to hymen	II	< 1 cm proximal or distal to hymen plane
3	Descent halfway past hymen	III	> 1 cm below hymen plane, protrudes < 2 cm from total vaginal length
4	Maximal descent	IV	Eversion of lower genital tract

CERVICAL CANCER SCREENING

 A 42-year-old married woman with no history of previous abnormal Pap smears has a ⊖ Pap smear and a ⊖ HPV test. When should she get another Pap smear?

If she has only 1 sexual partner, has no other risk factors for cervical cancer, and has had 3 negative tests, she can have her next Pap smear in 3 years.

Screening Guidelines

Current guidelines from ACOG recommend that Pap smears should begin at age 21, regardless of sexual activity. Screening should not be performed prior to 21 years of age to avoid unnecessary and harmful evaluation/treatment in women at low risk for cancer.

- According to ACOG, cervical cytology screening is recommended every 2 years between ages 21 and 29 years.
- ACOG recommends that women ≥ 30 years should be screened every 3 years once they have had 3 consecutive negative Pap tests.
- Annual screening after age 30 should continue for all women with a history of in utero DES exposure; HIV; treatment for CIN2, CIN3, or cancer; as well as for all other immunocompromised patients.
- After a total hysterectomy (involving both the uterus and cervix), women do not need to be screened unless the surgery was performed to treat cancer or a precancerous condition.
- After age 65–70, women with at least 3 or more ⊖ consecutive Pap smears without abnormal results in the past 10 years can consider stopping cervical cancer screening.
- Conventional and liquid-based methods for cervical screening are acceptable. Limitations of the conventional method include the need to avoid blood, discharge, and lubricant, and the possibility of artifact when drying. Limitations of liquid-based methods include increased probability of misinterpretation of results with presence of heavy bleeding from cycle and presence of lubricant on cervix; higher cost; and lower specificity, leading to higher rates of false ⊕ results. Advantages of the liquid-based methods include decreased presence of artifact and ease of testing for HPV, chlamydia, and gonorrhea.
- Women immunized with HPV vaccine should be screened according to the same guidelines as nonimmunized women.
- Sexually active adolescents (< 21 years old) should be counseled and tested for STIs, which may be performed without cervical cytology screening.

Management of Abnormal Cervical Cytology

- **Atypical squamous cells of undetermined significance (ASCUS):**
  - Associated with a 6%–12% risk of CIN 2–3+.
  - Options include colposcopy, triage to colposcopy via HPV testing (if HPV ⊕, there is a 15%–27% risk of CIN 2–3+; if HPV ⊖, there is less than a 2% risk), or repeat cytology at 6 and 12 months.
- **Low-grade squamous intraepithelial lesions (LSILs):**
  - Associated with a 15%–30% risk of CIN 2–3+.
  - Perform colposcopy (adolescents can be monitored as outlined above for ASCUS and HPV ⊕).

- If colposcopy is normal or shows CIN 1, repeat cytology at 6 and 12 months or HPV testing at 12 months; repeat colposcopy for ASC or higher or for those with HPV ⊕ status.
  - **ASC—cannot exclude high-grade intraepithelial lesion (ASC-H):**
    - Carries a 24%–94% risk of CIN 2–3+.
    - Perform colposcopy.
    - If colposcopy is normal or shows CIN 1, repeat cytology at 6 and 12 months or HPV testing at 12 months; repeat colposcopy for ASC or higher or for those with HPV ⊕ status.
  - **High-grade squamous intraepithelial lesions (HSILs):**
    - Associated with ≥ 70% risk of CIN 2–3+ and a 1%–2% risk of invasive cancer.
    - Immediate LEEP or colposcopy with biopsy of visible lesions and endocervical biopsy (unless the patient is pregnant).
    - If colposcopy is ⊖, excision with LEEP or conization is recommended to ensure that no high-grade lesions are missed.
    - Adolescents with adequate colposcopy and ⊖ endocervical curettage can be followed with repeat cytology and colposcopy at 6-month intervals for up to 2 years.
  - **Atypical glandular cells/adenocarcinoma in situ (AGC/AIS):**
    - Colposcopy with endocervical sampling for all patients; endometrial sampling is indicated if "atypical endometrial cells" are specified; and for all women ≥ 35 years of age and those < 35 years of age with abnormal bleeding, obesity, or oligomenorrhea.
    - In patients with AGC and both a ⊖ initial evaluation and ⊖ HPV status, repeat cytology and endocervical sampling in 1 year.
    - For AGC favoring neoplasia, AIS with a ⊖ initial evaluation, or a repeat AGC, excision with cold-knife conization is recommended.
  - **Cytology ⊖, HPV ⊕:**
    - Associated with a 4% risk of developing CIN 2–3+ (includes CIN 2, CIN 3, adenocarcinoma in situ, and cancer).
    - Cotesting with HPV is not recommended for women < 30 years old.
    - Women ≥ 30 years: repeat cytologic and HPV testing in 12 months, as transient HPV infection may resolve; perform colposcopy if the repeat test is abnormal. If repeat testing is ⊖, return to normal screening frequency (ie, every 3 years if 3 prior negatives).

Management of Colposcopy Results

- **CIN grade 1:**
  - Most cases remit spontaneously over time.
  - Options include treatment (LEEP or cryotherapy) or observation, including 2 cytology screening tests 6 months apart or a single HPV ⊕ test at 12 months, with colposcopy for ASC or higher or HPV status.
- **CIN grade 2 or 3:**
  - Although roughly 40% of CIN 2 cases regress over 2 years, regression of CIN 3 is rare.
  - Immediate treatment with excision or ablation is recommended in nonpregnant patients. Consider hysterectomy for persistent or recurrent CIN 2 or 3.

GYNECOLOGIC CANCERS

Ovarian Cancer

The leading cause of gynecologic cancer death, with its high mortality rate attributable primarily to its often late-stage presentation. Ovarian cancer develops from 3 types of tissue: epithelial, stromal, and germ cell. Epithelial cell tumors usually occur in women > 50 years, stromal cell tumors may occur in women of any age, and germ cell tumors occur in females age 15–19.

Risk factors include advancing age (greatest risk in postmenopausal females), family history of breast or ovarian cancer, early menarche, late menopause, and nulliparity. Use of hormonal contraception provides significant and long-lasting protection. A history of tubal ligation and, to a lesser degree, hysterectomy appears to be protective.

The U.S. Preventive Services Task Force (USPSTF) recommends **against** routine screening for ovarian cancer.

SYMPTOMS

- Initially asymptomatic, or may present with nonspecific symptoms such as pelvic fullness, increased abdominal size, bloating, urinary urgency, frequency, incontinence, early satiety, weight loss, fatigue, constipation, or dyspareunia.
- Rarely presents with acute abdominal pain from a torsed or ruptured mass.
- May lead to irregular menses or postmenopausal bleeding.
- Later, abdominal pain and swelling may result either from invasive tumor or from 2° ascites.

EXAM

Symptoms should be evaluated with bimanual and rectovaginal exams, which may reveal a solid, irregular, fixed pelvic mass.

DIFFERENTIAL

- Consider the broad differential diagnosis of abdominal pain and bloating.
- A palpable pelvic mass may be benign or may point to other malignancy.

DIAGNOSIS

- Pelvic ultrasound reveals a solid or cystic mass with extramural fluid, wall thickening, septa, and papillary projections, Doppler flow to the solid component of the mass with increased number and tortuosity of vessels, +/– presence of ascites.
- CA-125 ↑ in the presence of malignancy and is useful for tracking the course of disease, but it is nonspecific and therefore not useful for screening asymptomatic women.

TREATMENT

- Surgical excision and "debulking" of tumor burden.
- Chemotherapy if indicated.
- Women with a known hereditary syndrome may choose prophylactic oophorectomy.

Uterine Cancer

Endometrial cancer is the most common gynecologic malignancy in the United States. Since it often causes early symptoms, it tends to be diagnosed at a curable stage. Uterine sarcomas are rare but are more likely to be diagnosed late. No recommendations for universal population-based screening exist at this time. The American Cancer Society recommends annual screening with endometrial biopsy beginning at age 35 for women at risk or who have hereditary nonpolyposis colorectal cancer (HNPCC).

KEY FACT

There is no effective way to screen for ovarian cancer, but suspicious symptoms should be evaluated by pelvic exam +/– transvaginal ultrasonography and CA-125.

KEY FACT

The use of OCPs significantly reduces the risk of endometrial and ovarian cancer.

- Type I (endometrioid) accounts for > 75% of cases and has a good prognosis. Usually results from unopposed estrogen stimulation of the endometrium, leading to hyperplasia.
- Type II lesions are not related to estrogen exposure or endometrial hyperplasia. Usually diagnosed at a more advanced age and with a poorer prognosis. Includes serous, clear cell, mucinous, squamous, and adenosquamous carcinomas.

SYMPTOMS

- Commonly presents with postmenopausal bleeding, or in premenopausal women, with heavy or irregular menses.
- ACOG recommends ruling out cancer in women > 35 years of age with suspected anovulatory uterine bleeding and postmenopausal women with benign endometrial cells on Pap smear.

EXAM

The uterus may be enlarged or normal. On general physical exam, look for signs associated with ↑ risk.

DIFFERENTIAL

- Benign causes of irregular or postmenopausal bleeding, such as atrophic vaginitis, endometrial hyperplasia, polyps, fibroids, trauma, infection, and hormonal medications.
- Other gynecologic cancers.

DIAGNOSIS

- Suspicious symptoms should be evaluated with endometrial biopsy. Transvaginal ultrasound can be helpful in postmenopausal women, where an endometrial stripe < 4 mm is reassuring and need not be followed by endometrial biopsy.
- D&C +/− hysteroscopy may also assist in the workup.
- Pelvic masses suspicious on imaging but ⊖ on endometrial sampling should be excised to evaluate for sarcoma. Most are found incidentally at the time of surgery for fibroids or other benign indications.

TREATMENT

- Staging is surgically based.
- TAH-BSO is almost always indicated.
- Radiation, chemotherapy, and/or hormonal agents as indicated by the stage and type of cancer.

Cervical Cancer

Since the introduction of the Pap smear, mortality from cervical cancer has greatly ↓ in the United States; see the discussion of cervical cancer screening for more information on the management of an abnormal Pap smear. It is now known that infection with a high-risk subtype of HPV is necessary for the development of cervical cancer. Risk factors include early sexual activity, multiple sexual partners, partner with high number of sexual partners, STIs, previous history of squamous dysplasias of cervix/vagina/vulva, immunosuppression, and smoking. Two major histologic types of invasive cervical cancer are squamous cell carcinoma (80% of cases) and adenocarcinoma or adenosquamous carcinoma.

SYMPTOMS

- Preinvasive lesions (dysplasia and carcinoma in situ) are asymptomatic.
- Invasive carcinoma generally leads to abnormal vaginal bleeding +/− a foul-smelling discharge.
- Advanced disease may lead to pelvic pain, lower extremity edema, or urinary symptoms.

EXAM

- Even invasive lesions may be invisible to the naked eye on speculum exam.
- If visible, tumors may appear ulcerated, necrotic, or exophytic.
- Bimanual +/− rectovaginal exam may reveal cervical distortion or a frank mass.
- Look for signs of disease extension such as inguinal lymphadenopathy, leg edema, ascites, or hepatomegaly.

DIFFERENTIAL

- Benign causes of abnormal bleeding and discharge, such as atrophic vaginitis, endometrial hyperplasia, polyps, fibroids, trauma, infection, and hormonal medications.
- Other gynecologic cancers.

DIAGNOSIS

Colposcopy with directed biopsy and endocervical curettage.

TREATMENT

- Low-grade lesions can be followed without therapy, as > 90% will spontaneously regress.
- High-grade preinvasive lesions can be ablated or excised with cryotherapy, loop electrosurgical excision procedure (LEEP), or conization.
- Invasive disease requires radical hysterectomy and/or radiation therapy.

COMPLICATIONS

- Most superficial therapies are safe and have little or no effect on future pregnancies.
- LEEP may modestly ↑ the risk of PROM and preterm delivery in future pregnancies.
- Conization ↑ the risk for cervical stenosis or incompetence.
- Pelvic radiation and radical surgery may have serious adverse effects.

KEY FACT

All women who have had sex and who have a cervix should be routinely screened for cervical cancer. Cervical cytology (Pap smear) is the standard-of-care screening test.

Vulvar and Vaginal Cancer

A 60-year-old woman with a long-standing history of genital lichen sclerosus presents with ↑ vulvar itching, pain, and dysuria. What is the likely diagnosis, and how is it confirmed?
Biopsy of the lesion confirms squamous cell carcinoma in situ arising in an area of lichen sclerosus (Figure 16.16). Although itself a benign condition, lichen sclerosus leads to vulvar cancer in 4%–6% of affected women.

Vulvar and vaginal cancer is rare, but care should be taken not to miss the diagnosis, as the presenting symptoms can be nonspecific. In utero exposure

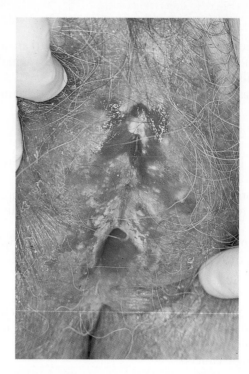

FIGURE 16.16. **Squamous cell carcinoma of the vulva arising in an area of lichen sclerosus.** (Reproduced, with permission, from Wolff K, et al. *Fitzpatrick's Color Atlas & Synopsis of Clinical Dermatology,* 5th ed. New York: McGraw Hill, 2005: 1047.)

to diethylstilbestrol (DES) is an important risk factor for clear cell adenocarcinoma of the vagina. Other risk factors include HPV exposure, smoking, and advancing age. Secondary cancers of the vagina are more common than primary vaginal cancer.

SYMPTOMS

- Many patients are asymptomatic.
- Vulvar itching is the most common presenting symptom in vulvar cancer. Vaginal discharge is the most common presenting symptom in vaginal cancer.
- Less commonly, patients will see or feel a lesion.

EXAM

- External genital and speculum exams may reveal a lesion that can vary in color, texture, and appearance.
- Paget disease of the vulva, which is often associated with an underlying adenocarcinoma, appears as a well-demarcated, scaly lesion that may look like eczema.
- Skin cancers, including melanoma, may present on the vulva.

DIFFERENTIAL

Genital warts; vaginitis; benign skin lesions, including lichen sclerosus and lichen planus.

DIAGNOSIS

- Vaginal malignancies may be detected on Pap smear.
- Biopsy, often guided by colposcopy, is required for definitive diagnosis.

KEY FACT

Malignant melanoma is the second most common vulvar cancer. In patients at ↑ risk for melanoma, the full-body skin check should truly include the entire body!

TREATMENT

Surgical excision +/– radiation.

Gestational Trophoblastic Neoplasia

A malignancy arising from fetal tissue. This diagnosis includes a persistent or invasive mole and malignant choriocarcinoma. The majority of cases are curable, but metastases may be fatal. Although gestational trophoblastic neoplasia is most likely to occur after a molar pregnancy, 50% of cases occur after a normal pregnancy.

SYMPTOMS

- Presents with persistent pregnancy symptoms and irregular vaginal bleeding for > 6 weeks following cessation of a term, preterm, ectopic, or molar pregnancy.
- Metastatic disease may present with pulmonary, GI, or neurologic symptoms.

EXAM

Exam reveals an enlarged uterus, adnexal fullness due to ovarian cysts, and RUQ pain from hepatic involvement.

DIFFERENTIAL

Normal pregnancy; other pelvic masses.

DIAGNOSIS

- Look for a rapidly rising β-hCG.
- Ultrasound reveals a "snowstorm" appearance.
- Pathologic diagnosis is made after surgical treatment. The characteristic "bunches of grapes" appearance is caused by hydropic villi (Figure 16.17).
- Staging is based on age, β-hCG level, type of previous pregnancy, duration of disease, site of metastasis, and number of metastases.

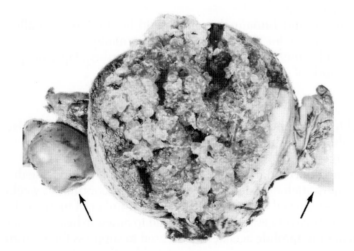

FIGURE 16.17. **Complete hydatidiform mole with multiple edematous villi ("bunches of grapes" appearance) and no fetus.** (Reproduced, with permission, from Cunningham FG, et al. *Williams Obstetrics,* 22nd ed. New York: McGraw-Hill, 2005: 275.)

TREATMENT

- D&C is curative in many cases. Rarely, hysterectomy is necessary.
- Methotrexate may be used in nonmetastatic disease.
- Combination chemotherapy is necessary in metastatic disease.
- Follow β-hCG levels to resolution; plateau or rise in β-hCG levels is a marker of persistent disease.

COMPLICATIONS

Molar pregnancy carries a 1% risk of recurrence with future pregnancies. Since choriocarcinoma may metastasize to the lungs, vagina, brain, liver, kidney, or GI tract, recommend CXR, CT of chest/abdomen/pelvis, and brain CT.

MENSTRUAL DISORDERS

Dysmenorrhea

Defined as pain during menses resulting from uterine contractions caused by the release of prostaglandins. Dysmenorrhea is the leading cause of recurrent short-term absence from school in adolescent girls. 1° dysmenorrhea affects women with normal pelvic anatomy; risk factors include age < 20, nulliparity, heavy menses, depression, and smoking. 2° dysmenorrhea can be caused by endometriosis, adenomyosis, pelvic infection, IUC use, cervical stenosis, congenital vaginal or uterine abnormalities, or fibroids.

SYMPTOMS/EXAM

- Presents with crampy pelvic pain beginning at the onset of menses and lasting 1–3 days.
- A pelvic mass, abnormal vaginal discharge, and pelvic tenderness not limited to the time of menses suggest 2° dysmenorrhea.

DIAGNOSIS

- Can be treated empirically if the history and physical are consistent with 1° dysmenorrhea.
- A **speculum and bimanual exam** should be done on sexually active patients to evaluate for STIs or anatomic abnormality.
- Ultrasound is useful in evaluating 2° dysmenorrhea; laparoscopy is best for the diagnosis of endometriosis.

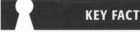

TREATMENT

- NSAIDs are the best first-line treatment, as they have an analgesic effect while also decreasing the volume of menstrual flow.
- Levonorgestrel IUCs ↓ dysmenorrhea.
- **Combined hormonal contraceptives** ↓ prostaglandin release during menses. Options include extended-cycle use (ie, 12 continuous weeks of active hormones followed by 1 week off) to ↓ the number of menstrual periods.
- Depot medroxyprogesterone acetate lead to amenorrhea in most women.
- Danazol or leuprolide acetate can be used to suppress the menstrual cycle, but both drugs are expensive and have side effects; thus, they are best reserved for refractory cases of 2° dysmenorrhea.
- Alternative therapies that may be effective include topical heat, vitamin E, thiamine, omega-3 fatty acids, and acupuncture.
- Hysterectomy is indicated only for severe, refractory cases.

Abnormal Uterine Bleeding

Bleeding that deviates from the patient's normal pattern. Prior to the onset of menses, any vaginal bleeding should be considered abnormal with the exception of self-limited, physiologic withdrawal bleeding in some newborns. In women of childbearing age, abnormal uterine bleeding encompasses bleeding between cycles as well as any change that may occur in menstrual frequency, duration, or amount of flow. As a whole, bleeding may be classified as ovulatory or anovulatory, based on the timing, duration, and amount of flow. Etiologies include the following:

- **Ovulatory bleeding:**
    - **Anatomic lesions:** Cervical disease (polyps, inflammation, cancer), PID, IUC use, uterine disease (fibroids, cancer).
    - **Concurrent disease:** Foreign body; coagulopathy; thyroid, hepatic, or renal disease.
    - **Medications:** Anticoagulants, antipsychotics, corticosteroids, herbal supplements (ginseng, gingko, soy), SSRIs, tamoxifen.
- **Anovulatory bleeding:**
    - **Endocrine dysfunction:** PCOS; hypothyroidism; excess androgen, cortisol, or prolactin.
    - **Hypothalamic cause:** Situational stress; excess exercise or weight loss.
    - **Functional cause:** Puberty; perimenopause.
- **Dysfunctional uterine bleeding:** A diagnosis of exclusion that may be due to hormonal imbalances either at the pituitary level (anovulatory bleeding) or at the level of the endometrial lining (ovulatory bleeding). Pregnancy, iatrogenic causes, genital tract pathology, and systemic conditions must be ruled out before dysfunctional uterine bleeding is diagnosed.
- **Pregnancy:** Ectopic pregnancy, threatened abortion, incomplete abortion.
- **Postmenopausal bleeding:**
    - **Vaginal pathology:** Atrophic vaginitis.
    - **Cervical pathology:** Polyps, erosion, cancer.
    - **Uterine pathology:** Polyps, fibroids, cancer.

KEY FACT

Dysfunctional uterine bleeding is a diagnosis of exclusion and is due to hormonal imbalances.

SYMPTOMS

Clinical presentation varies according to the pattern of abnormal bleeding.

- **Ovulatory patterns:**
    - **Menorrhagia:** Excessive or prolonged bleeding during times of expected menstrual flow.
- **Anovulatory patterns:**
    - **Metrorrhagia:** Irregular bleeding that occurs between ovulatory cycles.
    - **Menometrorrhagia:** Irregular, noncyclic bleeding characterized by heavy flow or duration.
    - **Oligomenorrhea:** Cycles lasting > 35 days.
    - **Amenorrhea:** Bleeding that is absent for at least 6 months.
- **Other:** Additional abnormalities of menstruation are defined as follows:
    - **Polymenorrhea:** Cycles < 21 days; usually due to luteal phase dysfunction.
    - **Midcycle spotting:** Physiologic spotting just before ovulation.
    - **Postmenopausal bleeding:** Bleeding that occurs in a menopausal woman more than 1 year after cessation of menses or unpredictable bleeding in menopausal women who have been receiving hormone therapy for 12 months or more.

EXAM

Note patient's weight and height, and Tanner stage of breast and pubic hair. Exam may reveal postural signs, weight gain or loss, thyromegaly or thyroid tenderness, hirsutism, edema, petechiae, bruising, jaundice, enlargement of the liver or spleen, breast tenderness or discharge, an enlarged uterus, a firm or fixed uterus, cervical motion or uterine tenderness, or an adnexal mass (Table 16.16).

DIAGNOSIS

- **Always rule out pregnancy.**
- **Labs:** hCG, CBC, LFTs, PT, PTT, TSH, prolactin, blood glucose, DHEA, free testosterone, Pap smear, gonorrhea and chlamydia cultures.
- **Imaging:** Transvaginal ultrasound, hysteroscopy for cases unresponsive to empiric treatment.
- Endometrial assessment (endometrial biopsy or D&C) is indicated for women < 35 years old with 2–3 years of untreated anovulatory bleeding, especially if they are obese; for any woman > 35 years of age with a change in bleeding pattern; and for all women with postmenopausal bleeding.

TREATMENT

- **Acute anovulatory bleeding:** To stop bleeding, give high-dose oral or IV estrogen to build up the endometrial lining. Oral medroxyprogesterone or IM progesterone can also be used to convert proliferative endometrium to secretory endometrium. D&C or hysteroscopy is appropriate in refractory cases.
- **Chronic anovulatory bleeding:** Treat the underlying cause, and add monthly progesterone therapy or combination hormonal contraceptives both to promote regular endometrial shedding and to prevent endometrial hyperplasia.
- **Ovulatory bleeding:** Treat the underlying cause and associated anemia. NSAIDs, combined hormonal contraceptives, or a levonorgestrel-releasing

TABLE 16.16. **Exam Findings Associated with Abnormal Uterine Bleeding**

SYMPTOMS	CONDITION
Weight loss, stress	Hypothalamic suppression
Galactorrhea, headache, visual disturbance	Pituitary adenoma
Pelvic pain	Ectopic pregnancy, PID, trauma, miscarriage
Nausea, weight gain, fatigue, urinary frequency	Pregnancy
Weight gain, fatigue, constipation, cold intolerance	Hypothyroidism
Weight loss, palpitations, heat intolerance	Hyperthyroidism
Bleeding tendency, easy bruising	Coagulopathy
Jaundice, abdominal pain	Liver disease
Hirsutism, acne, acanthosis nigricans, +/− obesity	PCOS
Postcoital bleeding	Cervical dysplasia, endocervical polyp

IUC can ↓ the duration and quantity of bleeding. Consider myomectomy in refractory cases associated with fibroids.

- In severe cases, surgical options such as endometrial ablation or hysterectomy may be indicated.

Amenorrhea

Defined as the absence of menstrual periods. **1° amenorrhea** is defined as failure of menses to appear by age 16 in a patient with normal 2° sexual characteristics or by age 14 in a patient with no 2° sexual characteristics. **2° amenorrhea** is defined as the absence of menses for 3 consecutive months in women with previous normal menstruation or for 9 months in women with prior oligomenorrhea. Etiologies of **1° amenorrhea** include the following:

- **Hypothalamic/pituitary:**
  - **Hypothalamic dysfunction:** May be due to organic illness, vigorous exercise, stressful life events, or anorexia nervosa.
  - **Genetic gonadotropin deficiency:** Kallmann syndrome.
  - **Hypothalamic lesions:** Craniopharyngioma.
  - **Pituitary tumors:** Prolactinoma.
  - **Endocrinopathies:** Cushing syndrome, hypothyroidism.
  - **Hyperandrogenism:** From adrenal, ovarian, or exogenous sources.
- **Ovarian:** Turner syndrome, ovarian failure due to autoimmunity, ovarian steroidogenic enzyme deficiencies.
- **Uterine:** Congenital absence or malformation of the uterus; imperforate hymen.
- **Pseudohermaphroditism:** Absent uterus and intra-abdominal or cryptorchid testes due either to an enzymatic defect in testosterone synthesis or to complete androgen resistance (testicular feminization).

Etiologies of **2° amenorrhea** are as follows:

- Pregnancy.
- **Hypothalamic/pituitary:**
  - Emotional stress, illness, dieting, exercise, medications (phenothiazine, OCPs), anorexia nervosa, intensive exercise leading to extreme weight loss.
  - Cushing syndrome; hypothyroidism.
  - Pituitary tumor (eg, prolactinoma); pituitary infarction (eg, Sheehan syndrome).
  - Granulomatous disease (sarcoidosis).
- **Ovarian:**
  - PCOS.
  - Premature ovarian failure (autoimmune, radiation therapy, chemotherapy, endometriosis, oophoritis, idiopathic).
  - Hyperandrogenism (from adrenal, ovarian, or exogenous sources).
- **Uterine:** Asherman syndrome (involves extensive intrauterine scarring and synechia formation); cervical scarring leads to closure of the os.

HISTORY

- Obtain a detailed menstrual history, including age at menarche, the character of normal cycles, and the timing of missed cycles, as well as a pregnancy history.
- Ask about the patient's psychosocial history, including situational stresses, emotional problems, dieting and nutritional issues, bulimia, weight loss, and exercise.
- Determine the patient's history of medication use, especially use of antipsychotics and OCPs.

MNEMONIC

Causes of 2 ° amenorrhea:

SOAP

Stress
OCPs
Anorexia
Pregnancy

- Ask about hormonal symptoms, including hot flashes, skin changes, hirsutism, headaches, breast changes, galactorrhea, and changes in libido.
- Inquire about previous CNS or pelvic chemoradiation.
- Determine if there is a family history of genetic defects or infertility; ask about the menstrual and pubertal history of the patient's mother and sisters.

EXAM

Table 16.17 outlines physical exam findings that commonly occur in association with amenorrhea.

DIAGNOSIS

- 1° amenorrhea:
  - **Labs:** FSH, LH, prolactin, testosterone, TSH, free T_4, hCG. Virilized or hypertensive patients should have serum electrolytes and further hormonal evaluation.
  - **Imaging:** MRI of the hypothalamus and pituitary is indicated in girls with low to normal FSH and LH as well as high prolactin levels.
  - Karyotyping can diagnose X chromosome mosaicism in patients with a normal uterus and high FSH without classic features of Turner syndrome.
- 2° amenorrhea:
  - Measure urine or serum hCG; if ↑, the most likely cause is pregnancy (although false ⊕ results are possible with ectopic hCG secretion, as occurs in choriocarcinoma or bronchogenic carcinoma).
  - Progestin challenge can be attempted; if withdrawal bleed occurs, the patient is likely anovulatory. If no withdrawal bleed occurs, an estrogen/progestin challenge can be used to distinguish a hypothalamic/pituitary disorder from outflow tract obstruction.
  - Labs that can be helpful include prolactin, FSH, LH, TSH, potassium, and renal and liver function tests.
  - MRI is indicated for ↑ prolactin or hypopituitarism.

TABLE 16.17. **Exam Findings Associated with Amenorrhea**

FINDING	RELATED DIAGNOSIS
Obesity, hirsutism, acne	PCOS
Webbed neck, widely spaced nipples, short stature	Turner syndrome
Hypertension, buffalo hump, central obesity, easy bruising, striae	Cushing syndrome
Pubic hair with absent uterus	Müllerian agenesis
Virilization, clitoral hypertrophy	Androgen-secreting tumor
Galactorrhea, visual field defects	Pituitary tumor
Enlarged thyroid	Hypothyroidism
Imperforate hymen, transverse vaginal septum	Outflow tract obstruction
Anosmia	Kallmann syndrome

- In hirsute or virilized women, check serum testosterone.
- In patients with signs of hypercortisolism, a 1-mg overnight dexamethasone suppression test is needed.

TREATMENT

- **1° amenorrhea:** Treatment is based on the underlying cause.
- **2° amenorrhea:** Also directed at the cause. For reversible conditions, withholding therapy periodically is recommended to determine if periods return.
  - **Hypothalamic dysfunction:** Periods usually return when precipitants (exercise, dieting, situational stress) are withdrawn. Patients with anorexia nervosa often need to reach 90% of their normal weight prior to the return of menses. Chronic amenorrhea can be treated with medroxyprogesterone or combined hormones to bring on withdrawal bleeding every 1–3 months.
  - **Pituitary disease:** Bromocriptine, a dopamine agonist, is used for hyperprolactinemia; larger pituitary tumors may require surgical intervention. Patients with destructive pituitary lesions may need replacement of estrogen, progesterone, thyroid hormone, or adrenal steroids.
  - **Ovarian causes:** Estrogen/progesterone replacement is indicated for ovarian failure.
  - **Uterine disease:** Asherman syndrome can be treated with dilation and recurettage to sever bridging synechiae and with glucocorticoids to inhibit the formation of new scar tissue.

COMPLICATIONS

Infertility, endometrial cancer, osteoporosis, heart disease.

Polycystic Ovarian Syndrome (PCOS)

Characterized by androgen excess, insulin resistance, and gonadotropin abnormalities, PCOS is the most frequent cause of anovulatory infertility. Etiology of PCOS is unknown.

SYMPTOMS/EXAM

May present with menstrual irregularities, infertility, hirsutism, acne, obesity, possible ovarian enlargement, and acanthosis nigricans.

DIFFERENTIAL

- Pregnancy, premature ovarian failure, medications (progestational agents), pituitary adenoma, thyroid disorders, adrenal tumors, Cushing syndrome, congenital adrenal hyperplasia.
- In patients with rapidly progressive hirsutism, ↑ DHEAS levels suggest a virilizing adrenal tumor.
- If congenital adrenal hyperplasia is suspected in patients with hypertension and potassium abnormalities, check serum 17-hydroxyprogesterone levels at 8 A.M.
- Patients with physical findings of cortisol excess (eg, hypertension, easy bruising, central obesity, proximal muscle weakness) should have an overnight dexamethasone suppression test to rule out Cushing syndrome.

DIAGNOSIS

- Primarily a clinical diagnosis consisting of a combination of oligomenorrhea and hyperandrogenism. Laboratory tests are not necessary if clinical diagnosis is clear, though pregnancy must be ruled out.

- Laboratory findings can include ↑ testosterone, androstenedione, LH, estradiol, estrone, and fasting insulin; an ↑ ratio of LH to FSH (> 3:1); and ↓ sex hormone-binding globulin.
- Other useful labs include hCG to rule out pregnancy, TSH, prolactin, fasting glucose, and a lipid panel.
- Diagnosis by ultrasound consists of 1 or both ovaries with 12 or more follicles < 10 mm in diameter, but imaging is not necessary or sufficient for the diagnosis.

TREATMENT

- **Oligomenorrhea:**
  - Combination OCPs (choose the least androgenic progestins; avoid norgestrel and levonorgestrel) prevent pregnancy and endometrial hyperplasia, normalize menstrual cycles, and treat hirsutism and acne.
  - Monthly DMPA is an option for contraception and endometrial protection, but does not suppress ovarian androgen production.
- **Hirsutism:** Treat with antiandrogens such as spironolactone in combination with OCPs, or use OCPs with a progestin with antimineralocorticoid activity. Topical eflornithine cream is FDA approved for management of hirsutism. Management with shaving, waxing, plucking, bleaching, thermolysis, electrolysis, depilatory creams, and laser removal may be helpful.
- **Anovulation/infertility:** Weight loss; clomiphene citrate +/− metformin. Surgical options (which are rarely used) include ovarian cautery and laser vaporization.
- **Weight loss:** ↓ serum androgen, insulin, and LH. Diet and exercise are recommended for all patients; metformin can help with weight loss.

COMPLICATIONS

Chronic anovulation and amenorrhea, with associated long-term exposure to unopposed estrogen, can lead to endometrial hyperplasia and endometrial cancer. Women with PCOS have ↑ risk of diabetes (check fasting glucose or glucose tolerance test), metabolic syndrome, insulin resistance, and nonalcoholic fatty liver disease.

OTHER GYNECOLOGIC CONDITIONS

A healthy 25-year-old woman asks you for a CA-125 test to screen for ovarian cancer. Should you order one?

No. The positive predictive value (PPV) in this patient is only 2.3%.

Ovarian Mass

Most ovarian masses are found on physical exam in both symptomatic and asymptomatic women or are discovered incidentally on imaging. Types of benign ovarian masses include ovarian cysts, germ cell tumors (mature teratomas = dermoid cysts), stromal cell tumors (thecomas, fibromas), and epithelial cell tumors (serous or mucinous adenomas and Brenner tumors). The risk of malignancy ↑ significantly with age, from 13% in premenopausal women to 45% following the onset of menopause. Malignant adnexal lesions include 1° ovarian carcinoma and metastatic disease from the uterus, breast, or GI tract. Additional considerations are as follows:

- Newborns can have small functional cysts due to maternal hormones for a few months.

- In girls < 9 years of age, 80% of adnexal masses are malignant (usually germ cell tumors).
- In reproductive-age women, most adnexal masses are follicular and corpus luteum cysts of the ovary and benign tumors such as mature teratomas, endometriomas, and serous or mucinous cystadenomas.
- Nonmalignant masses in postmenopausal women include ovarian fibromas.

SYMPTOMS

Many patients are asymptomatic, but symptoms may include urinary frequency, pelvic pressure or pain, dyspepsia, abdominal bloating, early satiety, constipation, and changes in stool caliber. Patients with ovarian cancer often complain of vague GI symptoms.

EXAM

Evaluate for cervical, supraclavicular, and groin lymphadenopathy. Perform a breast exam, as the ovary is a common site of metastasis for breast carcinoma. Perform bimanual and rectovaginal exams as well.

DIAGNOSIS

- **Imaging:** Ultrasound is the most important diagnostic study. Important characteristics include size, whether cystic or solid, and other signs suggestive of malignancy, such as internal septae/papillae or the presence of ascites. Signs suggestive of benign mass include unilocular, thin-walled sonolucent cysts with smooth, regular borders.
- **Labs:** Lab tests include β-**hCG level** to rule out ectopic pregnancy. Serum tumor markers are useful in certain instances.
- **α-fetoprotein:** For endodermal sinus tumors.
- **LDH:** For dysgerminomas.
- **β-hCG:** For nongestational choriocarcinomas.
- **Serum CA-125:** ↑ in malignant conditions such as serous epithelial ovarian, breast, colon, lung, and pancreatic cancers. In the setting of a postmenopausal woman with an ultrasonographically suspicious pelvic mass, the PPV for malignancy is 97%. Because it can be ↑ in benign conditions, CA-125 is not recommended as a routine screening test (the PPV in healthy patients is only 2.3%).

TREATMENT

- **Prepubertal patients:** All adnexal masses in prepubertal girls must be evaluated with ultrasound and referral.
- **Premenopausal patients:** Premenopausal women with cysts < 10 cm can be followed. If cyst persists > 12 weeks, referral is recommended. Monophasic OCPs can suppress symptomatic functional cysts. All solid adnexal masses call for immediate surgical exploration, as does the presence of ascites.
- **Postmenopausal patients:**
  - Postmenopausal women with asymptomatic ovarian cysts < 5–10 cm in diameter and a normal serum CA-125 can be followed with serial ultrasounds, as such patients have a very low risk of malignancy. Larger cysts should be evaluated laparoscopically.
  - Symptomatic patients with an ultrasonographically suspicious mass and ↑ serum CA-125 should be referred for surgical evaluation.

KEY FACT

Ultrasound is the most important diagnostic test used in evaluating adnexal masses.

Fibroids

 A 36-year-old woman with mild pelvic pain and moderately heavy periods but no anemia is found on pelvic ultrasound to have multiple small uterine fibroids. How would you manage this patient?

As her symptoms are mild, the patient can be reassured and treated conservatively with pain medication and OCPs to ↓ menstrual flow. If she develops more severe symptoms, the ultrasound should be repeated and surgery considered.

The most common benign neoplasm of the female genital tract. Also called uterine leiomyomas, fibroids are discrete, round, firm uterine tumors composed of smooth muscle and connective tissue. They are classified by anatomic location as intramural, submucosal, subserosa, intraligamentous, parasitic (deriving its blood supply from an organ to which it becomes attached), and cervical. Risk factors include nulliparity, advanced age, obesity, family history, and African American race.

SYMPTOMS

- Often asymptomatic, but may present with pelvic pain, dysmenorrhea, or menorrhagia (which may lead to anemia), as well as with urinary frequency, incontinence, or other complications stemming from the presence of an abdominal mass.
- Fibroids that distort the uterine cavity may lead to infertility or recurrent pregnancy loss.

EXAM

Irregular enlargement of the uterus.

DIFFERENTIAL

Pregnancy, adenomyosis, ovarian tumor, leiomyosarcoma.

DIAGNOSIS

- **Labs:** Low hemoglobin results from blood loss, with rare cases of polycythemia from production of erythropoietin by the myomas.
- **Imaging:** Ultrasound can confirm the presence of fibroids and monitor their growth, and it can also be used to exclude ovarian masses. MRI is accurate in delineating intramural and submucous fibroids; hysteroscopy can confirm cervical or submucous fibroids.

TREATMENT

- No treatment is necessary for small, asymptomatic fibroids. Most fibroids grow slowly until menopause, when they start to shrink.
- OCPs or progestins (including the levonorgestrel-releasing IUD) can be used to control menstrual bleeding, but they do not ↓ the size of fibroids.
- For severe anemia, ↓ bleeding with monthly depot medroxyprogesterone acetate or daily danazol.
- Surgery is indicated for rapid growth, severe bleeding leading to anemia, or pressure on the ureters, bladder, or bowel.
- Surgical options include myomectomy (preferable during childbearing years), hysterectomy, uterine artery embolization, and MRI-guided focused ultrasound surgery.
- Given that the risk of surgical complications ↑ with larger myomas, GnRH analogs (depot leuprolide, nafarelin) can be given preoperatively to ↓ the size of myomas.

Endometriosis

The presence of endometrial tissue on the ovaries, fallopian tubes, or other abnormal sites leads to pain or infertility. Endometriosis is a progressive disease affecting 5%–10% of women. Although its exact cause is not known, theories on its etiology include retrograde menstruation, transformation of peritoneal epithelium into endometrial tissue, and the differentiation of müllerian remnants into endometrial tissue. Risk factors include early menarche, increased frequency of cycles, heavy prolonged cycles, and low parity.

SYMPTOMS

Dysmenorrhea, menorrhagia, dyspareunia, and low back pain that worsens during menses. Rectal pain and painful defecation may also be seen. Infertility is often the presenting complaint. Many patients are asymptomatic. Pain is not correlated with the stage of disease.

EXAM

- Exam is best performed during early menses, when implants are largest and most tender.
- Although most patients have normal pelvic exams, findings can include tenderness on bimanual exam, nodularity in the posterior cul-de-sac or along the uterosacral ligament, ↓ uterine mobility or retroversion, and adnexal masses.

DIAGNOSIS

- No lab tests can help make the diagnosis, although CA-125 levels are sometimes ↑.
- If masses are present, CT, MRI, or ultrasound can be useful. Transvaginal ultrasound is the imaging modality of choice. Endometriomas appear as homogeneous cysts on ultrasound.
- Laparoscopy is required for definitive diagnosis, although lesions must be histologically confirmed, as they can be confused with a variety of lesions. Histologic appearance consists of endometrial glands and stroma. Visual appearance includes black powder burn lesions (classic) and red/white lesions (nonclassic).
- Clinical manifestations and surgical findings often correlate poorly.

KEY FACT

Laparoscopy with histologic confirmation is needed for a definitive diagnosis of endometriosis.

TREATMENT

- Medical treatment should be reserved for patients with symptoms other than infertility, as such treatment does not restore fertility.
- Combined hormonal contraceptives or progestin-only methods suppress LH and FSH and prevent ovulation, also lead to thinning of endometrial tissue and ↓ menstrual volume. May be used continuously.
- Danazol is an androgen derivative that inhibits LH and FSH and leads to endometrial atrophy. Androgenic side effects include acne, edema, hirsutism, and voice deepening; estrogen deficiency can lead to headache, flushing, sweating, and atrophic vaginitis.
- GnRH agonists (IM leuprolide, SQ goserelin, nasal nafarelin) inhibit gonadotropin secretion and produce pain relief in 90% of patients. Hypoestrogenic side effects, including bone loss, can be minimized by supplementing with low doses of estrogen.
- Surgical treatment is indicated for infertile patients with advanced endometriosis. Surgical ablation of lesions is often performed at the time of diagnostic laparoscopy. A combination of medical and surgical therapy may improve outcomes. Excision of endometrioma is recommended rather than simple drainage, as it is associated with a high recurrence rate.

- Hysterectomy with oophorectomy can be performed in women with intractable pain who no longer want to become pregnant.
- Alternative therapies include heat, exercise, acupuncture, and dietary modification.

COMPLICATIONS

Without treatment, endometriosis progressively worsens in 65%–80% of patients. Implants may grow and spread throughout the pelvis and to the urinary and intestinal tracts, leading to pain, infertility, and obstruction.

Ovarian Torsion

Usually occurs in a pathologically enlarged ovary. Most common in the early reproductive years, with more than half of all cases affecting patients with ovarian masses. (The masses are usually benign; malignant tumors often have adhesions that fix the ovary.) Pregnant women with enlarged corpus luteum cysts, women undergoing ovulation induction, and patients with a history of pelvic surgery, especially tubal ligation, are at ↑ risk for ovarian torsion. Prepubertal patients with congenitally elongated fallopian tubes and normal ovaries are also at ↑ risk.

SYMPTOMS

Sudden-onset, severe, unilateral pelvic pain that radiates to the back or thigh. Pain can also be mild or bilateral. Most patients complain of nausea and vomiting. Onset often occurs during exercise.

EXAM

Most patients have a unilateral, tender adnexal mass, but up to 30% can have no tenderness on exam. In advanced cases, fever and peritoneal signs can be present.

DIFFERENTIAL

Appendicitis, diverticulitis, endometriosis, mesenteric ischemia, bowel obstruction, ovarian cyst, PID, tubal ovarian abscess, ectopic pregnancy, renal calculi, UTI.

DIAGNOSIS

- **Labs:** Rule out other diagnoses with a pregnancy test, UA, and gonorrhea and chlamydia cultures.
- **Imaging:** Ultrasound usually shows ovarian enlargement or an ovarian mass. Doppler flow imaging can be useful, but flow can be normal during transient periods of detorsing. CT can be used to rule out other causes of pain.

TREATMENT

- Laparoscopy can be used for confirmation of diagnosis as well as for treatment; conservative treatment consists of uncoiling the torsed ovary.
- Salpingo-oophorectomy is necessary in cases with severe vascular compromise, peritonitis, or tissue necrosis.

COMPLICATIONS

Delayed diagnosis and treatment can lead to infarction and necrosis of the ovary.

Vulvodynia

> A 35-year-old woman comes to your office complaining of chronic vulvar pain and itching. On exam, she is found to have a $\oplus$ swab test for vestibular point tenderness, and there are no signs of fungal or bacterial infection. How should you manage this patient?
>
> Treatment for vulvar vestibulitis includes oral calcium citrate, topical estradiol cream, and in severe cases, intralesional interferon injection.

A syndrome of unexplained vulvar pain, often accompanied by physical disabilities, limitations in daily activities such as sitting or walking, sexual dysfunction, and psychological distress. Subtypes include the following:

- **Vulvar vestibulitis syndrome:** Usually premenopausal.
- **Cyclic vulvovaginitis:** Associated with pain that worsens during menses.
- **Dysesthetic or essential vulvodynia:** Usually peri- or postmenopausal.
- **Vulvar dermatoses.**
- **Papulosquamous vulvar dermatoses:** Itching is prominent.
- **Vesiculobullous vulvar dermatoses:** May present with itching or burning.
- **Vestibular papillomatosis:** A normal anatomic variant that is often asymptomatic.

SYMPTOMS

- Usually acute in onset, becoming chronic and lasting months or years.
- Discomfort is often described as stinging or burning, or, alternatively, a feeling of rawness or irritation. Itching may be prominent, and pain may be associated with menses, intercourse, or tampon use.
- Any history of vaginal infections, cryotherapy or laser therapy, and use of medications must be obtained.

EXAM

- Some women have minimal findings.
- On pelvic exam, assess for **erythema, edema,** and **vaginal discharge,** and perform a swab test for vestibular point tenderness (vulvar vestibulitis).
- Also look for thickened or scaly lesions (papulosquamous vulvar dermatoses), blisters or ulcers (vesiculobullous vulvar dermatoses), or plaques (possible neoplasms), and assess for skin lesions elsewhere on the body.

DIFFERENTIAL

Allergic vulvitis, chronic candidal vulvitis, lichen planus, lichen sclerosus, vulvar atrophy, vulvar intraepithelial neoplasia.

DIAGNOSIS

- Fungal and bacterial cultures; KOH microscopic exam; biopsy of suspicious areas with acetowhitening and colposcopy to rule out dermatoses or neoplasm.
- The swab test involves palpation of the vestibulum with a moist, cotton-tipped swab to assess for point tenderness.

TREATMENT

- **Oral medications:** Fluconazole for cyclic vulvovaginitis; TCAs, SSRIs, or gabapentin for essential vulvodynia; calcium citrate for cyclic vulvovaginitis or vulvar vestibulitis.

- **Topical medications:** Lidocaine or cromolyn cream; estradiol cream for vulvar vestibulitis; corticosteroids for papulosquamous dermatoses.
- Intralesional interferon injection for **vulvar vestibulitis.**
- Low-oxalate diet; physical therapy with biofeedback to ↓ vaginal spasms and strengthen weakened pelvic floor muscles; support groups.
- **Surgical treatment:** Vulvar vestibulectomy and excited dye laser surgery are reserved for severe cases in which all medical therapies have failed.

VULVAR CUTANEOUS CONDITIONS

Lichen Sclerosus

Chronic, progressive, inflammatory disorder of skin commonly seen on the vulva with extragenital lesions. Onset commonly seen in postmenopausal women, but may occur at all ages. Etiology is unclear. ↑ risk of developing squamous cell carcinoma.

SYMPTOMS

May be asymptomatic, but commonly presents with intense vulvar pruritus. May be associated with dyspareunia, burning sensation, and irritation.

EXAM

May initially appear as white, thickened, and excoriated with edema of labia minora; progresses to thinned and crinkling "cigarette paper" appearance on skin. Vaginal epithelium usually spared. Perianal involvement usually observed (figure-of-eight appearance). May observe clitoral hood phimosis and labia minora fusion.

DIFFERENTIAL

Atopic and contact dermatitis, lichen planus, lichen simplex chronicus, genital atrophy, vulvodynia, psoriasis, vulvar intraepithelial neoplasia, vulvar cancer, contact dermatitis, scabies, pediculosis, vulvovaginal candidiasis, tinea cruris.

DIAGNOSIS

Shave vulvar biopsy.

TREATMENT

- High-potency topical steroid (clobetasol propionate) to reduce symptoms, prevent architectural damage, and reverse histologic changes.
- Immunosuppressants (tacrolimus) are considered second-line therapy.
- Surgery is not curative; reserved for treatment of malignancy or release of labial adhesions.

Lichen Planus

Inflammatory autoimmune disorder of keratinized and mucosal surfaces. Vulvovaginal lichen planus is a chronic and recurring disease. Three types include erosive, papulosquamous, and hypertrophic form. Erosive type is the most common form and may lead to destruction of vulvar architecture. Peaks between ages 30 and 60 years.

SYMPTOMS

Itching, dyspareunia, burning, vaginal discharge, postcoital bleeding, pain.

EXAM

- White, lacy, or fernlike striae (Wickham striae) on mucosal membranes. May observe typical pruritic, purple, shiny papules. Genital skin may appear dusky pink without scales.
- In erosive form, may observe painful, erythematous erosions and denuded epithelium.

DIFFERENTIAL

Lichen sclerosus, mucous membrane pemphigoid, pemphigus vulgaris, Behçet syndrome, desquamative inflammatory vaginitis.

DIAGNOSIS

Punch biopsy.

TREATMENT

- High-potency topical steroids, oral steroids, topical and oral cyclosporine, topical immunosuppressant (tacrolimus).
- Surgery reserved for release of labial adhesion.

Vulvar Lichen Simplex Chronicus

Eczematous disease caused by chronic scratching that may occur consciously or unconsciously while sleeping. Usually a response from heat, excessive sweating, irritation from clothing or lotions, soaps, perfumes. May also occur as a secondary reaction from candidiasis, tinea, HPV, psoriasis, scabies, or neoplasia.

SYMPTOMS

Intense pruritus in vulvar area.

EXAM

Itchy, scaling, lichenified plaques. In chronic conditions, skin may appear thickened and leathery, associated with hypo/hyperpigmentation.

DIFFERENTIAL

Lichen sclerosus, psoriasis, neoplasia, contact dermatitis.

DIAGNOSIS

Vulvar biopsy.

TREATMENT

- Treat the underlying disorder.
- Moderate-potency topical steroids, oral steroids. Must break the itch-scratch cycle.
- Amitriptyline and SSRIs may be effective in controlling subconscious scratching.

MENOPAUSE

Defined as cessation of menses for 12 months without another pathologic cause. It occurs from gradual depletion of functioning ovarian follicles. After menopause, ovaries lose the ability to produce estrogen. The average age of menopause is 51 years. Most women experience vasomotor symptoms for about 2 years after their LMP, but 25% of women are asymptomatic.

SYMPTOMS

- **Hot flashes:** Worsened by eating, exertion, emotional stress, and alcohol.
- **GU symptoms:** Vaginal atrophy leading to dryness, pruritus, and dyspareunia; urethral atrophy leading to stress incontinence, frequency, urgency, and dysuria.
- **Mood changes:** Irritability, anxiety, depression, sleep disturbance.
- **Perimenopause:** Precedes actual menopause; characterized by variable cycle length, often accompanied by the symptoms of menopause.

EXAM

Exam reveals ↓ breast size, vaginal dryness, and urogenital atrophy.

DIFFERENTIAL

Premature ovarian failure (cessation of menses in women < 40); infections such as TB; malignancy.

DIAGNOSIS

↑ serum FSH can be indicative of menopause, although it is insensitive and is rarely needed for diagnosis.

TREATMENT

KEY FACT

HRT is best used as short-term treatment at the lowest effective dosage for menopausal symptom relief, as it ↑ the risk of coronary disease and breast cancer.

KEY FACT

Alternatives to HRT in the treatment of hot flashes include lifestyle changes, SSRIs, gabapentin, and clonidine.

- **Hormone replacement therapy (HRT):**
  - Associated with a significant ↓ in hot flash severity and frequency; also improves GU symptoms and can prevent osteoporosis.
  - HRT ↑ a woman's risk of coronary disease, stroke, DVT, and breast cancer, and therefore it is most appropriately used as a short-term treatment aimed at symptom relief. In order to prevent endometrial cancer, women with a uterus must be treated with a combination of estrogen and progestin.
  - HRT is contraindicated in patients with a history of breast cancer, premalignant breast lesions, endometrial cancer, unexplained vaginal bleeding, DVT or pulmonary embolism, liver disease, or CAD.
- Symptoms of **vaginal atrophy** can be controlled with topical estrogen cream, vaginal estradiol rings, and vaginal lubricants.
- **Other oral medications** that may ↓ hot flashes are SSRIs, including paroxetine, fluoxetine, and venlafaxine, as well as gabapentin and clonidine.
- Phytoestrogens, including soy and red clover, have not consistently been shown to help relieve menopausal symptoms, and studies of black cohosh have also yielded conflicting results.
- **Lifestyle interventions** to ↓ vasomotor symptoms include lowering room temperatures, consuming cold food and drinks, weight control, regular physical activity, tobacco avoidance, and relaxation techniques.

COMPLICATIONS

Long-term complications related to menopause and ↓ estrogen include cardiovascular disease and osteoporosis.

FAMILY AND INTIMATE PARTNER VIOLENCE

Affects individuals from all socioeconomic and cultural backgrounds and all family structures, including same-sex relationships, and is vastly underreported by victims and overlooked by physicians. Victims are more commonly women, and children of abused mothers are at ↑ risk for abuse or neglect. Additional risk factors include marital stress or instability, alcohol or drug abuse, social stressors (eg, unemployment, poverty), and a family history of violence. The highest risk of injury or death occurs during the time and after the victim leaves the perpetrator.

SYMPTOMS

- Although there is insufficient evidence of the benefit of **universal screening,** experts recommend screening all women in the course of prenatal and routine well woman care. The incidence of domestic violence increases during pregnancy and postpartum.
- In the outpatient setting, abuse may present as vague, recurrent somatic complaints, depressive symptoms, or ↑ use of medical services.
- Physical abuse is often preceded or accompanied by psychological abuse (insulting, controlling financial and social life, denying of basic needs) and/or sexual abuse.
- Use the patient's own words when documenting symptoms. Document name of abuser, type of violence (emotional, physical, verbal, or sexual), and if weapons are used.

EXAM

- Look for patterns of injuries, such as bruises in various stages of healing.
- If physical signs of abuse are present, document them in detail and take identifying photographs.

DIFFERENTIAL

Bleeding disorder; affective, anxiety, and somatoform disorders.

TREATMENT

- Validate the patient's right to be free from abuse (eg, "You don't deserve to be hurt like this") and offer support.
- Recognize that abuse often occurs in repeated cycles: escalating tension → violence → remorse and reconciliation (honeymoon period). Do not expect victims to leave right away, and avoid blaming or giving up on them if they return to the abuser.
- Help the patient establish a safety plan.
- If you suspect that children are being harmed or neglected, report to Child Protective Services.
- Know your state's laws with respect to reporting requirements for suspected abuse.

COMPLICATIONS

Learned helplessness, low self-esteem, depression, anxiety, substance abuse, and PTSD; physical injury and disability; exacerbation of chronic medical conditions; death by suicide or homicide.

SEXUAL VIOLENCE

Includes any actual or attempted sexual contact that is against the victim's will or that occurs when the victim is unable to consent because of age, disability, or impairment. At least 1 in 3 women and 1 in 33 men have been victims of rape or attempted rape. More than half of lifetime rapes occur before age 18. Certain groups are more vulnerable, including adolescents, survivors of childhood sexual or physical abuse, disabled persons, persons with substance abuse, and sex workers.

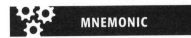

MNEMONIC

Questions for detecting domestic violence:

SAFE

Stress/**S**afety?
Afraid/**A**bused?
Friends/**F**amily aware?
Emergency plan?

KEY FACT

Pregnancy and attempted separation are especially high-risk times for abuse victims.

SYMPTOMS

- Patients who present acutely after sexual assault may have symptoms of trauma that are physical (**bruises, broken bones**), sexual (**genital lacerations, abrasions, bruises**), and/or psychological (**feeling fearful, withdrawn, angry**).
- Patients with a past or ongoing history of sexual violence may have symptoms of psychological sequelae such as **depression** or **PTSD**, or they may present with chronic somatic complaints such as **headache, nausea,** or **fatigue.**

EXAM

- After an acute sexual assault, care should be taken to conduct the exam in a way that allows for adequate collection of forensic evidence and avoids retraumatizing the victim. If available, call on a certified sexual assault nurse examiner (SANE) or a rape victim's advocate.
- Document all signs of trauma and abuse.
- Patients with a past or ongoing history of sexual violence may experience added fear and anxiety with the routine physical (especially pelvic) exam. Limit invasive exams to those absolutely necessary, and offer to have a support person present.

DIAGNOSIS

- Although there is insufficient evidence to recommend routine screening, all patients with suggestive signs or symptoms (physical or psychological) should be asked about their exposure to sexual violence.
- All victims of sexual assault should be offered testing for STIs (including oropharyngeal and anal sites if applicable) and pregnancy.

TREATMENT

- In the setting of acute assault, if clinically applicable, make sure to offer **emergency contraception** to prevent pregnancy, **postexposure HIV prophylaxis and HBV vaccination,** and **empiric STI treatment.**
- Compassion and advocacy throughout the clinical encounter tell victims that you are there to help. An independent victim's advocate, if available, should be provided.
- Work with law enforcement when applicable.
- Offer acute and ongoing psychological counseling.

COMPLICATIONS

Undesired pregnancy; STIs; depression, anxiety, eating disorders, PTSD, and substance abuse; chronic headaches, sleep disturbance, and GI complaints; suicidal behavior.

SEXUAL DYSFUNCTION

Female Sexual Dysfunction

Distress and impairment resulting from a disturbance in sexual desire and/or from emotional and physiologic changes in the sexual response cycle. Affects approximately 25%–40% of women. Factors that predict sexual functioning

KEY FACT

Emergency contraception is the standard of care for women who are capable of becoming pregnant at the time they are raped. The sooner they get it, the more effective it will be at preventing pregnancy as a result of the assault.

include a general state of well-being and a quality relationship with a partner; dysfunction is generally **not** related to hormone levels. Subtypes include the following:

- **Hypoactive sexual desire disorder/low libido:** Absence of sexual fantasies and lack of desire to engage in sexual activity.
- **Sexual arousal disorder/excitement phase dysfunction:** Inability to respond to sexual stimulation despite genital vasocongestion and lubrication.
- **Orgasmic dysfunction:** Inability to have an orgasm despite normal sexual desire and ability to enjoy intercourse.
- **Pain associated with sex:** Dyspareunia, vaginitis, incompletely ruptured hymen, Bartholin gland cyst, postepisiotomy pain, vulvovaginal atrophy, vulvar vestibulitis, vaginismus (involuntary spasm of musculature of the outer third of the vagina, making penetration impossible or painful), PID, ovarian cyst, endometriosis, fibroids, relaxation of pelvic support.

SYMPTOMS

- Obtain a complete sexual history, including concerns, degree of satisfaction, sexual orientation, relationship issues, partner performance and satisfaction, contraception, and safe sex practices. Also elicit a psychiatric history (major depression, anxiety disorder, somatization disorder).
- Obtain a complete medical and surgical history to rule out 2° causes of sexual dysfunction (eg, Cushing disease, Addison disease, DM, hyperprolactinemia, hypothyroidism, hypopituitarism, degenerative joint disease, MS, temporal lobe lesions, CAD).
- Explore the following:
  - **Interpersonal relationships:** Relationship quality and conflict.
  - **Psychology:** Depression, anxiety, past sexual or physical abuse, substance abuse.
  - **Sociocultural influences:** Stress, fatigue, lack of privacy, religion, lack of education about sex and sexuality.
  - **Physiology:** Medications, medical/neurologic problems, gynecologic/urologic problems, estrogen or androgen deficiency.

EXAM

Perform a pelvic exam to evaluate for vulvovaginitis, cervicitis, uterine masses or tenderness, cervical motion tenderness, and rectocele or cystocele.

DIAGNOSIS

Diagnosis is primarily based on history, but some of the following may be indicated:

- **Labs:** CBC, ESR, FSH, estradiol, testosterone, TSH, prolactin, cervical cultures.
- **Imaging:** Pelvic ultrasound if exam is suspicious for a pelvic mass.

TREATMENT

- Treat the underlying cause; counseling, sex therapy, and adjustment of life situation may be of benefit.
- **Estrogen** may be helpful for women with vaginal dryness or atrophy. Options include low-dose estrogen cream, an estradiol vaginal ring for postmenopausal vaginal dryness.

KEY FACT

Female sexual function is more commonly related more to a state of well-being and relationship quality than to hormone levels.

MNEMONIC

Sexual response cycle:

EXPLORE

EXcitement
PLateau
Orgasm
REsolution

Erectile Dysfunction (ED)

> A 68-year-old male smoker with hypertension and diabetes asks you to prescribe sildenafil for erectile dysfunction. The patient takes an ACEI, a diuretic, aspirin, a statin, metformin, and insulin. What do you tell him? Although sildenafil is absolutely contraindicated only in patients taking nitrates, before writing the prescription, you should make sure that the patient understands the risks of sexual activity with his multiple cardiac risk factors.

Repeated inability to achieve or sustain a penile erection sufficient for sexual intercourse. Affects up to 10% of men; more common in older men and smokers. Screen for cardiovascular risk factors in men with ED; symptoms of ED present 3 years earlier than symptoms of CAD on average (increased risk of coronary, cerebrovascular, and peripheral vascular diseases). Up to 50% of ED is due to organic causes (Table 16.18).

SYMPTOMS

- Obtain a thorough sexual history as well as a history of medications and substance abuse.
- Elicit a psychiatric, medical, and surgical history.
- Preservation of morning erections suggests psychogenic disease.
- Assess for atherosclerotic risk factors.

EXAM

- **Vital signs:** Look for orthostatic changes in BP; BMI (obesity is a risk factor).
- **Skin:** Signs of endocrinopathies include palmar erythema, dryness, hyperpigmentation, and spider angiomata.

TABLE 16.18. Etiologies of Erectile Dysfunction

DISORDER	EXAMPLES/COMMENTS
Psychogenic disorders	Performance anxiety, depression, mental stress.
Diabetes mellitus	ED is seen in up to 50% of DM cases.
Peripheral vascular disease	
Endocrine disorders	Hypogonadism, hyperprolactinemia, thyroid abnormalities, Addison disease, Cushing disease, acromegaly.
Pelvic surgery, spinal cord injury	
Drugs of abuse	Amphetamines, cocaine, marijuana, chronic alcoholism, tobacco, opiates, barbiturates.
Medications	Antihypertensives (thiazides, β-blockers, clonidine, methyldopa), antiandrogens (spironolactone, H_2 blockers, finasteride), antidepressants (TCAs, SSRIs, MAOIs, lithium), antipsychotics, benzodiazepines, opiates, antihistamines.
Prostate cancer	
Penile and urethral lesions	Pelvic fracture, hypospadias, priapism, Peyronie disease, phimosis.

- **GU exam:** Inspect the penis for tumors, inflammation, discharge, phimosis, testicular masses, atrophy, or asymmetry; perform a prostate exam.
- **Vascular exam:** Assess peripheral pulses and evaluate for femoral and aortic bruits.
- **Neurologic exam:** Assess for pain sensation in the genital and perianal areas; test the bulbocavernosus reflex to evaluate the 2nd, 3rd, and 4th sacral segments of the spinal cord (the anal sphincter contracts around the examining finger as the glans is squeezed).
- **Other:** Thyroid exam; palpate the spine for tenderness and evidence of cord compression; examine for gynecomastia.

DIAGNOSIS

- **Labs:** Depending on clinical presentation, consider checking fasting glucose and lipids, TSH, and morning total testosterone.
- Nocturnal penile tumescence testing; Doppler ultrasonography.

TREATMENT

- Offer psychological support.
- Adjust medications that may be contributing to ED.
- Address the underlying cause, especially nicotine dependence.
- 1st-line medications include oral phosphodiesterase type 5 inhibitors (sildenafil, vardenafil, and tadalafil, which has the longest duration of action). Side effects include flushing, headache, dyspepsia, and visual disturbance (sildenafil only); contraindicated if patients are on nitrates because of the risk of hypotension.
- Phosphodiesterase type 5 inhibitors are effective in the treatment of ED associated with diabetes and spinal cord injury and in treatment associated with sexual dysfunction with antidepressants.
- Men with hypogonadism may benefit from testosterone to improve ED and libido. Because of increased risk of adenocarcinoma of prostate, monitor hemoglobin, serum transaminase, and PSA levels and perform digital rectal exam.
- Other treatments include intracavernosal injection with alprostadil and/or papaverine, transurethral alprostadil, penile prostheses, and vacuum constriction devices.
- Inform patients about potential risk of prolonged erections and seek immediate medication evaluation for erections lasting > 4 hours.

KEY FACT

Patients on nitrates should not take sildenafil, vardenafil, or tadalafil owing to the risk of hypotension.

INFERTILITY

A husband and wife present to your clinic appearing very anxious. They state that they have been married for almost 2 years and are eager to have a child but so far have not conceived. The woman, who is 33 years old, has been pregnant once and had an abortion. She reports regular menses every 30 days. The man, who is 38 years old, has 2 children from a previous marriage. Both travel frequently for work and report that they may go for 2–3 weeks at a time without having intercourse. What is the likely diagnosis, and how would you proceed?

This couple is probably not experiencing true infertility, since they are not having regular intercourse reliably during fertile periods. They may have 2° or acquired infertility, but that diagnosis is not yet merited. Given that they have both been able to conceive in the past and that the woman has regular menstrual cycles, they have a high likelihood of being able to conceive together. Provide education about fertile times of the month, and encourage them to keep a journal of fertile periods and sexual activity to assist in the workup. At this visit, it would also be appropriate to provide the couple with preconception counseling regarding genetic risks, infection exposure, and nutrition.

Defined as the inability to conceive after 1 year of regular, unprotected vaginal intercourse. In 20% of cases, no cause is found. Among the rest, 40% are due to male factors, 40% to female factors, and 20% combined (Table 16.19).

SYMPTOMS

- Patients may present with a wide array of concerns that they associate with impaired fertility. Inquire about the frequency and timing of intercourse and how long the couple has been trying to conceive.
- Take a complete menstrual and reproductive history. Irregular menses may indicate anovulatory cycles; prior conception rules out 1° infertility. A history of STIs or endometriosis predisposes women to 2° infertility.

EXAM

- Perform a complete GU exam to look for anatomic abnormalities such as undescended testis or varicocele in men or large fibroids in women.
- Examine patients for 2° sexual characteristics as well as for signs of endocrine/metabolic disorders such as gynecomastia in men or hirsutism or extreme body weight in women.

TABLE 16.19. Causes of Infertility

	MALE FACTORS	FEMALE FACTORS
Anatomic (congenital or acquired)	Varicocele Cryptorchidism History of orchitis	Gonadal dysgenesis Uterine anomalies Endometriosis Prior surgery affecting the reproductive organs Prior tubal inflammation such as that associated with PID Asherman syndrome (uterine synechiae)
Endocrine/metabolic	Hypothalamic or pituitary dysfunction Hyperprolactinemia Thyroid disease Adrenal disease	Hypothalamic or pituitary dysfunction Hyperprolactinemia Thyroid disease Premature ovarian failure Androgen excess Extremes of body weight
Functional	Erectile dysfunction Ejaculatory dysfunction ↓ libido	Sexual dysfunction ↓ libido
Exposures	Chemical, radiation, or heat effects on testes Exogenous androgens	DES in utero Exogenous androgens Chemical or radiation effects on ovaries

DIAGNOSIS

- Order a semen analysis to evaluate the male partner for ejaculatory function, sperm count, morphology, and motility.
- If hormonal/metabolic causes in the female partner are considered, check TSH, FSH, free testosterone, DHEAS, and an oral glucose tolerance test.
- If it is unclear whether the woman is ovulating, obtain a midcycle progesterone or home luteinizing hormone urine test kit. Daily basal body temperature readings can also be of benefit; a sustained rise of ≥ 0.4°F suggests that ovulation has occurred.
- If there is a concern for ↓ ovarian reserve, **obtain a day-3 FSH.**
- If anatomic causes in the female partner are considered, refer for appropriate imaging, which may include ultrasound, hysterosalpingography, hysteroscopy, and laparoscopy.

TREATMENT

- Treatment should be targeted to the couple-specific cause of infertility.
- All couples should be advised to maximize fertility through lifestyle changes, including decreasing caffeine, alcohol, and tobacco, and optimizing weight, as well as timing intercourse to ovulation.
- Anovulation can be treated with clomiphene citrate.
- PCOS-related infertility should be addressed with weight loss. If this is unsuccessful, clomiphene citrate +/– metformin may be useful.
- Couples with irreversible or unidentified causes of infertility may still be able to conceive using intrauterine insemination, in vitro fertilization, or other assisted reproductive therapies.
- Couples may consider adoption as an alternative.
- Infertility and assisted reproductive therapy can be stressful and emotionally trying. For this reason, psychosocial support should be provided throughout the workup and treatment.

KEY FACT

Women with PCOS or metabolic syndrome ↑ their chance of conceiving by improving their insulin sensitivity.

Men's Health

EPIDIDYMITIS

The most common cause of scrotal inflammation in adults. The usual route of infection is retrograde ascent of bacteria. Usually sexually transmitted in men < 35 years (usually chlamydia but sometimes gonorrhea); usually 2° to UTI or prostatitis in older men (usually *Escherichia coli*, sometimes other coliforms).

SYMPTOMS

- Painful, swollen scrotum that is usually acute in onset (< 6 weeks). Pain is localized to the posterior testis but may radiate to the groin, abdomen, or flank.
- Dysuria and urinary frequency are common.
- Fever, chills, and malaise are common.
- Urethral discharge is possible.

EXAM

- Exam reveals a swollen, tender mass attached to the testicle and tender spermatic cord. Inflammation may extend locally.
- Exam may reveal swollen and tender lymph nodes.
- Normal cremasteric muscle reflex.

MNEMONIC

Differential diagnosis of scrotal swelling:

THE THEATRES

Torsion
Hernia
Epididymitis/orchitis
Trauma
Hydrocele, varicocele, hematoma
Edema
Appendix testes (torsion, hemorrhage)
Tumor
Recurrent leukemia
Epididymal cyst
Syphilis, TB

- Positive Prehn sign (relief of pain with elevation of testis).
- Reactive hydrocele may be seen.
- Fever may be present, and patients may occasionally appear toxic.

DIAGNOSIS

- UA and culture may reveal bacteriuria, pyuria, and hematuria, though they are sometimes normal.
- CBC and blood culture are indicated if the patient is febrile or toxic.
- Urine nucleic acid amplification tests or urethral culture for gonorrhea and chlamydia; offer testing for other STIs.
- Ultrasound with Doppler is not necessary for diagnosis, but reveals enlarged, thickened epididymis with increased blood flow.

TREATMENT

- Empiric treatment should be started, based on likely pathogens, before test results return. If patient is 14–35 years old with suspicion of sexual transmission, antibiotics to cover *Neisseria gonorrhoeae* (ceftriaxone) and *Chlamydia trachomatis* (doxycycline or azithromycin) should be prescribed; TMP-SMX or a fluoroquinolone if enteric gram-$\ominus$ organisms or staph are suspected.
- Hospitalization for IV therapy if the patient has intractable pain, is vomiting, experiences failure of outpatient therapy, or is febrile or toxic.
- NSAIDs, scrotal elevation, limitation of activity, and cold packs are of benefit.

COMPLICATIONS

Sepsis, abscess, infertility, and extension of infection. Follow with periodic exams to exclude an underlying testicular mass. Prepubescent boys need urology referral to rule out urogenital abnormalities. Evaluate for urethral obstruction 2° to enlargement of prostate in men > 50 years.

PROSTATITIS

A 65-year-old man comes to your office complaining of dysuria and deep rectal pain for the past 2 months. He is generally healthy and has no new sexual partners and no other urinary symptoms. On DRE, his prostate is found to be normal in size, shape, and consistency, and is nontender. Urine culture is $\ominus$. Exam of expressed prostatic secretions reveals multiple WBCs, but culture is $\ominus$. What is the likely diagnosis, and how would you treat this patient?

The patient has chronic nonbacterial prostatitis. Treatment is symptomatic, consisting of NSAIDs and sitz baths. α-blockers or antispasmodics may provide additional relief.

An inflammatory disorder of the prostate that may be irritative or infectious. It may present as an acute febrile illness with risk of sepsis or may have a chronic, lingering course. Bacterial prostatitis stems from enteric gram-$\ominus$ organisms (*E coli, Klebsiella, Proteus, Pseudomonas*), gram-$\oplus$ organisms (*Staphylococcus, Enterococcus*), and/or gonorrhea or chlamydia.

SYMPTOMS

- Patients present with perineal, rectal, and/or low back pain.
- May be acute in onset, with fever, chills, malaise, and myalgias, or chronic, with fewer systemic symptoms.

- Urinary urgency, frequency, retention, nocturia, hesitancy, straining to void, incomplete voiding, and dysuria are seen.
- Painful ejaculation is common.

EXAM

- In acute prostatitis, the prostate feels boggy, swollen, warm, and tender, and the patient is febrile and appears toxic.
- Chronic prostatitis may present with a normal exam.

DIFFERENTIAL

- Voiding symptoms may indicate UTI or BPH.
- Pain may be isolated prostatodynia with no exam or lab findings.
- Prostatic abscess, which is rare in nondiabetics, presents with high fever and nonresponse to treatment and requires surgical drainage.
- If the patient is not responding to antibacterial therapy, consider TB and *Cryptococcus*, especially in immunocompromised patients.
- Consider fistula, foreign body within urinary tract, stones, and bladder cancer.

DIAGNOSIS

- In bacterial prostatitis, UA reveals bacteriuria, hematuria, and pyuria.
- Urine culture and sensitivity identifies the causal organism. If ⊖ in chronic prostatitis, prostatic secretions may be expressed by massage.
- In acute prostatitis, CBC reveals leukocytosis, and blood cultures may be ⊕.

TREATMENT

- Acutely ill patients may require hospitalization and IV antibiotics. Ampicillin and an aminoglycoside are recommended until cultures can guide therapy.
- If infectious but IV therapy is not required, treat for at least 4–6 weeks with TMP-SMX, amoxicillin, or a fluoroquinolone.
- Adjuvant therapy includes analgesics (usually NSAIDs) and stool softeners for comfort.
- If chronic symptoms persist and cultures are ⊖, treatment is symptomatic with analgesics, anti-inflammatory agents, α-blockers, and sitz baths.

COMPLICATIONS

- Acute prostatitis can seed the blood and lead to sepsis.
- Acute episodes may recur or become low-grade chronic prostatitis. A full month of therapy may ↓ the risk of recurrence. Occasionally, patients may require chronic suppressive antibiotic therapy.
- Chronic prostatitis is the most common cause of recurrent UTI in men.

URETHRITIS

Classified as gonoccocal or nongonoccocal. Primary pathogens are *C trachomatis* and *N gonorrhoeae*. Common nongonoccocal organisms include *Mycoplasma genitalium* and *Ureaplasma*; less common organisms include *Trichomonas*, HSV, and adenovirus.

SYMPTOMS

Urethral discharge, penile itching or tingling, dysuria, urgency, hematuria.

KEY FACT

If you suspect acute prostatitis, avoid prostate massage and urethral catheterization if possible, as they may ↑ the risk of bacteremia.

EXAM

Examine for urethral discharge, ulcers, inguinal lymphadenopathy.

DIFFERENTIAL

UTI, pyelonephritis, HSV, prostatitis, epididymitis, orchitis.

DIAGNOSIS

- Presence of urethral discharge.
- UA with positive leukocyte esterase or ≥ 10 WBCs present.
- Urine nucleic acid amplification tests or urethral culture for gonorrhea and chlamydia; offer testing for other STIs.
- Consider *Mycoplasma*, *Trichomonas*, or *Ureaplasma* cultures from urethra or urine for recurrent infection.

TREATMENT

- Treat gonorrhea with ceftriaxone and chlamydia, *Mycoplasma*, *Ureaplasma* with azithromycin. Chlamydia may also be treated with doxycycline. *Trichomoniasis* may be treated with metronidazole.
- If infections are not present, suggest fragrance-free soaps and lotions; ↑ water intake and ↓ carbonated beverages; ↓ frequency of masturbation or intercourse; no spermicide use.
- Treat partner for STIs. Abstain from sex for at least 1 week following therapy initiation.
- CDC recommends annual screening for men who have sex with men, including urethral/urine DNA testing for chlamydia and gonorrhea, rectal testing for chlamydia and gonorrhea, and DNA swab or culture for pharyngeal gonorrhea. Pharyngeal chlamydia testing is not recommended.
- CDC recommends annual screening in both men and women < age 25 years with urine, urethral, or vaginal GC/CT DNA testing.

BALANITIS

Inflammation of the glans penis, usually related to fungal organisms but sometimes due to bacteria from skin or sexually transmitted organisms. The condition is more common in uncircumcised men and diabetics.

SYMPTOMS

- Presents with burning, irritation, and redness of the head of the penis.
- Dysuria may be present.
- A white, cheesy discharge may be seen if the cause is fungal.

EXAM

- Exam reveals a tender, erythematous, and swollen glans, prepuce, and urethral opening.
- Papules, pustules, or ulcerations may be seen (Figure 16.18).
- If the patient is uncircumcised, retract the foreskin to reveal an adherent, cheesy discharge.

DIFFERENTIAL

In prepubertal boys, rule out sexual abuse.

DIAGNOSIS

- The history and exam are usually diagnostic.
- Consider skin culture for fungus and bacteria; consider testing for STIs.

KEY FACT

Diabetes is the most common condition underlying balanitis. Don't miss an opportunity to diagnose diabetes or motivate good glycemic control!

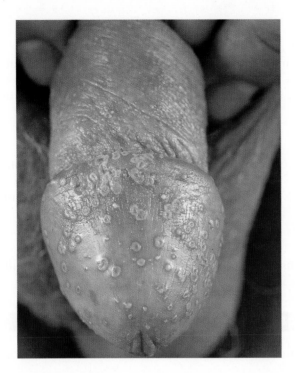

FIGURE 16.18.   Candidal balanitis. (Reproduced, with permission, from Wolff K, et al. *Fitzpatrick's Color Atlas & Synopsis of Clinical Dermatology,* 5th ed. New York: McGraw-Hill, 2005: 727.)

TREATMENT

- Topical antifungals if a fungal source is suspected or proven.
- Recommend hygiene measures (keep the area clean and dry; avoid unnecessary foreskin manipulation) to prevent recurrence.
- Aggressive glycemic control in diabetics.
- Antibacterials against skin or STI organisms.
- If fungal infection recurs, consider treating the sexual partner to prevent reinfection.

COMPLICATIONS

If balanitis recurs frequently in an uncircumcised patient, consider circumcision.

ORCHITIS

Infection of the testes, primarily caused by the mumps virus. Other causes include non-mumps viruses, or, rarely, TB, fungi, or local bacterial spread from epididymitis.

SYMPTOMS

- Presents with abrupt onset of painful, swollen testicle.
- If the infection is caused by mumps, associated symptoms include parotitis, fever, and malaise.

EXAM

- The testicle is tensely swollen and tender. Reactive hydrocele may be present.
- Normal cremasteric muscle reflex.

DIAGNOSIS

- The history and exam are usually diagnostic.
- Testicular masses of unknown etiology should be evaluated with ultrasound.
- In mumps, generalized symptoms and parotitis precede orchitis by 4–6 days.

TREATMENT

- Supportive care with analgesics, limitation of activity, scrotal support, and cold packs.
- If symptoms do not improve, consider abscess or other causes of testicular mass.

COMPLICATIONS

Mumps orchitis leading to impaired fertility in 10% of men affected and testicular atrophy in 30%–50%.

BENIGN SCROTAL MASSES

Hydrocele, varicocele, and spermatocele are relatively common scrotal swellings.

SYMPTOMS

- Patients present with a scrotal swelling or lump.
- Also presents with scrotal discomfort or heaviness, occasionally with inguinal or low back pain.

EXAM

- Hydrocele surrounds or sits below the testis and can be separated from it on exam. Hydrocele is painless, unilateral, fluctuant, nontender scrotal swelling.
- Spermatocele consists of 1 or several cysts of the epididymis and sits just above and attached to the testis.
- Varicocele consists of dilated veins of the spermatic cord, more commonly on the left side, and feels like a "bag of worms" on palpation. The mass enlarges when standing or with Valsalva and may disappear if the scrotum is elevated or when the man is lying down.
- Hydrocele and spermatocele transilluminate; varicocele does not.

DIFFERENTIAL

Inguinal hernia and malignancy must be considered as sources of a scrotal mass.

DIAGNOSIS

If the exam is not definitive, imaging (usually ultrasound) is required to rule out testicular cancer.

TREATMENT

- **Hydrocele and spermatocele** usually do not require treatment. If they become large or uncomfortable, surgical repair is offered.
- **Varicocele repair** is considered part of infertility treatment. If the mass was detected incidentally, repair may be advised to prevent infertility; watchful waiting may be appropriate if semen parameters are normal.

COMPLICATIONS

By reducing spermatogenesis, varicocele may contribute to male fertility problems.

TESTICULAR TORSION

A surgical emergency, as cessation of blood supply for 4–6 hours will lead to permanent loss of the testicle. Most common in infants, teens, and men < 30 years of age.

SYMPTOMS

May present with testicular pain, abdominal pain, nausea, and vomiting. Scrotal pain is not always present.

EXAM

- Affected testicle is tender and swollen, which may progress to reactive hydrocele and scrotal wall erythema.
- Cremasteric muscle reflex is absent.
- High-riding testicle, may be transversely oriented.
- Pain with testicular elevation.

DIFFERENTIAL

Torsion of the appendix testis, appendicitis, epididymitis.

DIAGNOSIS

- If torsion is considered, **do not delay consulting urology.**
- Ultrasound may help distinguish among the causes of scrotal pain but can be falsely ⊖ for torsion (approximately 10% of the time). Ultrasound with Doppler may reveal normal-appearing testis with decreased blood flow.
- UA is ⊖.

TREATMENT

- Immediate surgical repair is the definitive treatment.
- Bilateral surgical fixation may be done to prevent recurrence.
- If surgical treatment is not available, manual detorsion may be attempted.
- Torsion of the appendix testis does not require treatment, but surgical exploration may be needed to rule out testicular torsion.

COMPLICATIONS

- May lead to testicular infarction and impaired fertility if not corrected in time.
- If not surgically fixed, the testes have ↑ risk of recurrent torsion on the ipsilateral or contralateral side.

BENIGN PROSTATIC HYPERTROPHY (BPH)

Enlargement of the prostate gland. BPH is common as men age and can cause partial urethral obstruction, leading to urinary symptoms and occasionally impaired renal function. The severity of symptoms may not correlate with the size of the gland felt on exam.

KEY FACT

Since testicular torsion can lead to complete loss of blood supply to the testicle if not surgically corrected, the "acute scrotum" should be treated as an emergency.

MNEMONIC

Symptoms of BPH or "prostatism":

HI FUN

Hesitancy
Intermittence, **I**ncontinence
Frequency, **F**ullness
Urgency
Nocturia

SYMPTOMS

- Presents with urinary frequency (≤ every 2 hours) due to incomplete emptying; urinary hesitancy (difficulty initiating stream) or weak stream; and urinary dribbling or incontinence. Nocturia is common.
- Intermittence of voiding (starting and stopping urine flow during voiding) is also seen.

EXAM

The gland feels smooth and symmetrically enlarged on DRE, and the bladder may be distended.

DIFFERENTIAL

Prostate cancer, UTI, prostatitis, neurogenic bladder, medications (antihistamines, diuretics, opiates, TCAs).

DIAGNOSIS

- The history and exam are usually diagnostic.
- Postvoid residual urine volume and urodynamic studies can be used to indicate the degree of obstruction.
- PSA may be ↑ but is nonspecific.
- Serum creatinine and other signs of renal impairment may be ↑ due to obstruction and resultant hydronephrosis.

TREATMENT

- Treatment is primarily symptomatic and is aimed at preventing or treating clinically significant urinary obstruction.
- α-blockers (doxazosin, terazosin, prazosin, tamsulosin) relieve symptoms by relaxing the smooth muscles of the bladder neck.
- 5α-reductase inhibitors (finasteride, dutasteride) shrink the prostate medically, although they do not acutely relieve symptoms.
- These 2 classes of medications can safely be used in combination.
- Transurethral resection of the prostate (TURP) and other minimally invasive surgical techniques have proven effective. Side effects of TURP include sexual dysfunction, hemorrhage, strictures, and hyponatremia associated with hypotonic saline during the procedure.
- Open prostatectomy is the treatment of last resort.

COMPLICATIONS

- Obstruction, leading to hydronephrosis and chronic renal insufficiency; recurrent UTI may result from incomplete bladder emptying.
- Complete inability to urinate that requires urgent bladder catheterization may occur.

BENIGN PENILE CONDITIONS

Peyronie disease, leading to "crooked" erections that may be painful due to thickening of the corpora tunica. **Priapism** is a prolonged, painful erection. It is most commonly related to medications such as chlorpromazine and sildenafil or to hematologic conditions such as sickle cell disease and leukemia. **Penile trauma** during erection can lead to rupture of the tunica albuginea, sometimes called penile fracture.

SYMPTOMS

- Peyronie disease presents as a bent angle of the shaft that is often accompanied by pain during erection. The patient may also note subcutaneous nodules.
- The painful, prolonged erection of priapism may be accompanied by fever and inability to urinate.
- Penile fracture is an acutely painful sensation that usually occurs during sexual activity and may be accompanied by a popping sound.

EXAM

- Peyronie disease includes palpable, nontender plaques just beneath the skin of the penile shaft, usually on the dorsum.
- Priapism presents with an erect or semierect penis that may last for hours to days.
- Penile fracture is usually accompanied by a subcutaneous hematoma and by swollen "eggplant deformity" of the penis.

DIAGNOSIS

- The history and exam are diagnostic.
- With penile injury, surgical exploration may be required to determine the extent of trauma.

TREATMENT

- Peyronie disease can be managed with verapamil injection, shock wave therapy, radiotherapy, or surgery. Many cases resolve without treatment.
- Priapism should be relieved as quickly as possibly to prevent cellular damage that can lead to functional impairment. Treatment is intracavernosal injection of a sympathomimetic drug and/or aspiration and irrigation. Surgical shunting is an option if these therapies are not successful.
- Penile trauma may require surgical repair. Rupture of the tunica albuginea is a surgical emergency.

COMPLICATIONS

- Peyronie disease may progress and lead to worsening pain and sexual dysfunction.
- Prolonged priapism can lead to erectile dysfunction.
- Untreated trauma to the corpora cavernosa or urethra can lead to permanent sexual and urinary dysfunction.

PENILE CUTANEOUS CONDITIONS

Noninfectious lesions are categorized as inflammatory and papulosquamous lesions.

Psoriasis

Genital involvement occurs in up to 40% of patients. Commonly seen in males age 16–22 years and 57–60 years. Triggers include stress, alcohol and tobacco use, acute infections, β-blockers, and lithium.

SYMPTOMS

Penile pruritus.

EXAM

Red or salmon-colored papules or plaques, white or silvery scales. May note extragenital psoriasis on extensor surfaces of elbows and knees, scalp, and lumbosacral region, and nail pitting.

DIFFERENTIAL

Carcinoma in situ.

DIAGNOSIS

Based on physical exam. Biopsy performed if lesions are atypical.

TREATMENT

Topical corticosteroids, tacrolimus, pimecrolimus, vitamin D_3 analogs.

Lichen Sclerosus

Also known as balanitis xerotica obliterans. May occur at all ages; average is 42 years old. Associated with squamous cell carcinoma. Primarily affects the glans penis and prepuce.

SYMPTOMS

Asymptomatic or complaint of urinary retention, painful erections, phimosis, pain, itching, bleeding.

EXAM

Hypopigmented lesion with skin similar to crinkled paper. May note erosions, atrophy, or bullae.

DIFFERENTIAL

Carcinoma in situ, scleroderma, leukoplakia.

DIAGNOSIS

Based on physical exam. Perform biopsy if squamous cell carcinoma is suspected.

TREATMENT

- Topical corticosteroids, circumcision if limited to glans penis and prepuce, surgery if patient has persistent disease. Retinoids reserved when local therapy fails.
- Lifelong monitoring for possible malignancy.

Lichen Nitidus

A harmless papular rash that generally appears in children and young adults. It can be of cosmetic concern to patients but does not have malignant potential.

SYMPTOMS

Usually asymptomatic, or, rarely, pruritus.

EXAM

Discrete hypopigmented papules.

DIFFERENTIAL

Pearly papules, HSV.

DIAGNOSIS

Based on physical exam.

TREATMENT

- Observation; may resolve spontaneously.
- Treatment for cosmesis includes corticosteroids, vitamin A analogues, cyclosporine, itraconazole, and phototherapy.
- Laser ablation not recommended because of potential for scarring.

Lichen Planus

Typically systemic condition affecting mucous membranes, nails, and scalp; 25% of patients have genital lesions. Relatively uncommon.

SYMPTOMS

Pruritus, soreness, and occasionally ulceration.

EXAM

Raised, violaceous, flat-topped, polygonal papules. May observe fine white streaks (Wickham straie).

DIFFERENTIAL

Secondary syphilis.

DIAGNOSIS

Based on physical exam.

TREATMENT

Topical corticosteroids or circumcision if isolated only on prepuce.

Angiokeratomas

Common in white men > 40 years of age. Benign lesions.

SYMPTOMS

Asymptomatic, or, rarely, pruritus, pain, intermittent bleeding.

EXAM

Well-circumscribed red or blue papules on glans penis, scrotum, thighs, and abdominal wall.

DIFFERENTIAL

Pearly papules, penile cancer.

DIAGNOSIS

Based on physical exam.

TREATMENT

- Observation.
- If patient is symptomatic or bleeding, treat with surgery, cryoablation, electrocautery, and laser ablation.

PROSTATE CANCER

The most common malignancy among U.S. men, and the second most common cause of cancer death. Most cases remain latent, with only 10% progressing to clinically significant disease. Risk factors include advancing age, African American ethnicity, and a ⊕ family history of 1st-degree relatives.

SYMPTOMS

- Often asymptomatic, or may lead to urinary obstruction with symptoms of prostatism.
- Bony metastases can lead to vertebral or hip pain.

EXAM

- DRE reveals areas of induration or nodules if the tumor is on the posterior aspect of the prostate.
- Anterior tumors will produce a normal exam.
- Palpate vertebrae for bony tenderness from metastases.

DIFFERENTIAL

BPH.

DIAGNOSIS

- There is insufficient evidence to support routine screening, but experts recommend discussing the risks and benefits of screening with all men starting at age 50 years, or at a younger age if risk factors are present.
- If PSA or DRE raises concern, ultrasound-guided biopsy is indicated.

TREATMENT

- Treatment depends on the stage at diagnosis and on the patient's comorbidities and may include surgery, radiation, hormonal therapy, or watchful waiting.
- Close attention to pain control is essential, including management of bone pain from metastases with analgesics and bisphosphonates.

COMPLICATIONS

Treatment (surgery or radiation) may lead to impaired sexual function and/or incontinence.

KEY FACT

Discuss the risks and benefits of prostate cancer screening with all men starting at age 50, or younger in African American men or those with a family history.

TESTICULAR CANCER

Can occur at any age, but most commonly seen at ages 20–35 years. Risk factors include cryptorchidism (undescended testicle), family history, infertility, tobacco use, white race, and exposure to DES in utero. USPSTF and American Cancer Society recommend against routine screening and self-examination in low- and high-risk asymptomatic men. All scrotal masses should be evaluated to rule out cancer.

SYMPTOMS

- May be asymptomatic, or may present with a painless mass in the scrotum.
- Patients may have a dull ache/pain, swelling, or hardness in the lower abdomen or scrotum.
- Symptoms of metastasis include neck mass, abdominal mass, lumbar back pain, hemoptysis, dyspnea, cough, or GI symptoms.

EXAM

Exam reveals a firm, hard, or fixed nodular mass on the testis that does **not** transilluminate. May be accompanied by epididymitis. Palpate for inguinal lymphandenopathy.

DIFFERENTIAL

Isolated epididymitis; benign scrotal mass; hydrocele; swelling of testicular appendix; varicocele.

DIAGNOSIS

- Any suspicious history or exam findings should be evaluated with ultrasound and possible referral to urology.
- Serum tumor markers include β-hCG, LDH, and α-fetoprotein.
  - Nonseminoma: Elevated α-fetoprotein and β-hCG.
  - Seminoma: Normal α-fetoprotein and usually elevated β-hCG.
  - Metastasis: Elevated LDH.

TREATMENT

- Staging determined by TNMS (tumor, regional nodes, metastasis, serum tumor markers) system.
- Depends on the tumor type. Orchiectomy +/– lymph node dissection in most cases. May include chemotherapy.
- Cure rates are high, with roughly 95% 5-year survival.
- After diagnosis, CT of chest/abdomen/pelvis to detect metastasis.

COMPLICATIONS

Impaired fertility after germ cell tumor; ↑ risk of cardiovascular disease and 2° malignancies (leukemia and gastric cancer 2° to chemotherapy and radiation). Due to ↑ risk of infertility from therapy, recommend sperm banking. ↑ risk of cancer in contralateral testicle.

PENILE CANCER

A rare squamous cell cancer occurring largely in uncircumcised men. Incidence peaks in men > 70 years old. Appears to be associated with high-risk HPV infection. Risk factors include smoking, advanced age, presence of foreskin, phimosis, smegma, poor hygiene, and lichen sclerosus.

SYMPTOMS

Presents with an ulcer, erosion, or nodule on the glans or prepuce or, rarely, on the shaft. Often accompanied by phimosis, which masks the lesion.

EXAM

Retract the foreskin to thoroughly examine the glans, prepuce, and shaft.

DIFFERENTIAL

Genital warts, HSV, Peyronie disease.

DIAGNOSIS

Any suspicious lesion should be referred for biopsy.

TREATMENT

- Depends on the stage at diagnosis.
- Local excision +/– lymph node dissection +/– radiation.
- Adjuvant chemotherapy may be advised.
- Amputation of the penis is standard treatment for higher-staged tumors.

COMPLICATIONS

Urinary and sexual function after treatment depends on the extent of surgery and radiation required.

CHAPTER 17

Sports Medicine and Musculoskeletal Disorders

Andres Marin, MD

The Preparticipation Physical Evaluation (PPE)

The PPE is used to screen athletes for injuries, illness, and other factors that might place them or others at risk during sports.

SYMPTOMS/EXAM

- **History:** The history is the most important and highest-yield part of the PPE. Screen for the following conditions:
    - A history of sudden death in a family member < 50 years of age (hypertrophic cardiomyopathy is autosomal dominant).
    - A history of dizziness, palpitations, chest pain, or syncope with exertion.
    - A history of concussion, including confusion, memory loss, or headache with exertion (recent concussion ↑ the risk of recurrence).
    - A history of asthma or coughing/shortness of breath during or after exercise (may point to exercise-induced bronchospasm).
    - Rashes or skin problems, especially in close-contact sports such as wrestling.
    - Recent or current illnesses, infections, or fever.
- **Exam:**
    - Table 17.1 describes the standard components of a PPE.
    - Further testing is indicated for the following:
        - Systolic murmurs of grade 3/6 or more (atrial stenosis, mitral regurgitation).
        - Any diastolic murmur.
        - Any murmur that grows louder with ↓ venous return.

KEY FACT

Because of the risk of splenic injury that occurs with mononucleosis (even in the absence of splenomegaly), sports should be avoided for 21–28 days from the start of infection.

KEY FACT

If a murmur ↑ with the Valsalva maneuver or when the patient stands up from a squatting position, worry about hypertrophic cardiomyopathy.

T A B L E 1 7 . 1 .   Components of the PPE

SYSTEM	COMPONENT
Vitals	Take routine vital signs (height, weight, pulse, BP, lungs).
Cardiovascular	Palpate pulses, auscultate for murmurs in both sitting and standing positions, and evaluate the effects of exercise on the individual.
Musculoskeletal	Determine previous injuries, strength, flexibility and range of motion (general, neck, shoulder/upper extremity, and back), gait/lower extremity, and asymmetry of muscle bulk/scarring/posture.
Skin	Check for contagious lesions and rashes.
Vision	General screening; look for evidence of retinal problems or eye injury.
Abdomen	Check for masses and evidence of hepatosplenomegaly.
Genitourinary—Males only	Check for testicular abnormalities and hernias; note Tanner stage.
Neurologic	Rule out problems with coordination, gait, and mental processing.

Based on data from Wilson PE, Matthews DJ. Rehabilitation and Sports Medicine. In Hay WW, et al. *Current Pediatric Diagnosis and Treatment,* 18th ed. New York: McGraw-Hill, 2007.

DIAGNOSIS

- No routine diagnostic testing is recommended.
- If the history and physical exam suggest structural heart disease, the standard evaluation generally includes a 12-lead ECG, stress echocardiography, and graded exercise testing.

KEY FACT

Myocarditis is an absolute contraindication to any sport because of the risk of sudden death with exertion.

Concussion Management

You are serving as team physician for a high school football game. One of the players sustains a forceful tackle and falls to the ground unresponsive. You run onto the field and find him dazed but coherent. He reports a headache and dizziness. His teammates report that the player appeared to be unconscious for a few seconds before you reached him on the field. After clearing his C-spine, you help the player off the field and conduct a neurologic exam, which is normal. After 10 minutes, the player states that he feels fine and that his headache and dizziness are gone. He asks to return to the game. What do you do?

You inform the player and his coach that although the player may feel better, he is at risk for sustaining a more severe head injury if he is hit again, so it is not safe for him to resume playing football today. You explain that you and the trainer will monitor him for symptoms over the next few days and will slowly ↑ his activity level if he remains symptom free. He will need to be able to exercise at game intensity without inducing any symptoms before he is safe to play again.

A concussion, also known as mild traumatic brain injury (MTBI), is defined as an alteration in cerebral function 2° to a direct or indirect (rotational) force on the brain. Concussions are classified as follows:

- **Simple concussion:** Symptoms progressively resolve without complications in 7–10 days.
- **Complex concussion:** Symptoms persist > 10 days and involve symptom recurrence with exertion, prolonged loss of consciousness (> 1 minute), and/or prolonged cognitive impairment after the injury.

SYMPTOMS/EXAM

- May present with headache, dizziness, nausea, confusion, irritability, double or blurry vision, sensitivity to light or noise, changes in sleep pattern, difficulty concentrating, memory problems, ↑ emotionality, and easy fatigability.
- Exam may reveal delayed verbal and motor responses, a vacant stare, disorientation, slurred or incoherent speech, incoordination, and memory deficits.

KEY FACT

Amnesia is thought to be a better indicator of concussion severity than loss of consciousness.

DIFFERENTIAL

Structural injury or abnormalities such as cerebral hemorrhage or infection.

DIAGNOSIS

- A clinical diagnosis.
- Any abnormalities found on neurologic exam are not normal for a concussion and should be emergently evaluated in the emergency department.

■ Consider head CT or MRI if patient has worsening of symptoms such as headache, persistent vomiting, increasing disorientation or deteriorating level of consciousness, seizures, or unequal pupil size.

TREATMENT

■ Recommend complete mental and physical rest while the patient is symptomatic (including no homework or video games).
■ Allow slow progression of activity from light aerobic exercise through the following stages: sport-specific exercise, noncontact drills, full-contact drills, and then game play. Each stage should last at least 1 day. Athletes must remain asymptomatic to progress to the next stage.

Supplements and Steroids

Table 17.2 outlines the uses and mechanisms of action of commonly used supplements.

TABLE 17.2. Common Sports Supplements

	DESCRIPTION	SIDE EFFECTS
Glucosamine and chondroitin	Shown in some clinical trials to ↓ the symptoms of osteoarthritis, although a recent meta-analysis shows them to be no more effective than placebo. Glucosamine is thought to promote the formation and repair of cartilage. Chondroitin is a component of cartilage that is thought to promote water retention and elasticity and inhibit the enzymes that break down cartilage.	Considered safe, without significant side effects.
Creatine	A nutritional supplement used to promote protein synthesis and provide a quick source of energy for muscle contraction. Thought to enhance performance in short-duration, high-intensity exercise such as sprinting and weight lifting.	Associated with weight gain due to intracellular water retention. This can also lead to intravascular dehydration and possible renal injury.
Androgens	"Nutritional supplements" (eg, DHEA, a precursor to androgenic steroids) and synthetic agents used to stimulate muscle growth and strength. Banned by most competitive sports organizations.	Suppression of endogenous testicular function; diminishing spermatogenesis and fertility. Chronic use (over years) can cause loss of testicular size. Also associated with gynecomastia, erythrocytosis, hepatotoxicity, adverse effects on serum lipids, virilization of female athletes, premature epiphyseal fusion and stunting of growth, and psychological disorders, including major mood disorders and aggressive behavior ("roid rage").
International Olympic Committee (IOC) doping classes	Stimulants, narcotics, anabolic agents, β_2-agonists, β-blockers (used to calm, stop trembling, and ↓ BP and heart rate), diuretics (used to meet weight goals), peptide hormones and analogs (eg, GH and erythropoietin), street drugs.	Banned by the IOC for use in athletic competition (except β_2-agonists in the setting of documented asthma).

Overuse Injuries

Repetitive stress across a bone, tendon, or muscle without adequate healing time can lead to tissue injury and degradation. The process can be largely inflammatory, as in carpal tunnel syndrome and de Quervain tenosynovitis; largely degenerative, as in lateral epicondylitis; or due to incomplete remodeling, as seen in stress fractures.

MEDIAL TIBIAL STRESS SYNDROME (SHIN SPLINTS)

 A 28-year-old woman presents to your office complaining of pain and tenderness over her tibia when she runs. Previously, she had pain only at the end of her runs, but now is having symptoms with walking. She is training for a marathon and has increased her mileage significantly in the past several weeks. She runs only on pavement. On physical exam you find focal tenderness at her mid-tibia and ↑ pain when you place a tuning fork over the area. X-ray is negative, but you still suspect a stress fracture, so you order an MRI, which shows a small hairline fracture in the anterior tibia. How do you counsel this patient?

You tell her that rest is the only option for complete healing of the stress fracture. You give her a walking boot and crutches to use for 4–8 weeks (healing times vary according to location, severity, and the body's healing response). After she is pain free with ambulation, activities may be gradually resumed as long as she remains pain free. You advise her to avoid running on pavement (vs. in parks) and tell her not to increase her mileage more than 10% a week. You also tell her that if she continues to run with this stress fracture she is at risk for progression to a complete fracture.

- Diffuse stress reaction along the tibia; seen in runners and jumpers (basketball, dancing, racket sports).
- **Sx:** The onset of symptoms is insidious and is similar to that of tibial stress fractures, but pain often occurs at the beginning of a run, resolves as workout continues, and recurs after the workout. Alternatively, it may occur only at the end of the run.
- **Exam:** Reveals a more diffuse pattern of pain and tenderness along the medial border of the middle and distal thirds of the tibia (muscle attachment sites). Pain is noted with resisted plantar flexion and toe walking.
- **Differential:** Stress fracture; chronic exertional compartment syndrome (suggested by localized calf pain that progressively worsens with persistent running and is relieved with cessation of exercise); bony tumor (suggested by unusually severe bone pain and/or night pain).
- **Dx:** Triple-phase bone scan or MRI can distinguish the injury from stress fracture if the exam is unclear.
- **Tx:** Treatment is similar to that of tibial stress fractures, but is shorter and may begin with relative rest and cross-training (no immobilization). Cryotherapy/ice, NSAIDs, and physical therapy (for stretching exercises of calf and plantar flexors of the foot) can also be used.

KEY FACT

If you encounter multiple stress fractures, especially in a female athlete, you should do a prompt workup for osteoporosis along with questioning regarding the female athlete triad (disordered eating, amenorrhea, osteoporosis).

KEY FACT

For athletes, the tibia is the most commonly involved bone in stress fractures, whereas in military recruits, fractures of the metatarsal and calcaneal bones are more common because of the biomechanics of running vs. marching.

TENDINOPATHIES

- Repetitive stress along a tendon (Achilles, patellar, medial and lateral elbow, rotator cuff) can lead to collagen degeneration or tendinosis. Many studies have cast doubt on the role of inflammation (tendinitis). Overloading of the tendon due to poor biomechanics (eg, muscle imbalances, foot overpronation) and repetitive stress can cause collagen breakdown and/or inflammation.
- Tx:
  - Includes rest, cryotherapy/ice, unloading devices (eg, counterforce straps for the elbow and patellar tendon; heel lifts for the Achilles tendon), and physical therapy.
  - The role of NSAIDs and corticosteroid injections is controversial, but treatment can often afford short-term relief.
  - Healing is slow and can take 6 months or longer.
  - Surgical debridement is a last resort but is usually effective.

General Approach to the Joint Exam

- **Terms:** In the forearm and hand, different terms are used to specify location. Volar = anterior; dorsal = posterior; ulnar = medial; and radial = lateral (remember the anatomic position of the hand). Axial alignment is described in terms of the angle made by the proximal and distal segments.
  - **Valgus alignment:** Two limb segments create an angle that points toward midline.
  - **Varus alignment:** The angle formed by the 2 segments points away from midline.
- **Inspection:** Involves surface anatomy (muscle wasting, symmetry), alignment (eg, genu valgum), gait, and active and passive ROM.
- **Palpation:** Performed to identify landmarks, localize tenderness, compare temperature with the contralateral side (to detect the warmth of infection or posttraumatic inflammation or to gauge the coolness of vasoconstriction or vascular compromise), and check pulses.
- **Manipulation:** Tests muscle strength, sensation, reflexes, stability, and special tests. Muscle strength is graded 0–5.

MNEMONIC

In genu val**GUM,** the knees are stuck together with **GUM.**

KEY FACT

A fracture with any overlying laceration or abrasion should be considered an open fracture and requires further evaluation (the old term for this was a compound fracture).

Principles of Imaging

STANDARD VIEWS

Radiographs must include a minimum of 2 views, AP and lateral, to fully evaluate patients for fractures. Table 17.3 describes additional views that may be useful (see Figure 17.1).

IMAGING OF FRACTURES

Fracture Categories

Fractures are categorized by location (eg, distal radius, tibial plateau), type (see Table 17.4 and Figure 17.2), and degree of displacement (see Table 17.5).

TABLE 17.3.   Radiologic Views and Key Points

REGION	VIEWS
Wrist	AP view of clenched fist with ulnar deviation to evaluate the scaphoid.
Elbow	Comparison views may be helpful. Look for an anterior **sail sign** (fat pad displaced by effusion), which suggests fracture (Figure 17.1).
Cervical spine	The lateral view must include C1–C7 to fully clear C-spine. The swimmer's view (arm overhead) may help visualize C7.
Hip/pelvis	AP and frog-leg views.
Knee	Weight-bearing AP in full extension and 40° of flexion (notch view) if osteoarthritis is suspected; axial (merchant or sunrise) view to evaluate the patellofemoral joint.
Ankle	The mortise view allows for the evaluation of ankle joint integrity (symmetry of the mortise space).

Imaging of Pediatric Fractures

Until late adolescence, tendons and ligaments are stronger than bones, so fractures are more common and true sprains are infrequent. Children's bones are also more malleable, creating a few fracture terms specific to pediatrics (see Figure 17.3):

- **Torus or buckle fracture:** An impaction fracture identified by a focal widening (or outward buckling) of the cortex. The periosteum bends but does not break.

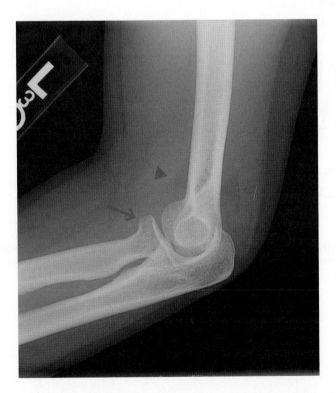

FIGURE 17.1.   Elbow effusion and fracture. Displacement of the anterior and posterior fat pads (*arrowheads*) at the elbow joint on a lateral radiograph indicates the presence of a joint effusion, raising concern for fracture. The arrow denotes a subtle associated fracture of the head. (Reproduced, with permission, from USMLERx.com.)

TABLE 17.4. Fracture Types

TYPE	DESCRIPTION
Transverse	Perpendicular to the shaft of the bone.
Oblique	Slanting or inclined fracture line.
Spiral	Multiplanar fracture line, caused by a torsional force.
Comminuted	Multiple fragments.
Segmental	Large, well-defined fragments (a type of comminuted fracture).
Intra-articular	Extends into the joint space. The general rule is that if the fracture includes more than one third of the joint space, it requires surgical evaluation for possible fixation.
Avulsion	Bony fragment pulled away from its native bone.
Compression	Impaction of bone, such as in the vertebrae or proximal tibia.
Pathologic	Fracture through bone weakened by tumor or disease (eg, osteoporosis).

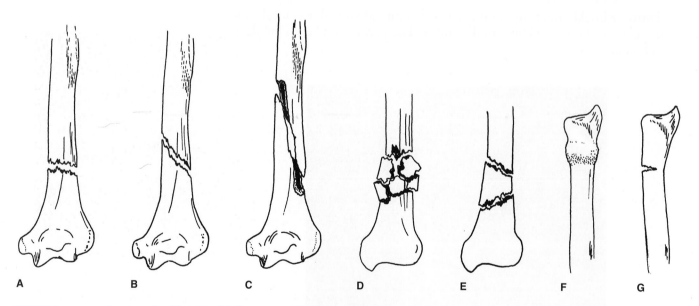

A B C D E F G

FIGURE 17.2. Fracture classification. (A) Transverse. (B) Oblique. (C) Spiral. (D) Comminuted. (E) Segmental. (F) Buckle (torus). (G) Greenstick. (Reproduced, with permission, from Tintinalli JE, et al. *Tintinalli's Emergency Medicine*: *A Comprehensive Study Guide*, 6th ed. New York: McGraw-Hill, 2004, Fig. 267-2.)

TABLE 17.5. **Degrees of Fracture Displacement**

TERM	DEFINITION
Displaced	When one fragment shifts in relation to the other through translation, angulation, shortening, or rotation.
Nondisplaced	A fracture in which the fragments are in anatomic alignment.
Translation	Movement in the AP (volar/dorsal in the forearm) or medial-lateral plane (ulnar/radial in the forearm).
Angulated	Malalignment described using the direction the apex is pointing—eg, apex dorsal angulation.
Bayonetted	The distal fragment longitudinally overlaps the proximal fragment.
Distracted	The distal fragment is separated from the proximal fragment by a gap.

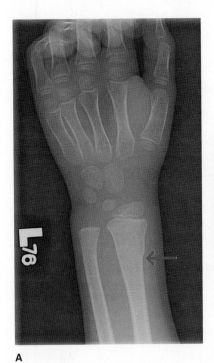

A

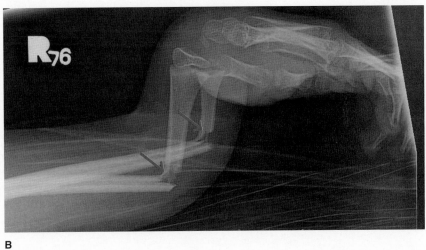

B

FIGURE 17.3. **Pediatric fractures.** (**A**) Buckle (torus) fracture *(arrow)* of the distal radius after trauma. (**B**) Greenstick fractures of the distal radius and ulna after a motor vehicle accident. Note the intact periosteum and cortex *(arrows)* opposite the side of fracture through the cortex and periosteum. (Reproduced, with permission, from USMLERx.com.)

TABLE 17.6. Salter-Harris Classification of Fractures

Type	Location	Outcome	Image
I	Through the physis.	Associated with the best prognosis (difficult to distinguish from normal growth plate).	
II	Through the physis and metaphysis.	Growth arrest may occur.	
III	Through the physis and epiphysis.	Growth arrest is rare, but joint surface involvement requires close maintenance of anatomic reduction (referral).	
IV	Through the metaphysis, across the physis, and through the epiphysis.	Associated with a risk for both growth arrest and articular cartilage damage (referral).	
V	Crush injury to the physis.	Usually diagnosed retrospectively if growth arrest or angular deformity has occurred.	

- **Greenstick fracture:** The periosteum buckles on one side and breaks on the other, which can allow for angulation that may need to be reduced.
- **Salter-Harris classification:** Physeal injuries are unique to children, as their open growth plates allow for more fractures. Such fractures are classified using the Salter-Harris system (see Table 17.6).

Shoulder Injuries

Guidelines for the evaluation of shoulder injuries:

- **Inspection:** Note supraspinatus and infraspinatus atrophy seen on the posterior shoulder with **suprascapular nerve entrapment** or chronic rotator cuff tears.
- **Palpation:** Check for acromioclavicular (AC) joint tenderness (separation, arthritis).
- **ROM:** Watch for scapular dyskinesis or winging on abduction and forward flexion (rotator cuff dysfunction).

Table 17.7 outlines special tests that can aid in the evaluation of injuries to the shoulder.

ROTATOR CUFF TEARS AND IMPINGEMENT SYNDROME

- The rotator cuff is made up of the supraspinatus (abduction), infraspinatus (external rotation), teres minor (external rotation), and subscapularis (internal rotation) muscles (**"SITS"** muscles).
- **Sx/Exam:** Rotator cuff impingement and tearing usually begin in the supraspinatus tendon as it passes under the acromion. Patients are usually

MNEMONIC

Salter-Harris categories:

SALTER

I **S = Slipped:** Separation physis
II **A = Above:** Fracture lies above the physis
III **L = Lower:** Fracture below the physis in the epiphysis
IV **T = Through:** Fracture through the metaphysis, physis, and epiphysis
V **ER = Erased/Crushed:** The physis has been crushed

KEY FACT

Cervical disk disease, apical lung tumor, pleural disease, myocardial ischemia, and subdiaphragmatic processes should all be considered as causes of referred shoulder pain.

TABLE 17.7. Special Tests for the Diagnosis of Shoulder Injury

EXAM	TECHNIQUE	INDICATIONS
Hawkins test	With the patient's elbow and shoulder flexed to 90°, the examiner passively internally rotates the shoulder by stabilizing the elbow and pushing down on the wrist.	Pain points to rotator cuff tendinosis/impingement.
Neer impingement sign	The examiner performs maximal passive forward flexion with internal rotation while stabilizing the patient's scapula with the other hand.	Pain points to rotator cuff tendinosis/impingement.
Jobe test (empty can)	The arms are abducted 90° and brought forward 30°, thumbs down. The patient resists downward pressure.	Pain points to supraspinatus tendinosis; weakness suggests tear.
O'Brien test	Forward flex the shoulder to 90° with the elbow extended and the arm 15° toward the midline. The patient resists downward force with the thumb down and the thumb up.	Deep pain with the thumb down that improves with the thumb up suggests superior glenoid labrum (SLAP) lesions.
Apprehension test (crank test)	The shoulder is in 90° abduction and slight extension with the elbow flexed. The examiner externally rotates the arm.	Simulates the most common position of subluxation/dislocation. Pain or anxiety suggests anterior instability.

> 50 years of age and will often have significant pain with abduction above the head and internal rotation (reaching up the back). Can occur in young athletes. Will often hear a "pop" (eg, baseball pitchers). **Hawkins** and **Neer** tests are ⊕.

- **Dx/Tx:** If there is weakness on exam and lack of full improvement with rehabilitative exercises and subacromial corticosteroid injection, you should suspect a tear rather than isolated impingement. Tears are diagnosed with MRI and often require surgical repair.

ADHESIVE CAPSULITIS (FROZEN SHOULDER)

- Idiopathic loss of both active and passive motion of the shoulder that usually resolves over a period of **6 months to 2 years.**
- Usually results from prolonged immobility due to another shoulder injury. Significant association with **diabetes, especially type 1;** 40%–50% of people with diabetes will develop bilateral disease. People without diabetes are also at ↑ risk for occurrence in the other shoulder.
- **Sx/Exam:** The initial "freezing" phase is progressive and painful, presenting with complaints similar to those of rotator cuff pathology (differentiated by loss of **passive** ROM). This is followed by a "thawing" phase with improvement in pain and ROM.
- **Tx:** Treat initially with NSAIDs and stretching exercises (such as arm pendulum and wall push-ups). Can use glenohumeral corticosteroid injections and rarely will need surgery.

ACROMIOCLAVICULAR (AC) JOINT PATHOLOGY

- Degenerative **arthritis** of the AC joint is often a component of rotator cuff pathology and shoulder pain seen in patients > 50 years of age. For this reason, a distal clavicle resection often accompanies surgical repair of the rotator cuff.
- AC injuries (**shoulder separations**) usually occur from a fall onto the lateral aspect of the shoulder, causing stress and tearing of the AC ligaments and sometimes the coracoclavicular (CC) ligaments as well. Remember, this is not the same thing as a shoulder dislocation, which involves the glenohumeral joint (see Glenohumeral Dislocations below). AC injuries are graded as types I–III (Figure 17.4).
    - **Type I:** Partial or full disruption of the AC ligaments with CC ligaments intact, causing tenderness but no step-off on palpation.
    - **Type II:** The AC ligaments are torn and the CC ligaments are partially disrupted, allowing for partial separation of the clavicle from the acromion on stress radiographs and palpation.
    - **Type III:** Complete disruption of the AC and CC ligaments, causing complete separation of the clavicle from the acromion superiorly.
- **Tx:** Type I and II injuries are treated nonoperatively with a sling, analgesics, and ice, followed by rehabilitative exercises. Type III injuries can be treated conservatively or surgically. Type II may take up to 8 weeks to heal, whereas type III may take up to 12 weeks.

GLENOHUMERAL DISLOCATIONS

- The shoulder is at its most vulnerable when abducted and externally rotated. A fall or tackle with the arm in this position can cause an anterior dislocation. Posterior dislocations are less common, but can occur with a grand mal seizure or an electrical shock.

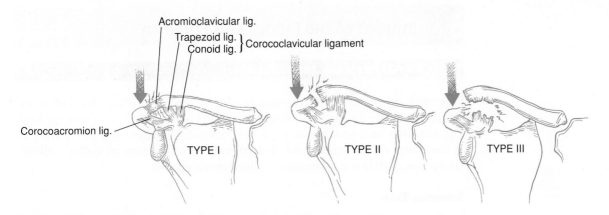

FIGURE 17.4. **Classification of AC joint separation.** (Reproduced, with permission, from Knoop KJ, et al. *The Atlas of Emergency Medicine*, 3rd ed. New York: McGraw-Hill, 2010, Fig. 11.2.)

- Recurrence rates after 1° traumatic dislocation are 65%–95% in patients < 20 years of age; 60% in patients 20–40 years of age; and 10% in patients > 40 years of age.
- **Tx:**
  - After reduction, treat initially with a sling and then physical therapy for strengthening.
  - Surgical repair of the capsule integrity is required for recurrent dislocations.

SLAP LESIONS

- Defined as an injury or tear of the **S**uperior **L**abrum from **A**nterior to **P**osterior. The superior labrum is the upper portion of the cartilaginous ring that surrounds the glenoid fossa, increasing its depth and adding to shoulder stability.
- **Sx/Exam:** SLAP lesions are most common in throwing athletes such as baseball pitchers. Patients experience a sense of catching or popping in the shoulder, with loss of force +/– pain.
- **Dx/Tx:** Diagnosed with MRI or MR arthrography. Requires surgical repair.

FRACTURES OF THE SHOULDER

- **Fractures of the clavicle:** Usually due to a fall onto the lateral aspect of the shoulder or a direct blow. Eighty percent affect the middle third of the clavicle. You can treat most nonoperatively with either an arm sling or a figure-of-eight harness for 4–6 weeks (or 3–4 weeks for children < 12 years of age). Surgical referral is indicated for displacements greater than the width of the clavicle or for shortening > 20 mm.
- **Fractures of the scapula:** Usually due to high-energy trauma such as significant falls and motorcycle accidents. Ninety percent are associated with other injuries, such as rib fractures, pneumothorax, pulmonary contusion, and injuries of the head, spinal cord, and brachial plexus. Most are treated with a sling for comfort and early ROM.
- **Fractures of the proximal humerus:** Commonly occur in elderly patients with osteoporosis, especially women. Most are minimally displaced and can be treated with a sling and early mobilization.

Injuries of the Elbow and Forearm

EPICONDYLITIS/ELBOW TENDINOSIS

Repetitive stress across the common tendon of the wrist flexors (medial) or extensors (lateral) can lead to collagen breakdown and a failure of tendon healing, resulting in a tendinosis. It's a degenerative problem, not inflammation, as the name would suggest. Medial epicondylitis is known as **golfer's elbow;** lateral epicondylitis is commonly called **tennis elbow.**

SYMPTOMS/EXAM

- Presents with activity-related pain progressing to pain at rest and functional strength loss.
- Exam reveals tenderness over the medial or lateral tendon origins and pain with resisted wrist flexion/pronation (medial) or resisted wrist and middle finger extension/supination (lateral).

DIAGNOSIS

Clinical diagnosis is based on the history and exam. Can do MRI for nonresolving cases.

TREATMENT

- Patient must rest and avoid aggravating activities.
- NSAIDs can control pain and allow for rehabilitative exercises. Can use corticosteroid injection if necessary.
- Therapeutic modalities such as ice or heat, high-voltage electrical stimulation, and ultrasound can aid in pain relief.
- Control of force loads across the tendon, with use of counterforce strap bracing and improvements in technique.
- Surgical debridement of the tendon is appropriate if conservative measures fail. With conservative measures, it may take weeks to months for symptoms to resolve.

ULNAR NERVE COMPRESSION

Chronic or posttraumatic compression of the ulnar nerve near or at the elbow, leading to an ulnar neuritis. May occur in multiple sites, the most common of which is the cubital tunnel ("funny bone"), where the nerve passes through the groove on the posterior aspect of the medial epicondyle.

SYMPTOMS/EXAM

- Presents with aching pain in the medial aspect of the elbow, along with numbness and tingling into the 4th and 5th fingers.
- A later finding is weakness of the intrinsic muscles, which can interfere with activities such as opening jars or turning a key.
- Exam reveals pain and paresthesias in an ulnar distribution with tapping on the nerve in the cubital tunnel (⊕ **Tinel test**) (there is also a Tinel test for carpal tunnel syndrome).

DIAGNOSIS

Nerve conduction velocity studies can confirm the clinical diagnosis and may provide an objective measure of nerve impairment.

TREATMENT

- Activity modification to limit elbow flexion and direct pressure on the ulnar nerve.
- A nighttime splint is used to prevent full flexion (nerve stretch).
- Surgical decompression or transposition of the nerve for failure of conservative measures after 3–4 months.

COMPLICATIONS

Loss of grip and pinch strength, with numbness in the ring and little fingers; can become permanent in long-standing cases.

PEDIATRIC INJURIES OF THE ELBOW AND FOREARM

A mother brings in her 2-year-old son and states that he is refusing to use his left arm. He is holding his hand in a slightly flexed and pronated position. He was having a tantrum in a store when she picked him up by his hands to get him off the floor. The child does not appear to be in severe pain, but he does not move his left arm despite attempts to have him reach for a toy with that arm. Given the history and exam, you suspect a subluxation of the radial head (nursemaid's elbow). What do you do?

The child's arm must be reduced. This is accomplished by holding the child's hand and stabilizing his elbow while supinating and flexing the forearm. Immediately, the child begins using his arm again. You let the mother know that he is at risk for this to recur and advise her to avoid pulling him by his arms.

Fractures

- Supracondylar fractures of the distal humerus are the most common elbow fractures in children, typically affecting those 2–12 years of age.
- Given the high incidence of neurovascular injuries, you should always refer.
- Medial and lateral epicondyle fractures are unique to pediatrics because of growth plate weakness.

Little League Elbow

- Medial epicondyle apophysitis is seen in young throwers because of the repetitive valgus stress across the elbow.
- **Dx:** Clinical; rule out ulnar nerve involvement and ligamentous instability.
- **Tx:** Responds well to rest and conservative measures. Indications for surgical intervention include ulnar neuropathy with displaced fracture and valgus instability.

Injuries of the Hand and Wrist

Table 17.8 outlines special tests that may facilitate the diagnosis of wrist and hand injuries. The presentation and treatment of specific wrist and hand injuries are described in the sections that follow.

TABLE 17.8.   Special Tests for the Diagnosis of Wrist and Hand Injuries

EXAM	TECHNIQUE	INDICATIONS
Finkelstein test	With the hand in a neutral position, the patient flexes the thumb across the palm and then ulnar-deviates the wrist.	Pain along the 1st dorsal compartment indicates de Quervain tenosynovitis.
Tinel test	The examiner taps over the median nerve in the wrist.	Pain and tingling into the hand suggests carpal tunnel syndrome.
Phalen test	The patient compresses the backs of the hands against each other so that the wrists are flexed 90° for 1 min.	Reproduction of the patient's symptoms and aching or tingling in a median nerve distribution suggest carpal tunnel syndrome.

CARPAL TUNNEL SYNDROME

Compression of the **median nerve** in the carpal tunnel at the wrist due to direct trauma, repetitive use, or anatomic anomalies. Most commonly affects middle-aged or pregnant women.

SYMPTOMS/EXAM

- Presents with a vague ache into the thenar eminence and sometimes the forearm.
- Numbness, tingling, and pain occur in a median nerve distribution (the thumb, index, long, and radial half of the ring fingers).
- Late symptoms include weakness, dropping objects, persistent numbness, and thenar atrophy.
- Reproduction of these symptoms with the Tinel and/or Phalen test is suggestive.
- ↓ 2-point discrimination can be seen on sensation testing.

DIFFERENTIAL

- **DM** with neuropathy.
- **Flexor carpi radialis tenosynovitis:** Presents with tenderness near the base of the thumb.
- **Cervical radiculopathy affecting the C6 nerve:** Presents with neck pain and numbness in the thumb and index finger only.
- **Hypothyroidism:** Detected by laboratory testing.
- **Arthritis of the wrist or carpometacarpal joint of the thumb:** Presents with painful, limited motion; evident on radiographs.

DIAGNOSIS

- EMG (median nerve conduction velocity study) confirms the diagnosis and indicates severity (important if surgery is being considered).
- Approximately 5%–10% of patients with carpal tunnel syndrome have normal EMG results.

TREATMENT

- Wrist splints at night and for provocative activities, with a short course of NSAIDs and ergonomic modifications if indicated.
- Corticosteroid injection into the carpal canal (avoid the median nerve).
- Surgical decompression is appropriate for patients who fail conservative treatment or who have weakness or atrophy.

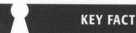

KEY FACT

If your patient awakens at night with wrist pain, you must consider carpal tunnel syndrome (due to sleeping with wrist in flexed position).

DE QUERVAIN TENOSYNOVITIS

Swelling and stenosis of the sheath that surrounds the thumb extensor tendons. More common in middle-aged women. Often precipitated by repetitive use of the thumb and activities requiring a forceful grip (eg, cleaning tasks, racket sports).

SYMPTOMS/EXAM/DIAGNOSIS

- Presents with pain and tenderness over the radial styloid, especially with use of the thumb and ulnar deviation of the wrist (pulls tendons through the inflamed sheath). There may also be some swelling and triggering symptoms.
- A ⊕ **Finkelstein** test is pathognomonic.

TREATMENT

- Treated with a thumb spica splint to immobilize both the wrist and the thumb, along with a 2-week course of NSAIDs.
- Corticosteroid injection into the tendon sheath.
- Surgical decompression is appropriate if no improvement is seen with conservative measures.

THUMB AND FINGER INJURIES

Ulnar Collateral Ligament (UCL) Tear

- A fall onto an abducted thumb, causing an acute rupture of the UCL of the thumb metacarpophalangeal (MCP) joint. Also known as **skier's** or **game-keeper's thumb.**
- **Sx/Exam:** Patients present with instability of the MCP joint of the thumb accompanied by pain and weakness with pinch grasp. Up to 70% of full ruptures are associated with a **Stener lesion,** in which the torn end of the UCL is displaced, preventing healing and requiring surgical repair. This is suggested by a palpable lump or gross instability.
- **Tx:** In the absence of a Stener lesion, many injuries heal well in a thumb spica cast for 4 weeks, followed by protective splinting during competitive activities for 2–4 months.

Mallet Finger

- Forced flexion of an actively extended distal interphalangeal (DIP) joint (eg, "jammed finger"), causing disruption of the extensor mechanism at its insertion into the distal phalanx (Figure 17.5).
- **Sx/Exam:** The patient will have full passive ROM but an inability to actively extend at the DIP joint.
- **Dx:** Based on physical exam, but x-rays should be obtained to evaluate for bony avulsion vs. tendon rupture as the cause.
- **Tx:** Treatment involves **continuous** extension splinting for at least 6 weeks, followed by 4 weeks of nighttime splinting. If the finger is bent at all during the initial 4 weeks, healing can be greatly affected. Surgical referral for large bony avulsion or failure to heal with splinting.

Jersey Finger

- Forced extension of an actively flexed DIP joint (eg, grabbing someone's jersey), causing an avulsion of the flexor digitorum profundus tendon from its insertion on the distal phalanx. Approximately 75% of cases involve the

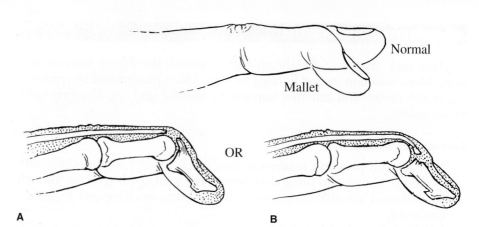

FIGURE 17.5.   Mallet finger. Disruption of the extensor mechanism can be due to extensor tendon injury (**A**) or avulsion of bone fragment (**B**) at the dorsal insertion of the extensor tendon. (Reproduced, with permission, from Knoop KJ, et al. *The Atlas of Emergency Medicine*, 3rd ed. New York: McGraw-Hill, 2010, Fig. 11.50.)

ring finger. The person will be unable to bend the finger down to the palm of the hand.

- **Tx:** All cases require surgical repair, but the urgency depends on the degree of tendon retraction (the more retracted, the more urgent).

Boutonnière Deformity

- Deformed position of a finger caused by acute injury or progressive arthritis. There is a disruption of the central slip of the extensor tendon where it inserts into the middle phalanx. If not properly treated, the head of the middle phalanx may buttonhole through the defect between the lateral bands of the extensor tendon mechanism, causing fixed flexion at the proximal interphalangeal (PIP) joint (Figure 17.6).
- **Dx:** Radiographs are required to rule out fracture.
- **Tx:** The finger is treated with extension splinting of the PIP while allowing DIP motion for 6 weeks. Surgical repair is required for large bony fragments or with lack of improvement with splinting.

Trigger Finger

- Inflammation of the flexor tendon, with thickening and stenosis of the 1st annular (A1) pulley, causing pain and catching with flexion/extension of the finger. Most cases are degenerative, although there is an association with rheumatoid arthritis.
- **Dx:** Can see catching as the patient extends a fully flexed finger. A nodule (the thickened A1 pulley) is often palpable by the distal palmar crease.

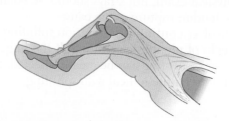

FIGURE 17.6.   Boutonnière deformity. Avulsion or laceration of the central extensor mechanism results in a flexion deformity at the PIP joint and hyperextension of the DIP joint—the boutonnière, or buttonhole, deformity. (Reproduced, with permission, from Doherty GM. *Current Diagnosis & Treatment: Surgery,* 13th ed. New York: McGraw-Hill, 2010, Fig. 42-15.)

■ **Tx:** Treatment is with corticosteroid injection into the tendon sheath at the level of the A1 pulley. Surgical release is appropriate for stubborn lesions.

Fractures of the Hand and Wrist

In a fall onto an outstretched hand, approximately 80% of the force goes through the radial side of the wrist. Subtypes of wrist fractures include the following:

■ **Distal radius fractures:** The most frequently occurring fracture in adults.
- ■ **Colles fracture:** Typically occurs from falling onto an extended wrist. The distal fragment of the radius is tilted dorsally. The most common type; may be associated with an ulnar styloid fracture.
- ■ **Smith fracture:** Occurs from falling onto a flexed wrist. The distal fragment of the radius is tilted volarly. Less angulation is tolerable in this direction.
■ **Scaphoid fractures:**
- ■ The most common carpal bone to be fractured. Young men are most likely to sustain this injury. Not as common in children and older adults because the distal radius is the weak point in these 2 populations.
- ■ Clinically presents with snuff box tenderness. If initial x-rays are negative for fracture, you should still immobilize the area and x-ray again in 2 weeks (many fractures are not initially apparent).
- ■ If pain persists and x-rays are nondiagnostic, an MRI or CT is indicated.
- ■ Many patients will require surgical fixation.
■ **Metacarpal fractures:**
- ■ More common in adults (vs. phalangeal fractures, which are more common in children).
- ■ **Boxer's fracture** is a fracture of the neck of the 5th metacarpal. It results from punching an object with a closed fist. Up to 40 degrees of angulation tolerated as long as there is no extensor lag (the patient can fully extend the finger). Treated with an ulnar gutter cast for 2–3 weeks.
- ■ Less angulation is tolerated in fractures of the other metacarpals 2° to less mobility of the bones in the hand structure.

KEY FACT

Scaphoid fractures have a high incidence of osteonecrosis.

Injuries of the Back and Spine

Lower back pain affects 60%–80% of adults at some point in their lives. Most episodes of back and neck pain resolve within a few weeks, but you should still fully evaluate each case.

EXAM

■ Exam includes inspection (eg, loss of normal lordosis), palpation (eg, midline tenderness vs. paraspinal tenderness), ROM, muscle testing, reflexes, and sensation (Table 17.9).
■ **Red flags** include night pain and weight loss (think tumor); fevers, chills, and sweats (think bone or disk infection); acute bony tenderness (think fracture); morning stiffness lasting > 30 minutes in young adults (think seronegative spondyloarthropathy); and any neurologic deficit or bowel/bladder involvement (think nerve root compromise).

TABLE 17.9.   Nerve Root Testing

Nerve Root	Motor Testing	Reflex	Sensation
C5	Deltoid, biceps.	Biceps.	Lateral shoulder.
C6	Biceps, wrist extensors.	Brachioradialis.	Radial side of the forearm, thumb, and index finger.
C7	Triceps, wrist flexors, finger extensors.	Triceps.	Middle finger.
C8	Finger abduction and adduction finger flexors.	–	Ulnar side of the forearm and ring and pinky fingers.
L4	Foot dorsiflexion.	Patellar.	Medial side of the big toe and lower leg.
L5	Big toe dorsiflexion.	–	Dorsum of the foot from the lateral side of the big toe to the medial side of the little toe.
S1	Foot eversion, plantar flexion.	Achilles tendon.	Lateral side of the little toe and lower leg.

- **Spurling test:** The patient extends the neck and tilts the head to the side while you press down on the head. This narrows the neural foramen, which worsens or reproduces radicular pain due to disk herniation or cervical spondylosis. It is very specific but not very sensitive.
- **Straight-leg raise:** With the patient supine, the straight leg is raised (many variations), placing the L5 and S1 nerve roots and the sciatic nerve under tension. ⊕ with reproduction or worsening of radicular symptoms. Dorsiflexion of the foot should worsen symptoms.

HERNIATED DISK

Bulging or herniation of the **nucleus pulposus** (a gel-like substance that cushions axial compression) through the surrounding **annulus fibrosus** (the outer, ligamentous portion of the intervertebral disk) into the spinal canal, causing nerve root irritation and compression. Also known as herniated nucleus pulposus. Lumbar disk herniations affect 2% of the population, but only 10%–25% of these patients have symptoms that persist > 6 weeks.

SYMPTOMS/EXAM

- Often presents with abrupt onset of unilateral radicular leg pain with low back pain that is worsened by sitting, walking, standing, coughing, or sneezing.
- Most commonly occurs at the L4–L5 or L5–S1 level.

DIFFERENTIAL

- **Lateral femoral cutaneous nerve entrapment:** Involves the lateral thigh; sensory only.
- **Spinal stenosis:** Affects the older population; associated with relief with flexion. Classic symptom is pseudoclaudication, which presents as leg and buttock pain that is exacerbated by walking (worse going downhill).
- **Cauda equina syndrome:** Bilateral involvement; presents with perianal numbness, with possible ↓ sphincter tone with urinary incontinence or retention. Remember, this is a surgical emergency!
- **Demyelinating conditions:** Can present with clonus.

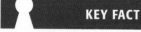

KEY FACT

In spinal stenosis, walking DOWN causes pain to go UP.

DIAGNOSIS

- Obtain plain radiographs to evaluate vertebral alignment and disk space. Imaging is likely to show degenerative changes in older patients.
- MRI is necessary only for progressive neurologic changes or preoperative planning.

TREATMENT

- Acute use of NSAIDs, muscle relaxants, and/or narcotics, with 1–3 days of bed rest if needed, followed by slow progression of activity.
- A short course of oral steroids or an epidural steroid injection may be necessary.
- Surgical evaluation is appropriate for patients who show no improvement or have progressive neurologic symptoms.

DEGENERATIVE DISK DISEASE

- Refers to age-related degenerative changes of the intervertebral disks. The amount of degeneration may be modified by factors such as injury, repetitive trauma, infection, heredity, and smoking.
- **Sx/Exam:** Presents with recurrent, episodic low back pain that radiates to 1 or both buttocks +/– intermittent sciatica.
- **Dx:** AP and lateral radiographs may reveal anterior osteophytes, loss of disk height, and a "vacuum sign" showing apparent air (nitrogen) in the disk space.
- **Tx:** Treat with intermittent NSAIDs, weight reduction, and core strengthening. You can also attempt spinal injections. If there is no improvement, you can refer for consideration of surgical repair (usually spinal fusion).

LUMBAR SPINAL STENOSIS (NEUROGENIC CLAUDICATION)

Narrowing of 1 or more levels of the spinal canal with resultant compression of the nerve roots. Up to 30% of adults > 60 years of age have lumbar stenosis anatomically, but many are asymptomatic.

SYMPTOMS/EXAM

- Presents with radicular symptoms in the calf, buttock, or thigh +/– back pain. It starts gradually or following a minor trauma and usually progresses from proximal to distal.
- Pain is aggravated by extension, and patients have poor walking tolerance.
- Walking and prolonged standing cause fatigue and leg weakness.
- Leg pain due to vascular claudication resolves when the patient stops walking, whereas neurogenic claudication does not immediately subside.

DIFFERENTIAL

Vascular claudication, DM with neuropathy, folic acid or vitamin B_{12} deficiency, infection, tumor, degenerative disk disease.

DIAGNOSIS

- Obtain AP and lateral x-rays to look for contributing degenerative factors such as spondylolisthesis, narrowing of the intervertebral disk spaces, osteoporosis, osteophytic changes, or an old burst fracture of a vertebral body.
- Usually diagnosed on MRI.

KEY FACT

In general, paresthesias and dysesthesias are found in neurogenic claudication but not in vascular claudication.

TREATMENT

- Physical therapy focusing on flexion exercises and core/abdominal strengthening.
- Surgical decompression is often needed.

PEDIATRIC INJURIES OF THE BACK AND SPINE

Back pain is uncommon in children and always warrants evaluation when it does not rapidly resolve.

Spondylolisthesis

- Slippage of 1 vertebral body forward in relation to the vertebral body below it. In children, this is most often a movement of L5 forward on S1 due to a congenital defect or stress fracture through the pars interarticularis of the vertebra (**spondylolysis**) (Figure 17.7).
- **Sx:** Presents with localized back pain at the site of spondylolysis. May have radicular symptoms if slippage is present. Pars injuries are more common in youth sports involving significant hyperextension, such as gymnastics and football.
- **Exam:** The "stork test" can localize a pars defect. Have the patient stand on 1 leg and perform extension of the back. Test is ⊕ if it causes localized pain on side of spondylolysis. ↑ lordosis, ↓ ROM, and tight hamstrings may also be seen.
- **Dx:** Oblique radiographs can show a break in the neck of the "**Scottie dog**," which represents the pars defect (spondylolysis). If radiographs are ⊖, bone scan and MRI are more sensitive. If spondylolisthesis (slippage) is present, it will be evident on lateral radiographs.
- **Tx:** Usually treat conservatively (with rest, core strengthening, and moni-

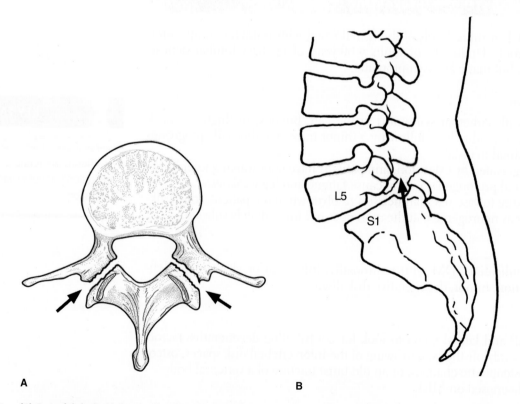

FIGURE 17.7.   (A) Spondylolysis (defect or fracture through the pars, can be unilateral). (B) Spondylolisthesis (slippage that can occur as a result of bilateral spondylolysis). (Reproduced, with permission, from Imboden J, et al. *Current Rheumatology Diagnosis & Treatment,* 2nd ed. New York: McGraw-Hill, 2007, Fig. 10-4.)

toring) unless patient has a documented progression of a slip > 50%, in which case bracing or spinal fusion may be considered.

Scoliosis

- Lateral curvature of the thoracic or lumbar spine > 10 degrees. Usually idiopathic, but can be 2° to neuromuscular disease (cerebral palsy, spinal muscular atrophy, myelomeningocele) or vertebral disease (tumor, infection). Can also be disease associated (eg, neurofibromatosis or Marfan syndrome).
- **Sx:** Usually develops in early adolescence. Mild cases (curves < 20 degrees) have an equal male-to-female ratio, but girls are 7 times more likely to have progressive disease requiring treatment. Usually asymptomatic unless there is underlying disease.
- **Exam:** Use a forward bending test to assess for vertebral and rib rotation. Evaluate for associated conditions such as skin lesions, cavus feet (high arches), limb-length discrepancy, abnormal joint laxity, and neuromuscular abnormalities.
- **Dx:** Order weight-bearing PA and lateral full-length spinal radiographs to measure the **Cobb angle.** Unusual findings such as pain, convex left thoracic curves, foot deformities, or neurologic abnormalities require evaluation for underlying etiologies.
- **Tx:** Monitor for progression of curvature (progression frequency depends on the degree of curvature and the amount of growth remaining). Bracing is appropriate for progressive curves in the range of 20–45 degrees; spinal fusion is indicated for curves > 50 degrees. If the curve is < 50 degrees at skeletal maturity, progression usually ceases.
- **Cx:** An idiopathic thoracic curve > 60 degrees often progresses in adulthood and can compromise respiratory function.

Injuries of the Hip and Thigh

Pain from actual hip pathology such as osteoarthritis localizes to the anterior groin or thigh and is exacerbated with internal rotation of the hip. Lateral hip pain is much more likely to be 2° to soft tissue pathology such as trochanteric bursitis/iliotibial band (ITB) tightness. ROM and resisted muscle testing will often identify the source of pain in soft tissue injuries. Special tests are listed in Table 17.10.

KEY FACT

When a patient has groin or thigh pain, remember to think about hip pathology.

TABLE 17.10.   Special Tests for the Diagnosis of Hip and Thigh Injuries

Exam	Technique	Indications
Ober test	The patient lies on his or her side with the affected side up. The knee is flexed 90° and the hip is abducted, extended, and then allowed to drop down toward the table.	⊕ if the knee does not drop past the midline, suggesting a tight ITB.
Trendelenburg test	The patient is observed from behind while standing on 1 foot and then the other. Pelvic stability is noted.	⊕ if an unsupported hemipelvis droops, suggesting hip abductor weakness on the other side (weakness on the side of the leg the patient is standing on).
FABER (**F**lexion, **AB**duction, **Ex**ternal **R**otation) test	The patient is supine and places the leg of the affected side into the figure-4 position, with the ankle resting above the contralateral knee. The examiner presses down on the ipsilateral knee, stressing the sacroiliac joint and stretching the psoas.	Posterior hip pain suggests sacroiliac pathology; anterior pull suggests psoas involvement.

ILIOTIBIAL BAND (ITB)–RELATED PATHOLOGY

 A 22-year-old professional ballet dancer complains about an audible popping sensation and pain across her thigh and lateral knee when she is dancing. She notices the feeling when she extends her legs quickly from a flexed position (eg, standing from a squat). She has increased the intensity of her workouts, as she is trying to join a dance troupe. On exam, you note a snapping sensation at the lateral hip with rotation of the hip. There is also tenderness to palpation at the trochanteric bursa. What do you tell her?

You tell her that her symptoms are likely due to tightness in her ITB and weakness in her hip abductors and external rotators. You suggest that she first try physical therapy for stretching and strengthening. You also prescribe NSAIDs for pain. Given that she has pain at the trochanteric bursa, you suspect it might be inflamed and offer a corticosteroid injection. You tell her that if she does not improve with initial conservative treatment, you will likely need an MRI to rule out other conditions like a labral tear or intra-articular loose body.

The ITB is a large, flat, fascial band that runs from the iliac crest down the lateral thigh and inserts onto the lateral condyle of the tibia at the knee (Gerdy tubercle). Tightness of this band can cause pain and bursitis as it rubs over bony prominences both proximally (at the greater trochanter) and distally at the lateral knee.

Iliotibial Band Syndrome

- An overuse tendinopathy of the ITB as it passes over the lateral femoral condyle.
- **Sx/Exam:** Presents with lateral knee pain and crepitus at the lateral femoral condyle or insertion on the Gerdy tubercle. A tight ITB is seen on the Ober test. Check for contributing mechanics such as genu varus, excessive foot pronation or supination, and weak hip abductors/pelvic stabilizers.
- **Tx:** ITB stretching, foam roller exercises for soft tissue work to relax the ITB, rest, ice, NSAIDs, iontophoresis.

Snapping Hip

- A snapping or popping sensation that occurs as a tendon "snaps" across a bony prominence. Most commonly due to the ITB snapping over the greater trochanter, but can also be due to the iliopsoas tendon sliding over the pectineal eminence of the pelvis or to labral tears of the acetabulum.
- **Sx/Exam:**
  - Presents with a snapping sensation at the lateral hip that can often be reproduced in the office with rotation of the hip. If the trochanteric bursa has become inflamed, there will be tenderness with palpation.
  - Snapping of the iliopsoas tendon is felt in the groin as the hip extends from a flexed position (eg, with rising from a chair).
- **Dx:** If not evident on exam, obtain AP pelvis and lateral hip radiographs to exclude bony pathology. If the diagnosis remains unclear, MR arthrography may be needed to rule out a labral tear or an intra-articular loose body.
- **Tx:** Physical therapy for stretching of the ITB, hip abductors, adductors, and flexors. If the injury is painful, corticosteroid injection into the trochanteric bursa or psoas sheath may be needed.

Trochanteric Bursitis (Greater Trochanteric Pain Syndrome)

- Inflammation, swelling, and hypertrophy of the greater trochanteric bursa. Can develop with direct injury, ITB tightness/overuse, or 2° to problems with hip mechanics (eg, lumbar spine disease, intra-articular hip pathology, or significant limb length inequalities).
- **Sx/Exam:** Presents with pain and tenderness at the lateral hip over the greater trochanter. Can make rising from a chair or sleeping on the affected side intensely painful. Point tenderness is diagnostic, but radiographs may be used to rule out bony and articular pathology.
- **DDx:** Osteoarthritis of the hip, trochanteric fracture, sciatica, tumor.
- **Tx:** Treated with stretching of the ITB, NSAIDs, rest, activity modification, and corticosteroid injection.

FRACTURES OF THE HIP AND THIGH

- Hip fractures are a common problem in the elderly, occurring with equal frequency in the femoral neck with twisting injuries and in the intertrochanteric region with a fall onto the side.
- Age is the most important risk factor, with the frequency of hip fractures doubling with each decade beyond 50 years. Other risk factors include being white, female, sedentary, a smoker, and an alcoholic.
- **Sx/Exam:** Patients with a displaced fracture will present with the limb externally rotated, abducted, and shortened. Femoral neck stress fractures will have gradual onset of groin pain, antalgic gait, and pain on internal rotation.
- **Dx:** AP pelvis and cross-table lateral radiographs are usually diagnostic for complete fractures. Stress fractures may require MRI for diagnosis (Figure 17.8).
- **Tx:**
  - Most hip fractures require operative management.
  - Compression-side stress fractures (those on the inferior surface) can be managed with non-weight-bearing status until there is radiographic evidence of healing.

KEY FACT

Patients with a stress fracture of the hip may present with diffuse aching pain in the thigh or groin that is worsened with weight-bearing activities.

KEY FACT

A femoral neck fracture in a patient < 60 years of age is a surgical emergency because nondisplaced hip fractures have the potential to displace, which can cause avascular necrosis of the femoral head.

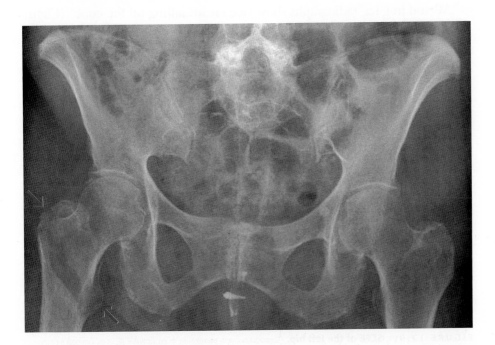

FIGURE 17.8. Right hip fracture. AP radiograph of the pelvis clearly demonstrates an intertrochanteric fracture of the right femur (*arrows*). (Reproduced, with permission, from USMLERx.com.)

PEDIATRIC INJURIES OF THE HIP AND THIGH

> A 13-year-old overweight boy is brought to your office for evaluation of anterior thigh and knee pain. He does not remember sustaining any injury, but his mother has noticed that he has been limping intermittently over the past few weeks. His knee exam is normal, but when you flex his hip and knee to 90 degrees and attempt to internally rotate the hip, he has pain and loss of internal rotation compared with the other side. What is the likely diagnosis?
>
> Slipped capital femoral epiphysis. Once the diagnosis is confirmed with radiographs, you make him non-weight-bearing and arrange for urgent surgical evaluation. You tell the patient and his mother that the same problem may develop on the other side at some point in the future.

Slipped Capital Femoral Epiphysis (SCFE)

A fracture in the physis (growth plate) of the femoral head can lead to slippage of the overlying epiphysis. It usually occurs during the adolescent growth spurt. Predisposing factors include obesity, male gender, and involvement in sports activities. The typical age range is 10–14 years for girls and 11–16 years for boys. If you have a patient who has onset outside the normal age range, you should consider an underlying endocrine disorder. Bilateral involvement over time is seen in 40%–50% of patients.

SYMPTOMS/EXAM

- Presents with pain in the anterior proximal knee or thigh that is exacerbated by activity. Knee exam will be normal.
- Loss of hip internal rotation, especially with the hip flexed, is both sensitive and specific.
- Patients typically walk with the involved extremity externally rotated.

DIAGNOSIS

- AP and frog-leg radiographs show "ice cream falling off the cone" (Figure 17.9).

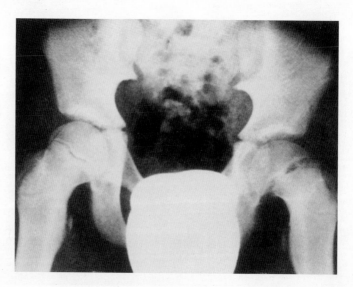

FIGURE 17.9. **SCFE of the left hip.** (Reproduced, with permission, from Tintinalli JE, et al. *Tintinalli's Emergency Medicine: A Comprehensive Study Guide,* 6th ed. New York: McGraw-Hill, 2004: 883.)

- Early diagnosis is critical, as the degree of displacement correlates with the duration of symptoms.

TREATMENT

- All cases warrant **urgent orthopedic evaluation** for stabilization surgery. Patient should be non-weight-bearing and restricted to bed rest until then.
- Inability to walk or severe pain after a fall suggests an unstable SCFE and requires emergent reduction and stabilization.

COMPLICATIONS

Surgically stabilized mild or moderate SCFEs usually have good long-term function. More severe disease can progress to arthritis, chondrolysis, and osteonecrosis.

Legg-Calvé-Perthes Disease

- Idiopathic osteonecrosis of the femoral head typically occurs in children 4–8 years of age, but range is 2–12 years of age. Ninety percent of cases are unilateral. The disorder is 4 times more common in boys and is uncommon in blacks.
- **Sx/Exam:** Presents with a limp that worsens with activity, possibly accompanied by an ache in the groin or proximal thigh. Restricted hip abduction is also seen (vs. the ↓ internal rotation seen in SCFE). Bilateral involvement should prompt screening for thyroid disease and epiphyseal dysplasia (AP radiographs of the hand and knee).
- **Dx:** AP and frog-leg radiographs of the pelvis show ↑ density of the femoral head early on and the crescent sign once a shear fracture has occurred in the subchondral bone. Obtain an MRI if radiographs are ⊖.
- **Tx:** The younger the patient, the better the healing process. Children < 6 years of age are usually monitored, whereas older children may need bed rest, abduction bracing, or osteotomy to alter the area of the weight-bearing surface of the femoral head.
- **Cx:** Residual deformity can progress to osteoarthritis of the hip.

KEY FACT

Failure to treat slipped capital femoral epiphysis can lead to avascular necrosis.

Knee Injuries

MENISCAL TEARS

The medial and lateral menisci are fibrocartilaginous disks that provide shock absorption and stability between the femur and tibia. The blood supply to the menisci is very poor, so tears don't usually heal, which can predispose the knee to degenerative arthritis.

SYMPTOMS/EXAM

- Traumatic tears usually occur with a sudden twisting injury and have **slow development** of swelling and stiffness over a few days. Symptoms can then wax and wane.
- Pain is localized to the medial (more common) or lateral joint line and often recurs with twisting or squatting motions such as getting out of a car.
- Mechanical symptoms such as locking, catching, and popping can also develop.
- Moderate effusion, joint line tenderness, pain with forced flexion, and meniscal rotation signs on exam (**McMurray sign**) are suggestive.

DIFFERENTIAL

- **Anterior cruciate ligament (ACL) tear:** Sudden; characterized by larger swelling and instability.
- **Medial collateral ligament (MCL) injury:** Presents with pain with valgus stress.
- **Osteoarthritis:** Loss of joint space is seen on weight-bearing radiographs.
- **Pes anserine bursitis:** Medial tenderness **below** the joint line at the attachment of the sartorius, gracilis, and semitendinosus tendon.
- **Bony pathology:** Tibial plateau fracture; osteonecrosis of the femoral condyle.
- **Patellar subluxation or dislocation:** Presents with tender patellar facets and apprehension sign (while patient is supine and leg is in full extension, you apply pressure to the medial patella; test is ⊕ if it causes pain or apprehension).

DIAGNOSIS

- Radiographs to rule out bony conditions.
- MRI is used for diagnosis, as it is highly sensitive and specific for meniscal pathology.

TREATMENT

- Arthroscopic debridement or repair is the treatment of choice for traumatic tears in the younger, active population.
- For degenerative tears (more likely in the older population) or in the absence of mechanical symptoms such as catching or locking, conservative measures (eg, rest, ice, NSAIDs, physical therapy, corticosteroid injection) can initially be tried.

LIGAMENTOUS INJURIES

Anterior Cruciate Ligament (ACL) Tear

The ACL is the 1° stabilizer of the knee. It resists anterior translation of the tibia on the femur and is the most frequently injured major ligament of the knee. A tear results from forced hyperflexion (common in skiing, football, soccer, and basketball). Seventy percent of ACL injuries occur during sporting activities.

SYMPTOMS/EXAM

- Forty percent of patients report feeling or hearing a pop (the most reliable factor).
- There is usually rapid development of hemarthrosis, causing significant swelling.
- There is usually instability of the knee or a "wobbly" feeling.
- The Lachman test is the most sensitive test (87%–98%), showing ↑ anterior tibial displacement and a soft end point.

DIAGNOSIS

The history and exam remain key diagnostic tools, but MRI is increasingly used for confirmation as well as for the evaluation of associated injuries, such as injury of the menisci, posterior cruciate ligament (PCL), and collateral ligaments.

TREATMENT

- Treatment decisions depend on patient preference, age, activity level, knee instability, and associated injuries.
- Some older, less active patients can have satisfactory outcomes with rehabilitation alone (the ACL does not heal, but patients can develop muscular stability). Younger, more active patients are more likely to need reconstruction to remain active.

Collateral Ligament (MCL and LCL) Injuries

- Most often caused by a direct blow to the lateral aspect of the knee, leading to valgus stress and MCL injury. Isolated lateral collateral ligament (LCL) injuries are rare.
- **Sx/Exam:**
  - Presents with pain +/– laxity on valgus (MCL) or varus (LCL) stress testing at 30 degrees of flexion (relaxes the cruciate ligaments).
  - LCL injuries should be thoroughly evaluated for accompanying injuries (ACL, PCL, posterolateral corner injuries).
- **Tx:** Nonoperative management with a hinged knee brace and ROM exercises usually suffices for isolated MCL or LCL injuries. Rehabilitation can take 6–8 weeks.

PATELLOFEMORAL PAIN SYNDROME

Patella-related pain is the single most common cause of knee pain. Patellofemoral pain syndrome is a multifactorial syndrome characterized by aching anterior knee pain that worsens with activities that stress the patellofemoral joint (eg, climbing stairs, kneeling).

SYMPTOMS/EXAM

- Presents with diffuse, aching anterior knee pain that is exacerbated by loaded flexion activities such as stair climbing, jumping, or prolonged sitting (theater sign).
- Note any patellar crepitation or tenderness of the patellar retinaculum or facets.
- Evaluate for contributing factors, including ↑ Q angle at the knee, (angle between the quadriceps and patellar tendon, more common in women because of wider pelvises), patellar tilt or malalignment, excessive lateral patellar mobility, tight hamstrings, weak quadriceps, and excessive femoral anteversion.

DIFFERENTIAL

- **Patellar tendinitis (jumper's knee):** Point tenderness over the inferior pole of the patella.
- **Patellofemoral osteoarthritis:** Diagnosed by radiographic changes on sunrise view; affects older patients.
- **Synovial plica:** A redundant fold of synovial lining that can become painfully inflamed and fibrotic, most commonly occurring along the medial border of the patella.
- **Chondromalacia patellae:** Disruption in the articular cartilage of the patella (painful or nonpainful), with possible etiologies including trauma, malalignment, and biomechanical or metabolic factors.
- **Patellar instability:** Transient displacement (usually laterally) of the patella, either partially (subluxation) or completely (dislocation), causing acute and/or chronic patellar pain. Associated with a ⊕ **apprehension sign** when displacing the patella laterally.

KEY FACT

The most common cause of an acute hemarthrosis after a sports-related knee injury is an ACL tear.

KEY FACT

The unhappy triad is a common constellation of knee injuries occurring during contact sports and includes the ACL, MCL, and meniscus.

DIAGNOSIS

A clinical diagnosis. AP, lateral, and sunrise radiographs can evaluate for articular cartilage loss, tilt, and subluxation.

TREATMENT

- Treated with activity modification and an exercise program consisting of quadriceps strengthening (especially the medial quadriceps) and hamstring flexibility. Should also attempt to fix contributing mechanical factors such as flat feet or overpronation with orthotic foot inserts. NSAIDs can alleviate discomfort.
- Use of a knee sleeve with patellar cutout or a patellar stabilizing brace.

QUADRICEPS AND PATELLAR TENDON RUPTURES

Typically occur with a fall onto a knee that is partially flexed while the quadriceps muscle is forcibly contracting to break the fall. Patellar tendon ruptures usually occur in younger patients (< 40 years of age) and are frequently associated with sporting activities. Quadriceps tendon ruptures typically occur in patients > 40 years of age and are 3 times more common than patellar tendon ruptures.

SYMPTOMS/EXAM

Patients often feel a pop at the time of injury and have a palpable defect in 1 tendon, with an inability to extend the knee against gravity or perform a straight-leg raise.

DIAGNOSIS

- Radiographs of the knee can rule out patellar fracture. In a patellar tendon rupture, radiograph will show patella alta (patella has moved up along the thigh; Figure 17.10), whereas in quadriceps tendon rupture it will show patella baja (patella has moved abnormally low).
- MRI to confirm the diagnosis and for surgical planning.

TREATMENT

- Immediate surgical repair is indicated for complete ruptures of either tendon.
- Partial tears with little loss of strength and maintenance of the ability to extend the knee can be treated conservatively with a cylinder cast in full extension for 4–6 weeks (uncommon).

PEDIATRIC KNEE INJURIES

Osgood-Schlatter Disease

- Rupture of the growth plate at the tibial tuberosity, which causes stress on the patellar tendon. It is a repetitive stress injury that occurs in rapidly growing adolescents. It is 5 times more common among those active in sports and 2–3 times more common in boys, typically occurring in those 10–15 years of age.
- **Sx/Exam:** Presents with pain and tenderness at the tibial tubercle that is exacerbated by running, jumping, and kneeling. May be bilateral, but 1 side is usually worse.
- **Dx:** Radiographs can be normal or may show small spicules of heterotopic ossification anterior to the tibial tuberosity.

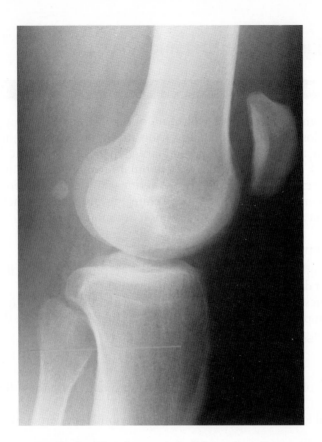

FIGURE 17.10. **Patella alta.** Note the superiorly dislocated patella. (Reproduced, with permission, from Tintinalli JE, et al. *Tintinalli's Emergency Medicine: A Comprehensive Study Guide,* 6th ed. New York: McGraw-Hill, 2004, Fig. 274-11.)

- **Tx:** Relative rest/activity modification; quadriceps stretching and strengthening; icing after activity; analgesics. Will resolve once growth is complete.

Osteochondritis Dissecans

- Osteonecrosis of subchondral bone (most commonly on the medial femoral condyle) that causes separation from underlying well-vascularized bone, leading to fragmentation of bone and cartilage in the joint. Thought to be due to repetitive small stresses to the subchondral bone.
- Onset in most cases is during childhood, although patients may not become symptomatic until late adolescence or early adulthood. Early diagnosis is critical, as the injury has a better potential to heal while the bones are still growing.
- **Sx/Exam:** Presents with gradual onset of vague knee pain and intermittent swelling after running and sports activities.
- **Dx:** Usually visible on plain radiographs (especially the tunnel view). MRI is used to assess the stability of the fragment as well as the viability of subchondral bone.
- **Tx:**
  - Younger patients with smaller, stable lesions are most likely to heal well with conservative measures. Activity modification (no running or jumping; possible crutch use) minimizes shear forces and allows for new bone formation.
  - If the overlying articular cartilage is disrupted, a loose body is present, or the patient is skeletally mature, evaluation for operative management is appropriate.

Injuries of the Foot and Ankle

ANKLE SPRAINS

Partial or complete tearing of 1 or more of the ligaments that support the ankle joint. Most often due to an inversion mechanism, causing injury to the lateral ligaments. The anterior talofibular ligament (ATFL) is the 1st ligament to be injured, followed by the calcaneofibular ligament (CFL) and, finally, in the most severe lateral sprains, the posterior talofibular ligament (PTFL). A syndesmotic ankle sprain (high ankle sprain), involves the ligaments that connect the tibia and fibula; it is less common but more severe.

KEY FACT

The ATFL is the most commonly sprained ligament in the ankle or foot.

SYMPTOMS/EXAM

- Lateral ankle swelling and ecchymosis are proportional to the degree of ligament damage and the number of ligaments involved.
- Tenderness of the anterior tibiofibular ligament and pain with the **squeeze test** (compressing the tibia and fibula at midcalf stresses the distal syndesmosis) suggest a high ankle sprain.

DIFFERENTIAL

- Fracture of the lateral malleolus, calcaneus, talus, or base of the 5th metatarsal.
- Peroneal tendon tear or subluxation (retrofibular tenderness and swelling).

DIAGNOSIS

The need for radiographs to rule out fracture is based on the **Ottawa ankle rules** (Figure 17.11). Indicated if the patient is unable to bear weight for 4 steps immediately after injury or in the office, or if there is lateral or medial malleolar bone tenderness; does not apply to patients < 18 years of age.

TREATMENT

- Acutely treat with **RICE** therapy (rest, ice, compression, elevation). Can use NSAIDs for pain. Can use a brace, an air cast, or crutches, depending on severity, with early mobilization and strengthening exercises as swelling ↓.
- The speed of recovery depends on the degree of injury (Table 17.11).
- Residual symptoms can occur in up to 40% of patients.

KEY FACT

The most common eversion ankle fracture is a fracture of the lateral malleolus.

ACHILLES TENDON RUPTURE

- Disruption of the Achilles tendon, which most commonly affects middle-aged men who play quick stop-and-go sports such as tennis, squash, and basketball.
- **Sx/Exam:** Presents with sudden, severe calf pain, with swelling and a palpable defect in the tendon. Patients will say they felt like they were kicked or shot in the back of the ankle. Exam shows lack of plantar flexion with manual squeezing of the calf (⊕ **Thompson test**).
- **DDx:** Achilles tendinosis (gradual onset), medial gastrocnemius tear (more proximal tenderness), DVT (no history of injury; ⊖ Thompson test).
- **Tx:** Nonoperative or surgical repair. Both require a program of graduated casting or bracing to allow for healing.

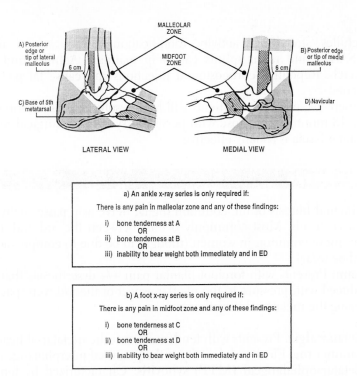

a) An ankle x-ray series is only required if:

There is any pain in malleolar zone and any of these findings:

i) bone tenderness at A
        OR
ii) bone tenderness at B
        OR
iii) inability to bear weight both immediately and in ED

b) A foot x-ray series is only required if:

There is any pain in midfoot zone and any of these findings:

i) bone tenderness at C
        OR
ii) bone tenderness at D
        OR
iii) inability to bear weight both immediately and in ED

FIGURE 17.11. **Ottawa ankle rules for ankle and midfoot injuries.** (Reproduced, with permission, from Tintinalli JE, et al. *Tintinalli's Emergency Medicine: A Comprehensive Study Guide*, 6th ed. New York: McGraw-Hill, 2004: 1738.)

PLANTAR FASCIITIS

- An overload injury (inflammation, degeneration, and tearing) of the plantar fascia, most commonly occurring at its calcaneal insertion. Contributing factors include a tight gastrocnemius–soleus complex, tight plantar fascia, a rigid rear foot, and overpronation or supination.
- **Sx/Exam:** Presents with pain and tenderness at the plantar medial heel that worsens with the **1st few steps in the morning,** after rest, and with extended walking.
- **Dx:** A clinical diagnosis, but radiographs show a plantar heel spur in 50% of patients with plantar fasciitis and in 15% of asymptomatic patients. A bone scan can differentiate plantar fasciitis from calcaneal stress fracture.

TABLE 17.11.   **West Point Ankle Sprain Grading System**

	GRADE 1	GRADE 2	GRADE 3
Edema/ecchymosis	Localized/slight	Localized/moderate	Diffuse/significant
Weight-bearing ability	Full or partial without significant pain	Difficult without crutches	Impossible
Ligament pathology	Ligament stretch	Partial tear	Complete tear
Instability testing	None	None or slight	Definite
Time to return to sports	11 days	2–6 weeks	4–26 weeks

- **Tx:**
    - Achilles stretching, activity modification, orthotics, ice massage, NSAIDs, and night splints can help maintain Achilles and plantar stretch. Repetitive corticosteroid injections can cause fat pad insufficiency.
    - Ninety-five percent of patients will have resolution of symptoms within 12–18 months. For those with persistent symptoms, surgical release of plantar fascia is usually effective.

MORTON NEUROMA

- A perineural fibrosis of the common digital nerve as it passes between the metatarsal heads. Most commonly occurs between the 3rd and 4th toes; 5 times more common in women (thought to be due to compression from tight shoe wear).
- **Sx/Exam:** Presents with forefoot plantar pain +/– dysesthesias that can be reproduced with pressure to the plantar aspect of the 3rd web space while squeezing the metatarsals together.
- **DDx:**
    - **Metatarsalgia:** Presents with tenderness over the metatarsal heads.
    - **Hammer toe:** Flexion deformity of the proximal interphalangeal joint.
    - **Metatarsophalangeal (MTP) synovitis:** Characterized by tenderness and swelling over the MTP joint.
    - **Stress fracture:** Dorsal metatarsal tenderness.
- **Tx:** Use of shoes with low heels and a wide toe box; metatarsal pads to spread the metatarsal heads; lidocaine/corticosteroid injection.

FRACTURES OF THE FOOT AND ANKLE

Malleolar Fractures

- The ankle joint is considered stable with an isolated malleolar fracture (usually lateral). When combined with an injury to the other side of the ankle (eg, lateral malleolus fracture and deltoid ligament disruption), the ankle joint becomes unstable.
- **Sx/Exam:** Patients present with a history of trauma with swelling, tenderness, and possible deformity at the site of the fracture.
- **Dx:** AP, lateral, and mortise views can evaluate for fracture and widening of the mortise, which suggest an unstable ankle joint.
- **Tx:**
    - **Stable fractures of the distal fibula:** Use of a weight-bearing cast or a brace for 4–6 weeks.
    - **Unstable, nondisplaced fractures:** Use of a non-weight-bearing short- or long-leg cast for a longer period, with close orthopedic follow-up.
    - **Unstable, displaced** fractures usually require open reduction.

Maisonneuve Fracture

- A spiral fracture of the proximal fibula that is associated with a tear of the tibia–fibula syndesmosis. Associated with fracture of the medial malleolus or rupture of the deltoid ligament. Often occurs in athletes who reinjure an inadequately healed ankle sprain.
- Occurs with significant torsional force to the ankle, which is transmitted up the syndesmosis to the proximal fibula.
- **Dx:** Patient will have pain at the medial malleolus and proximal fibula.

Fracture of the Base of the 5th Metatarsal

There are 3 types of proximal 5th metatarsal fractures:

- **Avulsion fracture of the tuberosity:** The most common type. Usually occurs with high lateral ankle sprains. Generally treated with weight bearing in a walking cast or hard-soled shoes until pain subsides.
- **Jones fracture:** Fracture just distal to the tuberosity at the neck. Associated with higher rates of nonunion; treated with intramedullary fixation or a non-weight-bearing short-leg cast for 6–8 weeks.
- **Diaphyseal stress fracture:** Treated with a non-weight-bearing short-leg cast for 6–8 weeks.

Rheumatology

SYSTEMIC LUPUS ERYTHEMATOSUS (SLE)

A chronic inflammatory disease that can affect multiple organ systems, including the skin, joints, kidneys, lungs, nervous system, and serous membranes. The disease course can include episodes of remission as well as chronic or acute flare-ups. The female-to-male ratio is 9:1, with onset often occurring in the 20s and 30s. Three times more common among African Americans.

SYMPTOMS/EXAM

Nearly 90% of patients have joint symptoms.

DIAGNOSIS

- Diagnostic criteria can be summarized with the mnemonic **DOPAMINE RASH.** At least 4 of the 11 criteria listed must be present for diagnosis.
- ANA testing is highly sensitive but is not specific, whereas antibodies to dsDNA and Smith are specific but not sensitive. Titers of dsDNA antibodies generally correlate with disease activity.

TREATMENT

- Sun and stress avoidance; skin protection.
- Pharmacologic treatment depends on the severity of the disease and the degree of organ involvement; can include NSAIDs, topical and systemic steroids, antimalarials, methotrexate, and IVIG.

COMPLICATIONS

Organ-specific damage plus accelerated atherosclerosis and opportunistic infections.

Drug-Induced Lupus

- Similar presentation to that of SLE, but with equal prevalence among men and women. Symptoms resolve with withdrawal of the offending medication.
- The most commonly associated drugs are hydralazine, procainamide, INH, quinidine, methyldopa, and chlorpromazine.

KEY FACT

SLE can have multiple clinical presentations and is known as one of "the great imitators."

MNEMONIC

Diagnostic Criteria for SLE:

DOPAMINE RASH

Discoid rash (thick, scaly patches)
Oral ulcers
Photosensitivity rash
Arthritis
Malar rash (butterfly rash)
Immunologic criteria (⊕ anti-dsDNA or ⊕ anti-Sm)
NEurologic or psychiatric symptoms
Renal disease
ANA ⊕
Serositis (pleural, peritoneal, or pericardial)
Hematologic disorders (thrombocytopenia, anemia, or leukopenia)

RHEUMATOID ARTHRITIS

A chronic systemic inflammatory disease that primarily affects the joints. Affects 1%–2% of the U.S. population, with a female-to-male ratio of 3:1 and a typical age of onset of 20–40 years.

SYMPTOMS/EXAM

- Presents with **symmetric,** inflammatory joint pain, most commonly of the PIP and MTP joints, wrists, ankles, and knees (Figure 17.12). Inflammatory characteristics include morning stiffness and pain; improvement of symptoms with use of the joint; and possible erythema, warmth, and/or swelling of the joint.
- Patients with long-standing, erosive, RF-⊕ disease can also develop extra-articular disease, including vasculitis, interstitial lung disease, serositis, ocular disease, Sjögren syndrome, and amyloidosis.

DIFFERENTIAL

Osteoarthritis (affects the DIP joints; lacks inflammatory characteristics). Table 17.12 outlines features that distinguish rheumatoid arthritis from osteoarthritis.

DIAGNOSIS

- Diagnostic criteria are as follows (4 of 7 criteria lasting > 6 weeks must be met for diagnosis):
  - Morning stiffness.
  - Arthritis in 3 or more joint areas.
  - Arthritis involving the hands.
  - Symmetric arthritis.
  - Serum RF ⊕.
  - Radiographic changes consistent with disease.
  - Rheumatoid nodules (subcutaneous nodules over the extensor surfaces or bony prominences).
- Classic radiographic findings include periarticular osteopenia, joint space narrowing, and juxta-articular erosions (Figure 17.13). X-rays may be normal in early stages.
- RF is ⊕ in 70%–80% of patients but is not specific.

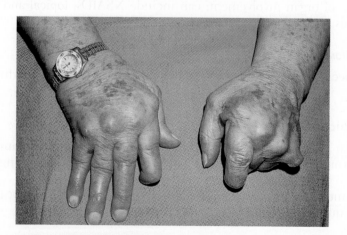

FIGURE 17.12.   Rheumatoid arthritis. Typical ulnar deviation of the MCP joints and swelling of the PIP joints in a patient with rheumatoid arthritis. Multiple subcutaneous rheumatoid nodules are also seen. (Reproduced, with permission, from Wolff K, et al. *Fitzpatrick's Dermatology in General Medicine,* 7th ed. New York: McGraw-Hill, 2008, Fig. 161-1A.)

TABLE 17.12. **Rheumatoid Arthritis vs. Osteoarthritis**

	RHEUMATOID ARTHRITIS	OSTEOARTHRITIS
Age of onset	Generally 20s to 40s.	Usually old age.
Speed of onset	Rapid: weeks to months.	Over years.
Joints affected	Small and large joints on both sides (symmetrical).	Often begins on 1 side of body and usually limited to 1 set of joints (fingers or knees).
Morning stiffness	Lasts longer than 1 hr.	Usually worsens as day progresses.
Systemic symptoms	Fatigue and general malaise.	No systemic symptoms.

TREATMENT

The American College of Rheumatology recommends starting disease-modifying anti-rheumatic drugs (DMARDs) within 3 months of diagnosis. Examples of DMARDs include systemic and injected steroids, methotrexate, plaquenil, cyclophosphamide, and many other immunomodulators. NSAIDs are appropriate for symptom flares.

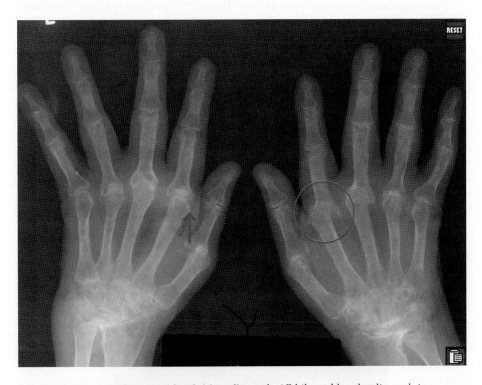

FIGURE 17.13. **Rheumatoid arthritis radiograph.** AP bilateral hand radiograph in a patient with advanced rheumatoid arthritis shows joint space narrowing involving carpal, MCP, and PIP joints as well as subluxation at multiple MCP joints *(circle)* and periarticular erosions *(arrow)*. (Reproduced, with permission, from USMLERx.com.)

SERONEGATIVE SPONDYLOARTHROPATHIES

A group of disorders characterized by $\ominus$ serologies for ANA and RF, a strong association with the HLA-B27 antigen, and spinal arthritis. Include ankylosing spondylitis, psoriatic arthritis, reactive arthritis (Reiter syndrome), and IBD-associated arthritis.

Ankylosing Spondylitis

- Particularly involves the sacroiliac joints and spine.
- Affects 1 in 2000 people, with men having more severe disease than women.
- **Sx:** Presents with progressive pain and stiffening of the spine, with low back pain that is worse in the morning and with inactivity but improves with exercise.
- **Exam:** Exam reveals tenderness of the sacroiliac joints with $\downarrow$ lumbar lordosis and cervical motion.
- **Dx:** Diagnosed by the classic "bamboo-like" appearance of the spine on radiographs and/or sacroiliitis on radiographs or MRI. $\ominus$ RF with $\uparrow$ ESR (Figure 17.14).
- **Tx:** NSAIDs, physical therapy, methotrexate, and spinal fusion in severe cases.

Psoriatic Arthritis

- Affects 10%–20% of patients with psoriasis.
- Has significant association with nail disorders (pitting, ridging, onycholysis).
- **Sx/Exam:** Has multiple patterns of presentation, including mono- and polyarticular types.

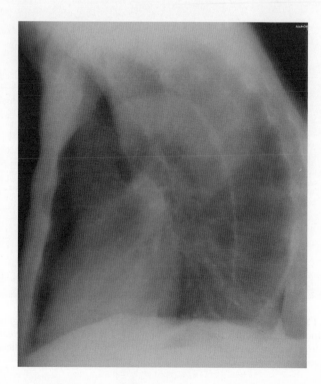

FIGURE 17.14. **Ankylosing spondylitis.** Cropped view of the spine from a lateral chest radiograph demonstrates the classic "bamboo spine" of ankylosing spondylitis. (Reproduced, with permission, from USMLERx.com.)

- **Dx:** Characteristic radiographic changes are seen, such as marginal erosions and "pencil-in-cup" deformities of the distal digits.
- **Tx:** NSAIDs, DMARDs.

Reactive Arthritis (Reiter Syndrome)

- Develops as autoimmune response to infection with *Salmonella, Shigella, Campylobacter, Yersinia, Chlamydia,* or other pathogens.
- **Sx/Exam:** Presents with the classic triad of **conjunctivitis, urethritis, and arthritis** (more commonly of the larger peripheral joints than of the spine). Patients may also have systemic symptoms such as fever and weight loss.
- **Dx:** Arthrocentesis with an inflammatory pattern and a ⊖ culture.
- **Tx:** NSAIDs; antibiotics as indicated; DMARDs if arthritis does not improve.
- **Cx:** Rare aortitis and aortic regurgitation.

IBD-Associated Arthritis

- Twenty percent of patients with IBD (Crohn disease > ulcerative colitis) will develop associated arthritis.
- **Sx/Exam:** Peripheral arthritic flares are associated with GI disease. Presents with peripheral, asymmetric, oligoarticular, large-joint involvement. Spinal involvement mimics ankylosing spondylitis and is independent of intestinal disease.
- **Tx:** NSAIDs. Treatment of GI disease can control peripheral arthritis.

KEY FACT

To remember the symptoms of Reiter syndrome, think "can't see, can't pee, can't climb a tree."

CRYSTALLINE-INDUCED ARTHROPATHIES

Deposition of crystals in the synovium and other tissues triggers an inflammatory response. Characterized by episodes of abrupt-onset, severe, and usually monoarticular joint pain.

Hyperuricemia

- ↑ the risk of gout, but the majority of patients do not actually develop gout.
- Due to **overproduction** of uric acid (glycogen storage diseases, psoriasis, myeloproliferative disorders, large tumor burden) or **underexcretion** of uric acid (renal disease, thiazide or loop diuretics, lactic acidosis, alcoholism, ketoacidosis). More than 90% of people are underexcretors.
- More common in men, patients with DM, HTN, hyperlipidemia, obesity, and patients of Pacific Islander ancestry.

Gout

- Deposition of uric acid crystals in the synovium, bursae, tendon sheaths, skin, heart valves, and kidneys, which can cause arthritis, tophi, renal stones, and gouty nephropathy.
- Onset is usually after age 30 years. Women affected are almost always postmenopausal.
- **Sx/Exam:** Typically presents with acute, exquisitely tender, monoarticular arthritis. Usually is a "red-hot" swollen joint. The 1st MTP joint is most commonly affected, but the knees, ankles, feet, elbows, and hands may also be involved. Nodular deposits of uric acid crystals, or **tophi,** may be seen in subcutaneous tissues, tendons, cartilage, and bone.

- **Dx:** Negatively birefringent, needle-like crystals are seen in synovial fluid aspiration. Cultures are sterile. "Rat-bite" erosions may be seen on joint radiographs (but typically normal in 1st 10 years) (Figure 17.15). Serum uric acid is ↑ in 95% of cases, but this is not diagnostic and is not required for the diagnosis.
- **Tx:**
  - For acute attacks, use an NSAID such as indomethacin as 1st-line therapy. If patient is not an NSAID candidate (renal insufficiency, heart failure, PUD), use colchicine. Can also use intra-articular or systemic corticosteroids.
  - Diet modification, including alcohol avoidance, to ↓ purine intake is also recommended.
  - Patients with recurrent attacks can be treated with daily allopurinol or colchicine (for both overproducers and underexcretors) or probenecid for underexcretors.

Calcium Pyrophosphate Deposition Disease (CPPD)

- Crystalline arthropathy can lead to a spectrum of disease, ranging from asymptomatic chondrocalcinosis (calcification of the articular cartilage surface) to **pseudogout.**
- **Sx/Exam:** Presents with a monoarticular inflammatory arthropathy similar to gout.
- **Dx:** Weakly ⊕ birefringent rhomboid-shaped crystals are seen on synovial fluid aspiration. Radiographs can show the white lines of chondrocalcinosis in joint spaces.
- **Tx: NSAIDs;** corticosteroid injections; colchicine for chronic cases.

KEY FACT

Rapid or unusual distribution of degenerative joint disease should raise suspicion of CPPD.

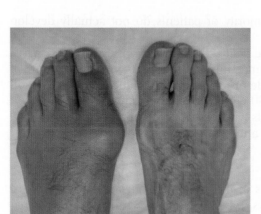
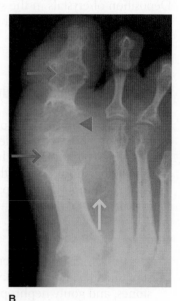

A   B

FIGURE 17.15. **Gout.** (A) A swollen left 1st MTP joint with overlying erythema and warmth, characteristic of an acute gout attack (podagra). (B) An AP radiograph showing the severe consequences of long-standing gout, including large, nonmarginal erosions with overhanging edges of bone (*red arrows*), soft tissue swelling, and destruction of the 1st MTP joint (*arrowhead*). Note the subtle calcification of a gouty tophus (*yellow arrow*). (Image A reproduced, with permission, from LeBlond RF, et al. *DeGowin's Diagnostic Examination*, 9th ed. New York: McGraw-Hill, 2009, Plate 30. Image B reproduced, with permission, from USMLERx.com.)

INFECTIOUS ARTHRITIS

Gonococcal Arthritis (Disseminated Infection)

- Arthritis and arthralgias are the principal manifestations of disseminated gonococcal infection, which occurs in 1%–3% of patients infected with *Neisseria gonorrhoeae*. Most common in patients < 40 years of age.
- **Sx/Exam:** Presents with migratory polyarthralgias and tenosynovitis with fever and a papulopustular rash that can involve the **palms and soles.**
- **Dx:** Blood, rectal, throat, and urethral cultures are 70%–80% sensitive, whereas synovial fluid culture is < 50% sensitive.
- **Tx:** Treat with IV antibiotics (3rd-generation cephalosporin) until clinical improvement is seen, followed by oral antibiotics for a 7- to 10-day total course. Treat empirically for chlamydia.

Nongonococcal Arthritis (Septic Joint)

- Inoculation of bacteria into a joint from hematogenous spread, direct penetration of the joint, or spread from an adjacent focus of infection. The most common organisms are gram-⊕ species (*Staphylococcus aureus*, *Streptococcus*). Gram-⊖ organisms such as *Escherichia coli* or *Pseudomonas* are less common. There is an ↑ risk with previous joint damage, IV drug use, endocarditis, and prosthetic joints.
- **Sx/Exam:** Presents with acute-onset, monoarticular joint pain with swelling, warmth, and erythema. Patients usually have fevers and chills. Passive ROM of the joint is exquisitely painful.
- **Dx:** Joint aspiration reveals > 50,000 WBC, predominantly neutrophils. Fifty percent of patients have ⊕ blood cultures, and 75% have ⊕ synovial fluid cultures and a ⊕ Gram stain. Radiographs can show joint erosions, osteomyelitis, demineralization, or periostitis.
- **Tx:** IV antibiotics (often needed for up to 6 weeks).
- **Cx:** Articular destruction; septicemia.

KEY FACT

When considering prosthetic infections, think *Staphylococcus epidermidis.*

INFLAMMATORY MYOPATHIES

Polymyositis

- A systemic inflammatory disease characterized by proximal muscle weakness. Women are affected twice as often as men; average age of onset is 40–60 years.
- **Sx/Exam:** Presents with progressive muscle weakness of the neck and proximal musculature of the limbs along with difficulty swallowing. **Pain is not pronounced.**
- **DDx:** Inclusion body myositis (distal muscles are more affected), polymyalgia rheumatica (pain is more common), myopathy or myositis 2° to malignancy, medications, toxins, endocrine/metabolic disorders.
- **Dx:** ↑ muscle enzyme markers (CK and/or aldolase); muscle biopsy. EMG shows nonspecific changes.
- **Tx:** Corticosteroids, DMARDs.

KEY FACT

The 1st presentation of polymyositis is often early fatigue when walking or difficulty rising from a chair.

Dermatomyositis

- A systemic inflammatory disease with proximal muscle weakness and characteristic skin rashes. Often associated with occult malignancy.
- **Sx/Exam:** Similar to polymyositis plus rashes.
  - **Gottron papules:** A scaly rash over the extensor surfaces.
  - **Shawl sign:** Erythema in a sun-exposed V-neck or shoulder distribution.

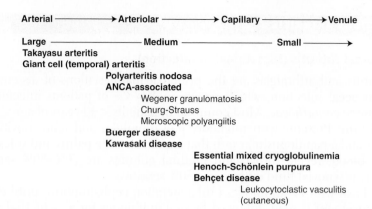

FIGURE 17.16. **Classification of 1° vasculitis according to size of vessel involved.** (Reproduced, with permission, from Le T, et al. *First Aid for the Internal Medicine Boards*, 2nd ed. New York: McGraw-Hill, 2008: 653.)

- **Heliotrope rash:** A violaceous rash over the eyelids +/– periorbital edema.
- **Facial erythema:** A diffuse, dusky facial rash.
- **Dx:** Similar to polymyositis, with a different inflammatory pattern on muscle biopsy.
- **Tx:** Corticosteroids, DMARDs, IVIG for refractory cases.

SYSTEMIC SCLEROSIS (SCLERODERMA)

- An autoimmune disorder characterized by **CREST** syndrome (Calcinosis, Raynaud phenomenon, Esophageal dysmotility, Sclerodactyly, and Telangiectasias). The majority of cases (80%) are limited scleroderma, which has a better prognosis; progressive systemic sclerosis can also have kidney, heart, lung, and GI tract involvement.
- Both types are ANA ⊕, with anticentromere antibodies in limited scleroderma and anti-SCL-70 antibodies in the progressive type.
- **Tx:** Treatment of CREST syndrome is symptomatic; progressive disease also requires corticosteroids and immunosuppressants.

VASCULITIS

- A group of disorders that is characterized by inflammatory destruction of blood vessels. Can be 1° or 2°.
- **Sx/Exam:**
  - Presentation depends on the structures involved.
  - 1° vasculitis can be categorized according to the size of the involved vessels (see Figure 17.16).
  - 2° vasculitis can be due to infection (especially indolent infections such as bacterial endocarditis and HCV), medications, collagen vascular disease, or malignancy.
- **Tx:** Treatment usually includes corticosteroids and/or immunosuppressants.

Emergency/Urgent Care

Diana Coffa, MD

Shock

A 78-year-old woman with a history of dementia and DM is sent to the ER from her nursing home because of fever, lethargy, and hypotension. Her caregiver reports a recent history of foul-smelling urine, ↓ mentation, and urinary incontinence. In the ER, the patient is found to have a temperature of 39.2°C (102.5°F) and a BP of 72/35. What is her most likely diagnosis?

Distributive shock due to urosepsis. If diagnosed early, fluid resuscitation, prompt initiation of IV antibiotics, and pressor support may resolve her symptoms.

KEY FACT

Types of shock:

- Hypovolemic: blood **volume** problem
- Cardiogenic: blood **pump** problem
- Distributive: blood **vessel** problem

A physiologic state in which alterations in tissue perfusion lead to ↓ tissue O_2 delivery. Although initially reversible, untreated or refractory shock can cause permanent organ damage, failure of multiple organ systems, and eventually death. Shock can be classified into three categories: **hypovolemic, cardiogenic,** and **distributive** (vasodilatory) (Table 18.1).

SYMPTOMS

Presents with hypotension (SBP < 90 mmHg or ↓ in SBP > 40 mmHg), oliguria, and changes in mental status.

EXAM

- Findings depend on the etiology, but almost all patients have tachycardia, tachypnea, altered mental status, and cool, clammy skin (except in distributive shock).
- The history may reveal food and medicine allergies, recent changes in medications, drug intoxication, preexisting illnesses, immunosuppressed states, or hypercoagulable conditions.

DIFFERENTIAL

See Table 18.1 for the different etiologies of shock.

TABLE 18.1. Etiologies and Mechanisms of Shock

TYPE	MECHANISM OF ACTION	COMMON ETIOLOGIES
Hypovolemic	Absolute deficiency in intravascular blood volume caused by hemorrhage or fluid loss.	Trauma, GI bleed, ruptured aneurysm, fractures, diarrhea, vomiting, heat stroke, inadequate replacement of insensible losses, burns, "third spacing" (seen in intestinal obstruction, pancreatitis, and cirrhosis).
Cardiogenic	Impaired cardiac contractility and pump failure.	Cardiomyopathies; arrhythmias; ischemic heart disease; mechanical (valvular) abnormalities; extracardiac (obstructive) disorders such as massive pulmonary embolus, tension pneumothorax, or pericardial tamponade.
Distributive	Inappropriate relaxation of peripheral vascular tone, often associated initially with ↑ cardiac output.	Sepsis, anaphylaxis, neurologic injury, drug-related causes.

TABLE 18.2.   Hemodynamic Features of Shock[a]

TYPE OF SHOCK	PRELOAD (PCWP)	PUMP FUNCTION (CO)	AFTERLOAD (SVR)	TISSUE PERFUSION (SvO$_2$)
Hypovolemic	↓	↓	↑	↓
Cardiogenic	↑	↓	↑	↓
Distributive	↓ or ↔	↑	↓	↑ (peripheral) and ↓ (central)

[a]PCWP = pulmonary capillary wedge pressure; SVR = systemic vascular resistance; CO = cardiac output; SvO$_2$ = mixed venous O$_2$ saturation.

DIAGNOSIS

- Generally diagnosed through the history and physical exam.
- CBC with differential, complete metabolic panel, amylase/lipase, cardiac enzymes, lactate, toxicology screen, UA, CXR, ABG, and blood cultures can help determine the etiology.
- Mixed venous O$_2$ saturation (SvO$_2$) and pulmonary artery catheterization (PCWP, CO/CI, SVR) can also help distinguish hypovolemic from cardiogenic and distributive shock (Table 18.2).

TREATMENT

- Always start with ABCs.
- Consider intubation and mechanical ventilation, which can facilitate elimination of CO$_2$ and compensate for any coexisting metabolic acidosis.
- Aggressive volume resuscitation with isotonic fluids and blood products if indicated. Once volume resuscitation is complete, begin vasopressors or cardiac inotropic agents (Table 18.3).

TABLE 18.3.   Pharmacologic Agents Used in Shock

PHARMACOLOGIC AGENT	RECEPTOR ACTIVITY				PREDOMINANT EFFECTS	INDICATIONS
	α$_1$	β$_1$	β$_2$	DA		
Phenylephrine	+++	0	0	0	SVR ↑↑, CO ↔/↑	Sepsis, neurogenic shock
Norepinephrine	++++++	++++	0	0	SVR ↑↑, CO ↔↓↑	Sepsis
Epinephrine	++++++	++++++	++	0	CO ↑↑, SVR ↓ (low dose); SVR ↔/↑ (high dose)	Anaphylaxis, ACLS, sepsis
Dopamine						
Low-dose (0.5–2 mcg/kg/min)	0	+	0	++	CO ↑, SVR ↑↓	Sepsis, cardiogenic shock
Mid-dose (5–10 mcg/kg/min)	+	++	0	++	CO ↑	
High-dose (10–20 mcg/kg/min)	++	++	0	++	SVR ↑↑	
Dobutamine	0/+	+++	++	0	CO ↑, SVR ↓	Cardiogenic shock
Isoproterenol	0	+++	+++	0	CO ↑, SVR ↓	Cardiogenic shock with bradycardia

- ■ If sepsis is a concern, begin early coverage with empiric broad-spectrum antibiotics.
- ■ Sodium bicarbonate may be indicated in patients with marked hypoperfusion causing lactic acidosis and a pH < 7.1.
- ■ Pharmacotherapy depends on the etiology. Table 18.3 lists the common pharmacologic agents used in shock, along with their indications and predominant effects.

Toxicology

COMMON INGESTIONS

Ingestions may be asymptomatic on initial presentation, depending on the time and the amount of ingestion. Timely consultation with a regional poison control center (1-800-222-1222), gut decontamination, and administration of an antidote (if available) can ↓ morbidity and mortality. Table 18.4 lists common ingestions and their treatment. Gut decontamination measures include the following:

TABLE 18.4. Common Ingestions and Toxidromes

Ingestion	Symptoms/Exam	Diagnosis	Treatment	Complications
Acetaminophen	Nausea, vomiting, jaundice.	History of overdose (> 140 mg/kg) or chronic overuse (> 4 g/day). ↑ liver enzymes; toxic serum level.	Activated charcoal if within 1–2 hr of ingestion. N-acetylcysteine (PO or IV) for 72 hr if serum level is toxic.	Metabolic acidosis, hepatic encephalopathy, fulminant hepatic failure, renal failure, death.
Acids or alkalis (commonly found in household cleaners)	Throat pain, abdominal pain, bloody emesis or stools, nausea, vomiting, difficulty swallowing or breathing, discoloration of skin and oral mucosa.	History of ingestion; prompt EGD to determine the extent of injury; CXR and abdominal x-ray (AXR) to evaluate for esophageal or gastric perforation.	Do **not** induce emesis. Dilute with milk or water to drink. Gastric lavage for liquid acid ingestion.	Respiratory failure, ARDS, local tissue necrosis, burns, death.
Anticholinergics (atropine, scopolamine, belladonna alkaloids, antihistamines, antipsychotics)	Mydriasis, dry mucous membranes, urinary retention, flushing, altered mental status ("dry as a bone, red as a beet, mad as a hatter").	History of ingestion.	Activated charcoal, gastric lavage. Benzodiazepines for agitation; physostigmine in severe cases (may induce seizures or arrhythmias).	Status epilepticus, hyperthermia, hypertension, coma, respiratory failure, death.
Carbon monoxide	Confusion, coma, seizures, headache, fatigue, nausea.	History of exposure to furnace or car exhaust. ↑ carboxyhemoglobin level; normal O_2 saturation.	Give 100% O_2 or hyperbaric O_2 in patients with CNS impairment, myocardial ischemia, or carboxyhemoglobin level > 30%.	Arrhythmias, myocardial ischemia, rhabdomyolysis, death.

TABLE 18.4. **Common Ingestions and Toxidromes** *(continued)*

INGESTION	SYMPTOMS/EXAM	DIAGNOSIS	TREATMENT	COMPLICATIONS
Cholinergics (organophosphates, pilocarpine, carbamates)	Diaphoresis, salivation, lacrimation, defecation, urination, miosis, nausea, altered mental status, weakness ("blind as a mole, moist as a slug, weak as a kitten").	Found in fertilizers. History of ingestion; farming or industrial work exposure; ↑ serum cholinesterase levels.	Skin decontamination with alkaline soap, then ethanol. Activated charcoal, gastric lavage. Atropine to dry secretions (may cause ileus); pralidoxime in symptomatic patients.	Seizures; respiratory failure; cranial nerve palsies; impaired hearing, visual memory, reaction time, dexterity, and problem solving; delayed peripheral neuropathy; death.
Iron	Nausea, vomiting, diarrhea, hypotension, acidosis.	History of ingestion. Serum levels > 350–500 µg/dL.	IV fluids, whole bowel irrigation. Deferoxamine to chelate the iron.	GI bleeding, metabolic acidosis, peritonitis, sepsis, fulminant hepatic failure, death.
Lead	Colicky abdominal pain, constipation, headache, irritability, seizures, motor neuropathy, learning disorders, microcytic anemia with basophilic stippling.	History of chronic repeated exposure (rare in acute ingestions). **Mild:** 10–50 µg/dL. **Moderate:** 50–70 µg/dL. **Severe:** 70–100 µg/dL.	Edetate calcium disodium (EDTA) +/– dimercaprol (BAL) for severe toxicity. Dimercaptosuccinic acid (DMSA) or EDTA for chelation in mild to moderate toxicity.	Learning disorders, motor neuropathy, anemia.
Salicylates	Nausea, vomiting, hyperventilation, tachycardia, tinnitus, coma, seizures, anion-gap metabolic acidosis, hyperthermia.	History of acute overdose (> 200 mg/kg) or chronic overmedication. Serum level > 100 mg/dL in acute, 60–70 mg/dL in chronic.	Activated charcoal, gastric lavage, hemodialysis. Sodium bicarbonate to treat metabolic acidosis and alkalinize the urine.	Coma, cardiovascular collapse, pulmonary edema, death.
Theophylline	Nausea, vomiting, tachycardia, tremulousness, hypotension, seizures, hypokalemia, hyperglycemia, metabolic acidosis.	History of acute overdose or chronic overmedication. Serum level > 100 mg/dL in acute, 40–60 mg/dL in chronic.	Activated charcoal, whole bowel irrigation, hemodialysis. Benzodiazepines or barbiturates for seizure treatment.	Ventricular arrhythmias, status epilepticus, death.
TCAs	Mydriasis, tachycardia, dry mouth, flushing, muscle twitching, ↓ peristalsis, QRS widening and QT prolongation, seizures, diaphoresis, hypotension.	History of ingestion.	Do **not** induce emesis. Activated charcoal, gastric lavage. Sodium bicarbonate boluses to reverse cardiotoxicity.	Ventricular arrhythmias, hyperthermia, status epilepticus, death.

- **Gastric lavage:** Not effective beyond 1.0–1.5 hours after ingestion, but may be useful in severely ill patients. Should be combined with activated charcoal and used only in patients who are intubated or able to protect their airway.
- **Activated charcoal:** The treatment of choice for most ingestions (except metals). Best if used within the first hour of overdose, but may be administered in all ingestions unless the agent is nontoxic or not bound by activated charcoal. Usual dose is 50–100 g in adults and 10–25 g in pediatric patients.
- **Whole bowel irrigation:** May be useful after the ingestion of enteric-coated and timed-release medications and in body packers. Usual dose is 3–8 L of GoLytely.
- **Ipecac:** Not useful for gut decontamination and no longer recommended for ingestions.

FOOD POISONING

An acute illness caused by ingestion of food contaminated by bacteria, bacterial toxins, viruses, parasites, natural poisons, or harmful chemical substances. Characterized by a short incubation period of hours up to 1 week, most cases of food poisoning are mild and improve with supportive care, antiperistaltic or antisecretory agents, absorbents, and volume repletion. Some patients, however, may have severe disease requiring hospitalization, aggressive rehydration therapy, antibiotic treatment, and avoidance of antiperistaltic agents. Table 18.5 lists the common etiologies of food poisoning.

TABLE 18.5.   Common Causes of Food Poisoning

SUBSTANCE	FOODS	SX/EXAM	ONSET	TREATMENT
Bacillus cereus	Fried rice.	Vomiting, diarrhea.	1–6 hr.	Supportive care.
Ciguatera	Red snapper, grouper, warm-water fish.	GI symptoms followed by perioral numbness, hot–cold reversal on the face, cranial nerve palsies, hallucinations, and hypotension.	Minutes to hours.	Supportive care, gut decontamination, calcium gluconate or atropine as needed.
Campylobacter jejuni	Untreated water; undercooked meat, milk, or shellfish.	Foul-smelling watery diarrhea, followed by bloody diarrhea, cramps, fever, and headache.	2–10 days.	Supportive care; erythromycin for invasive disease.
Clostridium perfringens	Undercooked meat or poultry.	Watery diarrhea, nausea, cramps.	6–12 hr.	Supportive care.

TABLE 18.5.   Common Causes of Food Poisoning *(continued)*

Substance	Foods	Sx/Exam	Onset	Treatment
Clostridium botulinum	Improperly canned foods, honey.	Diplopia, ptosis, descending weakness and paralysis, respiratory difficulties.	4–72 hr.	Supportive care, airway management, antitoxin.
Enterotoxic *E coli*	Contaminated water and food.	Watery diarrhea, vomiting, cramps.	8–12 hr.	Supportive care.
E coli O157:H7	Untreated water, raw beef, unpasteurized milk.	Cramps, bloody diarrhea, nausea, vomiting, fever.	3–4 days.	Supportive care; treatment of hemolytic-uremic syndrome if present.
Salmonella	Eggs, poultry.	Bloody diarrhea, cramps, low-grade fever, vomiting.	8–48 hr.	Supportive care; antibiotics for systemic infection.
Shigella	Undercooked food, egg salad.	Nausea, vomiting, fever, bloody diarrhea, neurologic symptoms, tenesmus.	36–72 hr.	Supportive care; antibiotics for severe infection.
Staphylococcus spp.	Improperly stored meats, dairy, or bakery products.	Vomiting, cramps, mild diarrhea.	1–2 hr.	Supportive care.
Hepatitis A virus	Contaminated food.	Fatigue, fever, nausea, vomiting, cramps, anorexia, jaundice, darkened urine.	14–50 days.	Supportive care; prophylaxis with immunization; liver transplantation for liver failure.
Vibrio cholerae	Contaminated water and food.	Profuse rice-water stools, cramps.	8–24 hr.	Supportive care, tetracycline.
Giardia lamblia	Contaminated groundwater.	Watery diarrhea +/– bloody diarrhea, cramps, fatigue, bloating, weight loss.	2–3 days.	Supportive care, metronidazole.

BIOTERRORISM

Bioterrorism refers to a spectrum of natural organisms or toxins that can be used to incapacitate, kill, or otherwise harm individuals. Characterized by low visibility, high potency, substantial accessibility, and easy delivery, biological weapons can cause widespread destruction. Typical biological weapons and the syndromes they cause are listed in Table 18.6.

TABLE 18.6. **Effects of Exposure to Biological Agents**

AGENT	DESCRIPTION	SYMPTOMS/EXAM	DIAGNOSIS	TREATMENT
Anthrax (*Bacillus anthracis*)	A large, aerobic, gram-⊕, spore-forming nonmotile bacillus causing a zoonotic disease in domesticated and wild animals.	**Cutaneous infection (> 95% of cases):** Fever, malaise, and headache; a painless papule or vesicle that later turns into a necrotic ulcer with a characteristic 1- to 5-cm black eschar; extensive surrounding edema; local lymphadenitis. **Inhalation infection:** Headache, fever, myalgias, fatigue, nonproductive cough, chest discomfort, respiratory distress. **Oropharyngeal/GI infection:** Oral ulcer from ingestion of infected or undercooked meat; fever, neck swelling, dysphagia, nausea and vomiting, respiratory distress, hematemesis, massive ascites, diarrhea.	⊕ Gram stain or culture of cutaneous lesion or peripheral blood; mediastinal widening and pleural effusion on CXR.	Penicillin and doxycycline are FDA approved (but may have resistance in terrorist attacks); fluoroquinolones in suspected inhalation anthrax infections.
Brucellosis (*Brucella* spp.)	A small, aerobic, nonmotile, gram-⊖ coccobacillus causing a zoonotic disease in wild and domesticated animals; transmitted via skin abrasions, the conjunctivae, and the GI or respiratory tract.	May present as an acute, systemic febrile illness, an insidious chronic illness, or a localized inflammatory process. Fever, diaphoresis, fatigue, anorexia, arthralgias, depression, headache, irritability, cough; focal pain in the bones, joints, or GU tract with localized infection.	⊕ tube agglutination test; ⊕ cultures of blood, bone marrow, or body fluid samples.	Relapse is common, so combined regimens are recommended: doxycycline + streptomycin or rifampin.
Plague (*Yersinia pestis*)	A gram-⊖ nonmotile coccobacillus causing a zoonotic disease spread by the flea bites of an infected animal (usually a rat) or inhalation of an infectious aerosol.	**Bubonic (85%–90%):** High fevers, chills, headache, nausea, vomiting, painful lymphadenopathy, severe malaise, altered mental status, cough, presence of buboes (swelling of lymph nodes). **Septicemic (10%–15%):** Fevers, chills, nausea, vomiting, diarrhea, DIC, acrocyanosis, purpura. **Pneumonic (1%):** Cough with blood-tinged sputum; bilateral alveolar infiltrates on CXR.	Presence of the organism in bubo aspiration; ⊕ cultures of blood, bubo aspirate, sputum, and CXR; fourfold rise in antibody titers.	Isolation; streptomycin +/– chloramphenicol (in patients with meningitis or hemodynamic instability).

TABLE 18.6. **Effects of Exposure to Biological Agents** *(continued)*

AGENT	DESCRIPTION	SYMPTOMS/EXAM	DIAGNOSIS	TREATMENT
Tularemia (*Francisella tularensis*)	A gram-$\ominus$, nonmotile, intracellular coccobacillus causing a zoonotic disease spread by the tick bites of an infected animal (usually a rabbit).	**Ulceroglandular (75%):** Fever, localized skin or mucous membrane ulceration, regional lymphadenopathy > 1 cm, cough, malaise. **Typhoidal (25%):** Fever, cough, shortness of breath, malaise, hemoptysis.	$\oplus$ cultures of blood, sputum, ulcers, pharyngeal and conjunctival exudates, and gastric washings; $\oplus$ ELISA or bacterial agglutination.	Streptomycin (drug of choice), gentamicin, tetracycline, chloramphenicol.
Q fever (*Coxiella burnetii*)	A rickettsia-like organism with high infectivity causing illnesses in livestock and humans who are exposed to them.	May present acutely or insidiously. Fever, chills, headache, diaphoresis, malaise, fatigue, anorexia, pneumonia, acute hepatitis, heart failure, clubbing, and splenomegaly in acute endocarditis.	$\oplus$ serologic studies (ELISA is the most sensitive method).	Tetracycline (drug of choice), erythromycin, azithromycin.
Botulism (*Clostridium botulinum*)	An anaerobic, gram-$\oplus$, spore-forming bacillus that produces toxins causing neuromuscular blockade.	Diplopia, mydriasis, ptosis, dysphagia, dysphonia, muscle weakness, symmetric descending flaccid paralasis, cranial nerve palsies, respiratory failure.	$\oplus$ ELISA analysis of nasal swabs.	Trivalent antitoxin, supportive care, botulinum immunization.
Smallpox (variola)	A highly infectious member of the poxvirus family that is spread to humans by aerosol.	High fever, headache, rigors, vomiting, malaise, abdominal pain, altered mental status, synchronous exanthem with a centrifugal distribution.	Demonstration of virions on electron microscopy of vesicular scrapings; $\oplus$ silver stain or gel diffusion test.	Respiratory isolation, supportive treatment, prophylaxis with smallpox vaccine.
Ricin	Plant protein toxin derived from beans of the castor plant.	**Inhalation:** Sudden onset of nasopharyngeal congestion, nausea, vomiting, urticaria, chest tightness, and respiratory distress. **Ingestion:** Less toxic due to poor absorption; nausua, vomiting, diarrhea, fever, cramps, hematochezia, shock.	$\oplus$ ELISA analysis of nasal swab sample; bilateral infiltrates on CXR.	Supportive treatment; activated charcoal and gastric lavage.

Intoxication/Withdrawal

Common presentations of substance use disorders in the acute setting. Drug dependency ranges from habituation to addiction and can encompass a spectrum of symptoms, depending on the amount of drug used, the duration of usage, and the presence of polysubstance abuse. Tables 18.7 and 18.8 outline the intoxication and withdrawal syndromes of the most commonly abused substances.

TABLE 18.7. Common Intoxication Syndromes[a]

	OPIOID	SEDATIVE	STIMULANT	HALLUCINOGEN
Symptoms	Altered mental status, euphoria, drowsiness, pruritus, nausea, abdominal pain, constipation, vomiting, urinary retention.	Altered mental status, slurred speech, ataxia, ↓ fine motor function, disinhibition, anxiety, drowsiness, hallucinations, coma.	Altered mental status, paranoia, seizures, hypervigilance, euphoria, chest pain, agitation, flushing, stroke symptoms, epistaxis, cough with black sputum.	Altered mental status, visual hallucinations, disorientation, sweating, mood lability, acute panic symptoms.
Exam	Respiratory depression, miosis, hypoxia, pulmonary rales.	Nystagmus, hypotonia, respiratory depression.	Seizures, diaphoresis, hyperthermia, dyspnea, tachycardia, mydriasis, hypertension.	Diaphoresis, tachycardia, mydriasis, tachypnea.
Treatment	Airway management and supportive care; naloxone for reversal; activated charcoal if recent oral overdose.	Airway management and supportive care; activated charcoal for acute benzodiazepine ingestion; flumazenil for benzodiazepine reversal; seizure and hypoglycemia treatment.	Airway management and supportive care; benzodiazepines for seizures and sedation; cooling measures; sedation; avoidance of nonselective β-blockers; activated charcoal for acute ingestion.	Supportive care in a nonstimulating environment; benzodiazepines if needed for sedation; cooling measures.
Complications	Pulmonary edema, hypotension, respiratory failure, death.	**Benzodiazepines:** Aspiration pneumonia, respiratory failure, death. **Alcohol:** Holiday heart, DTs, hypoglycemia, cardiomyopathy, liver failure, behavioral toxicity.	MI, cardiomyopathy, hypertensive crisis, pulmonary edema, behavioral toxicity, death.	Respiratory arrest, coma, hyperthermia, behavioral toxicity.

[a]Examples of opioids include morphine and heroin; sedatives, benzodiazepine and alcohol; stimulants, cocaine and amphetamine; and hallucinogens, LSD.

TABLE 18.8.   Common Withdrawal Syndromes[a]

	OPIOID	**SEDATIVE**	**STIMULANT**	**HALLUCINOGEN**
Symptoms	Sneezing, yawning, lacrimation, leg and abdominal cramps, nausea, vomiting, diarrhea.	Tremor, anxiety, nausea, disorientation, agitation, insomnia, hallucinations, sensory hyperacuity, seizures.	Dysphoria, craving, sleep disturbances, hunger, depression.	No true withdrawal state, but dysphoria may occur after discontinuation of chronic use.
Exam	Rhinorrhea, mydriasis, tachycardia, tachypnea, hypertension, piloerection, hyperthermia.	Tachypnea, tachycardia, diaphoresis, hyperthermia, hyperreflexia.	Psychomotor retardation.	
Treatment	Long-acting opioid agonist (methadone) or buprenorphine taper; clonidine, naltrexone for maintenance.	Benzodiazepines or barbiturates for withdrawal symptoms and seizures; dextrose, thiamine, clonidine, β-blockers.	Bromocriptine for withdrawal symptoms; desipramine for maintenance.	

[a]Examples of opioids include morphine and heroin; sedatives, benzodiazepine and alcohol; stimulants, cocaine and amphetamine; and hallucinogens, LSD.

Altered Mental Status

Acute change in mental status; may range from mild confusion to severe delirium to coma (see Table 18.9).

SYMPTOMS/EXAM

Presentation depends on the underlying disorder, but almost all patients exhibit disorientation, confusion, irritability, fluctuating levels of consciousness, mental slowing, agitation, and inattention.

DIAGNOSIS

Generally diagnosed through comprehensive history and physical exam, including the Mini-Mental Status Exam to assess cognitive function and rule out dementia.

- **Routine laboratory testing:** Comprehensive chemistry panel, LFTs, TFTs, ABGs, CBC, blood cultures, UA, LP if febrile, and toxicology screen.
- **Imaging studies:** EEG, CT, MRI, CXR, ECG.

TREATMENT

- Begin with ABCs and stabilize the patient.
- Give glucose and thiamine and consider naloxone. Other treatment is based on most likely cause.
- General principles include discontinuation of medications that may exacerbate the problem; establishment of a comfortable, nonthreatening environment with adequate nursing; fluid resuscitation; and behavioral control with medications (haloperidol, risperidone) or physical restraints (should not substitute for a diagnostic workup).

    MNEMONIC

Causes of altered mental status:

MOVE STUPID

Metabolic
Oxygen (hypoxia or hypercarbia)
Vascular
Electrolyte/Endocrine
Seizure
Trauma/Tumor
Uremia
Psychiatric
Infection
Drug ingestion or withdrawal

TABLE 18.9. **Causes of Altered Mental Status**

	ETIOLOGIES	TREATMENT
Metabolic	1. Hypo-/hyperglycemia. 2. Hepatic encephalopathy. 3. Wernicke encephalopathy. 4. Nutritional deficiencies: vitamin B_1 (beriberi) vitamin B_{12} (pernicious anemia), folate, nicotinic acid (pellagra). 5. Hypo-/hyperthermia.	1. Fluids, glucose, and thiamine/insulin. 2. Lactulose. 3. Thiamine. 4. Correct nutritional deficiency. 5. Maintenance of euthermia.
Oxygen	1. Hypercapnia. 2. Hypoxia.	1. Correct underlying cause (ie, bronchodialators). Consider BIPAP, intubation. 2. O_2 supplementation.
Vascular	1. Hypertensive encephalopathy. 2. Arrhythmias. 3. Stroke/TIA. 4. Thrombotic thrombocytopenic purpura. 5. CNS vasculitis. 6. Subarachnoid hemorrhage.	1. BP control to DBP < 100 mmHg. 2. Antiarrhythmic agents or cardioversion. 3. Evaluate for embolic source +/– anticoagulation. 4. Plasma exchange transfusion +/– prednisone, immunosuppressants, aspirin. 5. Glucocorticoids +/– cyclophosphamide. 6. Surgical drainage +/– clipping.
Electrolyte/ Endocrine	1. Hypo-/hypernatremia. 2. Hypercalcemia. 3. Hypo-/hypermagnesemia. 4. Thyroid dysfunction.	1–3. Correct electrolyte disturbance. 4. Replete thyroid hormone or treat hyperthyroid with cooling measures, propranolol, PTU; consider prednisone, iodine compounds.
Seizure	1. Postictal state. 2. Nonconvulsive status epilepticus.	1–2. Anticonvulsant therapy.
Trauma/ Tumor	1. Tumors may be primary or metastatic, malignant or benign. 2. Hydrocephalus. 3. Subdural hematoma.	1. Surgical decompression, radiation, chemotherapy; consider steroids for reduction of mass effect. 2. Ventriculoperitoneal shunt. 3. Craniotomy and evacuation.
Uremia	Can be due to any cause of renal failure.	Treat renal failure.
Psychiatric	1. Psychosis (due to schizophrenia, depression, bipolar, schizotypal, or other causes). 2. Alzheimer, parkinsonism, Huntington chorea, Pick disease, other dementias. 3. Sundowning. 4. ICU psychosis.	1. Psychiatric medications. 2. Neurologic medications as indicated. 3. Antipsychotics (eg, haloperidol). 4. Normal sleep–wake cycle, calm environment, +/– sedatives.
Infection	1. Meningitis/encephalitis. 2. Bacteremia, pyelonephritis, pneumonia. 3. AIDS, neurosyphillis. 4. Toxoplasmosis; brain abscesses can present with focal neurologic findings.	1–4. Treat underlying infection in all cases.
Drugs	1. Ingestion. 2. Withdrawal.	1–2. See toxicology and intoxication/withdrawal sections.

Headache

A common chief complaint seen in the ER or urgent care setting. Structural headaches caused by head trauma that cause space-occupying hematomas and elevation of ICP are considered neurosurgical emergencies.

EPIDURAL HEMATOMA

An accumulation of blood in the potential space between the dura and bone due to disruption of interposed vessels. Intracranial epidural hematomas are the most serious complication of head injury and are usually due to tearing of the middle meningeal artery. Associated with skull fractures in 85%–95% of adult cases.

SYMPTOMS

Headache, nausea, vomiting, seizures, focal neurologic deficits occurring within hours of the injury.

EXAM

Findings include bradycardia and/or hypertension due to ↑ ICP, anisocoria, skull fractures or lacerations, CSF rhinorrhea or otorrhea, hemotympanum, altered mental status, facial nerve injury, focal neurologic deficits, and vertebral column instability.

DIAGNOSIS

- Noncontrast head CT shows a hyperdense, lens-shaped mass between the brain and skull (Figure 18.1).
- Conventional angiography, MRA, or CT angiography may be used to confirm the presence of an underlying vascular malformation.

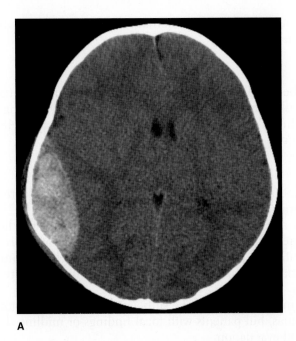
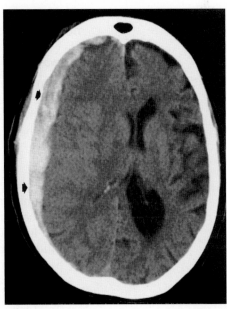

FIGURE 18.1.   Acute epidural and acute subdural hematoma. (A) Noncontrast transaxial CT showing a right temporal acute epidural hematoma. Note the characteristic biconvex shape. **(B)** Noncontrast transaxial CT demonstrating a right acute holohemispheric subdural hematoma *(arrows)*. Note the characteristic crescentic shape. (Image A reproduced, with permission, from Doherty GM. *Current Diagnosis & Treatment: Surgery,* 13th ed. New York: McGraw-Hill, 2010, Fig. 36-8. Image B reproduced, with permission, from Chen MY, et al. *Basic Radiology.* New York: McGraw-Hill, 2004, Fig. 12-32.)

TREATMENT

- Establish ABCs and immobilize patient.
- Additional measures include correction of any coexisting coagulopathy; osmotic diuretics; hyperventilation to achieve a P_{CO_2} of 28–32 mmHg; and elevation of the head of the bed to 30 degrees for patients with ↑ ICP.
- Systemic arterial BP control; isotonic fluids; seizure treatment or prophylaxis.
- Although conservative management may be a reasonable option in mild cases, craniotomy followed by evacuation of the hematoma is the definitive treatment.

COMPLICATIONS

Posttraumatic seizures, postconcussion syndrome, neurologic deficits, death.

SUBDURAL HEMATOMA

A collection of venous blood below the inner layer of the dura but external to the brain and arachnoid membrane. Usually caused by blunt head trauma that leads to disruption of bridging veins; more frequently found in patients > 60 years of age. If untreated, acute subdural hematomas can progress to subacute (3–7 days after injury) and chronic (2–3 weeks after injury) stages. Alcoholics, hemophiliacs, and patients on chronic anticoagulation therapy are at risk because of their ↑ risk of bleeding.

SYMPTOMS/EXAM

- Headache, loss of consciousness, mental status changes, and a history of blunt head trauma.
- Exam reveals impaired mental status, focal neurologic deficits, and a Glasgow Coma Scale (GCS) score of < 15.

DIFFERENTIAL

Child or elder abuse, epidural hematoma, meningitis, stroke, subarachnoid hemorrhage, dementia.

DIAGNOSIS

- Noncontrast head CT shows a hyperdense crescentic mass along the inner table of the skull, most commonly in the parietal region (see Figure 18.1).
- Contrast-enhanced CT or MRI is recommended for imaging 48–72 hours after head injury.

TREATMENT

- Consider endotracheal intubation in patients with a GCS score of < 10 to guarantee airway protection.
- Correction of any coexisting coagulopathy; elevation of the head of the bed to 30 degrees for patients with ↑ ICP; and, if the patient is intubated, mild hyperventilation to achieve a P_{CO_2} of approximately 30 mmHg.
- Systemic arterial blood pressure control; isotonic fluids; seizure treatment or prophylaxis.
- Conservative management may be sufficient for small, asymptomatic subdural hematomas, but patients with focal findings or midline shift require craniotomy and evacuation.
- Burr holes are a temporizing option before definitive surgery if herniation syndrome is evident.

COMPLICATIONS

↑ ICP, brain edema, recurrent hematoma, infection, seizures.

SUBARACHNOID HEMORRHAGE (SAH)

The presence of blood within the subarachnoid space resulting from a pathologic process, usually rupture of a berry aneurysm or an AVM. SAH carries a significant risk of morbidity and mortality and is commonly associated with uncontrolled hypertension, smoking, alcohol use, and cerebral AVMs.

SYMPTOMS

- Sudden onset of a severe headache that may be accompanied by loss of consciousness, nausea and vomiting, focal neurologic deficits, signs of meningeal irritation such as neck stiffness or low back pain, photophobia, and seizure activity.
- Prodromal symptoms from minor blood leakage ("sentinel" headache) are reported in 30%–50% of aneurysmal SAHs and are not due to ↑ ICP.

EXAM

Global or focal neurologic abnormalities, syndromes of cranial nerve compression, seizures, papilledema, retinal hemorrhages, ↑ BP.

DIFFERENTIAL

Encephalitis, hypertensive emergency, meningitis, stroke, TIA, temporal arteritis, tension/migraine/cluster headache.

DIAGNOSIS

- Noncontrast head CT is most sensitive within 24 hours of the event and shows SAH +/− evidence of associated hydrocephalus (Figure 18.2).
- If CT is ⊖, LP should be performed to look for the presence of RBCs and xanthochromia in the CSF.
- Cerebral angiography, CT angiography, or MRA may be used to evaluate the vascular anatomy and localize the site of the bleed.

TREATMENT

- Stabilize the patient and establish the ABCs; avoid sedation if possible.
- Additional measures include osmotic diuretics; elevation of the head of the bed to 30 degrees to ↓ ICP in patients with signs of herniation; and, if the patient is intubated, mild hyperventilation to achieve a P_{CO_2} of approximately 30 mmHg.
- Systemic arterial BP control to keep mean arterial pressure < 130, seizure prophylaxis, calcium channel blockers (nimodipine) to ↓ cerebral vasospasm, isotonic fluids.
- Ventriculostomy placement to address coexisting hydrocephalus.
- Definitive treatment involves surgical clipping or endovascular treatment (coiling) of the ruptured berry aneurysm.

COMPLICATIONS

Hydrocephalus, rebleeding, intraventricular or intracerebral hemorrhage, cerebral ischemia, hyponatremia from cerebral salt wasting, hypothalamic dysfunction, seizures, ↑ ICP, neurologic deficits, death.

KEY FACT

A patient complaining of "the worst headache of my life" or sudden onset like a "thunderclap" should make you think of subarachnoid hemorrhage.

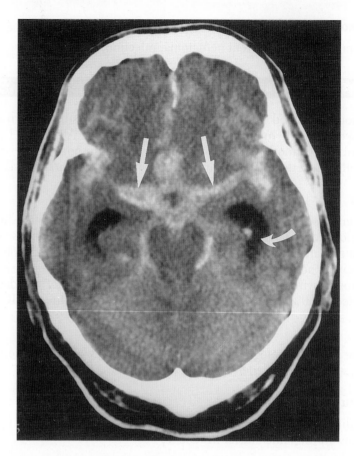

FIGURE 18.2. **Subarachnoid hemorrhage.** Transaxial noncontrast CT showing subarachnoid hemorrhage filling the basilar cisterns and sylvian fissures (*straight arrows*). The curved arrow shows the dilated temporal horns of the lateral ventricles/hydrocephalus. (Reproduced, with permission, from Tintinalli JE, et al. *Tintinalli's Emergency Medicine: A Comprehensive Study Guide,* 6th ed. New York: McGraw-Hill, 2004, Fig. 237-4.)

INCREASED INTRACRANIAL PRESSURE

- A pathologic state that indicates an ↑ in normal brain pressure (8–18 mmHg in adults); often caused by intracranial hematomas or cerebral edema. Can cause midline shift of brain structures and herniation syndrome, leading to an ischemic cascade that may eventually end in death.
- Common etiologies include severe head injury, epidural hematoma, subdural hematoma, hydrocephalus, brain tumor, hypertensive hemorrhage, intraventricular hemorrhage, meningitis, encephalitis, SAH, status epilepticus, and stroke.
- **Sx:** Nausea, vomiting, headache, mental status changes.
- **Exam/Dx:** Papilledema on funduscopic exam (see Figure 11.2 in the Neurology chapter for an image of papilledema), papillary dilation, global neurologic abnormalities, ↑ opening pressure on LP, Cushing response (hypertension and bradycardia), respiratory changes.
- **Tx:** Removal of the underlying cause. Temporizing measures include osmotic diuretics (mannitol); adequate analgesia; elevation of the head of the bed to 30 degrees; and, if the patient is intubated, mild hyperventilation to achieve a P_{CO_2} of approximately 30 mmHg.
- **Cx:** Permanent neurologic deficits, death.

Chest Pain

AORTIC DISSECTION

Most common in men > 60 years of age. Uncontrolled hypertension is the most important risk factor; less common associations include Marfan syndrome, congenital bicuspid aortic valves, aortic coarctation, pregnancy, and cocaine use.

SYMPTOMS

- Sudden, tearing pain in the anterior chest (ascending dissection) or posterior chest (descending dissection), neck, throat, or jaw.
- May be associated with syncope, CVA symptoms, CHF, MI, or abdominal pain.

EXAM

Exam reveals hypertension or hypotension, asymmetrical pulses, asymmetrical BP, syncope, altered mental status, dyspnea, dysphagia, a new diastolic murmur, and findings suggestive of cardiac tamponade.

DIFFERENTIAL

Myocardial ischemia, pericarditis, pulmonary embolus, aortic regurgitation, aortic aneurysm, musculoskeletal pain, mediastinal tumors, pleuritis, cholecystitis, PUD, acute pancreatitis, acute coronary syndrome.

DIAGNOSIS

- Diagnosed by clinical symptoms suggestive of aortic dissection, mediastinal widening on CXR, variation in pulse (absence of a proximal extremity pulse), and a BP difference of > 20 mmHg between the right and the left arm. If clinical suspicion is high but CXR is normal, order a CT.
- Thoracic MRI or CT, transesophageal echocardiography (TEE), aortography (Figure 18.3).

TREATMENT

- Admit to the ICU and administer medications to ↓ cardiac contractility and control systemic arterial pressure (nitroprusside, β-blockers, calcium channel blockers).
- Ascending aortic dissections are treated with immediate surgical correction, whereas surgery for descending aortic dissections is indicated only in patients with persistent pain, aneurysmal dilation > 5 cm, end-organ ischemia, or evidence of retrograde dissection to the ascending aorta.

COMPLICATIONS

MI, stroke, pericardial tamponade, claudication, compressive symptoms, acute aortic regurgitation, aortic rupture, aneurysmal dilation, mesenteric or renal ischemia, death.

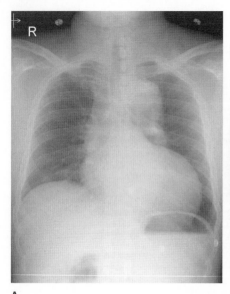
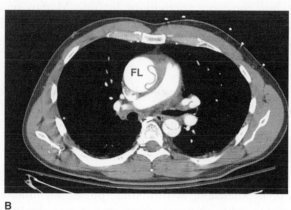
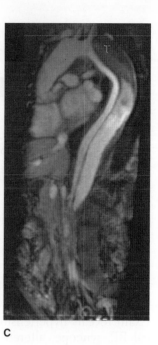

A   **B**   **C**

FIGURE 18.3. **Mediastinal widening on CXR and CT.** (A) Frontal CXR showing a widened mediastinum in a patient with an aortic dissection. (B) Transaxial contrast-enhanced CT showing a dissection involving the ascending and descending aorta (FL = false lumen). (C) Sagittal MRA image showing a dissection involving the descending aorta, with a thrombus (T) in the false lumen. (Images A and C reproduced, with permission, from USMLERx.com. Image B reproduced, with permission, from Doherty GM. *Current Diagnosis & Treatment: Surgery*, 13th ed. New York: McGraw-Hill, 2010, Fig. 19-17.)

MNEMONIC

Treat suspected acute coronary syndrome with MONA-B:

Morphine
Oxygen
Nitroglycerine
Aspirin
β-blocker

MYOCARDIAL INFARCTION (MI)

Rapid development of myocardial necrosis caused by an imbalance between myocardial O_2 supply and demand. Usually results from plaque rupture with thrombus formation in a coronary vessel. Considered part of the acute coronary syndrome spectrum that includes ST-segment elevation MI (STEMI), non-ST-segment elevation MI (NSTEMI), and unstable angina.

SYMPTOMS

Presents with prolonged substernal pressure radiating to the left arm or neck associated with nausea, vomiting, diaphoresis, or dyspnea. However, some patients, especially women and those with diabetes, may present atypically with only nausea, dyspnea, or neck pain.

EXAM

Exam reveals hypotension or hypertension, cool and clammy skin, systolic murmur (if valvular defects develop), S4, and signs of CHF.

DIFFERENTIAL

Cardiac ischemia without infarction, aortic dissection, aortic stenosis, cholecystitis, esophageal spasm, esophagitis, gastritis, GERD, pneumothorax, pulmonary embolism, acute pericarditis, anxiety disorder, pneumonia, pancreatitis.

DIAGNOSIS

- ↑ cardiac enzymes measured serially over a 24-hour period (CK-MB and troponin are most specific).
- ECG; echocardiogram showing wall motion abnormalities; myocardial perfusion imaging or cardiac angiography showing ↓ blood flow to portions of the myocardium.

TREATMENT

- Antiplatelet therapy with aspirin and/or clopidogrel; β-blockers; nitrates (contraindicated in RV infarction, hypotension, and phosphodiesterase inhibitor use within the past 24 hours).
- Morphine for pain control; supplemental O$_2$; ACEIs within the first 24 hours of STEMI in the absence of hypotension and as long-term therapy if LV dysfunction is present (can use an ARB if intolerant to ACE inhibitor).
- Glycoprotein IIb/IIIa receptor antagonists and heparin are appropriate in patients with continuing ischemia and in whom percutaneous intervention (PCI) is planned.
- Thrombolytic therapy is appropriate in patients with ST-segment elevation, new left bundle branch block, or anterior ST-segment depression consistent with posterior infarction if presenting within 12 hours of onset of symptoms and if PCI is not readily available within 90 minutes.
- PCI is considered the treatment of choice assuming a door-to-needle time of < 90 minutes.
- Coronary artery bypass graft (CABG) surgery is appropriate for patients who fail PCI or who develop mechanical complications.

COMPLICATIONS

Arrhythmias, recurrent ischemia, CHF, cardiogenic shock, acute valvular abnormalities, pericarditis, ventricular aneurysms, mural thrombi, hypertension.

Note: See the Pulmonary chapter for a discussion of pulmonary embolism and the Cardiology chapter for a discussion of pericarditis, 2 other important causes of chest pain.

Abdominal Pain

APPENDICITIS

Acute inflammation of the vermiform appendix.

SYMPTOMS

Abdominal pain, initially periumbilical and then migrating to the RLQ, along with anorexia, nausea, and vomiting.

EXAM

Low-grade fever, maximal tenderness at the McBurney point, Rovsing sign, psoas sign, and obturator sign. Peritoneal signs (guarding and rebound tenderness) are seen in appendiceal perforation; inability to jump up and down is a fairly sensitive test for peritonitis.

DIFFERENTIAL

Cholecystitis, biliary colic, constipation, diverticular disease, gastroenteritis, mesenteric ischemia, IBD, endometriosis, ovarian cysts or torsion, intussusception, PID.

DIAGNOSIS

- Generally diagnosed clinically, as lab studies are not specific for appendicitis.
- Look for leukocytosis, mild pyuria, and ↑ inflammatory markers.

- Abdominal ultrasound is the 1st-line test in pediatric and pregnant patients. Otherwise, CT scan with IV contrast (see Figure 12.2 in the Surgery chapter).

TREATMENT

Appendectomy with antibiotic treatment until the patient is afebrile and WBC count normalizes.

COMPLICATIONS

Although the prognosis is usually excellent, wound infections, abscess formation, persistent ileus, or cecal fistulas can occur.

ISCHEMIC BOWEL

Also called mesenteric ischemia; caused by a ↓ in intestinal blood flow, usually arising from occlusion, vasospasm, or hypoperfusion of the mesenteric vasculature. It can be categorized as acute or chronic, based on the rapidity and degree to which blood flow is impaired. Clinical consequences of acute mesenteric ischemia can be catastrophic, making rapid diagnosis and treatment imperative. Risk factors include advanced age, atherosclerosis, low cardiac output states, cardiac arrhythmias, recent MI, severe cardiac valvular disease, and intra-abdominal malignancy.

SYMPTOMS

- Rapid onset of severe periumbilical pain out of proportion to findings on the physical exam.
- Nausea, vomiting, anorexia, and diarrhea progressing to obstipation.
- Presentation may be more insidious in patients with chronic mesenteric ischemia or in those with thrombotic causes, vasculitis, or nonocclusive ischemia.
- Colonic (vs. small bowel) ischemia is usually associated with hematochezia and less pain.

EXAM

- Exam may initially be normal or may reveal only mild abdominal distention or occult blood in the stool.
- As ischemia progresses and infarction occurs, peritoneal signs develop and a feculent odor to the breath may be noted.

DIFFERENTIAL

Abdominal abscess, abdominal aneurysm, aortic dissection, appendicitis, biliary disease, diverticular disease, ectopic pregnancy, MI, pancreatitis, renal calculi, acute intermittent porphyria, bowel obstruction.

DIAGNOSIS

- Accurate diagnosis depends on a high index of suspicion in patients with known risk factors, as early signs are nonspecific and definitive diagnosis often requires invasive testing.
- Check CBC, ABG, lactate. Often associated with leukocytosis, metabolic acidosis.
- MRA, CT angiography, or duplex sonography.
- Angiography, although invasive, remains the gold standard.

TREATMENT

The goal is to restore intestinal blood flow as quickly as possible using the following measures:

- Aggressive hemodynamic monitoring and support, correction of metabolic acidosis, initiation of broad-spectrum antibiotics, and placement of an NG tube for gastric decompression.
- Systemic anticoagulation to prevent thrombus formation or propagation unless contraindicated.
- Medical treatment with close observation may be considered for patients without peritoneal signs and with good mesenteric blood flow on angiography.
- Intra-arterial vasodilators or thrombolytic agents, angioplasty, stent placement, embolectomy, or exploratory laparotomy with resection of necrotic bowel may be necessary.

COMPLICATIONS

Bowel necrosis, septic shock, death.

RUPTURED ABDOMINAL AORTIC ANEURYSM (AAA)

A degenerative process of the abdominal aorta due to atherosclerosis, leading to focal dilation with at least a 50% ↑ over normal arterial diameter. An estimated 65% of patients with ruptured AAAs die of sudden cardiovascular collapse before arriving at a hospital.

SYMPTOMS

- Sudden onset of abdominal, back, or flank pain associated with hypotension, tachycardia, or temporary loss of consciousness.
- Symptoms may be milder if the rupture is contained.

EXAM

Exam reveals hypotension, tachycardia, the presence of an abdominal bruit, or a pulsatile abdominal mass.

DIFFERENTIAL

Appendicitis, biliary disease, diverticular disease, gastritis, PUD, MI, bowel obstruction or infarction, pancreatitis, URI, nephrolithiasis.

DIAGNOSIS

Abdominal CT or MRI (Figure 18.4).

TREATMENT

Initial management includes hemodynamic support, blood transfusions, and immediate consultation for surgical repair.

COMPLICATIONS

Hemorrhage; death from exsanguination.

Note: See the Gastroenterology chapter for a discussion of other urgent and emergent etiologies of abdominal pain.

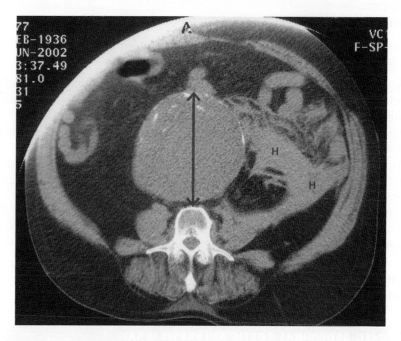

FIGURE 18.4. Ruptured abdominal aortic aneurysm. Transaxial image from noncontrast CT shows very large abdominal aortic aneurysm (*arrow*) with hemorrhage (H) extending into the left retroperitoneum, indicating rupture. (Reproduced, with permission, from Tintinalli JE, et al. *Tintinalli's Emergency Medicine: A Comprehensive Study Guide*, 6th ed. New York: McGraw-Hill, 2004, Fig. 58-3.)

Anaphylaxis

A severe allergic reaction involving more than 1 organ system; caused by the release of mediators from mast cells and basophils. Requires prior sensitization to an allergen with later reexposure, and symptoms can range from urticaria (hives) to angioedema with hypotension and bronchospasm (Table 18.10).

TABLE 18.10. Common Classes of Allergens Causing Anaphylaxis

ALLERGEN	COMMON OFFENDERS	SYMPTOMS/DIAGNOSIS
Medications	Penicillin and cephalosporin antibiotics (most common). IV radiocontrast; aspirin and NSAIDs.	May occur without a prior history of drug exposure. Desensitization or prophylactic pretreatment protocols may be instituted if there is no alternative to the particular allergenic medication.
Foods	Tree nuts, legumes, fish, shellfish, milk, soy, eggs.	Common and usually limited to mild GI symptoms, although full-blown anaphylaxis can occur.
Bites/stings	Insect stings (*Hymenoptera* venom).	Local reactions and urticaria are much more common than full-blown anaphylactic reactions. Consider referral to an allergist for desensitization or a treatment kit with epinephrine and oral antihistamines for patients with a history of anaphylaxis or generalized urticaria following insect stings.
Latex	Surgical gloves, Foley catheters.	Reactions are usually cutaneous or involve the mucous membranes, although anaphylactic reactions can occur.

SYMPTOMS

- Urticaria, flushing, conjunctival and/or cutaneous pruritus, angioedema, warmth, nasal congestion, rhinorrhea, dyspnea, throat tightness, wheezing, weakness, dizziness, chest pain, palpitations, nausea and vomiting (particularly in cases of food allergy).
- Symptoms usually begin within 5–30 minutes of allergen exposure, although in rare cases symptom onset can be delayed for several hours.

EXAM

Although exam findings depend on the affected organ systems and on the severity of the attack, common findings include nonpitting angioedema, hoarseness, wheezing, stridor, hypoxia, tachycardia, hypotension, flushing, urticaria, frank cardiovascular collapse, and respiratory arrest.

DIFFERENTIAL

Angioedema, anxiety, asthma, conversion disorder, carcinoid syndrome, epiglottitis, tracheal foreign bodies, MI, pulmonary embolism, idiopathic urticaria.

DIAGNOSIS

- Diagnosed by clinical history and exam; does not rely on laboratory testing.
- Skin testing and/or in vitro IgE testing may help confirm clinical reactivity.

TREATMENT

- As in all medical emergencies, establish ABCs and stabilize the patient.
- Remove the antigen source or place tourniquet on the extremity with the antigen source (do not leave in place > 30 minutes), then immediately administer IM epinephrine into a different extremity.
- Adjuvant medications include antihistamines (both H_1 and H_2 blockers), inhaled β-agonists, corticosteroids (to prevent late-phase reactions), and IV fluids for BP support.
- In cases of respiratory failure, endotracheal intubation, cricothyrotomy, or tracheotomy may be required.
- Discharge with an epinephrine pen and instructions for self-injection.

Advanced Cardiac Life Support (ACLS)

An algorithm used to treat adult cardiopulmonary arrest. There are four components of the ACLS algorithm: ventricular fibrillation (VF) and ventricular tachycardia (VT); pulseless electrical activity (PEA); bradycardia; and asystole. Figure 18.5 shows the ACLS algorithms for each case.

AIRWAY MANAGEMENT

- Adequate ventilation and oxygenation are crucial. Start with proper airway opening techniques such as head tilt and chin lift, or jaw thrust if trauma is suspected.
- Start bag-mask ventilation immediately, with the use of oropharyngeal or nasopharyngeal airway adjuncts as necessary.
- If bag-mask ventilation is inadequate, consider an advanced airway (endotracheal tube, Combitube, or laryngeal mask airway). Confirm placement

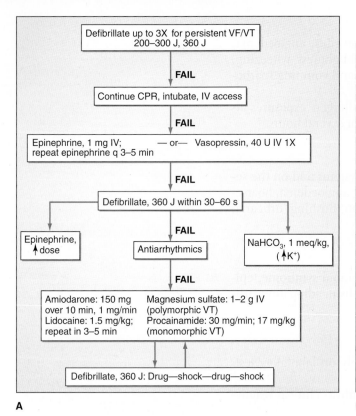

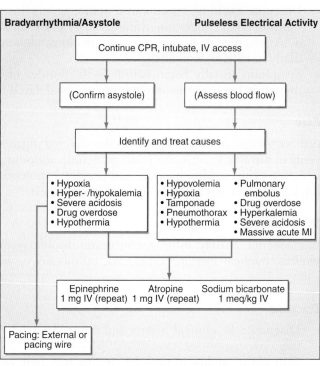

A   B

FIGURE 18.5. **Advanced cardiac life support algorithms.** (**A**) ACLS algorithm for ventricular fibrillation and ventricular tachycardia. (**B**) ACLS algorithm for bradycardia and pulseless electrical activity. (Reproduced, with permission, from Kasper DL, et al. *Harrison's Principles of Internal Medicine*, 16th ed. New York: McGraw-Hill, 2005: 1623.)

with both clinical assessment and confirmatory devices such as exhaled CO_2 detectors or esophageal detector devices.

■ Rapid sequence intubation (Table 18.11) should be used only in patients in whom control of the airway is certain, as the patient will be paralyzed and unable to breathe. Indications include respiratory failure, acute intracranial lesions, some drug overdoses, status epilepticus, and combative trauma patients.

TABLE 18.11. **Rapid Sequence Intubation**

PREPARATION	INDUCTION	PARALYSIS	INTUBATION
Preoxygenation, IV lines, monitor, oximetry, equipment.	Etomidate 0.3 mg/kg (20 mg usual adult dose), **or**	Succinylcholine 1.5 mg (100 mg usual adult dose), **or**	Endotracheal tube, laryngeal mask airway, or Combitube.
Lidocaine 1–2 mg/kg (100 mg usual adult dose)—may be omitted in non–head injury cases.	midazolam 0.1 mg/kg (7 mg usual adult dose).	rocuronium 0.6–1.2 mg/kg (70 mg usual adult dose), **or**	Approximate endotracheal tube size for children = (age/4) ++ 4.
Atropine 0.01 mg/kg (0.5 mg usual adult dose)—may be omitted if bradycardia is absent or if the patient is > 8 years of age.		vecuronium 0.1 mg/kg (10 mg usual adult dose).	Confirm tube placement after intubation.
Sellick maneuver (cricothyroid pressure to prevent vomiting and aspiration).			

Pediatric Advanced Life Support (PALS)

An algorithm used to treat pediatric cardiopulmonary arrest (Figure 18.6). Unlike adult cardiac arrest, the main cause of pediatric arrest is respiratory failure. Therefore, a lone rescuer for an unresponsive child should begin with five cycles of 30 compressions and two breaths and should then activate the emergency medical services system. The ratio of compressions to breaths is 15:2, and the dose of defibrillation is 2 J/kg.

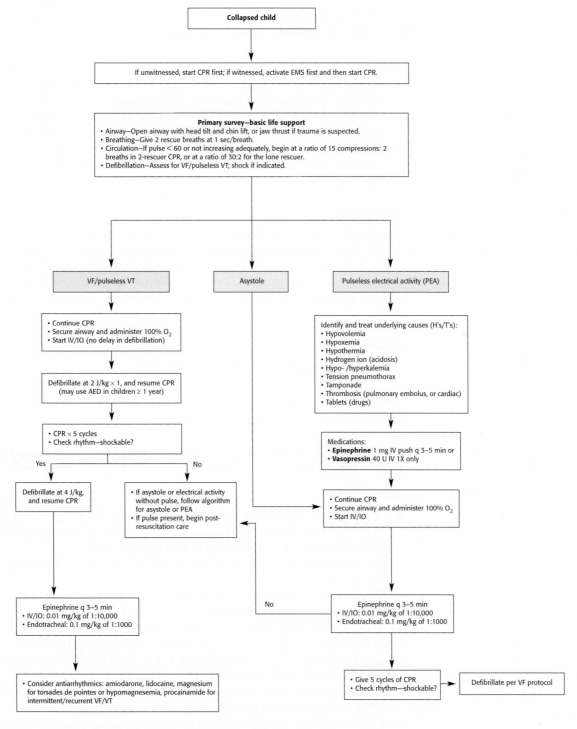

FIGURE 18.6. **PALS algorithm.** (Reproduced, with permission, from USMLERx.com.)

Ocular Disorders

THE RED EYE

A cardinal sign of ocular inflammation; caused by dilation of blood vessels in the eye. Most cases are benign and may be managed effectively by the patient's primary care physician.

SYMPTOMS

Clinical manifestations depend on the underlying etiology but may range from mild discomfort to severe pain with vision loss.

EXAM

- Eyelid inspection; visual acuity testing; examination for extraocular movements, pupil shape and reactivity, photophobia, presence of pain, and discharge; eversion of the upper lid to look for foreign body; fluorescein exam. A thorough exam is best done after application of topical anesthetic drops.
- If available, slit-lamp examination of the cornea, anterior chamber evaluation, ophthalmoscopy, and intraocular pressure measurements can facilitate diagnosis.

DIFFERENTIAL

Blepharitis, chemical burns, orbital or preseptal cellulitis, chalazion or hordeolum, conjunctivitis (allergic, bacterial, viral, and giant papillary types), corneal abrasion, corneal erosion, foreign body, dacryocystitis, dry eye syndrome, ectropion, entropion, endophthalmitis, episcleritis, iritis, acute angle-closure glaucoma, HSV, herpes zoster, pterygium, subconjunctival hemorrhage.

DIAGNOSIS

Usually diagnosed by clinical history and exam.

TREATMENT

Depends on the underlying disease process.

COMMON OCULAR EMERGENCIES

Orbital Cellulitis

- A potentially devastating infection that can rapidly progress to blindness, meningitis, or death. Most cases develop from the direct spread of untreated sinusitis. Considered an **ocular emergency.**
- **Sx:** Erythema, eye pain, fever, photophobia, chemosis, lid edema, visual loss, proptosis.
- **Exam:** Pain may be present with movement of extraocular muscles. Focus the exam on localizing the source of infection.
- **DDx:** Distinguished from preseptal or periorbital cellulitis by involvement of the orbit, which can lead to chemosis, proptosis, or visual loss.
- **Dx:** Leukocytosis; ⊕ blood cultures; CT scan of the orbit, sinus, and head (see Figure 6.4 in the Infectious Diseases chapter).
- **Tx:** IV antibiotics or antifungals; nasal decongestants; ophthalmologic or ENT consultation for possible surgical drainage.
- **Cx:** Visual loss, cavernous sinus thrombosis, brain abscess or meningitis, and death.

Angle-Closure Glaucoma

- A rare condition in which the iris blocks the aqueous humor outflow tract when the pupil becomes mid-dilated, causing an abrupt ↑ in intraocular pressure. Susceptible eyes have a shallow anterior chamber (more common in patients of East Asian origin). Also known as acute narrow-angle glaucoma.
- Considered an **ocular emergency;** prompt treatment is essential to prevent permanent optic nerve damage and vision loss.
- **Sx:** Sudden onset of severe eye pain, blurred vision, nausea/vomiting, and headache.
- **Exam:** Shallow, occluded anterior chamber on gonioscopy; ↑ intraocular pressure; diffuse lacrimation; swollen optic disk; mid-dilated pupil. May be precipitated by pupillary dilation.
- **Tx:** Topical agents to constrict the pupil and ↓ intraocular pressure until the patient can get laser iridotomy or surgical iridectomy.
- **Cx:** Visual loss.

Corneal Abrasion

- Disruption of the integrity of the corneal epithelium, often as a result of external physical forces. Frequently caused by dry eye, foreign body injuries, and wearing of contact lenses. One of the most common, yet often overlooked, eye injuries.
- **Sx:** Eye pain, foreign body sensation, photophobia, tearing, history of traumatic injury or contact lens use.
- **Exam:** A defect in the corneal epithelium is seen with fluorescein staining and Wood's lamp. Slit-lamp examination is helpful but not necessary to diagnose corneal abrasions. Also characterized by bulbar conjunctival injection, normal visual acuity, and possible foreign body seen on eversion of the eyelids.
- **Tx:**
  - Local anesthetic +/– cycoplegic agents, tetanus immunization, topical antibiotics.
  - Ophthalmologic referral if a retained foreign body or corneal ulcer is suspected; follow-up every 2 days until resolved.
  - Eye patching is no longer routinely recommended because of the ↑ risk of infection, especially among contact lens wearers.
  - Systemic analgesics are preferred over local anesthetic drops for patient use because of the potential for causing inadvertent damage to an insensate cornea.
- **Cx:** Usually minimal, although recurrent epithelial erosions or corneal ulcers may occur, leading to permanent loss of visual acuity.

Acute Uveitis

- Inflammation of one or all parts of the uveal tract, including the iris and anterior chamber (iritis), ciliary body (iridocyclitis), and posterior chamber (choroiditis or chorioretinitis).
- **Sx:** Unilateral, painful red eye; blurred vision; tearing; photophobia.
- **Exam:**
  - Perilimbal injection increasing toward the limbus (vs. conjunctivitis); normal or slightly ↓ visual acuity; direct and consensual photophobia; constricted pupils; normal or slightly ↓ intraocular pressure; keratitic precipitates, cells, or flare on slit-lamp exam.
  - The presence of associated conjunctivitis, urethritis, and polyarthritis suggests Reiter syndrome.
- **Dx:** No further workup is indicated for the 1st episode of simple acute uveitis, although bilateral, granulomatous, or recurrent uveitis merits a

workup (CBC, ESR, ANA, RPR, PPD, CXR, Lyme titer) to exclude uncommon etiologies.

■ **Tx:** Cycloplegics to ↓ pain and inflammation; ophthalmologic referral within 24 hours. Topical steroids should be initiated only by the consulting ophthalmologist.

■ **Cx:** An acute ↑ in intraocular pressure, leading to optic nerve atrophy and permanent vision loss.

Orbital Fracture

■ Fracture of any of the 6 facial bones composing the orbit: the frontal bone, zygoma, maxilla, maxillary sinus, lacrimal bone, ethmoid bone, and sphenoid bone. Due to traumatic injuries, blowout fractures occur when a blow to the eye ↑ pressure in the orbit, leading to a fracture of the weakest portion of the orbit, the thin orbital floor (maxilla), and lamina papyracea (ethmoid bone).

■ **Sx:** ↓ visual acuity; enophthalmos; paresthesia of the cheek on the affected side; periorbital ecchymosis and edema; diplopia; symptoms of associated eye injuries.

■ **Exam:** Full ophthalmologic exam plus evaluation for facial asymmetry, tenderness, or step-offs over the orbital bones, as well as for CSF leak and septal hematoma.

■ **Tx:** ABCs and trauma survey. Nasotracheal intubation may be contraindicated in severe facial injuries. Appropriate surgical referrals if indicated.

■ **Dx:** CT of the face and sinus is considered the test of choice (see Figure 18.7).

■ **Cx:** Corneal abrasion, lens dislocation, tears of the uveal tract, retinal detachment, hyphema, ocular muscle entrapment, globe rupture.

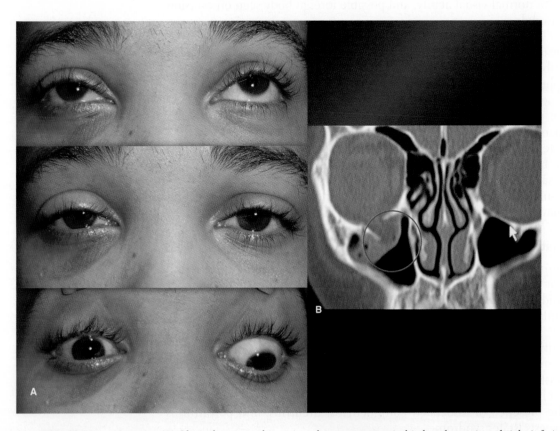

FIGURE 18.7. Orbital blowout fracture. (A) Clinical exam in this patient demonstrates periorbital ecchymosis and right inferior vertical gaze deficit. (B) Coronal reformat from a facial CT shows the fracture of the orbital floor (*red circle*) with herniation of orbital contents through the defect. (Reproduced, with permission, from USMLERx.com.)

Ear, Nose, and Throat Disorders

SEPTAL HEMATOMA

- A blood-filled cavity between the cartilage and supporting perichondrium resulting from nasal trauma. Left untreated, septal hematomas can easily become infected, causing necrosis of the underlying cartilage and permanent saddle nose deformity.
- **Sx/Exam:** Presents with a history of nasal trauma, pain, progressive nasal obstruction, and reddish-purple areas of fluctuance lying on one or both sides of the nasal septum, obstructing the nostril.
- **DDx:** Nasal polyps, deviated septum, enlarged nasal turbinates.
- **Dx:** Usually made clinically; requires a high index of suspicion.
- **Tx:** Aspiration +/– placement of a sterile drain; splints applied to both sides of the septum to provide pressure and support.
- **Cx:** Avascular necrosis of the cartilage; infection or abscess formation; saddle nose deformity.

EPISTAXIS

An acute hemorrhage from the nostril, nasopharynx, or nasal cavity that is frequently encountered in the ER or urgent care setting. Epistaxis may be due to anterior hemorrhage from the Kiesselbach plexus or from the anterior end of the inferior turbinate, or it may result from posterior hemorrhage from branches of the sphenopalatine artery in the posterior nasal cavity or nasopharynx.

SYMPTOMS/EXAM

- May present with a history of frequent epistaxis, anticoagulation use or coagulopathy, vascular abnormalities, or trauma.
- Bleeding from one or both nares is seen.
- Visualize anterior epistaxis using a nasal speculum or blood draining in the posterior pharynx, indicative of posterior epistaxis.

DIFFERENTIAL

Barotrauma, foreign bodies, hemophilia (or other coagulopathy), sinusitis, cocaine use, anticoagulation, hemoptysis, hematemesis.

DIAGNOSIS

- Usually made clinically, but a CT scan or nasopharyngoscopy may be indicated if a neoplasm is suspected.
- CBC, type and cross, bleeding time, and coagulation studies are warranted if the following are suspected: massive or recurrent epistaxis, anticoagulation use, liver failure, coagulopathy, neoplasm, or a platelet disorder.

TREATMENT

- Establish ABCs.
- Maintain continuous pressure over the entire nose for 10 minutes and insert pledgets soaked with anesthetic-vasoconstrictor solution into the nasal cavity. Gently cauterize using silver nitrate if the bleeding site is easily identified, and, if pressure or cautery fails, apply nasal packing using a compressed sponge, Vaseline gauze, or epistaxis balloons. Give empiric

antibiotics with staphylococcal and streptococcal coverage if nasal packing is placed.

■ ENT consultation and hospital admission are indicated in cases of posterior epistaxis that require packing.

COMPLICATIONS

■ Sinusitis, septal hematoma or perforation, aspiration, mucosal pressure necrosis, external nasal deformity.

Cardiac Disorders

MYOCARDIAL INFARCTION (MI)

See the discussion of chest pain for further details.

Fluids, Electrolytes, and Nutrition

DEHYDRATION

A loss of free water disproportionate to the loss of sodium. Dehydration may exist +/− volume depletion. Although dehydration can present in any age group, the highest rates of morbidity and mortality occur in the pediatric population, usually as a result of gastroenteritis and other diarrheal illnesses.

SYMPTOMS/EXAM

Table 18.12 lists the presenting symptoms and corresponding exam findings based on the degree of dehydration.

DIAGNOSIS

BUN-to-creatinine ratio > 20, ↑ urine specific gravity, ↑ serum osmolarity, ↓ arterial pH.

TREATMENT

■ **Mild to moderate dehydration:** Oral rehydration therapy given at doses of 50–100 mL/kg over 4 hours.

TABLE 18.12. Symptoms and Exam Findings of Dehydration

DEGREE OF DEHYDRATION	SYMPTOMS/EXAM
5%–6%	Slightly dry mucous membranes, thirst, concentrated urine, normal tear production, tachycardia 10%–15% above baseline.
7%–8%	Irritability, lethargy, dry skin, dizziness, flushing, headaches, very dry mucous membranes, ↓ tear production, resting tachycardia, weak peripheral pulses, ↓ skin turgor, oliguria, sunken eyeballs, sunken anterior fontanelle (in infants), tachypnea.
> 9%	Resting tachycardia or bradycardia, weak central pulses, cold and mottled skin, hypotension, delayed capillary refill, spastic muscles, lethargy, coma.

- **Severe dehydration:** IV rehydration (with calculation of electrolyte and free water deficits, maintenance requirements, and replacement of ongoing losses). Begin with isotonic fluids in 20 mL/kg boluses.
- Follow the "**4-2-1 rule**" for estimating maintenance fluid requirements: 4 mL/kg/hr for the first 10 kg of weight; 2 mL/kg/hr for the second 10 kg of weight; and 1 mL/kg/hr for each additional kilogram thereafter—eg, the maintenance rate for a child weighing 24 kg is $(4 \times 10) + (2 \times 10) + (1 \times 4) = 64$ mL/hr.

COMPLICATIONS

Iatrogenic electrolyte imbalances, CNS sequelae from overly aggressive replacement of volume deficits, coma, death.

Dermatologic Disorders

Erythema multiforme (EM), Stevens-Johnson syndrome (SJS), and toxic epidermal necrolysis (TEN) are thought to be variants of the same disease spectrum, whose features include widespread distribution of skin and mucosal lesions. Commonly affected sites include the torso, face, palms, soles, and extensor surfaces. SJS and TEN are the more serious variants and carry mortality rates of 5% and 40%, respectively (Table 18.13). The conditions are distinguished as follows:

- **Erythema multiforme:** A generally benign process characterized by target lesions in a symmetric distribution of the extremities (see Figure 10.33 in the Dermatology chapter for an image of EM), often involving the oral mucosa. Usually 2° to prior infection with a herpesvirus, EM has very low morbidity and is often recurrent.
- **SJS:** An immune complex–mediated hypersensitivity reaction involving the skin and mucous membranes (Figure 18.8). Also known as erythema

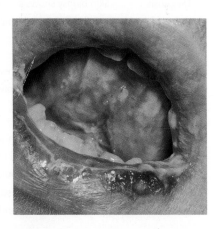

FIGURE 18.8. Stevens-Johnson syndrome involving the mucous membranes. (Reproduced, with permission, from Wolff K, et al. *Fitzpatrick's Dermatology in General Medicine*, 7th ed. New York: McGraw-Hill, 2008, Fig. 39-4A.)

TABLE 18.13. Stevens-Johnson Syndrome vs. Toxic Epidermal Necrolysis

	STEVENS-JOHNSON SYNDROME	TOXIC EPIDERMAL NECROLYSIS
Symptoms	**Chief complaint:** Pain associated with a rash. 1- to 14-day prodrome consisting of fever, sore throat, cough, malaise, arthralgias, chills, headache, vomiting, and diarrhea. Nonpruritic mucocutaneous lesions last 2–4 weeks.	**Chief complaint:** Pain associated with a rash. 2- to 3-day prodrome consisting of fever, sore throat, cough, malaise, arthralgias, and anorexia. 8- to 12-day acute phase consisting of persistent fevers, generalized epidermal sloughing, and mucosal involvement.
Exam	A nonpruritic macular rash develops into papules, vesicles, bullae, and confluent erythema with a characteristic target appearance. < 10% of body surface area (BSA) is affected. Associated findings include fever, tachycardia, orthostasis, hypotension, altered mental status, epistaxis, conjunctivitis, erosive vulvovaginitis or balanitis, seizures, and coma.	An erythematous maculopapular rash with bullae, erosions, and targetlike lesions, rapidly leading to confluent blisters that easily slough off. More than 30% of BSA is affected. ⊕ Nikolsky sign—epidermis separation when pressure is applied laterally to the epidermal surface. Associated findings are the same as those for SJS.

(continues)

TABLE 18.13.   **Stevens-Johnson Syndrome vs. Toxic Epidermal Necrolysis** *(continued)*

	STEVENS-JOHNSON SYNDROME	TOXIC EPIDERMAL NECROLYSIS
History	Drug exposure (sulfa, phenytoin, allopurinol, and penicillin are most commonly implicated), malignancies, vaccinations, and infections.	Same as that for SJS, but drugs are almost always the cause of TEN.
Differential	Chemical or thermal burns, exfoliative dermatitis, EM, pemphigus, cutaneous T-cell lymphoma, staphylococcal scalded skin syndrome, toxic shock syndrome.	Same as that for SJS.
Diagnosis	Skin biopsy shows subepidermal bullae +/− epidermal cell necrosis and lymphocytic infiltration of perivascular areas.	Skin biopsy shows full-thickness epidermal necrosis with little dermal and epidermal inflammation.
Treatment	Supportive treatment with airway management, fluid replacement, electrolyte correction, wound care, and pain control.	Same as that for SJS, but referral to a burn center and treatment with plasmapheresis or IVIG may also be indicated in TEN.
Complications	Depends on the organ system involved, but may include 2° infection, corneal ulceration, anterior uveitis, blindness, renal tubular necrosis, renal failure, vaginal or penile scarring, esophageal strictures, GI hemorrhage, respiratory failure, and cosmetic deformity.	Same as those for SJS.

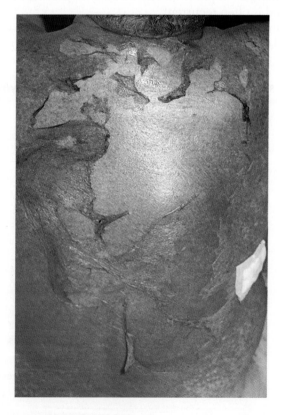

FIGURE 18.9.   **Toxic epidermal necrolysis.** Characterized by confluent rash with skin sloughing leading to extremely painful erosions. Patients with TEN have increased risk of infection and dehydration, much like burn patients. (Reproduced, with permission, from Wolff K, Johnson RA. *Fitzpatrick's Color Atlas and Synopsis of Clinical Dermatology,* 6th ed. New York: McGraw-Hill, 2009, Fig. 8-8.)

multiforme major, SJS is a serious systemic illness that can cause significant morbidity and mortality.

- **TEN:** A rapidly evolving mucocutaneous reaction characterized by widespread erythema, necrosis, and bullous detachment of the epidermis (Figure 18.9). More often seen in adults, TEN is potentially life threatening and is a true dermatologic emergency requiring prompt diagnosis and treatment.

Environmental Stressors

HYPOTHERMIA

A decline in core temperature < 35°C (95°F) due to either accidental exposure to cold (1°) or a failure of thermoregulatory function (2°). Most cases in the United States occur in an urban setting and are related to homelessness, coexisting psychiatric illness, trauma, substance abuse, or advanced age.

SYMPTOMS/EXAM

Table 18.14 lists the symptoms and exam findings for the different degrees of hypothermia. To ensure appropriate diagnosis, a true core temperature should be measured using a low-reading temperature probe in the bladder, esophagus, or rectum.

DIFFERENTIAL

Stroke, drug toxicity, hypothyroidism, hypopituitarism, frostbite, alcoholism, septic or hemorrhagic shock, delirium, anorexia nervosa, spinal cord injury, MI, CNS trauma.

DIAGNOSIS

↑ hematocrit (↑ 2% for each 1°C drop in core temperature) due to volume contraction; electrolyte abnormalities; hypoglycemia or hyperglycemia; ↑ pH and ↓ Pao_2 and $Paco_2$ on ABG; prolonged bleeding time; PR, QRS, and QTc prolongation and Osborn (J) waves on ECG.

TREATMENT

- **Rewarming measures:** Removal of wet clothing; heat packs or warmed blankets applied to the axillae, groin, and abdomen; provision of warmed, humidified O_2 and heated IV saline; warmed gastric, thoracic, and/or peri-

TABLE 18.14.   Symptoms and Exam Findings of Hypothermia

DEGREE OF HYPOTHERMIA	SYMPTOMS	EXAM
Mild 32°–35°C (89.6°–95°F)	Lethargy, confusion, shivering, loss of fine motor coordination.	Shivering, altered mental status, tachypnea, tachycardia, vasoconstriction, dysarthria, ataxia, lethargy.
Moderate 28°–32°C (82.4°–89.6°F)	Delirium, slowed reflexes.	Bradycardia, cessation of shivering, stupor, dilated pupils, arrhythmias.
Severe < 28°C (82.4°F)	Unresponsiveness, coma, respiratory difficulties.	Rigidity, apnea, hypotension, very cold skin, areflexia, fixed pupils, unresponsiveness, VF.

toneal lavage; warm water immersion; initiation of CPR as needed; hemodialysis; cardiopulmonary bypass.
■ Patients with hypothermia may appear dead; therefore, patients are not considered dead until they are warm and dead.

COMPLICATIONS

Cardiac arrhythmias, hypotension due to marked vasodilation during rewarming, aspiration pneumonia, pulmonary edema, peritonitis, acute tubular necrosis, metabolic acidosis, rhabdomyolysis, gangrene, compartment syndrome, death.

KEY FACT

Patients with hypothermia are not considered dead until they are warm and dead.

HYPERTHERMIA

Represents a continuum of illness ranging from heat exhaustion to heat stroke. Heat exhaustion, the most common heat-related illness, involves a mild to moderate dysfunction of temperature control caused by ↑ ambient temperatures and/or strenuous exercise, leading to dehydration and salt depletion. Heat stroke, which is associated with a systemic inflammatory response, is extreme hyperthermia (> 41.1°C [106°F]) that leads to end-organ damage and significant morbidity and mortality.

SYMPTOMS

Depends on the degree of heat illness, but may include fatigue, weakness, nausea and vomiting, headache, muscle cramps, irritability, altered mental status, coma, sweating, and, later, anhidrosis.

EXAM

↑ temperature (usually > 41°C [105.8°F]), tachycardia, orthostatic pulse and BP changes, piloerection, tachypnea, hyperventilation, CNS dysfunction, muscle tenderness, signs of DIC, and GU symptoms (hematuria, oliguria, or anuria) that may be due to concurrent acute renal failure.

DIFFERENTIAL

Delirium, DKA, DTs, hepatic or uremic encephalopathy, hyperthyroidism, encephalitis, meningitis, neuroleptic malignant syndrome, tetanus, status epilepticus, septic shock, cerebral malaria, drug toxicity (especially cocaine, amphetamine, phencyclidine, salicylates, anticholinergics, and MAOIs).

DIAGNOSIS

■ **Labs:** Laboratory studies are used primarily to detect end-organ damage and include CBC, coagulation panel (abnormal in concurrent DIC), metabolic panel, UA, hepatic enzymes (almost universally ↑ in heat stroke), CK (↑), serum glucose (reveals hypoglycemia), and ABG (reveals respiratory alkalosis and/or metabolic acidosis).
■ **Imaging:** CXR, head CT to rule out other causes of altered mental status.

TREATMENT

■ **Heat stroke is a medical emergency** requiring rapid reduction of core body temperature, as the duration of hyperthermia is the main determinant of outcome.
■ The ideal goal rate for decreasing core temperature is 0.2°C/min; the target goal is 39°C (102.2°F).
■ Rapid cooling measures include removal of clothing, covering the patient with ice water–soaked sheets or ice packs, ice water immersion, and evaporative techniques.

- Supportive measures include infusing $D_{50}W$ in IV lines to prevent hypoglycemia, placing an NG tube to monitor for GI bleeding and fluid losses, constant monitoring of core temperature, inserting a Foley catheter to monitor urine output, placing a Swan-Ganz catheter to guide fluid management, and mechanical ventilation if indicated.
- Useful adjunctive medications include benzodiazepines to stop agitation, shivering (caused by cooling measures), and seizures, as well as barbiturates for refractory seizures.
- Avoid anticholinergics, α-adrenergic agonists, and antipyretics.

COMPLICATIONS

Seizures, neurologic deficits, rhabdomyolysis, acute renal failure, hepatic failure, DIC, ARDS, pulmonary edema, respiratory alkalosis, electrolyte imbalances, death.

ALTITUDE SICKNESS

A 21-year-old medical student from New Orleans, Louisiana (below sea level), traveled to Cusco, Peru (approximately 11,000 feet), to hike the Inca trail to Machu Picchu. After spending a restless night at altitude, she awoke the next morning with a severe headache. Throughout the day, she felt lethargic and nauseated and vomited twice. By the next morning, her symptoms had resolved and she was able to hike the trail with no problems. What is her most likely diagnosis?

Acute mountain sickness. Gradual acclimatization and adjuvant treatment with acetazolamide result in timely resolution of symptoms.

One of a group of syndromes resulting from altitude-induced hypoxia. Acute mountain sickness (AMS) is caused by a fundamental lack of O_2 related to both the ascent rate and the maximum altitude achieved and represents the mildest and most common form of altitude illness. Other diseases in the spectrum include high-altitude pulmonary edema (HAPE) and high-altitude cerebral edema (HACE), which generally occur at elevations of 3500–5500 m (11,000–18,000 feet).

SYMPTOMS

Headache, anorexia, nausea, vomiting, weakness, lightheadedness, fluid retention with ↓ urination.

EXAM

There are no characteristic physical findings in AMS, but patients appear ill. Ataxia and altered mental status suggest HACE; cough, rales or wheezing, dyspnea, tachypnea, tachycardia, and low-grade fevers suggest HAPE.

DIFFERENTIAL

Anxiety, asthma, COPD, dehydration, MI, pneumonia, pulmonary embolism.

DIAGNOSIS

Usually made by clinical history and exam, but ↓ arterial O_2 saturation and a CXR showing unilateral or bilateral fluffy infiltrates are characteristic of HAPE.

TREATMENT

- For HAPE and HACE, definitive treatment is descent, but supplemental O_2, nifedipine, and portable hyperbaric chambers may be useful adjunctive treatments.
- For AMS, slow, gradual ascent with time for acclimatization, supplemental O_2, acetazolamide, and dexamethasone help both to prevent and to treat symptoms.

FROSTBITE

A cold-related injury due to formation of ice crystals within tissues and cellular death. Common sites of injury include the hands, feet, and exposed tissue such as the ears, nose, and lips.

SYMPTOMS

Coldness, stinging, numbness, burning, clumsiness, throbbing or burning pain on rewarming.

EXAM

- Findings depend on the degree of injury, but all injuries may cause joint pain, excessive sweating, bluish discoloration, hyperemia, skin necrosis, or gangrene (Figure 18.10).
- Severity of frostbite is distinguished as follows:
    - **First degree:** Erythema, edema, nonsensate white plaque with surrounding hyperemia.
    - **Second degree:** Clear blisters with surrounding erythema within 24 hours of injury.
    - **Third degree:** Hemorrhagic blisters followed by eschar formation over several weeks.
    - **Fourth degree:** Focal necrosis with tissue loss.

DIAGNOSIS

No routine lab tests or radiographs are indicated, but technetium scintigraphy or MRI may help visualize nonviable tissue earlier than clinical examination.

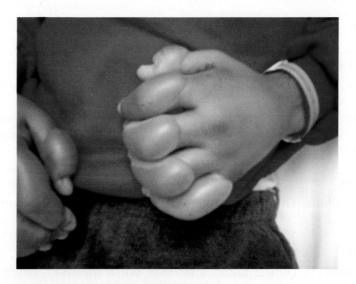

FIGURE 18.10. Frostbite. (Courtesy of Mark Sochor, MD.)

TREATMENT

- Rapid rewarming of affected parts (as long as it can be maintained) in circulating warm water at 40°–42°C (104°–108°F) for 15–30 minutes until thawing is complete.
- Topical application of aloe vera to debrided clear blisters and intact hemorrhagic blisters; elevation of affected parts; tetanus prophylaxis; analgesia as needed; daily hydrotherapy.
- Optional antibiotic coverage to prevent infection.
- Surgical debridement should be delayed for 3–4 weeks to prevent removal of viable tissue.

COMPLICATIONS

Sensory deficits, hyperhidrosis or anhidrosis, abnormal color changes, phantom pain of amputated extremities, cold sensitivity, joint pains, wound infection, tetanus, gangrene, death.

BURNS

May be classified by etiology into thermal, chemical, or radiation burns. Thermal burns are most common and occur when soft tissue is exposed to temperatures > 45.5°C (114°F). Regardless of the mechanism of thermal burn (scald, contact, steam, flame, gas, flash, or electrical), the injury involves ↑ capillary permeability, fluid loss, and ↑ plasma viscosity, leading to microthrombus formation.

SYMPTOMS/EXAM

As with frostbite, above, findings depend on the degree of injury:

- **First degree:** Red, warm, painful tissue involving the epidermis that blanches with pressure.
- **Second degree:** Red, wet, painful tissue +/− blisters involving the epidermis and portions of the dermis.
- **Third degree:** Dry, insensate, waxy, leathery tissue +/− overlying blisters involving the epidermis, dermis, and possibly underlying subcutaneous fat tissue, muscle, and bone.

DIAGNOSIS

- Evaluation of the extent (in BSA) and depth of burn is crucial for appropriate management.
- The extent of injury in adults may be estimated using the "rule of 9s" (Figure 18.11).
- Severe burns necessitate CBC, chemistry panel, ABG with carboxyhemoglobin, coagulation panel, UA, type and screen, CPK and urine myoglobin (in electrical burns), and CXR for suspected inhalational injuries.

TREATMENT

- Superficial burns may be managed in an outpatient setting with wound cleansing, pain control, topical dressing, and appropriate follow-up care.
- Deeper or more extensive burns should be managed in an inpatient setting (preferably a burn center) with establishment of the ABCs, fluid resuscitation using isotonic crystalloid solution for the first 24 hours (may use modified Brooke or Parkland formulas to calculate fluid deficit), wound excision and grafting if necessary, and rehabilitation.
- Topical medications include silver sulfadiazine, aqueous 0.5% silver nitrate, petrolatum, debriding enzymes, and topical antibiotic ointments.

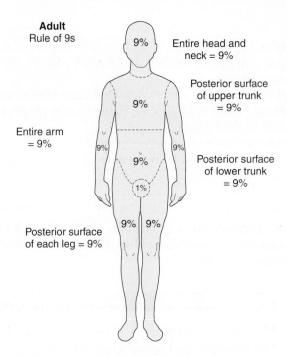

FIGURE 18.11. **Adult "rule of 9s" for burn evaluation.** (Reproduced, with permission, from McPhee SJ, Papadakis MA. *Current Medical Diagnosis and Treatment*, 49th ed. New York: McGraw-Hill, 2010, Fig. 37-2.)

COMPLICATIONS

Scarring, cosmetic deformity, burn infections, ARDS, sepsis, death.

Psychiatric Disorders

PSYCHOSIS

Defined as an impaired sense of reality, leading to an inability to communicate, emotional turmoil, and impaired cognitive abilities. Not a diagnosis in itself, psychosis is often linked to schizophrenia, severe clinical depression, bipolar disorder, drug intoxication and withdrawal (in particular, cocaine, amphetamines, PCP, and hallucinogens), SLE, dementia, traumatic brain injury, and electrolyte imbalances in the elderly.

SYMPTOMS/EXAM

Hallucinations, delusions, personality changes, disorganized thinking, lack of insight.

DIAGNOSIS

Usually made clinically, but laboratory testing and head imaging may be indicated to rule out organic causes of acute psychosis (eg, CBC, UA, LFTs, chemistry panel, TFTs, VDRL, HIV, and toxicology screen; heavy metal screen and ceruloplasmin level are rarely indicated).

TREATMENT

- Antipsychotics are given initially to control behavior, followed by hospitalization and long-term treatment directed toward the underlying etiology.

- Rapid tranquilization is necessary for violent, extremely agitated patients:
  - **Typical antipsychotics** (eg, droperidol, haloperidol, chlorpromazine): Given with diphenhydramine or benztropine to prevent extrapyramidal reactions.
  - **Atypical antipsychotics** (eg, olanzapine, risperidone).
  - **Benzodiazepines:** May be used as adjuncts to antipsychotics for sedative effects; the drugs of choice for alcohol and benzodiazepine withdrawal.

SUICIDAL IDEATION

Risk factors associated with completed suicide include male gender, white race, advancing age, widowed or divorced status, living alone, access to firearms, coexisting psychiatric disorders or substance abuse, major life stressors, and a prior personal or family history of suicide attempt.

SYMPTOMS/EXAM

Anhedonia, hopelessness, insomnia, anxiety, impaired concentration, psychomotor agitation.

DIAGNOSIS

Made clinically through a thorough psychiatric history, including discussion of the following factors:

- **Extent of suicidal ideation:** When suicidal thoughts began, precipitating factors, frequency of thoughts, aggravating/alleviating factors, formulation of suicidal plan, ability to control suicidal thoughts, deterrents to carrying out plan.
- **Lethality of suicidal plan:** Access to firearms and harmful medications, recent changes in will or life insurance policy, prior attempts.

TREATMENT

- Immediate hospitalization is indicated for all patients with a plan, access to lethal means, recent social stressors, and symptoms indicative of a psychiatric disorder.
- Involuntary commitment may be made if a person poses an imminent danger to self or others or displays an inability to care for self.
- Outpatient treatment may be an option if the patient is able to make a contract for safety, displays good judgment, and has adequate social support.
- Antidepressant therapy (in particular, SSRIs) and close monitoring are essential, as patients may be at ↑ risk for suicide as their energy level improves while the depressed mood persists. MAOIs are contraindicated in suicidal ideation because of their lethal potential in the event of an overdose.

HOMICIDAL IDEATION

SYMPTOMS/EXAM

Prior history of violence, coexisting psychiatric disorder, substance abuse, access to weapons.

KEY FACT

Although 80% of people who commit suicide are men, the majority of people who make nonfatal suicide attempts are women 25–44 years of age.

DIAGNOSIS

As with suicide, no clinician is able to predict what will happen. Thus, the goal is accurate risk assessment to develop a reasonable treatment plan and prevent injury.

TREATMENT

- Immediate hospitalization in all patients with a plan, access to lethal means, and symptoms indicative of a psychiatric disorder.
- Involuntary commitment may be made if a person poses an imminent danger to self or others or displays an inability to care for self.
- Initiation of appropriate psychiatric intervention, depending on the underlying diagnosis.

Trauma

The fourth-leading killer among Americans and the main cause of death in individuals < 45 years of age. Trauma care is predicated on the concepts of rapid triage, diagnosis, resuscitation, and therapeutic intervention. Evaluation of trauma is categorized by 2 main surveys: the 1° survey and the 2° survey.

- **1° survey (ABCDE):**
  - **Airway:** Establish an airway using a jaw thrust maneuver.
  - **Breathing:** Ventilate with 100% O_2 and check for breathing compromise.
  - **Circulation:** Apply pressure to sites of external bleeding, place 2 large-bore IV lines, assess blood volume status, and begin fluid resuscitation if hypovolemia is present.
  - **Disability:** Document functional status and perform a brief neurologic examination.
  - **Exposure:** Completely disrobe the patient and logroll to inspect the back.
- **2° survey:**
  - Perform a head-to-toe examination to search for other injuries and set further priorities.
  - May include trauma series imaging, Foley catheter placement, gastric tube placement, splinting of unstable fractures/dislocations, tetanus prophylaxis, surgical consultation, and medications.

HEAD TRAUMA

The cause of death in one-third of all traumatic deaths in persons < 45 years of age. Traumatic brain injury can result from **direct injury** caused by the force of an object striking the head or **indirect injury** from acceleration/deceleration forces. The GCS should be used to assess all patients with head trauma (Table 18.15).

SYMPTOMS/EXAM

- **Low-risk injuries:** Characterized by minor trauma, scalp wounds, a GCS score of 15, a normal neurologic exam, and the absence of signs of intracranial injury.
- **Moderate- to high-risk injuries:** Characterized by loss of consciousness, persistent nausea and vomiting, seizures, severe headaches, focal neurologic signs, presence of penetrating skull injuries, evidence of basilar skull

TABLE 18.15. **Glasgow Coma Scale for All Age Groups**

RESPONSE/SCORE	4 YEARS TO ADULT	CHILDREN < 4 YEARS	INFANTS
Eye opening			
4	Spontaneous.	Spontaneous.	Spontaneous.
3	To speech.	To speech.	To speech.
2	To pain.	To pain.	To pain.
1	No response.	No response.	No response.
Verbal response			
5	Alert and oriented.	Oriented, social, interacts.	Coos, babbles.
4	Disoriented conversation.	Confused speech, disoriented, consolable, aware.	Irritable cry.
3	Speaking but nonsensical.	Inappropriate words, inconsolable, unaware.	Cries to pain.
2	Moans or unintelligible sound.	Incomprehensible, agitated, restless, unaware.	Moans to pain.
1	No response.	No response.	No response.
Motor response			
6	Follows commands.	Normal, spontaneous movements.	Normal, spontaneous movements.
5	Localizes pain.	Localizes pain.	Withdraws to touch.
4	Withdraws to pain.	Withdraws to pain.	Withdraws to pain.
3	Decorticate flexion.	Decorticate flexion.	Decorticate flexion.
2	Decerebrate extension.	Decerebrate extension.	Decerebrate extension.
1	No response.	No response.	No response.

fracture (eg, CSF rhinorrhea, Battle sign, raccoon eyes, hemotympanum), a GCS score < 14, and altered mental status.

DIAGNOSIS

Head CT and skull radiographs are generally not indicated in adults unless depressed fracture is suspected and palpation of the skull is not possible or moderate- to high-risk features are present.

TREATMENT

- Establish ABCs, including cervical spine immobilization and intubation if the patient is unable to protect the airway.
- Prompt neurosurgical consultation if a high-risk injury is suspected.
- Hyperventilation to maintain a P_{CO_2} of 25–30, maintenance of normal cardiac output, mannitol, and elevation of the head of the bed to 30 degrees to ↓ ICP.

COMPLICATIONS

Postconcussion syndrome, seizures, neurologic deficits, death.

NECK TRAUMA

May be classified as penetrating or blunt trauma; one half of blunt trauma neck injuries are due to motor vehicle accidents. Optimal management of patients with neck trauma is challenging, as seemingly minor injuries can rapidly become life threatening.

SYMPTOMS/EXAM

- Depends on the type of injury, but may include active bleeding, large or expanding hematomas, diminished pulses or bruits, lateralizing signs, tracheal deviation, subcutaneous emphysema, cranial nerve palsies, stridor, hoarseness, vocal cord paralysis, hemoptysis, or hematemesis.
- To clear cervical spine fractures clinically, patients must meet all of the following criteria: no neck pain or tenderness on palpation, no history of loss of consciousness, no altered mental status, no symptoms referable to a neck injury (eg, paralysis, sensory changes), and no other distracting painful injuries.

DIAGNOSIS

- Three-view radiographs showing all 7 cervical vertebrae, the C7–T1 interspace, and a lateral view. If visualization of C-spine on x-ray is incomplete or equivocal findings are noted, CT imaging is indicated (Figure 18.12).
- A full spine series is indicated in patients with 1 spinal fracture.
- Consider CT angiography in the presence of a penetrating neck trauma close to the arterial blood supply.

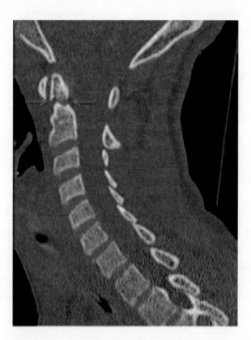

FIGURE 18.12. **Cervical spine fracture.** A sagittal reformation of a cervical spine CT shows a fracture through the base of the dens, a type 2 odontoid fracture *(red arrows)*. (Reproduced, with permission, from USMLERx.com.)

TREATMENT

Establish airway (orotracheal intubation, cricothyroidotomy, or tracheostomy); stop bleeding; stabilize the cervical spine until clearance can be definitively made.

SPINAL CORD TRAUMA

One of the most devastating trauma-related injuries. The majority of spinal cord trauma cases are caused by blunt trauma from motor vehicle accidents and occur most frequently on weekends and holidays and during the summer months.

SYMPTOMS/EXAM

Depends on the degree of injury, but may include flaccid paralysis and loss of sensation below the level of the lesion, urinary and fecal retention, loss of reflex activity, spastic paraplegia or quadriplegia, hyperreflexia and extensor plantar responses, priapism, paralytic ileus, vasomotor instability due to spinal neurogenic shock, loss of temperature and pain appreciation, or hypoventilation and hypoxia if above C5.

DIAGNOSIS

Complete spinal series, portable CXR and pelvic radiograph, CT for evaluation of bony elements, MRI for evaluation of the spinal cord.

TREATMENT

Prompt neurosurgical consultation, methylprednisolone 30 mg/kg within 8 hours of injury, anatomic realignment of the spinal cord, immobilization.

COMPLICATIONS

Decubitus ulcers, URI, depression, sensory deficits, incontinence, paralysis, death.

OPHTHALMOLOGIC TRAUMA

Commonly manifests as orbital floor ("blowout") fractures resulting from blunt anteroposterior force directed against the eyeball. See the discussion of common ocular emergencies, above, for more details.

Other common consequences of ocular trauma necessitating immediate consultation include hyphema (postinjury accumulation of blood in the anterior chamber) and ruptured globe (disruption of the integrity of its outer membranes by blunt or penetrating trauma).

MAXILLOFACIAL TRAUMA

Includes injuries to any bony or fleshy structure of the face caused by physical force, foreign objects, or burns. Maxillofacial trauma is most often due to athletic injuries, assaults, or motor vehicle accidents and should raise the question of domestic violence.

SYMPTOMS/EXAM

- Pain, swelling, bleeding, ecchymosis, bony deformity, paresthesias, epistaxis, CSF rhinorrhea, difficulty breathing.
- A patient's description of malaligned teeth is a sensitive indicator that a mandibular or maxillary fracture is present.

DIAGNOSIS

Can be made clinically, but plain film radiographs and CT scans may help diagnose fractures.

TREATMENT

Depends on the type of injury, but may include establishment of an airway; realignment and immobilization of fractures; pain control; and prompt referral to an otolaryngologist, a plastic surgeon, or an oral and maxillofacial surgeon if indicated.

COMPLICATIONS

Permanent facial deformity, chronic sinusitis, nonunion of fractures, hemorrhage, scars, nerve damage, infection, airway compromise, chronic pain.

ABDOMINAL TRAUMA

A leading cause of morbidity and mortality among all age groups. Abdominal trauma may be due to blunt injuries, the majority of which are due to motor vehicle accidents, or penetrating injuries, which are predominantly due to gunshot or stab wounds. Initial evaluation should be directed toward diagnosing hemorrhage, solid organ injury, or bowel rupture.

SYMPTOMS/EXAM

Lap-belt ecchymosis, abdominal pain, tenderness over the ribs, referred pain to the left (splenic injury) or right (liver injury) shoulder, hypotension, gross hematuria, flank discoloration, acute abdomen.

DIAGNOSIS

CXR, AXR, abdominal CT with contrast, FAST ultrasound, IVP, diagnostic peritoneal lavage (to detect the presence of intraperitoneal blood), exploratory laparotomy (Figures 18.13 and 18.14).

TREATMENT

Blood transfusions, pain control, fluid resuscitation, prompt surgical referrals if indicated.

COMPLICATIONS

Intra-abdominal sepsis, hemorrhage or abscess formation, delayed rupture of solid organs, infection, death.

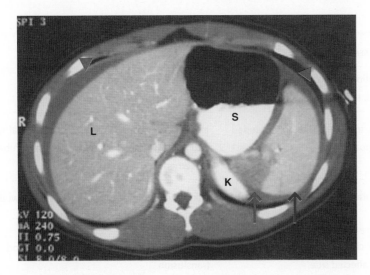

FIGURE 18.13. **Abdominal trauma.** A transaxial image from an abdominal CT in a trauma patient shows a splenic laceration (*red arrow*), which enhances less-than-normal splenic tissue (*blue arrow*), and hemoperitoneum (*red arrowheads*). L = liver; S = stomach; K = left kidney. (Reproduced, with permission, from Stone CK, Humphries RL. *Current Diagnosis & Treatment: Emergency Medicine,* 6th ed. New York: McGraw-Hill, 2008, Fig. 23-2.)

CHEST TRAUMA

Present in one-half of all patients with trauma-related injuries. Approximately 25% of all trauma deaths are directly attributable to chest trauma. Table 18.16 lists immediately and potentially life-threatening thoracic injuries.

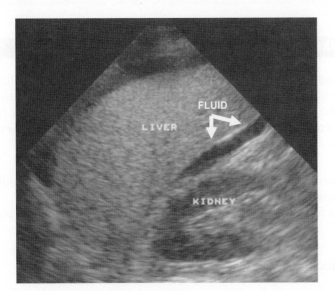

FIGURE 18.14. **FAST scan in abdominal trauma.** Longitudinal image from a trauma FAST ultrasound shows hemoperitoneum (labeled "fluid") in the hepatorenal space. (Reproduced, with permission, from Brunicardi FC, et al. *Schwartz's Principles of Surgery,* 9th ed. New York: McGraw-Hill, 2010, Fig. 7-28A.)

TABLE 18.16. Traumatic Chest Injuries

Type of Injury	Presentation	Treatment
Flail chest	Paradoxical chest wall motion due to multiple fractured ribs, chest pain, tachypnea, shallow respirations, crepitus.	Intubation if ventilation is compromised, supplemental O_2, pain control.
Tension pneumothorax	↓ breath sounds, dyspnea, tracheal deviation, distended neck veins, chest pain, hypotension.	Needle thoracostomy in the 2nd intercostal space and midclavicular line, followed by chest tube placement.
Open pneumothorax	↓ breath sounds, open thoracic wound, dyspnea, chest pain.	Occlusive dressing taped on 3 sides, followed by chest tube placement and wound closure.
Massive hemothorax	↓ breath sounds, dyspnea, chest pain, no midline shift, dullness to percussion on affected side.	Chest tube placement, surgical repair, blood transfusion.
Cardiac tamponade	JVD, muffled heart sounds, pulsus paradoxus, hypotension, tachycardia.	Pericardiocentesis, fluid infusion.
Myocardial contusion	Blunt trauma to the heart, causing episodes of chest pain, paroxysmal supraventricular tachycardia, or self-limited ventricular tachycardia; abnormal ECG.	Supportive care.
Aortic disruption	Chest and back pain, dyspnea, hypotension, enlarged aortic knob, widened mediastinum, and rightward esophageal deviation on CXR.	BP control, surgical repair.

CHEST WALL TRAUMA

A significant source of morbidity and mortality in the United States, blunt injury to the chest includes chest wall fractures, dislocations, barotraumas, or injuries to the pleurae, lungs, digestive tract, heart, great vessels, or lymphatics. The most common cause of blunt chest trauma is motor vehicle accidents.

SYMPTOMS

- Symptoms may range from minor pain to florid shock, depending on the mechanism of injury and the organ systems involved.
- Rib fractures (ribs 4–10) are the most common blunt thoracic injuries.

EXAM

Clinical findings depend on the organ systems affected.

DIAGNOSIS

ECG, CXR, chest CT, TEE or transthoracic echocardiography (TTE), esophagoscopy (if esophageal injury is suspected), bronchoscopy (if tracheobronchial injury is suspected), aortography (if aortic injury is suspected; Figure 18.15).

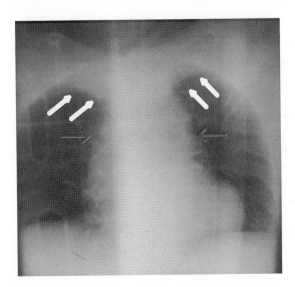

FIGURE 18.15. **Aortic injury.** A frontal CXR in a trauma patient shows widening of the superior mediastinum *(red arrows)*, with bilateral "apical caps" *(white arrows)* corresponding to mediastinal bleeding extending into the extrapleural spaces above the lung apices. (Reproduced, with permission, from Brunicardi FC, et al. *Schwartz's Principles of Surgery,* 9th ed. New York: McGraw-Hill, 2010, Fig. 7-23A.)

TREATMENT

- Most patients do not require surgical treatment and can be treated with supportive measures and simple interventions such as tube thoracostomy.
- Regardless of the type of injury, all patients require initial establishment of ABCs and a trauma survey.
- Immediate surgery is indicated for patients with loss of chest wall integrity; blunt diaphragmatic injuries; massive air leak following chest tube insertion; massive hemothorax; cardiac tamponade; pulmonary or cardiac emboli; or confirmed tracheal, major bronchial, esophageal, or great vessel injury.

COMPLICATIONS

Wound infection, MI, arrhythmias, septal defects, valvular insufficiency, aneurysm formation, respiratory infections, hemothorax, fistula formation, stroke, DVT.

HAND INJURIES

Common injuries seen in the ER or urgent care setting but seldom life threatening, hand injuries may cause significant disability and include soft tissue injuries, nerve damage, sprains, dislocations, and fractures. Hand injuries may be isolated or part of multisystem trauma.

SYMPTOMS/EXAM

- A full examination of the upper extremity is warranted, with special attention paid to asymmetry, anatomic deformities, color changes, ↓ range of motion against resistance, ↓ muscle strength, muscle wasting, and sensory deficits.
- Patients with injuries to the dorsum of the hand should be questioned about the possibility of a closed-fist injury with a human bite. Exam reveals a small laceration over the dorsal MCP joint +/– fracture of the 5th metacarpal bone.

> **KEY FACT**
>
> It is important to test resistance when assessing tendon function because up to 90% of a tendon can be lacerated with preservation of function.

> **KEY FACT**
>
> The combination of a 5th metacarpal fracture and lacerations over the dorsal MCP joints is a closed-fist injury until proven otherwise and should be treated as a human bite wound.

DIAGNOSIS

Plain film radiographs are indicated if fracture or occult foreign body is suspected; MRI may help detect tendon rupture, but not on an emergent basis.

TREATMENT

Depends on the type of injury, but may include laceration repair if the wound is < 12 hours old, antibiotic prophylaxis in closed-fist injuries and cat and human bites, irrigation and debridement of open wounds, analgesics and anti-inflammatory agents, reduction of dislocations, splinting, and prompt referral to a hand surgeon if indicated.

COMPLICATIONS

Pain, joint stiffness, nonunion of fractures, infection, scar formation, loss of extremity use.

TABLE 18.17. Management of Common Wounds

WOUND	HISTORY/PRESENTATION	TREATMENT
Animal bite	Type of animal and status, foreign body in wound, tendon or tendon sheath involvement, bone injury, joint space violation, neurovascular status.	Irrigation, debridement, 1° closure if clean or facial wound (otherwise delayed 1° closure), tetanus +/− rabies prophylaxis, antibiotics (amoxicillin-clavulanate) for cat bites.
Human bite	Tendon or tendon sheath involvement, crepitus, tissue loss, foreign body in wound.	Irrigation, tetanus prophylaxis, fracture treatment if necessary, delayed closure, IV antibiotics (amoxicillin-clavulanate).
Pressure ulcer, stage 1	Nonblanchable erythema of intact skin.	Transparent dressings.
Pressure ulcer, stage 2	Partial-thickness skin loss of epidermis, dermis, or both, with superficial ulcer formation.	Hydrocolloid or transparent dressings.
Pressure ulcer, stage 3	Full-thickness skin loss involving damage to subcutaneous tissue and extending into, but not through, underlying fascia.	Debridement, irrigation, hydrocolloid or transparent dressings.
Pressure ulcer, stage 4	Full-thickness skin loss with extensive involvement of underlying tissues, including muscle, bone, or supportive structures.	Surgical debridement, irrigation, advanced topical dressings +/− antibiotics, flap closure to cover defect.
Diabetic foot ulcer	Diabetes control, neurovascular status, presence of Charcot foot deformity.	Appropriate footwear and prevention, maintenance of moist wound environment, debridement, antibiotic therapy, blood glucose control.
Venous stasis ulcer	Due to ambulatory venous hypertension, brawny induration in extremities; shallow ulcer with weeping discharge.	Compression, debridement, maintenance of moist wound environment +/− skin grafting.
Arterial insufficiency ulcer	Pulselessness, cool skin, delayed capillary refill, atrophic skin, loss of hair, well-circumscribed punctate ulcers.	Debridement, maintenance of moist wound environment, surgical or medical treatment to ↑ arterial circulation.

WOUND CARE

Chronic wounds can arise from a number of causes, including pressure (decubitus) ulcers, diabetic foot ulcers, venous stasis ulcers, arterial insufficiency ulcers, neoplasms, atheroembolic disease, pyoderma gangrenosum, anticoagulant-induced skin necrosis, radiation damage, and various infections. Table 18.17 lists treatment strategies for common chronic wounds. Basic wound care guidelines are as follows:

- Accurately assess the entire patient.
- Ensure adequate oxygenation and nutrition.
- Treat underlying infections.
- Irrigate and remove foreign bodies.
- Provide a moist wound bed.
- Consider compression therapy.
- Provide proper pain control.

NOTES

Index

About the Authors

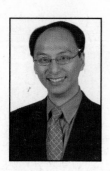

Tao Le, MD, MHS

Dr. Le developed his passion for medical education while still a medical student. He currently edits over 15 titles in the *First Aid* series. In addition, he is the founder of the *USMLERx* online video and test bank series as well as a cofounder of the *Underground Clinical Vignettes* series. As a medical student, he was editor-in-chief of the University of California, San Francisco (UCSF) *Synapse*, a university newspaper with a weekly circulation of 9000. Tao earned his medical degree from UCSF in 1996 and completed his residency training in internal medicine at Yale University and fellowship training at Johns Hopkins University. At Yale, he was a regular guest lecturer on the USMLE review courses and an adviser to the Yale University School of Medicine curriculum committee. Dr. Le subsequently went on to cofound Medsn, a medical education technology venture, and served as its chief medical officer. He is currently conducting research in asthma education at the University of Louisville.

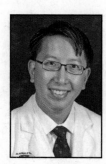

Michael Mendoza, MD, MPH

Dr. Mendoza is an assistant professor in the Department of Family Medicine at the University of Rochester School of Medicine and Dentistry and medical director of Highland Family Medicine. His education interests include teaching residents about quality improvement, practice innovation, and chronic illness management in underserved settings. Previously, he worked closely with medical students as a community preceptor on the South Side of Chicago. His teaching there earned him recognition as Teacher of the Year from the Illinois Academy of Family Physicians. Dr. Mendoza earned his medical degree from the University of Chicago and his master's degree in public health from the University of Illinois at Chicago. He completed his residency training and served an additional year as chief resident in family and community medicine at the University of California, San Francisco, and San Francisco General Hospital. A devoted father and husband, Dr. Mendoza devotes his free time to family, photography, and running.

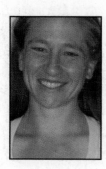

Diana Coffa, MD

Dr. Coffa is a clinical assistant professor in the Department of Family and Community Medicine at the University of California, San Francisco. After completing medical school and a residency at UCSF, she served as chief resident for a year and then joined the faculty. Currently, she is the assistant medical director of the Family Health Center at San Francisco General Hospital. She designs and implements curricula in the UCSF family medicine and internal medicine residencies, focused on substance abuse, chronic pain, care of underserved populations, and integrative medicine. In addition to running a chronic pain and addiction clinic and practicing primary care, Dr. Coffa practices consultative integrative medicine at the UCSF Osher Center for Integrative Medicine. In her free time, Dr. Coffa can be found bicycling in the Northern California countryside and turning herself upside down in various San Francisco yoga studios.